Hernia Surgery

Yuri W. Novitsky

Editor

Hernia Surgery

Current Principles

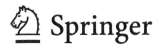

Editor
Yuri W. Novitsky
Case Comprehensive Hernia Center
University Hospitals Case Medical Center
Cleveland, OH, USA

Videos can also be accessed at
http://link.springer.com/book/10.1007/978-3-319-27470-6

ISBN 978-3-319-27468-3   ISBN 978-3-319-27470-6   (eBook)
DOI 10.1007/978-3-319-27470-6

Library of Congress Control Number: 2016935505

Printed on acid-free paper

This Springer imprint is published by Springer Nature
The registered company is Springer International Publishing AG Switzerland

Preface

Hernia repair remains one of the most common surgical procedures performed, but there is little consensus as to the best surgical technique, prosthetic material of choice, or most appropriate strategies to repair abdominal wall hernias. *Hernia Surgery: Current Principles* will serve as a state-of-the-art reference in the rapidly changing field of hernia surgery. With contributions by key opinion leaders in the field, this book will describe the latest trends and detailed technical nuances to approach both routine and complex of hernia scenarios. The reader will gain unique insights into a wide spectrum of hernia issues, including clinical anatomy and physiology of the abdominal wall, mesh selection, patient optimization, robotic and laparoscopic repairs, anterior and posterior component separations, parastomal, flank, suprapubic and other difficult hernia repairs, as well as reconstructions in the setting of contamination, enterocutaneous fistulas, and loss of abdominal domain. Furthermore, important issues in inguinal repairs, including open, laparoscopic and robotic repairs, postoperative groin pain, and treatment of sports hernias are extensively covered. Finally, important contributions from key reconstructive plastic surgeons will detail modern trends on how to deal with complex skin and soft tissue challenges, including concurrent panniculectomies, tissue expanders, and myofascial flaps. The textbook will provide unparalleled step-by-step instructions to perform both routine and complex repairs by using vivid illustrations and by highlighting operative details through intra-operative color photographs and a unique video collection of procedures performed and narrated by today's top hernia surgeons.

As a comprehensive and most up-to-date reference to modern trends in mesh science and technique selections, *Hernia Surgery: Current Principles* will be an invaluable resource to all residents and practicing general, plastic, and trauma surgeons to help them succeed in the field of Hernia surgery.

Cleveland, OH, USA   Yuri W. Novitsky

Contents

1   **Clinical Anatomy and Physiology of the Abdominal Wall** 1
    Arnab Majumder

2   **Classification of Hernias**. 15
    Clayton C. Petro and Yuri W. Novitsky

3   **Preoperative Imaging in Hernia Surgery** 23
    Richard A Pierce and Benjamin K Poulose

4   **Preoperative Preparation of the Patient Undergoing
    Incisional Hernia Repair: Optimizing Chances for Success** 31
    Robert G. Martindale and Clifford W. Deveney

5   **Wound Closure and Postoperative Hernia
    Prevention Strategies** 41
    An Jairam, Gabrielle H. van Ramshorst, and Johan F. Lange

6   **Synthetic Mesh: Making Educated Choices**. 53
    Issa Mirmehdi and Bruce Ramshaw

7   **Biologic Mesh: Classification and Evidence-Based
    Critical Appraisal** 61
    Corey R. Deeken

8   **Biodegradable Meshes in Abdominal Wall Surgery** 71
    Garth Jacobsen and Christopher DuCoin

9   **Abdominal Wall Spaces for Mesh Placement:
    Onlay, Sublay, Underlay**. 79
    Gina L. Adrales

10 **Reconstructive Options for Small Abdominal
    Wall Defects**. 89
    Parag Bhanot and Ryan Ter Louw

11 **Onlay Ventral Hernia Repair**. 99
    Nathaniel Stoikes, David Webb, and Guy Voeller

12 **Rives-Stoppa Retromuscular Repair** 107
    Alfredo M. Carbonell

**13 Posterior Component Separation Via Transversus
     Abdominis Muscle Release: The TAR Procedure** 117
     Yuri W. Novitsky

14 Open Anterior Component Separation 137
     Peter Thompson and Albert Losken

15 Endoscopic Anterior Component Separation 149
     David Earle

**16 Open Anterior Component Separation
     with Perforator Preservation** 159
     Gregory A. Dumanian

17 Open Parastomal Hernia Repair 169
     Matthew Z Wilson, Joshua S Winder, and Eric M Pauli

18 Open Flank Hernia Repair 183
     Melissa Phillips LaPinska and Austin Lewis

**19 Umbilical Hernia Repair: The Spectrum
     of Management Options** 195
     Kent W. Kercher

20 Managing Complications of Open Hernia Repair 207
     Eric M. Pauli and Ryan M. Juza

21 Laparoscopic Ventral Hernia Repair 223
     David M. Krpata and Yuri W. Novitsky

**22 Laparoscopic Ventral Hernia Repair
     with Defect Closures** 231
     Sean B. Orenstein and Yuri W. Novitsky

23 Laparoscopic Parastomal Hernia Repair 241
     Erin M. Garvey and Kristi L. Harold

**24 Laparoscopic Subxiphoid and Suprapubic
     Hernia Repair** 253
     William S. Cobb

25 Laparoscopic Repair of Flank Hernias 261
     Ciara R. Huntington and Vedra A. Augenstein

26 Robotic Ventral Hernia Repair 273
     Conrad Ballecer and Eduardo Parra-Davila

**27 Evidence-Based Optimal Fixation During Laparoscopic
     Hernia Repair: Sutures, Tacks, and Glues** 287
     H. Reza Zahiri and Igor Belyansky

28 Panniculectomy: Tips and Tricks to Maximize Outcomes 297
     Karan Chopra and Devinder Singh

29 Tissue Expansion During Abdominal Wall Reconstruction 307
     Lauren Chmielewski, Michelle Lee, and Hooman Soltanian

30 Flap Reconstruction of the Abdominal Wall 313
Donald P. Baumann and Charles E. Butler

31 Diagnosis and Management of Diastasis Recti 323
Maurice Y. Nahabedian

32 Negative Pressure Wound Therapy 337
Terri A. Zomerlei and Jeffrey E. Janis

**33 Adjuncts to Wound Healing for Abdominal
Wall Wounds** 351
Sarah Sher and Karen Evans

**34 Loss of Abdominal Domain: Definition
and Treatment Strategies** 361
Gregory J. Mancini and Hien N. Le

**35 Enterotomy During Hernia Repair:
Prevention and Management** 371
Brent D. Matthews

**36 Abdominal Wall Surgery in the Setting
of an Enterocutaneous Fistula: Combined Versus
Staged Definitive Repair** 379
Michael G. Sarr

37 Management of Infected Mesh in Ventral Hernias 387
Kamal M.F. Itani and C. Jeff Siegert

**38 Management of Ventral Hernia in the Morbidly
Obese Patient** 393
Jeffrey A. Blatnik and Ajita S. Prabhu

39 Emergent Surgical Management of Ventral Hernias 401
Phillip Chang and Levi D. Procter

40 Temporary Abdominal Closure 409
William W. Hope and William F. Powers

41 Chemical Component Separation Using Botulinum Toxin 421
Manuel López-Cano and Manuel Armengol-Carrasco

42 Groin Hernia Repair: Open Techniques 437
Sean M. O'Neill, David C. Chen, and Parviz K. Amid

43 Laparoscopic TAPP Inguinal Hernia Repair 451
Sergio Roll and James Skinovsky

**44 Laparoscopic Total Extra-Peritoneal (TEP) Inguinal
Hernia Repair** 461
Tammy Kindel and Dmitry Oleynikov

**45 The Extended-View Totally Extraperitoneal
(eTEP) Technique for Inguinal Hernia Repair** 467
Jorge Daes

46   **Inguinal Hernias: an Algorithmic Approach
      to Procedure Selection** 473
      Brian P. Jacob

47   **Evaluation and Treatment of Postoperative Groin Pain** 481
      Martin F. Bjurstrom, Parviz K. Amid, and David C. Chen

48   **Treating Inguinal Recurrences** 491
      Scott Roth and John E. Wennergren

49   **Nonoperative Treatment of Sports Hernia** 499
      Terra Blatnik

50   **The Surgical Approach to Sports Hernia** 509
      Thomas J. Wade and L. Michael Brunt

      Erratum to E1

      Index 521

List of Videos

Video 11.1 Onlay ventral hernia repair
Guy Voeller

Video 13.1 Posterior component separation via transversus abdominis release: the TAR procedure
Yuri Novitsky

Video 15.1 Endoscopic anterior component separation
J. Scott Roth

Video 15.2 Total laparoscopic (subcutaneous) abdominal wall reconstruction
Jorge Daes

Video 16.1 Perforator preserving anterior component separation hernia
Gregory Dumanian

Video 17.1 Open parastomal hernia repair with transversus abdominis release
Eric Pauli

Video 18.1 Open flank hernia repair
Yuri Novitsky

Video 22.1 Laparoscopic ventral hernia repair with defect closure
Yuri Novitsky

Video 23.1 Laparoscopic parastomal (Sugarbaker) hernia repair
Kristi Harold

Video 24.1 Laparoscopic subxiphoid hernia repair
Igor Belyansky

Video 24.2 Laparoscopic suprapubic hernia repair
Yuri Novitsky

Video 26.1 Robotic inguinal hernia repair
Conrad Ballacer

Video 26.2 Robotic retromuscular incisional hernia repair
Alfredo Carbonell

Video 28.1 Panniculectomy with ventral hernia repair
Devinder Singh

Video 41.1 Botulinum neurotoxin injection before incisional hernia repair
Manuel López-Cano

Video 42.1 Open Lichtenstein inguinal hernia repair
Parviz Amid

Video 43.1 Laparoscopic transabdominal preperitoneal (TAPP) inguinal hernia repair
Sergio Roll

Video 43.2 Laparoscopic transabdominal preperitoneal (TAPP) inguinal hernia repair
J. Scott Roth

Video 43.3 Laparoscopic transabdominal preperitoneal (TAPP) inguinal hernia repair
Yuri Novitsky

Video 44.1 Laparoscopic Total Extraperitoneal (TEP) Inguinal Hernia Repair
Brian Jacob

Video 45.1 Extended View Laparoscopic Total Extraperitoneal (eTEP) Repair
Jorge Daes

Video 50.1 Open Repair of Sports Hernia/Athletic Pubalgia
L. Michael Brunt

Contributors

Gina L. Adrales, M.D., M.P.H. Division of Minimally Invasive Surgery, The Johns Hopkins University School of Medicine, Baltimore, MD, USA

Parviz K. Amid, M.D. Department of Surgery, Lichtenstein Amid Hernia Clinic at UCLA, Santa Monica, CA, USA

Manuel Armengol-Carrasco, M.D., Ph.D. Department of Surgery, Hospital Universitari Vall d'Hebron, Barcelona, Spain

Vedra A. Augenstein, M.D. Division of Gastrointestinal and Minimally Invasive Surgery, Department of Surgery, Carolinas Medical Center, Charlotte, NC, USA

Conrad Ballecer, B.S., M.S., M.D. Arrowhead Medical Center, Banner Thunderbird Medical Center, Peoria, AZ, USA

Donald P. Baumann, M.D. Department of Plastic Surgery, University of Texas MD Anderson Cancer Center, Houston, TX, USA

Igor Belyansky, M.D. Department of Surgery, Anne Arundel Medical Center, Annapolis, MD, USA

Parag Bhanot, M.D. Department of Surgery, Medstar Georgetown University Hospital, Washington, DC, USA

Martin F. Bjurstrom, M.D. Department of Anesthesiology, Lichtenstein Amid Hernia Clinic at UCLA, Santa Monica, CA, USA

Terra R. Blatnik, M.D. Cleveland Clinic, Twinsburg, OH, USA

Jeffrey A. Blatnik, M.D. Department of Surgery, Section of Minimally Invasive Surgery, Washington University School of Medicine, St. Louis, MO, USA

L. Michael Brunt, M.D. Department of Surgery, Washington University School of Medicine, Saint Louis, MO, USA

Charles E. Butler, M.D. Department of Plastic Surgery, University of Texas MD Anderson Cancer Center, Houston, TX, USA

Alfredo M. Carbonell, D.O. Division of Minimal Access and Bariatric Surgery, Greenville Health System, University of South Carolina School of Medicine, Greenville, SC, USA

Phillip Chang, M.D. Department of Surgery, University of Kentucky, Lexington, KY, USA

David C. Chen, M.D. Department of Surgery, Lichtenstein Amid Hernia Clinic at UCLA, Santa Monica, CA, USA

Lauren Chmielewski, M.D. Department of Plastic Surgery, University Hospitals Case Medical Center, Cleveland, OH, USA

Karan Chopra, M.D. Department of Plastic Surgery, University of Maryland School of Medicine, Johns Hopkins University, Baltimore, MD, USA

William S. Cobb IV , M.D. Department of Surgery, The Hernia Center, Greenville Health System, Greenville, SC, USA

Jorge D. Daes, M.D., F.A.C.S. Department of Minimally Invasive Surgery, Clinica Bautista, Barranquilla, Columbia

Eduardo Parra Davila, M.D. General/Colorectal Surgery, Celebration, FL, USA

Corey R. Deeken, Ph.D. Covalent Bio, LLC, Eureka, MO, USA

Clifford Deveney, M.D. Department of Surgery, Oregon Health & Science University, Portland, OR, USA

Christopher DuCoin, M.D., M.P.H. Department of Surgery, University of California, San Diego, La Jolla, CA, USA

Gregory A. Dumanian, M.D. Department of Plastic Surgery, Northwestern Memorial Hospital, Chicago, IL, USA

David Earle, M.D. Department of Surgery, Tufts University School of Medicine, Springfield, MA, USA

Karen K. Evans, M.D. Department of Plastic Surgery, Georgetown University Hospital, Washington, DC, USA

Erin M. Garvey, M.D. Division of General Surgery, Mayo Clinic Arizona, Phoenix, AZ, USA

Kristi L. Harold, M.D. Division of General Surgery, Mayo Clinic Arizona, Phoenix, AZ, USA

William Hope, M.D. Department of Surgery, New Hanover Regional Medical Center, Wilmington, NC, USA

Ciara R. Huntington, M.D. Department of Surgery, Carolinas Medical Center, Charlotte, NC, USA

Kamal M.F. Itani, M.D. Department of Surgery, VA Boston Health Care System and Boston University, West Roxbury, MA, USA

Brian P. Jacob, M.D. Department of Surgery, Icahn School of Medicine at Mount Sinai, New York, NY, USA

Garth Jacobsen, M.D. University of California, San Diego, San Diego, CA, USA

An P. Jairam, M.D. Department of Surgery, Erasmus University Medical Center, Rotterdam, The Netherlands

Jeffrey E. Janis, M.D. Department of Plastic Surgery, University Hospital, Ohio State University Wexner Medical Center, Columbus, OH, USA

Ryan M. Juza, M.D. Department of Surgery, Penn State Milton S. Hershey Medical Center, Hershey, PA, USA

Kent W. Kercher, M.D. Division of Gastrointestinal and Minimally Invasive Surgery, Carolinas Medical Center, Charlotte, NC, USA

Tammy Kindel, M.D., Ph.D. Department of Surgery, University of Nebraska Medical Center, Omaha, NE, USA

David M. Krpata, M.D. General Surgery, Cleveland Clinic Comprehensive Hernia Center, Cleveland Clinic, Cleveland, OH, USA

Johan F. Lange, M.D., Ph.D. Department of Surgery, Erasmus University Medical Center, Rotterdam, The Netherlands

Melissa Phillips LaPinska, M.D. Department of Surgery, University of Tennessee Health Science Center, Knoxville, TN, USA

Hien Le, M.D. University of Tennessee Medical Center, Knoxville, TN, USA

Michelle Lee, M.D. Plastic and Reconstructive Surgery, Beth Israel Deaconess Medical Center, Harvard Medical School, Boston, MA, USA

Austin Lewis, M.D. Department of Surgery, University of Tennessee Health Science Center, Knoxville, TN, USA

Manuel Lopez-Cano, M.D., Ph.D. Abdominal Wall Surgery Unit, Universitary Hospital Vall D'hebron, Universidad Autonoma De Barcelona, Barcelona, Spain

Albert Losken, M.D. Department of Plastic Surgery, Emory University Hospital, Atlanta, GA, USA

Ryan P. Ter Louw, M.D. Georgetown University Hospital, Washington, DC, USA

Arnab Majumder, M.D. Department of Surgery, University Hospitals Case Medical Center, Cleveland, OH, USA

Gregory J. Mancini, M.D. Department of Surgery, University of Tennessee Health Science Center, Knoxville, TN, USA

Robert G. Martindale, M.D., Ph.D. Division of General Surgery, Oregon Health & Science University, Portland, OR, USA

Issa Mirmehdi, M.D. Halifax Health, General Surgery, Daytona Beach, FL, USA

Maurice Y. Nahabedian, M.D. Department of Plastic Surgery, Georgetown University, Washington, DC, USA

Yuri W. Novitsky, M.D. Department of Surgery, University Hospitals Case Medical Center, Cleveland, OH, USA

Sean M. O'Neill, M.D., Ph.D. Department of Surgery, Lichtenstein Amid Hernia Clinic at UCLA, Santa Monica, CA, USA

Dmitry Oleynikov, M.D. Department of Surgery, University of Nebraska Medical Center, Omaha, NE, USA

Sean B. Orenstein, M.D. Division of Gastrointestinal and General Surgery, Oregon Health & Science University, Portland, OR, USA

Eric M. Pauli, M.D. Division of Minimally Invasive and Bariatric Surgery, Department of Surgery, Penn State Hershey Medical Center, Hershey, PA, USA

Clayton C. Petro, M.D. Department of General Surgery, Case Comprehensive Hernia Center, University Hospitals Case Medical Center, Cleveland, OH, USA

Richard A. Pierce, M.D., Ph.D. Department of Surgery, Vanderbilt University Medical Center, Nashville, TN, USA

Benjamin K. Poulose, M.D., M.P.H. Department of Surgery, Vanderbilt University Medical Center, Nashville, TN, USA

William F. Powers IV, M.D. Department of Surgery, New Hanover Regional Medical Center, Wilmington, NC, USA

Ajita Prabhu, M.D. Department of Surgery, University Hospitals Case Medical Center, Cleveland, OH, USA

Levi D. Procter Department of Surgery, University of Kentucky, Lexington, KY, USA

Bruce Ramshaw, M.D. Department of Surgery, University of Tennessee Health Science Center, Knoxville, TN, USA

Gabrielle H. van Ramshorst, M.D., Ph.D. Department of Surgery, VU Medical Center, Erasmus University Medical Center, Amsterdam, The Netherlands

Sergio Roll, M.D., Ph.D. Department of Surgery, Santa Casa of Sao Paulo Hospital and Oswaldo Cruz German Hospital, Sao Paulo, Brazil

J. Scott Roth, M.D. Department of Surgery/General Surgery, A.B. Chandler Medical Center, University of Kentucky, Lexington, KY, USA

Michael G. Sarr, M.D. Department of Surgery, Mayo Clinic, Rochester, MN, USA

Sarah Sher, M.D. Department of Plastic Surgery, Georgetown University Hospital, Washington, DC, USA

C. Jeff Siegert, M.D. VA Boston Health care System, West Roxbury, MA, USA

Devinder Singh, M.D. Department of Surgery, Anne Arundel Medical Center, Annapolis, MD, USA

James Skinovsky, Ph.D. Positivo University, Curitiba, Curitiba, Paraná, Brazil; Department of Surgery, Red Cross University Hospital, Curitiba, Paraná, Brazil

Hooman Soltanian, M.D. Department of Plastic Surgery, Case Medical Center, Cleveland, OH, USA

Nathaniel Stoikes, M.D. Department of Surgery, University of Tennessee Health Science Center, Germantown, TN, USA

Peter W. Thompson, M.D. Plastic and Reconstructive Surgery, Emory University, Atlanta, GA, USA

Guy R. Voeller, M.D. Department of Surgery, University of Tennessee Health Science Center, Germantown, TN, USA

Thomas Wade, M.D. Department of Surgery, Washington University School of Medicine, St Louis, MO, USA

David Webb, M.D. Baptist Memphis and Methodist Germantown, Memphis, TN, USA

John E. Wennergren, M.D. Department of Surgery, University of Kentucky Chandler Hospital, Lexington, KY, USA

Matthew Z. Wilson, M.D. Department of Surgery, Section of Minimally Invasive Surgery, Washington University in St. Louis, St. Louis, MO, USA

Joshua S. Winder, M.D. Division of Minimally Invasive Surgery, Department of General Surgery, Penn State Milton S. Hershey Medical Center, Hershey, PA, USA

H. Reza Zahiri, D.O. Division of Minimally Invasive Surgery, Department of Surgery, Anne Arundel Medical Center, Annapolis, MD, USA

Terri A. Zomerlei, M.D. Department of Plastic Surgery, Wexner Medical Center, Ohio State University, Columbus, OH, USA

Clinical Anatomy and Physiology of the Abdominal Wall

Arnab Majumder

Introduction

The modern field of abdominal wall surgery relies on a thorough understanding of all components of the abdominal wall as well as their function and physiology. Advancements in technology have provided surgeons with a wide variety of mesh prosthetics along with novel tools to assist in hernia repair. As a result, improvements in recurrence rates and patient outcomes have been well documented [1, 2]. However, it is the steady progress in the understanding of the abdominal wall itself that has enabled the creation of more complex procedures including myofascial and musculocutaneous advancement flaps via component separation and muscle release [3–9]. Such advancements have allowed surgeons the technical ability to deploy prosthetics in novel manners and allow for closure of abdominal defects that were in the past considered impossible. Consequently, a comprehensive grasp of technical options should occur in tandem with a complete and systematic understanding of abdominal wall anatomy and physiology.

This chapter serves to provide a framework for understanding the clinical anatomy of the abdominal wall as well as the relevant physiol-

ogy and critical relationships that arise during surgery. A fundamental grasp of surface and deep anatomy is assumed with focus given to more subtle clinical findings based on these foundations. The chapter is framed to emphasize the importance in restoration of the linea alba during these repairs.

Boundaries

The anterior abdominal wall is a hexagonal area bounded by the xiphoid process superiorly with delineation of the superolateral edges by the costal margins. Inferiorly it extends along the iliac crests and narrows to the superior edge of the pubic bone of the pelvis in the midline. The inferolateral margins are defined by the inguinal ligaments bilaterally. Lateral extension occurs posteriorly to the erector spinae and quadratus lumborum muscles adjacent to the lumbar spine as these muscles contribute to the thoracolumbar fascia along with transversus abdominis [10] (Fig. 1.1).

The dynamic group of muscles contained in these boundaries is unique in that they are void of any bony structures aside from their attachments. However, given their broad area, the muscular groups serve a variety of purposes in coordination with other body systems. Integral roles include assistance with defecation and urination as well as respiration and coughing via an increase or decrease in intra-abdominal and intra-thoracic

A. Majumder, M.D. (✉)
Department of Surgery, University Hospitals Case Medical Center, 11100 Euclid Ave, Cleveland, OH 44106, USA
e-mail: arnab.majumder@uhhospitals.org

Fig. 1.1 Boundaries of the abdominal wall shown as a hexagonal area anteriorly with lateral extension around the flanks toward the muscles of the back

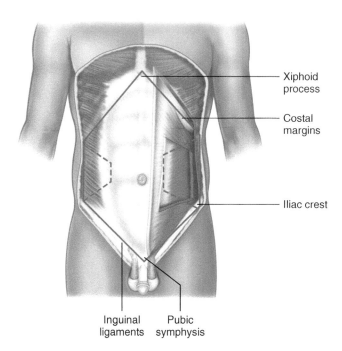

Xiphoid process

Costal margins

Iliac crest

Inguinal ligaments   Pubic symphysis

pressures. Additionally, in concert with muscles of the back the abdominal wall serves to flex, extend, and rotate the torso from the hips. Tension generated in the thoracolumbar fascia along with muscles of the back provides stabilization for the lumbosacral spine and pelvis, both playing a critical role in posture [11]. Finally, the robust overlap of the muscular girdle also provides physical protection for the underlying viscera when contracted. Given the large variety of roles of the abdominal wall, a critical understanding of each component and its function is paramount, with the ultimate goal of restoration or maintenance of these functions following surgery.

Components

The abdominal wall can be divided into midline and anterolateral groups of muscles comprising four main paired muscle groups and a variably present paired fifth muscle group. The muscular groups are covered by subcutaneous fat and skin along with superficial neurovascular structures which overlay the fascia. The rectus abdominis and the pyramidalis muscles comprise the midline group, although the presence of the pyrami-

dalis is not consistent among the population [12, 13] (Fig. 1.2). The bilateral anterolateral groups are composed of a trilaminar structure consisting of the external oblique muscles (EOMs), internal oblique muscles (IOMs), and transversus abdominis muscles (TAMs) (Fig. 1.3). In addition to the muscular groups and their associated neurovascular supply, there are a number of key tendinous structures and delineations including the linea alba, linea semilunaris, linea semicircularis (arcuate line of Douglas) as well as the anatomic spaces of Retzius and Bogros, formed from the interaction of these muscle groups, that are equally as important to understand.

Linea Alba

While the muscular components of abdominal wall are of crucial importance, the restoration of linea alba remains the goal of definitive abdominal wall reconstruction. This chapter begins with attention given to this oft-overlooked, but ultimately vital structure.

Literally translated as *the white line*, the linea alba is a completely fibrous structure composed of collagen and elastin traversing from the

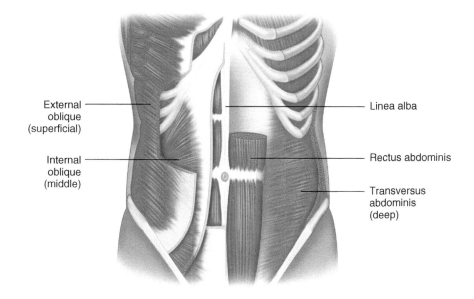

External oblique (superficial)

Internal oblique (middle)

Linea alba

Rectus abdominis

Transversus abdominis (deep)

Section from above arcuate line

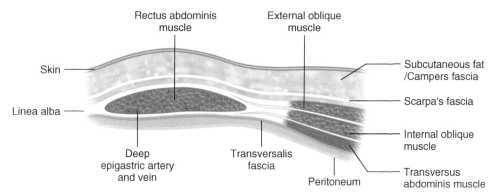

Rectus abdominis muscle

External oblique muscle

Skin

Linea alba

Deep epigastric artery and vein

Transversalis fascia

Peritoneum

Subcutaneous fat /Campers fascia

Scarpa's fascia

Internal oblique muscle

Transversus abdominis muscle

Section from below arcuate line

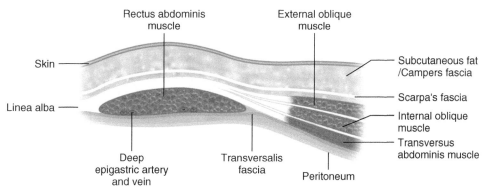

Rectus abdominis muscle

External oblique muscle

Skin

Linea alba

Deep epigastric artery and vein

Transversalis fascia

Peritoneum

Subcutaneous fat /Campers fascia

Scarpa's fascia

Internal oblique muscle

Transversus abdominis muscle

Fig. 1.2 Muscles of the abdominal wall with the antero-lateral group comprising the external and internal oblique along with the transversus abdominis extending medial to the linea semilunaris. The midline group is comprised of the rectus abdominis and pyramidalis muscles. Cross sections are illustrated above and below the arcuate line

Fig. 1.3 Transversus abdominis shown with relation to the rectus sheath, notably the fibers extend medial to the linea semilunaris superiorly with a more aponeurotic component inferiorly

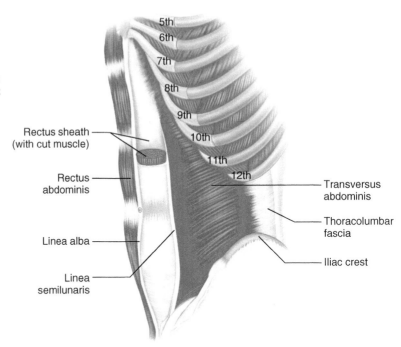

xiphoid process to the pubis symphysis. The linea alba varies in width among the population but generally is accepted as being approximately 15–22 mm along its course, widest at or just above the umbilicus and narrowing at superior and inferior extremes [14, 15]. It is formed as the aponeurosis of the EOMs, IOMs, and TAMs merge terminally in the midline, thus bisecting the paired rectus abdominis muscles. Given its completely avascular nature, it is a preferred location for incision and intra-abdominal access. However, the completely fibrous nature of this structure with implied lack of muscular coverage leads to weakness and the formation of the majority of de novo ventral hernias [16]. Additionally, as most intra-abdominal access occurs via a midline laparotomy, the linea alba is the location of most iatrogenic hernias as well.

Ultimately, the goal of abdominal wall reconstruction remains to restore linea alba by bringing the paired rectus muscles back to the midline. For patients with massive hernias and loss of domain, this is accomplished with various myofascial or musculocutaneous advancement techniques. Once complete, restoration of linea alba has been shown to improve isokinetic and isometric function of the abdominal wall and ulti-

mately quality of life [17]. In the modern era of abdominal wall reconstruction, this functional restoration is critical for not only a complete repair but one that maintains the integrity and actions of the whole abdominal wall unit.

Rectus Abdominis

The rectus abdominus muscles (RA) are the predominant component of the midline group, flanking the linea alba on each side. Occurring as paired strap-like muscles, they are distinctly unlike the broad muscles of the anterolateral group. The recti originate from the pubic crest and ligamentous portion of the pubic symphysis, the fibers course superiorly to insert onto the xiphoid process and anterior surface of the 5th–7th costal cartilages bilaterally. The linea alba bisects the two recti, where the aponeuroses of the anterolateral group decussate and fuse to form the tendinous line. There also exist approximately 3–4 separate tendinous bands that occur at variable points along the rectus in a transverse manner. These bands are irregular in nature and do not necessarily occur along regular intervals, but function as transverse anchor points along the muscle body allowing for flexion of the trunk. A strong attachment of the rectus is found to the anterior rectus sheath with posterior sheath attachment occurring more variably [18].

Vascular supply to the rectus muscles is distinctly different from the anterolateral group, with blood supply originating from paired superior epigastric arteries (SEAs) and deep inferior epigastric arteries (DIEAs), which run along the deep surface of the rectus after perforating the posterior sheath. Anastomotic connection between these two systems is generally found just above the umbilical area. The SEA vessels originate as terminal branches of the internal mammary artery around the level of the sixth costal cartilage. The SEAs enter the rectus sheath at the midpoint of the xiphoid process. The DIEAs arise as branches from the external iliac arteries just proximal to their course through the femoral ring where the external iliac arteries become the femoral arteries. The DIEAs serve as the pedicles for perforator techniques such as the TRAM (transverse rectus abdominis myocutaneous) and DIEP (deep inferior epigastric perforator) flaps seen in plastic surgery. Innervation, unlike vascular supply, is similar to that of the anterolateral group with the ventral rami of T6/7–L1 traveling in the transversus abdominis plane (TAP) to perforate the rectus sheath laterally. Sacrifice of these neurovascular perforating bundles during surgery can lead to atrophy of the rectus complex and should be avoided whenever possible. Ultimately, preservation of the neurovascular supply leads to maintenance of native rectus function and thus a more robust and functional repair.

The rectus abdominis is responsible primarily for flexion of the abdominal wall as well as assistance with increasing intra-abdominal pressure. Flexion of the abdominal wall can be the movement of the ribcage toward the pelvis, the pelvis toward the rib cage or both if neither point of flexion is fixed. The increase in abdominal pressure has contributions to various bodily functions including exhalation, defecation, and micturition. While the rectus is not necessarily engaged in any significant capacity during normal effort, it comes into play when these functions are forceful.

Clinically, it is important to return the rectus muscles back to the midline to recreate linea alba in order to allow for restoration of function. Without the central anchor point in the linea alba, the forces exerted by both the rectus muscles and the lateral abdominal wall are unlikely to translate to physiologic action that constitutes a truly functional repair.

Pyramidalis

The pyramidalis muscles are the second and most variable component of the midline group, with reported absence in 10–70% of the population on one or both sides [13]. The paired triangular muscles lie between the anterior surface of the rectus abdominis and associated anterior sheath caudal to the arcuate line. The fibers course superomedially, originating from the pubic crest and ligamentous portion of the pubic symphysis, inserting onto the linea alba. The function of the pyramidalis is not well understood, however it is thought to play a supplementary role in tensing the linea alba and increasing intra-abdominal pressure thus providing local compression of the bladder during micturition [12]. Given the variability in its occurrence in the population, the clinical significance of this muscle is essentially negligible.

Transversus Abdominis Muscle

The innermost muscle in the anterolateral group is the TAM. It lies directly under (dorsal to) the IOM and above (ventral to) the transversalis fascia. The muscle fibers originate from the inner surfaces of the 7th–12th costal cartilages, anterior leaflet of the thoracolumbar fascia, iliac crest, and lateral third of the inguinal ligament. These fibers course medially from their posterolateral origins in a largely horizontal manner until they insert onto the linea alba, pubic crest, and pectineal line. Superiorly, the fibers interdigitate with those of the diaphragm and travel in a more superior-medial manner. Moving inferiorly, there is a significant aponeurotic component to the muscle, which occurs closer to the midline at the inferior extreme, though clinically there is significant variation to the extension of the fibers toward the recti.

Generally, around the level of the umbilicus the aponeurotic component begins lateral to the rectus abdominis muscle. Clinically, however it is not uncommon to encounter muscle fibers themselves medial to the linea semilunaris when performing transversus abdominis release after reincision of the ventral portion of the posterior rectus sheath. Travelling inferiorly (caudad) the aponeurotic component occurs further medially, past linea semilunaris until the arctuate line.

Crucially, a major distinction occurs in the aponeurotic component of the TAM above and below the arcuate line. Above the arcuate line of Douglas, the transversus abdominis aponeurosis merges with the posterior lamella of the internal oblique aponeurosis forming the posterior rectus sheath, which then continues its path medially as it contributes to the linea alba. Below the arcuate line, the aponeurosis of the transversus is responsible for merging with the internal oblique, as it passes anterior to the rectus complex with eventual formation of the conjoint tendon as it reaches the pubic tubercle.

Blood supply and innervation is shared amongst the anterolateral group with a significant overlap in contributions to the trilaminar structure. Posteriorly the vascular supply arises as mirrored contributions from the aorto-subclavian and aorto-iliac system superiorly and inferiorly, respectively. Intercostal and lumbar arteries arising laterally anastomose to form a network running deep to the transversus muscle surface. This network pierces the transversus laterally to then run in the so-called TAP plane, between the TAM and the IOM. Extensions of this posterior network travel medially along the TAP as parallel neurovascular bundles medially until they perforate the posterior lamina of the internal oblique aponeurosis to innervate the rectus (Fig. 1.4). The vascular network arising posteriorly forms anastomotic connections with the anterior vascular supply, which is derived from descending branches of the intercostal and subcostal arteries. Medially, the SEAs and inferior epigastric arteries, which supply the rectus, also provide anastomotic connections to the posterolateral system creating a dense network with extensive collateralization.

Innervation to the TAM is also shared amongst the trilaminar group with nerves that arise from the ventral rami of T6/7–L1; traveling in parallel to the vascular supply in the TAP. During retrorectus ventral hernia repair, it is important to identify and spare these neurovascular branches as they perforate the posterior lamella of the internal oblique fascia and enter the rectus muscle. When the neurovascular bundles are encountered, dissection

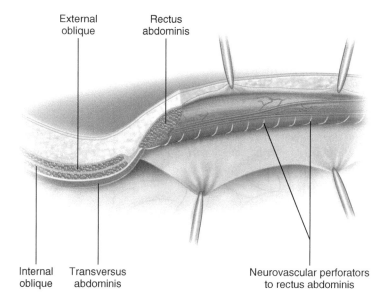

Fig. 1.4 Cross section of the anterior abdominal wall with posterior rectus sheath dissected away from the rectus abdominis revealing the perforating neurovascular bundles which pierce the posterior lamina of the internal oblique

External oblique

Rectus abdominis

Internal oblique   Transversus abdominis

Neurovascular perforators to rectus abdominis

should occur medial to the location of perforation to allow continued supply to the rectus abdominis, thus preventing atrophy. Although retrorectus dissection is traditionally thought of as limited by the linea semilunaris, in reality, it is just medial to this perimeter, as defined by the perforating vessels. These vessels may be dissected off the posterior sheath to be kept with the overlying muscle. If the neurovascular bundles are transected inadvertently and dissection is carried laterally past this threshold, one may find themselves transitioning from the posterior rectus sheath to the anterior one given enough tension.

TAM has significant functional role in the abdominal wall. Its main function occurs in concert with the internal oblique, acting as a "corset" around the visceral sac. The circumferential "hoop tension" created by this action is mainly through the synergistic action of the transversus and the posterior fibers of the IOMs [6]. The contraction not only provides rigidity to the anterior abdominal wall, it also serves to produce tension throughout the thoracolumbar fascia. The transversus exerts force primarily on the anterior (most ventrally positioned) leaflet of the thoracolumbar fascia. This occurs in concert with the quadratus lumborum on the middle leaflet and the sacrospinalis muscles on the posterior leaflet. This fascial tension serves to provide posterior support to the visceral sac and retroperitoneal organs as well as stabilization of the lumbosacral spine and pelvis with effects on posture.

Internal Oblique Muscle

IOM lies interleaved between the other components of the anterolateral group, above (ventral to) the TAM and just underneath (dorsal to) the EOM. It originates from the anterior leaflet of the thoracolumbar fascia, anterior two-thirds of the iliac crest, and lateral half of the inguinal ligament. Its fibers course in a superomedial manner to insert along the inferior border of ribs 10–12 as well as the linea alba. Just superior to the inguinal ligament, the lower most fibers of the internal oblique arch around the spermatic cord to give rise to the cremasteric fibers of the scrotum. In females, these fibers are attenuated and arch around the round ligament. Additionally, the aponeurotic component inferiorly merges with that of the transversus to insert onto the pectineal line as the conjoint tendon. The aponeurotic component of internal oblique also carries a crucial distinction occurring above and below the arcuate line similar to that of the transversus abdominis. Above the arcuate line, the aponeurosis splits to form two lamellae that encompass the rectus abdominis muscle, contributing to both the anterior and posterior sheaths. Inferior to the arcuate line however, the aponeurosis is only found above the rectus muscle where it fuses with that of the external oblique and TAM to contribute to the anterior sheath. Inferiorly, the posterior aspect of the rectus is only covered by the transversalis fascia (Fig. 1.5).

Neurovascular supply of the internal oblique is largely identical to that described for the transversus with posterior contributions traveling in the TAP and medial contributions from intercostal, subcostal, and epigastric arteries. As mentioned previously, the vessels of the posterolateral network perforate the posterior lamella of the internal oblique rather than the merged transversus and internal oblique sheaths. This anatomic distinction is crucial with attention given to ensure dissection occurs medial to the perforators during retrorectus plane development. Distinct to the internal oblique, the ilioinguinal and a branch of iliohypogastric nerve both pierce the muscle as they travel to their destinations. The ilioinguinal nerve perforates medially to travel with the spermatic cord as it traverses the inguinal canal. Laterally, the anterior cutaneous branch of the iliohypogastric, which travels in the TAP, transitions to a location between the internal and external oblique at the level of the anterior superior iliac spine (ASIS) on its way to the rectus muscle.

Functionally, the internal oblique serves a number of roles. As stated previously, it has a synergistic relationship with TAM, assisting with creation of circumferential hoop tension for the abdomen. It also works in tandem with the external oblique on the contralateral side to create ipsilateral rotation and torsion of the trunk.

Section from above arcuate line

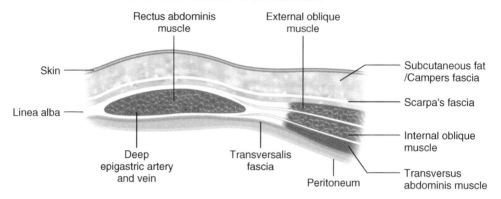

Rectus abdominis muscle

External oblique muscle

Skin

Subcutaneous fat /Campers fascia

Scarpa's fascia

Linea alba

Internal oblique muscle

Deep epigastric artery and vein

Transversalis fascia

Peritoneum

Transversus abdominis muscle

Section from below arcuate line

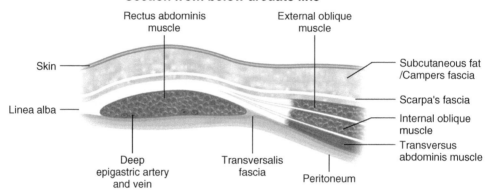

Rectus abdominis muscle

External oblique muscle

Skin

Subcutaneous fat /Campers fascia

Scarpa's fascia

Linea alba

Internal oblique muscle

Transversus abdominis muscle

Deep epigastric artery and vein

Transversalis fascia

Peritoneum

Fig. 1.5 Sections of the abdominal wall from above and below the arcuate line, importantly the posterior layer below the arcuate line consists only of the transversalis fascia

Lumbosacral stabilization occurs as a result of tension in the thoracolumbar fascia, once again a concerted effort from the IOM and TAM, although proportionally it is more so from the latter. Finally, the contraction of the IOM opposes that of the diaphragm assisting with exhalation by increasing intra-abdominal pressure.

Clinically, the fibers of internal oblique are seldom manipulated given their location between the external oblique and transversus abdominis. However, as mentioned previously, above the arcuate line the aponeurosis splits to form two lamellae encompassing the rectus muscles. The posterior lamella which merges with the transversus aponeurosis to form the posterior sheath is the location of the second incision made, albeit on the ventral aspect as one transitions from ret-rorectus dissection to posterior component separation. While the two aponeuroses do eventually merge without distinction medially as they contribute to the linea alba, the area covering the lateral portion of the rectus abdominis muscle medial to linea semilunaris still occurs as two distinct fascial planes. This is again dependent on the degree to which the transversus fibers course medially past the lateral edge of the rectus. This variability is important to recognize during posterior component separation because if dissection is not carefully done to separate the two layers, whether fascia from fascia or fascia from muscle fiber, fenestrations are created in the posterior sheath which subsequently need to be repaired to exclude the viscera from mesh placed as a sublay.

External Oblique

The EOM is the most superficial of the antero-lateral group of muscles, located directly on top of the IOM. Originating from the external surface of the 5th–12th ribs, the muscle fibers course inferomedially to insert along the linea alba, the pubic tubercle, and anteriorly along the iliac crest. The linea semilunaris is ultimately formed by the aponeurotic component of the muscle as it passes vertically downward from the ninth costal cartilage to the pubic tubercle along with the merger of the internal oblique and transversus abdominis aponeuroses lateral to the rectus abdominis muscles. The aponeurotic component of the EOM itself contributes heavily to the anterior rectus sheath along with the anterior lamella of the IOM above the arcuate line. Below this line, the transversus aponeurosis merges as well, leaving only the transversalis fascia and peritoneum between the rectus and the viscera. Inferior to the level of the ASIS, the muscle is completely aponeurotic in nature. This portion has clinical significance as it gives rise to the inguinal ligament between the ASIS and the pubic tubercle. A small triangular aperture approximately 1–1.5 cm superior and lateral to the pubic tubercle occurs as the superficial inguinal ring, allowing passage of the spermatic cord in males and round ligament in females. The external oblique aponeurosis also forms the regionally termed lacunar ligament as it inserts on the pectineal line as well as the reflected portion of the inguinal ligament termed the shelving edge.

Vascular supply of the EOM originates from the lower 6 or 7 intercostal arteries cranially and deep muscular branches of the deep circumflex iliac arteries caudally. Again, vascular arcades form with the deep epigastric system supplying the rectus abdominis. Innervation arises from the ventral rami of T7–T12 and L1 as with the remainder of the anterolateral group.

The EOM functions in conjunction with the remaining anterolateral group to provide compression for the visceral sac as well assisting with flexion and rotation of the trunk. By contracting the chest wall toward the abdomen, it is primarily responsible for lateral flexion as well as contralateral rotation. The EOM is distinct in that it does not function in tandem with the TAM to nearly the degree of the IOM in creating circumferential tension.

Traditional anterior component separation, as originally described by Ramirez [3, 19], involves the release of the EOM. Although there is morbidity associated with raising cutaneous flaps, this remains a widely used technique for myofascial advancement [5, 20]. Ultimately, while release of the EOM does reduce some circumferential tension, the TAM remains the primary contributor to generation of this force.

Arcuate Line

The arcuate line of Douglas or linea semicircularis is a critical landmark in abdominal wall anatomy which carries with it a number of clinical pearls. Located halfway between the umbilicus and pubic symphysis, the arcuate line represents the lower limit of the posterior rectus sheath. Inferior to this landmark, the posterior lamina of the internal oblique aponeurosis and that of the transversus pass anterior to the rectus muscle. While the arcuate line is generally regarded as a sharp cutoff to the posterior rectus sheath, in actuality it may occur as a much more gradual shift of the posterior sheath fibers toward the anterior sheath in a majority of the population [21]. Below the arcuate line only the transversalis fascia remains between the rectus abdominis and peritoneum, representing a layer with minimal strength (Fig. 1.5). Here, both Spigelian and exceedingly rare arcuate line hernias may occur [22]. Finally, the arcuate line also serves as a landmark where the inferior epigastric vessels perforate the rectus abdominis; care must be taken to identify these vessels while performing the retrorectus dissection. The arcuate line must be incised at its lateral-most point in order to enter the space of Retzius and Bogros from within the rectus sheath to carry out the caudal portion of the dissection during retrorectus repair and transversus abdominis release.

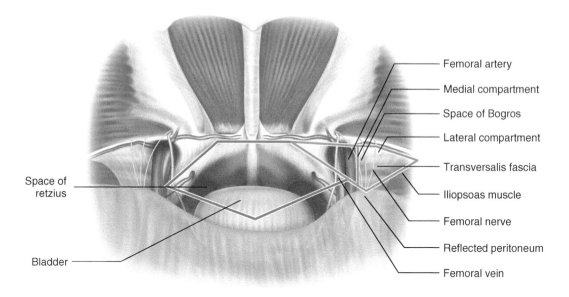

Femoral artery

Medial compartment

Space of Bogros

Lateral compartment

Transversalis fascia

Iliopsoas muscle

Femoral nerve

Reflected peritoneum

Femoral vein

Space of
retzius

Bladder

Fig. 1.6 Space of Retzius (*purple*) and Space of Bogros (*teal*) which is split into medial and lateral compartments with passing anatomic structures

Extraperitoneal Spaces

The space of Retzius is defined as the extraperitoneal space between the pubic symphysis and the bladder. This area is separated from the abdominal wall by the transversalis fascia and contains loose connective tissue and fat. Additionally, it may contain normal or aberrant variants of obturator vessels along with accessory pudendal vessels in 10% of patients. Appropriate dissection of this space is critical for the visualization of the pectineal ligament used for inferior mesh fixation in ventral and inguinal hernia repair (Fig. 1.6).

The space of Bogros is a similarly extraperitoneal space lying laterally to the space of Retzius and deep to the inguinal ligament. It is bound anteriorly by the transversalis fascia and posteriorly by the peritoneum. The space can be split into medial and lateral compartments with the medial compartment housing the femoral artery and vein while the lateral component allowing passage of the iliopsoas muscle and femoral nerve (Fig. 1.6).

Vascular Supply

The blood supply to the abdominal wall was previously described in a regional manner by Huger, consisting of three anatomically distinct zones [23] (Fig. 1.7). Zone I refers to the upper anterior midline of the abdominal wall with the SEAs and DIEAs as they supply the rectus abdominis and overlying subcutaneous tissue and skin. Zone II comprises the entirety of the caudal portion of the anterior abdominal wall. The blood supply in this region arises from four main arterial conduits with contributions from the femoral and iliac arteries. The superficial inferior epigastric and superficial external pudendal arteries originate from the femoral artery to supply the superficial fascia and skin in this area. The DIEAs and deep circumflex iliac arteries supply the musculature in this lower area. Zone III is located laterally past linea semilunaris with lumbar and intercostal arteries which arise from the aortic system. These arcades supply the lateral abdominal wall and eventually anastomose with the midline vascular structures.

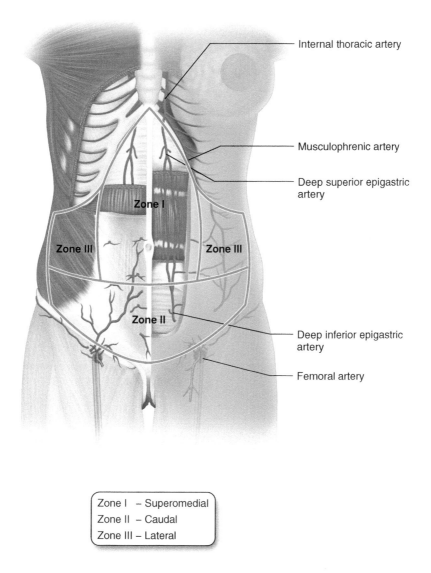

Internal thoracic artery

Musculophrenic artery

Deep superior epigastric artery

Zone I

Zone III

Zone III

Zone II

Deep inferior epigastric artery

Femoral artery

Zone I   – Superomedial
Zone II – Caudal
Zone III – Lateral

Fig. 1.7 Vascular supply to the abdominal wall with delineated Huger Zones I–III

Nerve Supply

As described before, the innervation to the abdominal wall is primarily derived from the ventral rami of T6/7–T12 and L1. Sensory innervation occurs from anterior branches of intercostal and subcostal nerves from the aforementioned spinal levels. Levels T6–9 are responsible for innervation of the area above the umbilicus while T10 innervates the umbilicus itself. The remainder including T11–L1 is responsible for the area below the umbilicus. Innervation to the overlying skin of the lateral abdominal wall arises as direct branches from the intercostal nerves. Motor innervation to the trilaminar and midline groups is provided by the intercostal branches as above along with named contributions from L1 as the

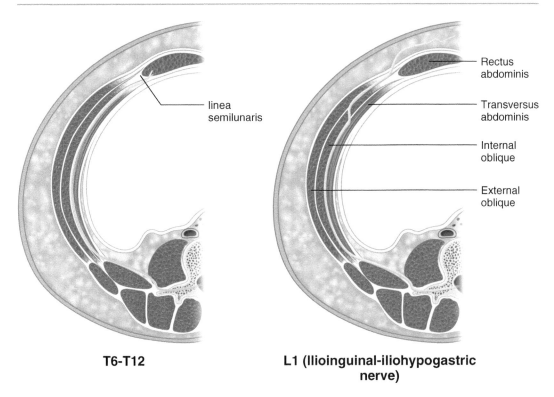

T6-T12

L1 (Ilioinguinal-iliohypogastric nerve)

Fig. 1.8 Nerves supplying the anterior abdominal wall traveling in the transversus abdominis plane (TAP). T6–T12 perforate the posterior lamina of the internal oblique fascia to supply the rectus abdominis. L1 perforates laterally to supply the skin and subcutaneous tissue of the lower abdomen

ilioinguinal and iliohypogastric nerves. The latter pair of nerves has isolated contributions to the IOMs and transversus muscles.

The lateral neurovascular structures travel in the TAP between the TAM and IOM (Fig 1.8). The so-called TAP block has gained favor in the surgical world as an adjunct for post-operative analgesia. Delivery of local anesthetic into this plane provides blockade to the sensory nerves that innervate the anterolateral group with reported improvements in post-operative pain scores, opioid use, and hospital stay [24–27].

References

1. Breuing K, Butler CE, Ferzoco S, Franz M, Hultman CS, Kilbridge JF, et al. Incisional ventral hernias: review of the literature and recommendations regarding the grading and technique of repair. Surgery. 2010;148(3):544–58.

2. Timmermans L, de Goede B, van Dijk SM, Kleinrensink G-J, Jeekel J, Lange JF. Meta-analysis of sublay versus onlay mesh repair in incisional hernia surgery. Am J Surg. 2014;207(6):980–8.

3. Ramirez OM, Ruas E, Dellon AL. "Components separation" method for closure of abdominal-wall defects: an anatomic and clinical study. Plast Reconstr Surg. 1990;86(3):519–26.

4. Novitsky YW, Porter JR, Rucho ZC, Getz SB, Pratt BL, Kercher KW, et al. Open preperitoneal retrofascial mesh repair for multiply recurrent ventral incisional hernias. J Am Coll Surg. 2006;203(3):283–9.

5. Krpata DM, Blatnik JA, Novitsky YW, Rosen MJ. Posterior and open anterior components separations: a comparative analysis. Am J Surg. 2012;203(3): 318–22.

6. Novitsky YW, Elliott HL, Orenstein SB, Rosen MJ. Transversus abdominis muscle release: a novel approach to posterior component separation during complex abdominal wall reconstruction. Am J Surg. 2012;204(5):709–16.

7. Bauer JJ, Harris MT, Gorfine SR, Kreel I. Rives-Stoppa procedure for repair of large incisional hernias: experience with 57 patients. Hernia. 2002;6(3):120–3.

8. Wheeler AA, Matz ST, Bachman SL, Thaler K, Miedema BW. Retrorectus polyester mesh repair for midline ventral hernias. Hernia. 2009;13(6): 597–603.

9. De Vries Reilingh TS, van Goor H, Charbon JA, Rosman C, Hesselink EJ, van der Wilt GJ, et al. Repair of giant midline abdominal wall hernias: "components separation technique" versus prosthetic repair: interim analysis of a randomized controlled trial. World J Surg. 2007;31(4):756–63.

10. Macintosh JE, Bogduk N, Gracovetsky S. The biomechanics of the thoracolumbar fascia. Clin Biomech (Bristol, Avon). 1987;2:78–83.

11. Willard FH, Vleeming A, Schuenke MD, Danneels L, Schleip R. The thoracolumbar fascia: anatomy, function and clinical considerations. J Anat. 2012;221(6): 507–36.

12. Van Landuyt K, Hamdi M, Blondeel P, Monstrey S. The pyramidalis muscle free flap. Br J Plast Surg. 2003;56(6):585–92.

13. Lovering RM, Anderson LD. Architecture and fiber type of the pyramidalis muscle. Anat Sci Int. 2008;83(4):294–7.

14. Rath AM, Attali P, Dumas JL, Goldlust D, Zhang J, Chevrel JP. The abdominal linea alba: an anatomo-radiologic and biomechanical study. Surg Radiol Anat. 1996;18(4):281–8.

15. Beer GM, Schuster A, Seifert B, Manestar M, Mihic-Probst D, Weber SA. The normal width of the linea alba in nulliparous women. Clin Anat. 2009;22(6): 706–11.

16. Johnson TG, Von SJ, Hope WW. Clinical anatomy of the abdominal wall: hernia surgery. OA Anatomy. 2014;2(1):3.

17. Criss CN, Petro CC, Krpata DM, Seafler CM, Lai N, Fiutem J, et al. Functional abdominal wall reconstruction improves core physiology and quality-of-life. Surgery. 2014;156(1):176–82.

18. Tran D, Mitton D, Voirin D, Turquier F, Beillas P. Contribution of the skin, rectus abdominis and their sheaths to the structural response of the abdominal wall ex vivo. J Biomech. 2014;47(12):3056–63.

19. Heller L, McNichols CH, Ramirez OM. Component separations. Semin Plast Surg. 2012;26(1):25–8.

20. Jones CM, Potochny JD, Pauli EM. Posterior component separation with transversus abdominis release: technique and utility in challenging abdominal wall reconstruction cases. Plast Reconstr Surg. 2014;134(4 Suppl 1):116.

21. Rizk NN. The arcuate line of the rectus sheath—does it exist? J Anat. 1991;175:1–6.

22. Montgomery A, Petersson U, Austrums E. The arcuate line hernia: operative treatment and a review of the literature. Hernia. 2013;17:391–6.

23. Huger WE. The anatomic rationale for abdominal lipectomy. Am Surg. 1979;45(9):612–7.

24. Yu N, Long X, Lujan-hernandez JR, Succar J, Xin X, Wang X. Transversus abdominis-plane block versus local anesthetic wound infiltration in lower abdominal surgery: a systematic review and meta-analysis of randomized controlled trials. BMC Anesthesiol. 2014;14:121.

25. Petersen PL, Mathiesen O, Torup H, Dahl JB. The transversus abdominis plane block: a valuable option for postoperative analgesia? A topical review. Acta Anaesthesiol Scand. 2010;54:529–35.

26. Keller DS, Ermlich BO. Demonstrating the benefits of transversus abdominis plane blocks on patient outcomes in laparoscopic colorectal surgery: review of 200 consecutive cases. J Am Coll Surg. 2014;219(6):1143–8.

27. Johns N, O'Neill S, Ventham NT, Barron F, Brady RR, Daniel T. Clinical effectiveness of transversus abdominis plane (TAP) block in abdominal surgery: a systematic review and meta-analysis. Colorectal Dis. 2012;14:635–42.

Classification of Hernias

Clayton C. Petro and Yuri W. Novitsky

Introduction

Ventral hernia repair is often culmination of a complex decision-making process by the surgeon. Defect size, location, patient comorbidities, the presence of contamination, acuity of the patient's presentation, necessity for an ostomy, and history of prior repairs with or without a prosthetic all weigh into the ultimate repair approach. The repertoire of operations available does nothing to simplify the matter. Laparoscopic and open approaches are complicated by innumerable prosthetic choices, and the choice of mesh is next met with a judgment regarding the location of its placement relative to the abdominal wall. Underlay, onlay, inlay, and sublay reinforcement are all viable options that typically compliment the approach. Finally, measurements of success can be equally ambiguous. Definitions for wound morbidity have only recently been defined and begun to penetrate the literature. Recurrence, which many would classify as a failure, can be convoluted by bulging or "pseudo recurrence" in the absence of a true fascial defect, while a true recurrence in an asymptomatic patient with significant improvement in quality-of-life can be a clinical achievement in the eyes of the surgeon.

Needless to say, the number of moving parts makes controlled clinical study challenging. Touted superiority of a particular technique can be met with skepticism regarding patient selection and hernia characteristics. The advantages of a prosthetic may only be applicable in the context of a particular technique, and expense cannot be ignored in an era of cost-awareness. The need for evidence-based guidance has never been more apparent. Conversely, evidence-based study necessitates a basic requirement that is noticeably absent in the field of ventral hernia repair: standardization. The absence of a uniform hernia classification scheme to describe a patient's preoperative state (Fig. 2.1a) has severely limited meaningful discussions regarding repair technique and prosthetic choice (Fig 2.1b). Fortunately, progress has been made in standardizing outcome measures (Fig 2.1c), creating a foundation on which to build. In order to adequately assess technique in a controlled fashion, the hernia, patient, and wound characteristics must be summarized in an organized way to allow standard inclusion and exclusion criterion. Here, we review and summarize previous attempts to address this disparity. We also present our approach to hernia classification generated from our data and experience.

C.C. Petro, M.D. • Y.W. Novitsky, M.D. (✉)
Department of General Surgery, Case Comprehensive Hernia Center, University Hospitals Case Medical Center, 11100 Euclid Ave, 7th Floor Lakeside, Cleveland, OH 44106, USA
e-mail: yuri.novitsky@uhhospitals.org

© Springer International Publishing Switzerland 2016
Y.W. Novitsky (ed.), *Hernia Surgery*, DOI 10.1007/978-3-319-27470-6_2

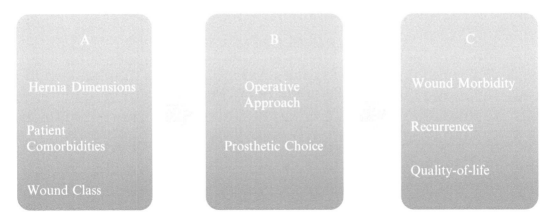

Fig. 2.1 Hernia, technique, and outcomes clinical investigation of any pillar theoretically requires standardized control of the remaining pillars (i.e., operative approach (**b**) cannot be properly studied (**c**) without controlling for the patient's preoperative state (**a**))

Wound Morbidity and Outcomes

The most effective efforts to standardize clinical study have come in the classification of wound morbidity. The designation surgical site occurrence (SSO)—originally coined by the Ventral Hernia Working Group (VHWG)—has been used as an umbrella term to encompass all perioperative wound events [1] (Fig 2.2). SSOs consist of infection, sterile fluid collections, wound dehiscence, and enterocutaneous fistulae. Infections are further subclassified by the CDC's definitions for surgical site infection (SSI) as superficial (skin/soft tissue), deep (adjacent to muscle, fascia, or a prosthetic), or organ space (intraperitoneal) [2]. Wound cellulitis—described as wound erythema treated with antibiotics but not requiring manipulation or opening of the incision—is not classified as an SSI by the CDC, and therefore would be itemized as an SSO. Sterile fluid collections are subclassified as seromas or hematomas based on the character of the fluid. Our practice is to further define collections or infections whether they require procedural interventions, such as bed-side drainage, interventional radiology drainage, or reoperation. Finally, the presence of an enterocutaneous fistula can be characterized by the nature of the fistula output or may be found to be an enteroprosthetic fistula as the underlying cause of a chronic mesh infection. Although the term SSO

being increasingly mentioned, the clinical significance of the "occurrences" is unclear and is likely less relevant than SSIs. As a result, we have been using and advocating a term SSE - surgical site events - the notion that includes all SSIs and clinically relevant SSOs. This term, we believe, is a more accurate reflector of true postoperative wound morbidity.

Efforts to identify predictors of SSO and SSI have naturally followed. In 2010, the VHWG generated an expert-based consensus statement that assigned risk of developing an SSO based on patient and wound characteristics [1]. This grading system is summarized in Table 2.1.

In 2012, our group attempted to validate the VHWG system using data from 299 hernia repairs, leading to several important findings. One was that immunosuppression was not statistically associated with development of an SSO and should therefore not be included in comorbid conditions under Grade 2. Next, while no statistical difference was demonstrated in our data between Grades 2–3 and 3–4, a statistical difference between Grades 2 and 4 was present when those patients with a history of wound infection were grouped with Grade 2, and those patients with stomas or GI tract violations included with other contaminated fields in Grade 4. As such, we proposed modifying the grading scheme into a 3-tiered system (Table 2.2). This simplification puts patients without comorbidities or wound

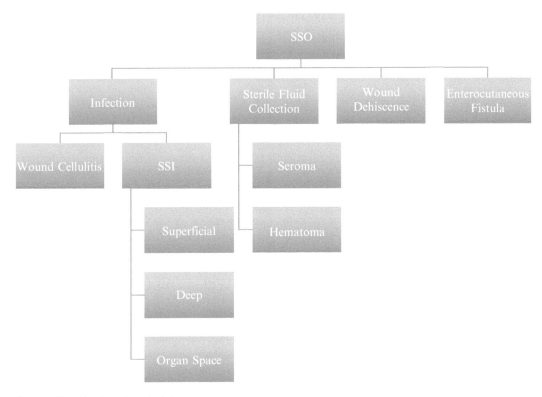

Fig. 2.2 Classification of surgical site occurrences

Table 2.1 VHWG grading system

Grade 1	Grade 2	Grade 3	Grade 4
Low risk	*Comorbid*	*Potentially contaminated*	*Infected*
• Low risk of complications	• Smoking	• Previous wound infection	• Grossly Infected mesh
• No history of wound infection	• Obesity	• Presence of ostomy	
	• Diabetes	• Violation of the GI tract	• Septic dehiscence
	• Immunosuppression		

Table 2.2 Modified ventral hernia working group grading system

Grade 1	Grade 2	Grade 3
Low risk	*Comorbid*	*Contaminated*
• Low risk of complications	• Smoking	• A. Clean-contaminated
• No history of wound infection	• Obesity	• B. Contaminated
	• Diabetes	• C. Active infection
	• Immunosuppression	
	• Previous wound infection	

contamination at low risk, comorbid patients in clean surgical fields at moderate risk, and contaminated cases at the highest risk. Grade 3 could be further stratified based on CDC wound class [3]. The important distinction is that Grade 3C includes chronic and/or active sinuses as well as frankly dirty wounds (CDC Wound Class IV) which makes that group quite heterogeneous.

In fact, one of the limitations of the Modified Grading System is that the studied cohort did not include sufficient number of Wound Class IV patients, limiting its accuracy.

While the aim was to validate the model proposed by the VHWG, some have appropriately pointed out that both systems exclude important hernia and operative characteristics. The presence of incarceration, concomitant surgery, acute presentation, and surgery-related factors, such as operative time, use of drains, and extent of tissue dissection, is not included in the aforementioned models. In an attempt to propose a more complete risk stratification system, Berger and colleagues proposed the Ventral Hernia Risk Score (VHRS) specifically for open ventral hernia repair using data from 888 patients. Odds ratios for those variables most closely associated with SSO and SSI were converted to a point system to stratify patient risk (Fig. 2.3) [4].

The use of operative characteristics in the VHRS system such as mesh implantation, concomitant procedure, or raising of skin flaps as variables for risk stratification becomes problematic, and underscores the difficulty in the creation of such systems. Ideally, if operative technique, mesh choice, and other surgical characteristics are to become dependent variables of study, then they should not be included in a *preoperative* risk-stratification system. While it is important to identify certain technique-dependent risk factors for wound morbidity, such as the association of skin flaps with SSE/SSI, this variable is not inherent to the presenting patient's preoperative state. Certainly, an area of study might be the need to raise skin flaps or not. However, inclu-

sion criterion that would generate patient cohorts with similar preoperative states would need to be defined first using standardized preoperative criteria. Paradoxically, if the preoperative criteria are identified using *no* control for technique—such as in the modified VHWG grading system—then one may incorrectly assume that identified risk factors for wound morbidity are independent of technique. Finally, while the VHWG Grading scheme, our proposed modification, and the VHRS effectively incorporate patient comorbidities and wound characteristics, any portrayal of the hernia itself is noticeably absent.

Hernia Characteristics

Classification of the hernia based on its dimensions and location has most effectively been done by European Hernia Society (EHS). In 2009, a group of international experts met to generate a consensus on hernia classification for future study [5]. For primary hernias, a cross-table was generated based on size and location (Fig. 2.4). As primary ventral hernias—not affiliated with a previous incision/operation—are typically concentric and in a limited number of locations, classification was able to be limited to two variables: diameter and location.

Incisional hernia classification is inherently more complex as defects can essentially take any theoretical configuration. While standard definitions for length and width were determined (Figs. 2.5 and 2.6), no single dimension could be agreed upon to generate a cross-table akin to pri-

Variable	VHRS for SSO			VHRS for SSI		
	OR	95% CI	Points	OR	95% CI	Points
Mesh implant	1.9	1.4–2.7	2	–	–	–
Concomitant hemia repair	2.2	1.5–3.4	2	2.1	1.4–3.3	2
Skin flaps created	2.2	1.6–3.1	2	2.3	1.6–3.4	2
ASA score ≥3	–	–	–	2.1	1.4–3.2	2
BMI ≥40	–	–	–	3.2	1.7–5.9	3
Wound class 4	8.7	3.7–24.1	9	6.8	3.2–15.4	7

ASA, American Society of Anesthesiologists; BMI, body mass index; OR, odds ratio; SSO, surgical site occurrence; SSI, surgical site infection; VHRS, Ventral Hernia Risk Score.

Fig. 2.3 Ventral hernia risk score for SSO and SSI

E H S Primary Abdominal Wall Hernia Classification		Diameter cm	Small <2cm	Medium ≥2-4cm	Large ≥4cm
Midline	Epigastric				
	Umbilical				
Lateral	Spigelian				
	Lumbar				

Fig. 2.4 EHS classification of primary ventral hernias

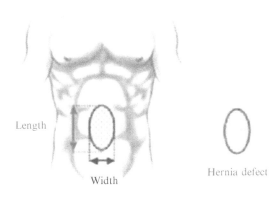

Fig. 2.5 Standardized measure of hernia length/width

mary ventral hernia system. As such, the final system incorporates both length and width, with arbitrary cutoffs (<4, 4–10, >10 cm). The supposition was that data would ultimately be used to make more meaningful designations and potentially validate and/or simplify this system.

Reciprocally, while these EHS classification schemes were an important step in the development of standardized descriptions of hernia dimensions, this does nothing to incorporate patient comorbidities and wound class. Certainly, one could conceive a comprehensive model that would incorporate any and every mentioned variable to accurately incorporate hernia, patient, and wound characteristics. Unfortunately, the result would likely generate a system so complex that it would not be easy to remember, and thus would not be embraced by the surgical community.

Other proposed systems have unfortunately met this fate [6, 7]. A classification scheme capable of accurately describing the patient's preoperative state, while not becoming hindered by its own completeness, is an ideal we sought to achieve.

Hernia, Patient, Wound: A TNM-Like Classification

We recently developed a hernia classification system akin to that of the TNM system for cancer staging. The TNM-model is enviable in its ability to amass large amounts of data with multiple variables and group permutations by prognosis. The outcomes of local recurrence and survival could be likened to wound morbidity and hernia recurrence. We therefore sought to generate such a system. The modified VHWG grading scale already stratifies patients' risk of developing wound morbidity using preoperative patient comorbidities and wound class. We next sought to identify hernia dimensions within the EHS classification system most closely associated with outcomes. The EHS classification system for incisional hernias includes nine potential locations on the abdominal wall, as well as length, width, and recurrent nature. In an attempt to validate these classification variables, we initially characterized patients by preoperative CT scan using this system. Crucially, with regards to both hernia recurrence and wound morbidity, we found no association

E H S Incisional Hernia Classification			
Midline	subxiphoidal	M1	
	epigastric	M2	
	umbilical	M3	
	infraumbilical	M4	
	suprapubic	M5	
Lateral	subcostal	L1	
	flank	L2	
	iliac	L3	
	lumbar	L4	
Recurrent incisional hernia ?		Yes O	No O
length:	cm	width:	cm

width cm	W1 <4cm O	W2 ≥4-10cm O	W3 ≥10cm O

Fig. 2.6 EHS incisional hernia classification

with hernia length, location, or recurrent nature. These findings are corroborated by data from Chevrel et al. [7]. Width cutoffs of 4 and 10 cm—as proposed by the EHS system—generate an intermediary group of 4–10 cm that is clinically indistinguishable from the smaller and larger counterparts. Interestingly, with width cutoffs of <10, 10–20, and ≥20 cm, we identified stepwise associations with hernia wound morbidity *and* recurrence. Therefore, width appears to be the incisional hernia dimension with the most meaningful ties to short- and long-term morbidity. Not only are these 10 and 20 cm cutoffs easy to remember, but they are clinically meaningful to us, as 10 cm represents the upper limit of what most would consider for laparoscopic repair. The second cutoff of 20 cm also triggers the potential need for myofascial release. As such, we characterize hernias (H) by width alone (H1 < 10 cm, H2 = 10–20 cm, H3 ≥ 20 cm), and patient (P) comorbidities (P0 = no comorbidities; P1 = presence of at least one of the following: morbid obesity, diabetes, smoking, and/or immunosuppression) and wound (W) status (W0 = clean, W1 = contaminated). This allows three important variables (Hernia, Patient, Wound) to be incorporated into a cross-table (Fig. 2.7). Permutations

Fig. 2.7 HPW—A "TNM-like" classification system

a

	HERNIA	PATIENT	WOUND	HPW STAGE
STAGE 1	1	0	0	H1, P0, W0
STAGE 2	1 or 2	any	0	H1, P1, W0 H2, any P, W0
STAGE 3	any	any	0 or 1	H1, any P, W1 H2, any P, W1 H3, P0, W0
STAGE 4	3	any	0 or 1	H3, P1, W0 H3, any P, W1

b

	H1	H2	H3
P0	STAGE 1	STAGE 2	STAGE 3
P1	STAGE 2	STAGE 3	STAGE 4
W1	STAGE 3	STAGE 3	STAGE 4

with similar complication profiles are grouped accordingly. The result is a Hernia, Patient, Wound (HPW) Staging system that ordinally ranks stages (I–IV) by risk of developing an SSE and hernia recurrence. This system is comprehensive, generated from evidence, easy to remember, and predicts both short-term wound morbidity (SSE) and long-term efficacy (recurrence). Two principles we hoped to convey in this effort were:

1. The INCLUSION of variables from all three important preoperative states—the hernia, the patient, and the wound class.
2. The EXCLUSION of intraoperative characteristics.

Our hernia–patient–wound model appears to accurately stratify outcomes using these three "TNM"-like variables (Table 2.3). Ultimately, we hope that all clinical trials involving hernia repair will include a hernia stage. In the future, the proposed system would be amendable to modification as more data are amassed, just as the TNM Classification is currently in its 7th edition. For instance, Grade 3 hernias might be further stratified into "a," "b," and "c" subgroups based on degree of contamination to make the system more precise (i.e., perhaps clean-contaminated hernias act more like clean cases than contaminated). While the first proposal may not be perfect, this model uniquely places key prognostic indicators on a platform that can be easily adjusted and, in our view is a necessary foundation to build upon. We anticipate as this classification is applied to other cohorts of patients, sub-staging like IIA and IIB and IIIA and IIIB will emerge. As a historical analogy, variations of the TNM cancer classification that arose in the 1940s were not unified on an international level until 1987. Seven years later, prognostic indicators were finally identified and published. The scope of this effort is daunting, and emphasizes that our proposal is merely a first step. As more investiga-

tors utilize this system on their practice/investigations, a more robust system may emerge using the current HPW system as a foundation.

In summary, a uniform classification system will provide the platform for inclusion/exclusion criteria in future investigations regarding technique, prosthetic choice, and perioperative optimization. The importance of defining our patients in a thoughtful and consistent manner will provide meaningful outcome research that is both widely accepted and widely applicable.

Table 2.3 Outcomes of our cohort of patients based on HPW characteristics

	SSE rate (%)	Recurrence rate (%)
Stage I	5.8	4.7
Stage II	12.6	9.2
Stage III	20.2	13.2
Stage IV	38.9	31.1

References

1. Ventral Hernia Working Group, et al. Incisional ventral hernias: review of the literature and recommendations regarding the grading and technique of repair. Surgery. 2010;148(3):544–58.
2. Horan TC, et al. CDC definitions of nosocomial surgical site infections, 1992: a modification of CDC definitions of surgical wound infections. Infect Control Hosp Epidemiol. 1992;13(10):606–8.
3. Kanters AE, et al. Modified hernia grading scale to stratify surgical site occurrence after open ventral hernia repairs. J Am Coll Surg. 2012;215(6):787–93.
4. Berger RL, et al. Development and validation of a risk-stratification score for surgical site occurrence and surgical site infection after open ventral hernia repair. J Am Coll Surg. 2013;217(6):974–82.
5. Muysoms FE, et al. Classification of primary and incisional abdominal wall hernias. Hernia. 2009;13(4):407–14.
6. Korenkov M, et al. Classification and surgical treatment of incisional hernia. Results of an experts' meeting. Langenbecks Arch Surg. 2001;386(1):65–73.
7. Chevrel JP, Rath AM. Classification of incisional hernias of the abdominal wall. Hernia. 2000;4:7–11.

Richard A. Pierce and Benjamin K. Poulose

Basics of Diagnostic Testing

In addition to a focused history and physical exam, several imaging modalities are useful for the detection and characterization of hernia defects, and frequently, more than a single study will be required. Ultrasound (US) has the advantages of being dynamic, in that the patient can be positioned either upright or supine, and that images can be obtained both while at rest and while performing a Valsalva maneuver [3]. It also avoids exposure to ionizing radiation, and can potentially be performed in the surgeon's office. However, ultrasound is very operator-dependent and can be limited by patient body habitus. Computed tomography (CT) is commonly used in the identification and characterization of ventral hernias, and somewhat less frequently in identifying inguinal hernias. It is rapid, and most surgeons are comfortable with interpreting the images obtained. CT is limited, in that the patient must be positioned either supine, or occasionally prone, which may lead to spontaneous reduction and lack of detection of small or easily reducible hernias. Exposure to ionizing radiation may also

be of concern in patients undergoing repeated evaluations. Magnetic resonance imaging (MRI) avoids the use of such radiation and gives excellent delineation of subtle tissue planes. Functional MRI also has the advantage of being dynamic in terms of allowing patients to perform a Valsalva maneuver. Similarly to CT, however, the patient must be either supine or prone, and the high cost of this imaging modality is often restrictive. Furthermore, most surgeons are generally not comfortable with image interpretation. Although not widely utilized in the United States, herniography can be beneficial in the diagnosis of inguinal hernias. The images are usually easily interpreted and the radiation exposure is significantly less than that of CT. Unfortunately, the procedure does carry with it the risks of visceral puncture and potential reaction to the intraperitoneal dye injection [3].

The metrics of diagnostic testing are usually described in terms of sensitivity, specificity, and predictive values (negative and positive). Sensitivity and specificity describe characteristics about the test itself. Given that the patient has the disease, the probability the test is positive describes sensitivity. Given that the patient does not have the disease, the probability the test is negative describes specificity. Predictive values reflect real-world performance and take into consideration the prevalence of the disease. When a test is positive, the probability that the patient actually has the disease in question is the positive predictive value (PPV). Conversely, when a test

R.A. Pierce, M.D., Ph.D., F.A.C.S. (✉)
B.K. Poulose, M.D., M.P.H., F.A.C.S.
Department of Surgery, Vanderbilt University
Medical Center,
D-5203 Medical Center North, 1161 21st Avenue
South, Nashville, TN 37232, USA
e-mail: Richard.Pierce@Vanderbilt.Edu

is negative, the probability that the patient does not have the disease is the negative predictive value.

Inguinal Hernia

Patients who present with a complaint of groin pain and an easily palpable bulge generally do not present a diagnostic dilemma to surgeons. The patient without a palpable bulge or impulse with Valsalva presents a more challenging clinical scenario. In cases of inguinal strain, osteitis pubis, athletic pubalgia, nerve entrapment, and even femoroacetabular joint disorders, no defect exists, and appropriate management will be different than a standard inguinal hernia repair. However, small yet symptomatic hernias, and even moderate-sized hernias in the obese can be difficult to detect clinically. It is these "occult hernias" that presented diagnostic challenges can benefit from the use of diagnostic imaging [4].

Ultrasound

Ultrasound is often considered the first-line diagnostic test for the occult inguinal hernia. Although quick, inexpensive, and noninvasive, US is subject to operator variability and may be limited by an obese patient's body habitus. A recent meta-analysis by Robinson et al. demonstrated US to have a sensitivity of 96.6%, specificity of 84.8%, and a PPV of 92.6% [5]. However, these values encompassed studies that included patients both with and without palpable groin bulges, and the authors note that both the sensitivity and PPV are significantly lower when only occult groin hernias were included [5]. In contrast, the specificity and negative predictive value were increased when evaluating occult, as opposed to clinically obvious, hernias. One such report from the United Kingdom (UK) examined 52 patients with a history suggestive of inguinal hernia, but with a normal or inconclusive clinical exam. When correlated with surgical findings, US showed a sensitivity of only 33%, and a specificity of 100% [6]. Thus, we advocate that, if an occult hernia is detected by US, then the diagno-

sis is confirmed, but if no hernia is seen, the surgeon should consider other imaging modalities before ruling out a true defect.

Computed Tomography

Despite its extremely widespread use in the United States and Europe, there are relatively few studies evaluating the use of CT in the diagnosis of occult inguinal hernias [7–9]. A systematic review and meta-analysis by Robinson and colleagues describe the overall sensitivity of CT as being approximately 80%, and the specificity being approximately 65% [4]. This was actually found to be inferior to both ultrasound and herniography in the same analysis. Additionally, CT performed after intraperitoneal injection of contrast did not give any significant improvement in the sensitivity or specificity versus standard herniography [5]. Nevertheless, despite its higher cost, CT has the distinct advantage of evaluating the entire abdomen, and thus may help identify other sources of pain such as soft tissue and/or skeletal abnormalities that might not be seen with US or herniography. CT is also useful in evaluation of the multiply recurrent inguinal hernia to assess potential involvement of adjacent structures and displaced mesh prostheses. Similarly, CT can be very helpful in delineating inguinal defects that do not contain a true hernia sac, but contain only herniated preperitoneal fat that can be a cause of significant pain if incarcerated (Fig. 3.1).

Thus, while US is the preferred first-line evaluation for the occult inguinal hernia, it is reasonable to proceed next to CT of the pelvis in the setting of a compelling history for inguinal hernia but a negative clinical exam and negative or equivocal ultrasound study.

Magnetic Resonance Imaging

Similarly to CT, there are few reports describing MRI in the diagnosis of occult inguinal hernias. Although noninvasive and safe, the modality is expensive and may be uncomfortable for patients with claustrophobia. Surgeons are typically not as comfortable with image interpretation as they are with those obtained by CT. In a study by Leander et al., MRI following herniography did not appear to be superior to herniography alone with respect to hernia detection. In the setting of a normal herniogram, however, MRI was able to identify other potential sources of groin pain in a limited number of patients [10]. A recent report by Miller et al. actually showed MRI (sensitivity=91%) to be superior to both US (sensitivity=33%) and CT (sensitivity= 54%) in the diagnosis of occult inguinal hernias [11] (Fig. 3.2). All patients underwent an operation, used as the gold standard reference, and the authors state that MRI correctly identified an occult hernia in 10 out of

11 cases where the hernia was not detected by CT. The single patient with a false positive MRI actually had a surgically correctable fascial tear of the external oblique but no true hernia [11]. Thus, although not a first- or second-line study, MRI can play a valuable role in patients with significant groin pain but an otherwise negative workup. In fact, MRI is likely the preferred modality in this setting, as it can not only rule out an occult hernia, but also elucidate other causes of groin pain such as osteitis pubis, femoral acetabular impingement (FAI) syndrome, and subtle abnormalities of the musculoskeletal attachments in the pelvis [3].

Herniography

First described in 1967 in Canada, herniography is a technique that uses intraperitoneal injection of radiopaque contrast followed by plain abdominal X-rays in the upright position to detect occult inguinal hernias (Fig. 3.3).

Although somewhat more commonly utilized in Scandinavia and the UK, it does not appear to have been widely adopted in the United States [4]. Nevertheless, herniography has been shown to be highly sensitive and specific in several reports [12, 13]. A recent systematic review out of the UK showed herniography to be superior to both CT and US, with a sensitivity of 91% and

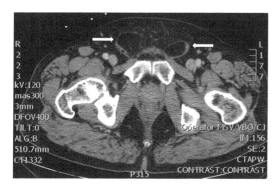

Fig. 3.1 Axial CT image of bilateral fat-containing inguinal hernias (*arrows*) without obvious hernia sac protrusion. Original image

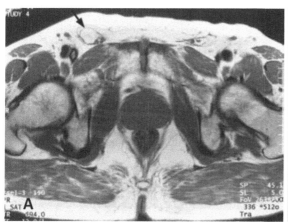
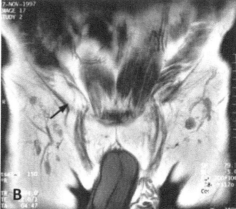

Fig. 3.2 MRI appearance of a small, fat-containing right inguinal hernia (*arrows*). (**a**) Axial, and (**b**) Coronal views. From Leander (2000), with permission

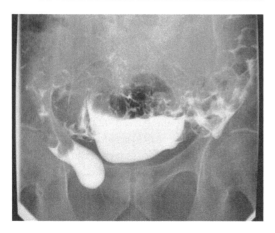

Fig. 3.3 Right inguinal hernia as seen on herniogram. From Alam (2005), with permission

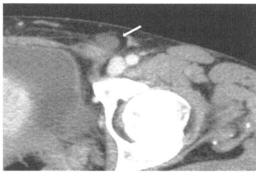

Fig. 3.4 Axial CT image of a small left femoral hernia (*arrow*). Modified from Burkhardt (2011), with permission

specificity of 83% [4]. Despite these excellent results, this invasive procedure carries with it the risk of injection site hematoma, visceral puncture, and vasovagal reaction to the intraperitoneal dye, which may explain its lack of widespread use in the United States [13].

Femoral and Obturator Hernias

Although only about 1/10 the incidence of inguinal hernias, femoral hernias are more prone to strangulation (20% vs. 3% at 3 months after diagnosis) [14, 15]. Thus, accurate diagnosis and prompt surgical correction are extremely important to prevent bowel ischemia and necrosis in an incarcerated femoral hernia. Clinical presentation is generally a mildly painful, nonreducible groin bulge below the inguinal ligament, however, differentiation of a femoral from an inguinal hernia on physical exam is not entirely reliable, regardless of the examining surgeon's experience [14]. Similarly to inguinal hernias, ultrasound should be the initial imaging study if there is ambiguity, with reported sensitivities and specificities of approximately 100% in two separate studies [16, 17]. As ultrasound does carry the variable of being operator-dependent, any equivocal study should be followed by a CT in order to confirm or rule out the diagnosis. On careful inspection, CT images will often display a subtle indentation of the ipsilateral femoral vein with

preservation of the inguinal canal and its contents [15]. In one retrospective study, CT correctly identified 74 out of 75 hernias (47 inguinal and 28 femoral) which were later confirmed at surgery [14]. In the setting of an acute abdomen with bowel obstruction, CT should be the first mode of imaging in order to evaluate for all possible sources of obstruction, even if a femoral hernia is the suspected culprit (Fig. 3.4).

Despite being the most frequently encountered pelvic floor hernias, obturator hernias are even less common than femoral hernias, with an incidence of 0.05–1.4% of all hernias [18, 19]. However, rapid and accurate diagnosis is again critical, as mortality can be as high as 70% when obturator hernias become acutely incarcerated [19]. Obturator hernias most commonly present as unexplained intestinal obstruction in an elderly, emaciated female patient without prior abdominal operations. Small bowel obstruction is the presenting complaint in nearly 90% of cases, with variable physical findings seen in the "classic triad" of obturator hernia (obturator neuralgia, Howship-Romberg sign, Hannington-Kiff sign). A palpable groin mass is a very uncommon finding [18, 19]. Ultrasound can occasionally be useful in the diagnosis, as it can display the level of bowel obstruction and distention. However, it can also be fraught with inaccuracy due to the relative depth of the obturator foramen within the pelvis. Therefore, CT is considered the initial imaging modality of choice, and several studies have shown a near 100% accuracy in diagnosing obturator hernia [19]. Again, CT has the added advantage of assessing the entire abdomen and pelvis, and can thus rule out other possible sources of obstruction, especially when oral contrast is used (Fig. 3.5).

Ventral Hernia

Similar to the occult groin hernia, detection of smaller, yet symptomatic ventral and incisional hernias can often be challenging, especially in the obese patient. In contrast, incisional and recurrent hernias of the ventral abdominal wall often have the propensity to be highly complex,

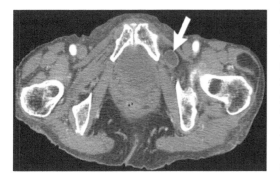

Fig. 3.5 Axial CT image of a left obturator hernia (*arrow*). Modified from Petrie (2011), with permission

involving significant adhesions to both omentum and abdominal viscera, abdominal muscle atrophy, and even loss of abdominal wall domain in the setting of a very large defect. Consequently, thorough evaluation and treatment of the ventral hernia can require both rapid and inexpensive modalities for detecting small defects, as well as high-resolution studies capable of predicting repair complexity in large recurrent defects.

Ultrasound

For detecting ventral abdominal hernias, US again has the advantage of being inexpensive, dynamic, and noninvasive. In the past, however, its utility has been limited by lack of standardize technique and operator variability, resulting in a sensitivity of only 71% [20]. Recently, Beck et al. have described a straightforward, standardized, and surgeon performed approach to using US and the detection of midline and lateral abdominal hernia defects [21]. Termed Dynamic Abdominal Sonography for Hernia (DASH), the technique uses a 12-MHz linear ultrasound probe in five sequential cranial-to-caudal passes of the ventral abdominal wall to detect even small fascial defects (Fig. 3.6).

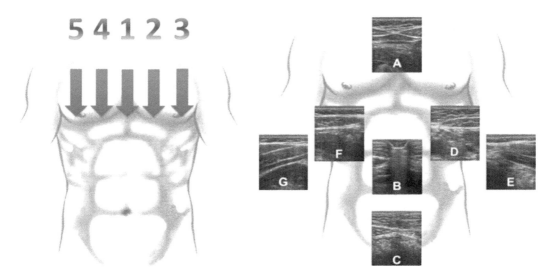

Fig. 3.6 Dynamic Abdominal Sonography for Hernia (DASH) schematic (*left panel*) and representative ultrasound images from the (**a**) midline epigastrium, (**b**) umbilicus, (**c**) midline below the arcuate line, (**d, f**) left and right linea semilunaris, (**e, g**) left and right oblique musculature (*right panel*). From Beck (2013), with permission

DASH has resulted in a highly sensitive (98%) and specific (88%) method for hernia detection, even exceeding that of CT, costing significantly less and avoiding a dedicated trip to the radiology suite [21]. Ultrasound evaluation can still be limited in the severely obese with a very thick layer of subcutaneous fat obscuring the fine detail of the underlying abdominal wall. Additionally, comprehensive evaluation of large defects by ultrasound can be challenging due to small probe size and the inability to perform three-dimensional reconstruction of the hernia sac. Both of these limitations can potentially be overcome by the use of an Automated Breast Volume Scanner (ABVS) as described in the recent report from Diao et al. [22]. At our institution, we typically rely on the use of DASH to assess for small primary defects or recurrences in patients presenting with new pain or bulge. We then standardly proceed to CT scanning for larger or more complex defects requiring further delineation of anatomic detail.

Computed Tomography

Due to its rapid image acquisition, demonstration of fine morphologic detail, 3-D reconstructability, and reproducibility, CT is generally the most popular imaging modality for the evaluation of known ventral abdominal hernias [3]. Although a non-contrasted study is sufficient in most situations, IV contrast should be used if there is a suspicion of infection or malignancy and the patient has satisfactory renal function. Perhaps most important is the ability to use CT imaging to preoperatively predict the surgeons ability to close a given hernia defect in an abdominal wall reconstruction scenario. Several algorithms are currently being developed for this purpose, such as the one described by Allen and colleagues. Their protocol allows for highly accurate length and volume calculations of the critical abdominal wall structures and compartments from otherwise standard axial and sagittal CT images [23] (Fig. 3.7).

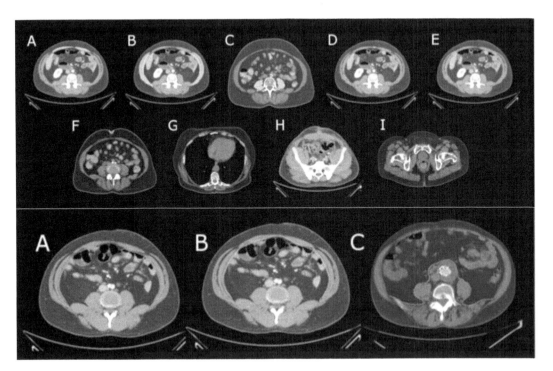

Fig. 3.7 Axial CT images showing abdominal wall segmentation and labeling. *Top panel*: (**a**) rectus abdominis/pyramidalis musculature, (**b**) oblique musculature, (**c**) psoas muscles, (**d**) linea alba, (**e**) linea semilunaris, (**f**) umbilicus, (**g**) xiphoid process, (**h**) anterior superior iliac spines, (**i**) pubic symphysis. *Bottom panel*: (**a**) outer abdominal wall, (**b**) inner abdominal wall, (**c**) posterior abdominal cavity. From Allen (2013), with permission

In a recent report, Franklin et al. retrospectively analyzed CT images from patients who underwent abdominal wall reconstruction with component separation over a 5-year period. Significant differences were seen with regard to transverse defect size, defect area, and the percentage of the total abdominal wall occupied by the defect in patients in whom fascial reapproximation was achieved as opposed to those two required a bridged repair [24]. Having such knowledge preoperatively can significantly influence surgical decision making in terms of an open versus laparoscopic approach, the type of mesh prosthetic used, and ultimately the placement of prosthetics. This is especially applicable in the setting of a recurrent hernia and a planned reoperation for abdominal wall reconstruction. Thus, it is commonplace to obtain preoperative CT scans on patients with large, complex, or recurrent defects. This allows for optimal operative planning and it maximizes the surgeon's chances of achieving fascial closure in these challenging patients.

Magnetic Resonance Imaging

Given the high degree of accuracy with which CT is able to characterize most ventral hernia defects, the use of MRI for this purpose is significantly limited. Although it does avoid radiation exposure of CT, additional cost of MRI is not typically justified to use as a routine imaging modality [3]. The one advantage that MRI can have over CT in the setting of recurrent hernia is an enhanced ability to visualize prosthetic mesh and its potential for dynamic assessment of the abdominal wall and visceral motion when using functional "cine" MRI. Namely, images can be obtained with the patient both at rest and during performance of a Valsalva maneuver. The motion of the abdominal viscera relative to that of the abdominal wall ("visceral slide") can then be ascertained and used to predict the degree of adhesion formation in a postoperative patient [25]. In May 2009 report by Kirchhoff et al., functional cine MRI was used to locate and quantify intra-abdominal adhesions in 43 patients who had undergone prior ventral hernia repair by either an open or laparoscopic approach. Twenty-five patients subsequently underwent reoperation, and after quantifying adhesions intraoperatively, the accuracy of MRI for predicting these adhesions was found to be approximately 86% [26]. The routine use of MRI for ventral hernia evaluation is not currently advocated outside the setting of a clinical trial. However, the imaging modality does show prominence for adhesion identification and could influence surgical decision making in patients without a detectable recurrence, but with significant abdominal pain after prior ventral hernia repair with mesh placement.

Conclusion

In terms of inguinal hernia detection, the initial use of US, possibly followed by CT, represents a sensitive and cost-effective progression for the evaluation of the patient with a clinical history suggestive of a hernia, but without evidence of a hernia on exam. Herniography is not widely utilized, but it does represent a sensitive and specific test in the hands of an experienced radiologist. MRI may be used to further evaluate other causes of groin pain in a patient with a negative US or CT study.

For ventral hernias, the use of DASH in the clinic is highly sensitive and specific if the diagnosis of a new or recurrent defect is in doubt. While MRI may be used in a research setting at this time, it should not supplant the use of CT. The use of CT is recommended in patients with large, recurrent, or complex ventral hernias in order to optimize preoperative planning and maximize the chance of obtaining abdominal wall defect closure.

References

1. Poulose BK, Shelton J, Phillips S, Moore D, Nealon W, Penson D, Beck W, Holzman MD. Epidemiology and cost of ventral hernia repair: making the case for hernia research. Hernia. 2012;16:179–83.
2. Baucom RB, Beck WC, Holzman MD, Sharp KW, Nealon WH, Poulose BK. Prospective evaluation of

surgeon physical examination for detection of incisional hernias. J Am Coll Surg. 2014;218:363–6.

3. Murphy KP, O'Connor OJ, Maher MM. Adult abdominal hernias. AJR Am J Roentgenol. 2014;202:W506–11.

4. Robinson A, Light D, Kasim A, Nice C. A systematic review and meta-analysis of the role of radiology in the diagnosis of occult inguinal hernia. Surg Endosc. 2013;27:11–8.

5. Robinson A, Light D, Nice C. Meta-analysis of sonography in the diagnosis of inguinal hernias. J Ultrasound Med. 2013;32:339–46.

6. Alam A, Nice C, Uberoi R. The accuracy of ultrasound in the diagnosis of clinically occult groin hernias in adults. Eur Radiol. 2005;15:2457–61.

7. Hojer AM, Rygaard H, Jess P. CT in the diagnosis of abdominal wall hernias: a preliminary study. Eur Radiol. 1997;7:1416–8.

8. Markos V, Brown EF. CT herniography in the diagnosis of occult groin hernias. Clin Radiol. 2005;60:251–6.

9. Garvey JF. Computed tomography scan diagnosis of occult groin hernia. Hernia. 2012;16:307–14.

10. Leander P, Ekberg O, Sjoberg S, Kesek P. MR imaging following herniography in patients with unclear groin pain. Eur Radiol. 2000;10:1691–6.

11. Miller J, Cho J, Michael MJ, Saouaf R, Towfigh S. Role of imaging in the diagnosis of occult hernias. JAMA Surg. 2014;149:1077–80.

12. Hachem MI, Saunders MP, Rix TE, Anderson HJ. Herniography: a reliable investigation avoiding needless groin exploration—a retrospective study. Hernia. 2009;13:57–60.

13. Hureibi KA, McLatchie GR, Kidambi AV. Is herniography useful and safe? Eur J Radiol. 2011;80:e86–90.

14. Whalen HR, Kidd GA, O'Dwyer PJ. Femoral hernias. BMJ. 2011;343:d7668.

15. Burkhardt JH, Arshanskiy Y, Munson JL, Scholz FJ. Diagnosis of inguinal region hernias with axial CT: the lateral crescent sign and other key findings. Radiographics. 2011;31:E1–12.

16. Bradley M, Morgan D, Pentlow B, Roe A. The groin hernia—an ultrasound diagnosis? Ann R Coll Surg Engl. 2003;85:178–80.

17. Djuric-Stefanovic A, Saranovic D, Ivanovic A, Masulovic D, Zuvela M, Bjelovic M, Pesko P. The accuracy of ultrasonography in classification of groin hernias according to the criteria of the unified classification system. Hernia. 2008;12:395–400.

18. Losanoff JE, Richman BW, Jones JW. Obturator hernia. J Am Coll Surg. 2002;194:657–63.

19. Petrie A, Tubbs RS, Matusz P, Shaffer K, Loukas M. Obturator hernia: anatomy, embryology, diagnosis, and treatment. Clin Anat. 2011;24:562–9.

20. den Hartog D, Dur AH, Kamphuis AG, Tuinebreijer WE, Kreis RW. Low recurrence rate of a two-layered closure repair for primary and recurrent midline incisional hernia without mesh. Hernia. 2009;13:45–8.

21. Beck WC, Holzman MD, Sharp KW, Nealon WH, Dupont WD, Poulose BK. Comparative effectiveness of dynamic abdominal sonography for hernia vs. computed tomography in the diagnosis of incisional hernia. J Am Coll Surg. 2013;216:447–53. quiz 510-441.

22. Diao X, Chen Y, Qiu Z, Pang Y, Zhan J, Chen L. Diagnostic value of an automated breast volume scanner for abdominal hernias. J Ultrasound Med. 2014;33:39–46.

23. Allen WM, Xu Z, Asman AJ, Poulose BK, Landman BA. Quantitative anatomical labeling of the anterior abdominal wall. Proc SPIE Int Soc Opt Eng. 2013;8673:867312.

24. Franklin BR, Patel KM, Nahabedian MY, Baldassari LE, Cohen EI, Bhanot P. Predicting abdominal closure after component separation for complex ventral hernias: maximizing the use of preoperative computed tomography. Ann Plast Surg. 2013;71:261–5.

25. Mussack T, Fischer T, Ladurner R, Gangkofer A, Bensler S, Hallfeldt KK, Reiser M, Lienemann A. Cine magnetic resonance imaging vs. high-resolution ultrasonography for detection of adhesions after laparoscopic and open incisional hernia repair: a matched pair pilot analysis. Surg Endosc. 2005;19:1538–43.

26. Kirchhoff S, Ladurner R, Kirchhoff C, Mussack T, Reiser MF, Lienemann A. Detection of recurrent hernia and intraabdominal adhesions following incisional hernia repair: a functional cine MRI-study. Abdom Imaging. 2010;35:224–31.

Preoperative Preparation of the Patient Undergoing Incisional Hernia Repair: Optimizing Chances for Success

Robert G. Martindale and Clifford W. Deveney

Introduction

The recurrence rate following a seemingly successful incisional hernia repair is reported to be between 10 and 60%. Although the majority of recurrences occur within 2 years of repair, these hernias can recur for up to 20 or 30 years following the index procedure [1]. Repairs of recurrent hernias have an even higher recurrence rate [1]. Although some causes of hernia recurrence are related to surgical technique, several patient factors contribute profoundly to hernia recurrence by delaying wound healing, or actually causing necrosis or absorption of connective tissue. It is also well-reported that perioperative surgical site occurrence (SSO), defined as infection, seroma, wound ischemia, and dehiscence increases the risk of recurrent hernia by at least threefold, if not more [2].

Because the success of hernia repair is often measured by the absence of recurrence, the focus of preoperative optimization aims at eliminating factors that inhibit wound healing. Well-documented factors of adverse effects on wound healing include smoking, obesity, hyperglycemia, nutritional deficiencies, and infection.

Modifiable factors should be addressed and corrected before elective repair, if possible. By correcting, eliminating, or reducing them if they are abnormal, one optimizes a patient's chance of undergoing successful hernia repair without recurrence, post-op infectious complications, or delayed wound healing [3].

Smoking

There are numerous studies that have documented the deleterious effects of smoking on wound healing and the role cessation has in the prevention of wound infections [4, 5]. Cigarette smoke contains myriad of compounds, such as nicotine, carbon monoxide, hydrogen cyanide, nitrogen oxides, nitrosamines, aldehydes, and polyaromatic hydrocarbons, all or some of which affect every aspect of wound healing. The adverse effects of smoking are well-summarized in two recent reviews [6, 7].

One of the principle effects of smoking is decreased tissue oxygenation. Low oxygen tension leads to tissue ischemia and necrosis in marginally perfused tissue, and is reversed within an hour of smoke inhalation. There are many other additional detrimental effects on the inflammatory and reparative processes of wound healing that predispose a patient to complications such as infection, dehiscence, and recurrent hernia.

Several clinical studies have demonstrated a maximal response to smoking cessation 3–4

R.G. Martindale (✉) • C.W. Deveney
Department of Surgery, Oregon Health and Science University,
3181 SW Sam Jackson Park Road, L223A, Portland, OR 97239, USA
e-mail: martindr@ohsu.edu; deveneyc@ohsu.edu

© Springer International Publishing Switzerland 2016
Y.W. Novitsky (ed.), *Hernia Surgery*, DOI 10.1007/978-3-319-27470-6_4

weeks post-operatively [8, 9]. After 4 weeks, the inflammatory components of wound healing normalize, but the proliferative phase of wound healing is still blunted. Nicotine attenuates the inflammatory phase of wound healing, but enhances the proliferative phase. In clinical trials, the effects of nicotine replacement therapy used in aiding smoking cessation do not seem to have detrimental significance [10].

With the abundance of information regarding the negative effects of smoking on wound healing, we require that all patients who will be undergoing elective herniorrhaphy cease smoking for at least 1 month before surgery. It is currently unclear whether or not nicotine patches alter wound healing or have adverse influence on post-operative physiology; as such, the use of nicotine patches as an aid to stop smoking is allowed. If the patient wears the patch, however, the physician will be unable to confirm abstinence from smoking with serum or urine nicotine levels. At our institution, we therefore reserve its use for those patients who seem most reliable, and have cohabitants that can corroborate their abstinence from smoking. It is also important to advise the patient that it will be necessary to abstain from smoking for at least 1 month following surgery, though permanent cessation is preferable because smoking will affect tissue healing, even after 1 month.

Obesity

Smoking cessation, glycemic control, and nutritional and metabolic support can all be achieved over a relatively short time (1–5 weeks), but obesity is a much weightier problem and unfortunately takes months to resolve in the best setting. It is probably the greatest concomitant factor influencing the development of incisional hernias and their recurrence. The effect of obesity on hernia formation is particularly pertinent in this era, where obesity rates have been increasing by epidemic proportions worldwide. With increasing weight, the probability of recurrence also increases almost exponentially. Presently, literature supports not performing routine elective hernia repairs in

patients with a BMI ≥ 50. In our prospective database (2300 patients), the recurrence rate following hernia repair in those patients with a BMI ≥ 50 approaches 100 %. It takes months for a patient to lose significant weight, even following a bariatric operation. If the surgeon has the luxury to delay (e.g., in the case of minimally or non-symptomatic reducible hernia), he or she should do so until the patient has lost a considerable amount of weight. Unfortunately, for those hernias which are symptomatic or incarcerated, the surgeon does not have this advantage.

Although it would be ideal for obese patients to lose weight perioperatively, in the majority of cases they do not. In the morbidly obese patient with an epigastric hernia who is to undergo a laparoscopic bariatric procedure, the hernia may or may not be repaired at the time of that procedure. If the bariatric procedure is an open one, it may be necessary to repair the hernia to safely close the abdomen. If the bariatric procedure can be done laparoscopically, the hernia may also be repaired laparoscopically [11]. If the hernia is symptomatic, or presents a threat of strangulation, the priority would be to repair the hernia and perform the bariatric procedure only if it can be done safely [12].

Glucose Control

It has been established that post-operative hyperglycemia is associated with an increase in surgical site infections (SSI). In a study of patients undergoing surgery in the Veterans Administration hospitals, an increased rate of SSI was seen in patients with HbA1c > 7%. The authors of this article recommended that, when possible, glycemic control should be used until the HbA1C is 7% or lower [13]. In another study, it was found that the rate of SSI increased in increments of 30% when the glucose level increased by 40 mg/dL, over a normal level of 110 mg/dL [14, 15]. The control of post-op glucose levels in the prevention of SSI seems to be most critical in the first 24 hours, because hyperglycemia impairs the ability of neutrophils to kill any bacteria in a wound.

Our policy is to reduce the Hb1C to less than 7.5% preoperatively, and to maintain blood glucose at 140 mg/dL or less in the post-op period.

Nutritional Intervention

In the current era of evidence-based surgical practice, recommendations for nutritional intervention in elective and emergent surgical practice are supported by a significant number of randomized clinical trials, observational studies, abundant meta-analyses, and systematic reviews [16]. The metabolic response to surgical insult is highly variable, and can now be manipulated to optimize fuel utilization and preserve lean body tissue [16]. Elective or semi-elective surgical procedures in the face of ongoing suboptimal nutritional status will result in poor outcome. This was convincingly demonstrated in the large Preoperative Risk Assessment Study conducted by the U.S. Department of Veterans Affairs. This prospective trial included >87,000 patients from 44 separate medical centers, where investigators collected 67 variables on each patient. It reported that the single most valuable predictor of poor outcome and increased morbidity was a serum albumin of less than 3.0 g/dL [17]. This large study plus several others support the concept of addressing nutrition prior to major surgical intervention.

The majority of patients undergoing major abdominal wall reconstruction (AWR) with an expected extended stay in the hospital and intensive care unit (ICU) at moderate to severe nutritional risk will gain significant outcome benefits from early attention to nutrition. While this has not been definitively shown in hernia surgery, it has been well-demonstrated for major visceral surgical procedures [18]. Patients with malnutrition going into AWR resulting from obstruction or infection, or an urgent or emergent major hernia repair will benefit from meticulous attention to nutritional issues even more [19]. Several factors will alter the realized benefit a patient receives from nutritional intervention, including route and timing of delivery, content of nutrient substrate, and efforts to promote patient mobility [16]. Recent data would support a preoperative

assessment and nutritional intervention if the patient meets high-risk criteria [19]. Several nutritional scoring systems or risk assessment methods have been proposed, with only one being validated in surgical population [20]. If the patient requires an ICU stay, the NUTRIC Score has been validated as an excellent predictor of nutritional risk [21].

Preoperative Metabolic Preparation for Surgical Intervention

The concept of metabolic manipulation in the preoperative time frame was popularized by now classic studies by Braga and Gianotti [22–24]. These investigators, using specific nutrients known to have metabolically active effects, demonstrated lowered perioperative complications by adding the amino acid arginine and omega-3 fatty acids, docohexanoic acid (DHA), and eicospentanoic acid (EPA) for 5 days preoperatively [22–24]. They reported major morbidity could be reduced by approximately 50% in patients undergoing major foregut surgery, including esophageal, stomach, or pancreas procedures. Surprisingly, the benefit was noted in both the well-nourished and malnourished patient populations [25, 26]. The finding that benefits were noted in well-nourished patients undergoing major GI oncologic surgery was new, and changed the concept of "metabolic manipulation" [26]. In these studies, the patients consumed approximately 750 mL per day of the metabolic-modulating formula, containing fish oils (EPA and DHA), arginine, and nucleic acids in addition to their regular diet. As noted above, this formula resulted in significant decreases in infectious morbidity, length of hospital stay (LOS), and hospital-related expenses [22–24]. In a contemporary meta-analysis and systematic review of the evidence including 35 strictly reviewed articles, Drover et al. reported that these metabolic manipulating supplements yielded a significant benefit in lowering infectious morbidity across several surgical specialties, and reported a decrease in hospital LOS [27].

It is believed that the arginine and fish oils are the largest contributors to the noted benefits. Fish oils, 20 carbon EPA, and 22 carbon DHA have many described mechanisms, including the attenuation of the metabolic response to stress, alteration of gene expression to minimize the proinflammatory cytokine production, beneficial modification of the Th1 to Th2 lymphocyte population to lower the inflammatory response, and an increase in the production of the lipid derivatives of EPA and DHA, which actively resolves tissues inflammation [28]. These compounds can allow apoptosis of macrophages and propagate macrophage class switches from the inflammatory M1 class to the less inflammatory M2 class [28–30]. Arginine was reported to have been of benefit in the enhancement of wound healing in the 1970s; since that time, additional benefits have been reported, including optimization of lymphocyte proliferation and enhancement of blood flow via nitric oxide vasodilation effects [31, 32]. The influence of the ribonucleic acid (RNA) found in these immune and metabolic formulations has theoretical benefits that have yet to be well-elucidated in mammalian trials [32].

Another area of importance in metabolic preparation is the concept of preoperative carbohydrate-loading of muscle, myocardium, and the liver to allow for immediate energy supply during a planned procedure [33]. This metabolic strategy employs an isotonic carbohydrate solution, containing approximately 150 g of carbohydrate to be given at midnight the night before surgery, with another 50 g to be given 3 hours preoperatively to "load" the muscle and liver with glycogen prior to the onset of surgical trauma [34]. In most Western surgical settings, "routine" management the night before surgery is for the patient to remain NPO after the evening meal until surgery. By following this "routine," glycogen stores are nearly depleted prior to the surgical insult. Soop et al. [35], Fearon et al. [36], and more recently, Awad et al. [37, 38] have demonstrated the beneficial metabolic effects of carbo-loading, primarily in reducing insulin resistance. Large multicenter randomized clinical trials in humans, however, are still required to solidify these concepts. It is difficult to make spe-

cific conclusions about preoperative carbohydrate loading because most of the supporting studies have been done as part of a bundle of items done as preoperative preparation in protocols. The Early Recovery After Surgery (ERAS) protocol is an example of how multiple issues are simultaneously evaluated, such as early mobilization, no use of nasogastric tubes, minimizing narcotics, avoidance of drains, tightly controlled perioperative fluid management, local, regional, and epidural anesthesia when possible, etc. [35]. In the studies currently published, carbohydrate loading has consistently demonstrated several metabolic benefits, including significantly reduced insulin resistance, decreased postoperative nitrogen loss, and better retention of muscle function, while reporting little to no increase in morbidity [35, 36].

Over the past 15 years, various nutritional agents, either alone or in combination, have been reported to improve outcomes in surgical practice. The reports of attenuating metabolic response to stress, enhancing lean body tissue, or preserving antioxidant capacity have proven too inconsistent, and have inadequate support from prospective randomized trials for its routine use [16]. The use of anabolic agents, such as oxandrolone and human recombinant growth hormone, has essentially no prospective data to support their use in anything other than experimental protocols [39].

Imaging

Virtually all of our patients with complex ventral (incisional) abdominal hernias get a preoperative CT scan. Cross-sectional imaging will accurately define the extent of the hernia, and reveal any hernias undiagnosed upon physical exam. The CT scan is essential in defining the hernia in obese patients, since physical exam is often not accurate for assessment of the presence of a hernia, amount and makeup of visceral content in the hernia sac, size of the hernia, or the width of the hernia sac [40]. In addition, the CT is very helpful in planning an approach to large hernias and, if necessary, other advanced techniques such as component separation [41]. The CT scan is particularly valuable in complex, infected, or recurrent hernias. It is also essential in defining the anatomy of enterocutaneous fistulas, when present. If there is a question of renal compromise with the use of contrast agents, the exam can be done without contrast to provide the majority of the information required. If the surgeon is planning a laparoscopic repair, it is essential to know the boundaries of the hernia sac, so that a trocar is not mistakenly placed through it and inserted within it.

Antibiotic Prophylaxis

Antibiotic prophylaxis is recommended for abdominal wall hernia repairs. The recommendations given in the Surgical Infection Society Guidelines are cost-effective and safe, while limiting excessive prophylaxis [42]. Antibiotics should be given 30–60 min before the incision is made, and should be re-dosed if the procedure lasts longer than their half-life. Achieving adequate tissue levels in obese patients requires larger doses of the antibiotic in most cases. When Ancef® is used in obese patients (BMI > 30), 2 g should be administered, and if BMI > 50, some have suggested dosing up to 3 g to reach the MIC at the tissue level prior to incision.

Wound infection following incisional hernia repair is associated with a significant increased incidence of hernia recurrence [43, 44]. Whether or not the infection rate is greater in patients who have had previously infected wounds is unknown. Nevertheless, when the patient has a previously infected wound, it is important that the surgeon try to determine the organisms involved, and include prophylactic antibodies that would be effective against them. Specifically, if the patient has previously had a wound infected with methicillin resistant *Staph aureus* (MRSA), vancomycin should be added along with cefazolin as prophylaxis.

For those patients with ongoing wound infections, infected mesh, or intestinal fistulas, staging of repairs is becoming more common. In these cases, extensive debridement of infected soft tissue, removal of mesh, and subsequent treatment of open abdomen followed in days, weeks, or even months for more extensive infections is indicated. These cases would be closed in a temporary manner, and then a formal AWR would be done on a subsequent date.

Preoperative Skin Preparation and Decolonization Protocols

The data on choice of skin preps for surgery continue to evolve. Two major trials have recently been published. Swenson et al. reported in a prospective trial in over >3200 patients, iodine skin preps were superior to chlorhexidine preps [45]. Within a year of the Swenson manuscript, a prospective randomized clinical trial with intention to treat analysis in over 800 patients was published, reporting that chlorhexidine was superior to iodine preps [46]. When these two papers were more intensely analyzed, it revealed the key to lower infections appeared to be the alcohol in the preps, that Duraprep® and Cloraprep® had nearly equivalent surgical infection risk, and that the iodine prep without alcohol was most commonly associated with infections [47].

Although shaving or removal of hair from the surgical site does not necessarily lower infection risk, it has been the standard of care for several years that clippers, rather than razors, be used to clear the surgical site hair that would interfere with the wound closure [48]. Surgical site barriers, such as adhesive skin covers and skin sealants, have not been prospectively studied in ventral hernia repair. The information available on these applications is inconsistent, with reports varying from beneficial to potentially detrimental. The data on skin sealants and surgical site barriers are far too inconsistent to make any data-driven recommendation for use. That being said, the concept of allowing mesh to be in contact with skin during placement could potentially contaminate the mesh. The use of preoperative showers with antiseptic soaps in hopes of decreasing SSI has not been well-supported by large randomized trials [49]. Showering with antiseptic agents, such as chlorhexidine or

Betadine, when compared to showering with standard soaps has not been proven to have a consistent benefit [50]. Most studies are underpowered, or were studied in a widely heterogeneous population, which makes consistent results near impossible. Many of the early studies do report a decrease in skin bacterial colonization at time of surgery, but have not shown a consistent decrease in SSI. A few [51, 52] of the smaller studies have shown the benefit of preoperative chlorhexidine shower in reducing SSI, but they are in the minority [53]. This inconsistency in the literature led the Cochrane analysis in 2012 to conclude preoperative showers with antiseptics have no significant benefit [50, 54]. Preoperative clearance of MRSA and methicillin-sensitive S. *aureus* (MSSA) in the preoperative has gained significant popularity in the last 4 years, following a landmark paper published by Bode et al. in the *New England Journal of Medicine*, 2010 [55]. The Bode manuscript was then supported by several other reports with similar outcomes [56]. In the Bode study, 6771 patients were screened on admission, with almost 20% being positive for S. *aureus*. The S. *aureus* patients were then prospectively randomized, with an intention to treat analysis, and mupirocin was applied twice daily to the nostrils with a chlorhexidine shower once daily vs placebo. They reported a 42% decrease in S. *aureus* post-operative infections in the treated group. The logistics of screening, then treating those patients that tested positive, has been reported to be difficult, and aggressive follow-up on positive screening cultures is required. Several recent studies have advocated just treating patients that are at high risk for MRSA colonization [57].

Miscellaneous Techniques and Treatments to Reduce Risk

Additional measures reported to decrease post-op infectious complications include antibiotic-impregnated suture, perioperative patient warming, as well as intraoperative and post-operative hyperoxygenation. Antibiotic-impregnated sutures, however, have very limited support in the literature [58]. Several moderately powered prospective randomized trials have now reported using Triclosan-impregnated sutures for reduced infection risk in a routine midline closure. Although results from the early reports are promising, more trials will be required before use of antibiotic-impregnated sutures becomes a standard of care [59, 60].

Intraoperative wound protectors are designed to protect from desiccation, contamination, and mechanical trauma. They have also been said to decrease wound infections. No hernia surgery-specific data on wound protectors are currently available. To date, at least six randomized clinical trials have been conducted, four of which reported no benefit in lowering SSI, and two of which showed a benefit. When weighing the quality of the studies, and using the Grade system to evaluate them, the review trends toward no benefit [61, 62].

The concept of perioperative warming, the use of forced air circulation to reduce SSI, has received significant attention in the past 10 years, with most operating rooms now using it as part of their quality improvement programs and protocols. Several observational studies in the early 2000s reported a significant correlation between hypothermia and SSI, which led to now numerous, well-controlled trials with very mixed results. The theoretical belief is that euthermia helps maintain better perfusion to skin, and that better oxygen tension at the skin level will decrease SSI [63]. Hypothermia has also been associated with adverse influence on the immune function, including T-cell-mediated antibody production, and a decrease in both oxidative and non-oxidative killing of bacteria by neutrophils [64]. These warming concepts were supported by two moderate-sized, randomized controlled trials, both showing relative hypothermia being significantly associated with increased SSI. A large nested, case-controlled study, using the NSQIP (National Surgery Quality Improvement Program) database, as well as several other trials specifically done on ventral hernias, appear to have not confirmed these earlier findings [65].

Supplemental perioperative oxygenation (hyperoxia) has been well investigated, primarily for colorectal surgery, but unfortunately not for complex ventral hernia surgery. The concept that adequate oxygenation is required for neutrophil and macrophage killing of bacteria, and the understanding that the tissue of surgical wounds has a much lower partial pressure of oxygen than that normal tissue makes this an attractive hypothesis for lowering SSI [66]. Two studies involving colorectal surgery patients reported benefit in reducing SSI led to multiple perioperative protocols that incorporated the use of supplemental oxygenation [67, 68]. These early results stimulated a large governmental-funded study of over 1400 patients that reported no significant benefit in perioperative hyperoxia [69]. A more recent meta-analysis of several large and small trials favors supplemental oxygen protocols in high-risk visceral surgical populations, such as colorectal surgery patients [70]. Although no studies have been conducted primarily for AWR and complex ventral hernia repair, this population has a risk of SSI almost identical to that of colorectal surgery patients, so it appears reasonable to extrapolate the colorectal data to ventral and incisional hernias.

Perioperative antibiotic use results in antibiotic-associated diarrhea (AAD) in an estimated 20% of patients [71]. Perioperative use of antibiotics is a major source for AAD and Clostridium *difficile* diarrhea [72, 73]. Numerous recent prospective trials have shown that appropriate selection and supplementation of probiotics (live viable bacteria, when given in adequate amounts show benefit in the host) are safe, and can significantly decrease both AAD and C. *difficile* diarrhea [72–74].

Over the past several years, many other techniques and/or trials have shown promise in the pre and intraoperative arena to optimize outcomes. Reviewing all of them is beyond the scope of this chapter. One concept that is rapidly gaining traction in major surgery, however, is the idea that a routinely scheduled preoperative physical activity program, or "prehabilitation" can both decrease length of stay and total complications associated with major surgery [75].

Conclusion

Each portion of the patient's surgical journey should be addressed and optimized when possible. This is especially true for major factors including smoking, obesity, and diabetes management. Other preoperative and perioperative interventions described above may be relatively minor, but have been shown to be safe and even cost-effective in most cases. The interventions performed in the immediate perioperative period, like the appropriate choosing and timing of prophylactic antibiotics, metabolic preparation with specific nutrients and/or carbohydrate-loading, choice of alcohol-containing skin preps, and preoperative decolonization of MRSA and MSSA from the nostrils and skin, are reasonable interventions, which, when implemented, should minimize perioperative morbidity.

References

1. Flum DR, Horvath K, Koepsell T. Have outcomes of incisional hernia repair improved with time? A population-based analysis. Ann Surg. 2003;237(1):129–35.
2. Slater NJ, Montgomery A, Berrevoet F, Carbonell AM, Chang A, Franklin M, et al. Criteria for definition of a complex abdominal wall hernia. Hernia. 2014;18(1):7–17.
3. Martindale RG, Deveney CW. Preoperative risk reduction: strategies to optimize outcomes. Surg Clin North Am. 2013;93(5):1041–55.
4. Khullar D, Maa J. The impact of smoking on surgical outcomes. J Am Coll Surg. 2012;215(3):418–26.
5. Mastracci TM, Carli F, Finley RJ, Muccio S, Warner DO. Members of the evidence-based reviews in surgery G. Effect of preoperative smoking cessation interventions on postoperative complications. J Am Coll Surg. 2011;212(6):1094–6.
6. Mills E, Eyawo O, Lockhart I, Kelly S, Wu P, Ebbert JO. Smoking cessation reduces postoperative complications: a systematic review and meta-analysis. Am J Med. 2011;124(2):144–54.
7. Sorensen LT. Wound healing and infection in surgery: the pathophysiological impact of smoking, smoking cessation, and nicotine replacement therapy: a systematic review. Ann Surg. 2012;255(6):1069–79.
8. Kuri M, Nakagawa M, Tanaka H, Hasuo S, Kishi Y. Determination of the duration of preoperative

smoking cessation to improve wound healing after head and neck surgery. Anesthesiology. 2005;102(5): 892–6.

9. Sorensen LT. Wound healing and infection in surgery. The clinical impact of smoking and smoking cessation: a systematic review and meta-analysis. Archiv Surg. 2012;147(4):373–83.

10. Sorensen LT, Toft BG, Rygaard J, Ladelund S, Paddon M, James T, et al. Effect of smoking, smoking cessation, and nicotine patch on wound dimension, vitamin C, and systemic markers of collagen metabolism. Surgery. 2010;148(5):982–90.

11. Praveen Raj P, Senthilnathan P, Kumaravel R, Rajpandian S, Rajan PS, Anand Vijay N, et al. Concomitant laparoscopic ventral hernia mesh repair and bariatric surgery: a retrospective study from a tertiary care center. Obesity Surg. 2012;22(5):685–9.

12. Eid GM, Wikiel KJ, Entabi F, Saleem M. Ventral hernias in morbidly obese patients: a suggested algorithm for operative repair. Obesity Surg. 2013;23(5):703–9.

13. Dronge AS, Perkal MF, Kancir S, Concato J, Aslan M, Rosenthal RA. Long-term glycemic control and postoperative infectious complications. Archiv Surg. 2006;141(4):375–80.

14. Berbari EF, Osmon DR, Lahr B, Eckel-Passow JE, Tsaras G, Hanssen AD, et al. The Mayo prosthetic joint infection risk score: implication for surgical site infection reporting and risk stratification. Infect Control Hosp Epidemiol. 2012;33(8):774–81.

15. Ramos M, Khalpey Z, Lipsitz S, Steinberg J, Panizales MT, Zinner M, et al. Relationship of perioperative hyperglycemia and postoperative infections in patients who undergo general and vascular surgery. Ann Surg. 2008;248(4):585–91.

16. Martindale RG, McClave SA, Taylor B, Lawson CM. Perioperative nutrition: what is the current landscape? J Parenter Enteral Nutr. 2013;37(5 Suppl):5S–20S.

17. Daley J, Khuri SF, Henderson W, Hur K, Gibbs JO, Barbour G, et al. Risk adjustment of the postoperative morbidity rate for the comparative assessment of the quality of surgical care: results of the National Veterans Affairs Surgical Risk Study. J Am Coll Surg. 1997;185(4):328–40.

18. Munroe C, Frantz D, Martindale RG, McClave SA. The optimal lipid formulation in enteral feeding in critical illness: clinical update and review of the literature. Curr Gastroenterol Rep. 2011;13(4):368–75.

19. Jie B, Jiang ZM, Nolan MT, Zhu SN, Yu K, Kondrup J. Impact of preoperative nutritional support on clinical outcome in abdominal surgical patients at nutritional risk. Nutrition. 2012;28(10):1022–7.

20. Kondrup J, Rasmussen HH, Hamberg O, Stanga Z, Ad Hoc EWG. Nutritional risk screening (NRS 2002): a new method based on an analysis of controlled clinical trials. Clin Nutr. 2003;22(3):321–36.

21. Heyland DK, Dhaliwal R, Jiang X, Day AG. Identifying critically ill patients who benefit the most from nutrition therapy: the development and initial validation of a novel risk assessment tool. Crit Care. 2011;15(6):R268.

22. Gianotti L, Braga M, Nespoli L, Radaelli G, Beneduce A, Di Carlo V. A randomized controlled trial of preoperative oral supplementation with a specialized diet in patients with gastrointestinal cancer. Gastroenterology. 2002;122(7):1763–70.

23. Braga M, Gianotti L, Vignali A, Schmid A, Nespoli L, Di Carlo V. Hospital resources consumed for surgical morbidity: effects of preoperative arginine and omega-3 fatty acid supplementation on costs. Nutrition. 2005;21(11–12):1078–86.

24. Braga M, Gianotti L, Nespoli L, Radaelli G, Di Carlo V. Nutritional approach in malnourished surgical patients: a prospective randomized study. Archiv Surg. 2002;137(2):174–80.

25. Manchio JV, Litchfield CR, Sati S, Bryan DJ, Weinzweig J, Vernadakis AJ. Duration of smoking cessation and its impact on skin flap survival. Plast Reconstr Surg. 2009;124(4):1105–17.

26. Braga M. Perioperative immunonutrition and gut function. Curr Opin Clin Nutr Metab Care. 2012;15(5):485–8.

27. Drover JW, Dhaliwal R, Weitzel L, Wischmeyer PE, Ochoa JB, Heyland DK. Perioperative use of arginine-supplemented diets: a systematic review of the evidence. J Am Coll Surg. 2011;212(3):385–99.

28. Serhan CN. Pro-resolving lipid mediators are leads for resolution physiology. Nature. 2014;510(7503): 92–101.

29. Pluess TT, Hayoz D, Berger MM, Tappy L, Revelly JP, Michaeli B, et al. Intravenous fish oil blunts the physiological response to endotoxin in healthy subjects. Intensive Care Med. 2007;33(5):789–97.

30. Calder PC. Fatty acids and inflammation: the cutting edge between food and pharma. Eur J Pharmacol. 2011;668 Suppl 1:S50–8.

31. Marik PE, Flemmer M. The immune response to surgery and trauma: implications for treatment. J Trauma Acute Care Surg. 2012;73(4):801–8.

32. Rudolph FB, Van Buren CT. The metabolic effects of enterally administered ribonucleic acids. Curr Opin Clin Nutr Metab Care. 1998;1(6):527–30.

33. Burden S, Todd C, Hill J, Lal S. Pre-operative nutrition support in patients undergoing gastrointestinal surgery. Cochrane Database Syst Rev. 2012;11:CD008879.

34. Svanfeldt M, Thorell A, Hausel J, Soop M, Nygren J, Ljungqvist O. Effect of "preoperative" oral carbohydrate treatment on insulin action—a randomised cross-over unblinded study in healthy subjects. Clin Nutr. 2005;24(5):815–21.

35. Soop M, Nygren J, Myrenfors P, Thorell A, Ljungqvist O. Preoperative oral carbohydrate treatment attenuates immediate postoperative insulin resistance. Am J Physiol Endocrinol Metab. 2001;280(4):E576–83.

36. Fearon KC, Ljungqvist O, Von Meyenfeldt M, Revhaug A, Dejong CH, Lassen K, et al. Enhanced recovery after surgery: a consensus review of clinical care for patients undergoing colonic resection. Clin Nutr. 2005;24(3):466–77.

37. Awad S, Constantin-Teodosiu D, Constantin D, Rowlands BJ, Fearon KC, Macdonald IA, et al. Cellular mechanisms underlying the protective effects of preoperative feeding: a randomized study investigating muscle and liver glycogen content, mitochondrial function, gene and protein expression. Ann Surg. 2010;252(2):247–53.

38. Awad S, Fearon KC, Macdonald IA, Lobo DN. A randomized cross-over study of the metabolic and hormonal responses following two preoperative conditioning drinks. Nutrition. 2011;27(9):938–42.

39. Maung AA, Davis KA. Perioperative nutritional support: immunonutrition, probiotics, and anabolic steroids. Surg Clin North Am. 2012;92(2):273–83.

40. Baucom RB, Beck WC, Holzman MD, Sharp KW, Nealon WH, Poulose BK. Prospective evaluation of surgeon physical examination for detection of incisional hernias. J Am Coll Surg. 2014;218(3):363–6.

41. Franklin BR, Patel KM, Nahabedian MY, Baldassari LE, Cohen EI, Bhanot P. Predicting abdominal closure after component separation for complex ventral hernias: maximizing the use of preoperative computed tomography. Ann Plast Surg. 2013;71(3):261–5.

42. Bratzler DW, Dellinger EP, Olsen KM, Perl TM, Auwaerter PG, Bolon MK, et al. Clinical practice guidelines for antimicrobial prophylaxis in surgery. Surg Infect. 2013;14(1):73–156.

43. Luijendijk RW, Hop WC, van den Tol MP, de Lange DC, Braaksma MM, IJzermans JN, et al. A comparison of suture repair with mesh repair for incisional hernia. N Engl J Med. 2000;343(6):392–8.

44. Cassar K, Munro A. Surgical treatment of incisional hernia. Br J Surg. 2002;89(5):534–45.

45. Swenson BR, Hedrick TL, Metzger R, Bonatti H, Pruett TL, Sawyer RG. Effects of preoperative skin preparation on postoperative wound infection rates: a prospective study of 3 skin preparation protocols. Infect Control Hosp Epidemiol. 2009;30(10):964–71.

46. Darouiche RO, Wall Jr MJ, Itani KM, Otterson MF, Webb AL, Carrick MM, et al. Chlorhexidine-alcohol versus povidone-iodine for surgical-site antisepsis. N Engl J Med. 2010;362(1):18–26.

47. Swenson BR, Sawyer RG. Importance of alcohol in skin preparation protocols. Infect Control Hosp Epidemiol. 2010;31(9):977.

48. Tanner J, Norrie P, Melen K. Preoperative hair removal to reduce surgical site infection. Cochrane Database Syst Rev. 2011;(11):CD004122.

49. Jakobsson J, Perlkvist A, Wann-Hansson C. Searching for evidence regarding using preoperative disinfection showers to prevent surgical site infections: a systematic review. Worldviews Evid Based Nurs. 2011;8(3):143–52.

50. Dumville JC, McFarlane E, Edwards P, Lipp A, Holmes A. Preoperative skin antiseptics for preventing surgical wound infections after clean surgery. Cochrane Database Syst Rev. 2013;3:CD003949.

51. Manunga Jr J, Olak J, Rivera C, Martin M. Prevalence of methicillin-resistant Staphylococcus aureus in elective surgical patients at a public teaching hospital: an analysis of 1039 patients. Am Surg. 2012;78(10):1096–9.

52. Savage JW, Anderson PA. An update on modifiable factors to reduce the risk of surgical site infections. Spine J. 2013;13(9):1017–29.

53. Edmiston Jr CE, Okoli O, Graham MB, Sinski S, Seabrook GR. Evidence for using chlorhexidine gluconate preoperative cleansing to reduce the risk of surgical site infection. AORN J. 2010;92(5):509–18.

54. Chlebicki MP, Safdar N, O'Horo JC, Maki DG. Preoperative chlorhexidine shower or bath for prevention of surgical site infection: a meta-analysis. Am J Infect Control. 2013;41(2):167–73.

55. Bode LG, Kluytmans JA, Wertheim HF, Bogaers D, Vandenbroucke-Grauls CM, Roosendaal R, et al. Preventing surgical-site infections in nasal carriers of Staphylococcus aureus. N Engl J Med. 2010;362(1): 9–17.

56. Kim DH, Spencer M, Davidson SM, Li L, Shaw JD, Gulczynski D, et al. Institutional prescreening for detection and eradication of methicillin-resistant Staphylococcus aureus in patients undergoing elective orthopaedic surgery. J Bone Joint Surg Am. 2010; 92(9):1820–6.

57. Huang SS, Septimus E, Kleinman K, Moody J, Hickok J, Avery TR, et al. Targeted versus universal decolonization to prevent ICU infection. N Engl J Med. 2013;368(24):2255–65.

58. Justinger C, Moussavian MR, Schlueter C, Kopp B, Kollmar O, Schilling MK. Antibacterial [corrected] coating of abdominal closure sutures and wound infection. Surgery. 2009;145(3):330–4.

59. Justinger C, Slotta JE, Ningel S, Graber S, Kollmar O, Schilling MK. Surgical-site infection after abdominal wall closure with triclosan-impregnated polydioxanone sutures: results of a randomized clinical pathway facilitated trial (NCT00998907). Surgery. 2013;154(3):589–95.

60. Chang WK, Srinivasa S, Morton R, Hill AG. Triclosan-impregnated sutures to decrease surgical site infections: systematic review and meta-analysis of randomized trials. Ann Surg. 2012;255(5):854–9.

61. Reid K, Pockney P, Draganic B, Smith SR. Barrier wound protection decreases surgical site infection in open elective colorectal surgery: a randomized clinical trial. Dis Colon Rectum. 2010;53(10): 1374–80.

62. Horiuchi T, Tanishima H, Tamagawa K, Matsuura I, Nakai H, Shouno Y, et al. Randomized, controlled investigation of the anti-infective properties of the Alexis retractor/protector of incision sites. J Trauma. 2007;62(1):212–5.

63. Flores-Maldonado A, Medina-Escobedo CE, Rios-Rodriguez HM, Fernandez-Dominguez R. Mild perioperative hypothermia and the risk of wound infection. Arch Med Res. 2001;32(3):227–31.

64. Qadan M, Gardner SA, Vitale DS, Lominadze D, Joshua IG, Polk Jr HC. Hypothermia and surgery: immunologic mechanisms for current practice. Ann Surg. 2009;250(1):134–40.

65. Bittner R, Bingener-Casey J, Dietz U, Fabian M, Ferzli G, Fortelny R, et al. Guidelines for laparoscopic treatment of ventral and incisional abdominal

wall hernias (International Endohernia Society [IEHS])-Part III. Surg Endosc. 2014;28(2):380–404.

66. Fakhry SM, Montgomery SC. Peri-operative oxygen and the risk of surgical infection. Surg Infect. 2012;13(4):228–33.

67. Greif R, Akca O, Horn EP, Kurz A, Sessler DI, Outcomes Research G. Supplemental perioperative oxygen to reduce the incidence of surgical-wound infection. N Engl J Med. 2000;342(3):161–7.

68. Belda FJ, Aguilera L, Garcia de la Asuncion J, Alberti J, Vicente R, Ferrandiz L, et al. Supplemental perioperative oxygen and the risk of surgical wound infection: a randomized controlled trial. JAMA. 2005;294(16):2035–42.

69. Meyhoff CS, Wetterslev J, Jorgensen LN, Henneberg SW, Hogdall C, Lundvall L, et al. Effect of high perioperative oxygen fraction on surgical site infection and pulmonary complications after abdominal surgery: the PROXI randomized clinical trial. JAMA. 2009;302(14):1543–50.

70. Al-Niaimi A, Safdar N. Supplemental perioperative oxygen for reducing surgical site infection: a meta-analysis. J Eval Clin Pract. 2009;15(2):360–5.

71. McFarland LV. Antibiotic-associated diarrhea: epidemiology, trends and treatment. Future Microbiol. 2008;3(5):563–78.

72. Hempel S, Newberry SJ, Maher AR, Wang Z, Miles JN, Shanman R, et al. Probiotics for the prevention and treatment of antibiotic-associated diarrhea: a systematic review and meta-analysis. JAMA. 2012;307(18):1959–69.

73. Johnston BC, Ma SS, Goldenberg JZ, Thorlund K, Vandvik PO, Loeb M, et al. Probiotics for the prevention of Clostridium difficile-associated diarrhea: a systematic review and meta-analysis. Ann Intern Med. 2012;157(12):878–88.

74. Goldenberg JZ, Ma SS, Saxton JD, Martzen MR, Vandvik PO, Thorlund K et al. Probiotics for the prevention of Clostridium difficile-associated diarrhea in adults and children. Cochrane Database Syst Rev. 2013;5:CD006095.

75. Valkenet K, van de Port IG, Dronkers JJ, de Vries WR, Lindeman E, Backx FJ. The effects of preoperative exercise therapy on postoperative outcome: a systematic review. Clin Rehabil. 2011;25(2):99–111.

Wound Closure and Postoperative Hernia Prevention Strategies

An Jairam*, Gabrielle H. van Ramshorst*, and Johan F. Lange

Introduction

Incisional hernia and abdominal wound dehiscence are common complications after laparotomy. Incidences of incisional hernia are 20% in the general population, increasing up to 50% in high-risk groups [1, 2]. Abdominal wound dehiscence, which can be considered as acute postoperative hernia, is less common than incisional hernia with incidences reported in the literature varying between 1 and 3.5% [3, 4]. These conditions are highly correlated as up to 69% of patients with abdominal wound dehiscence develop incisional hernia at long-term follow-up [5–8]. Numerous studies searched for risk factors for postoperative hernia and abdominal wound dehiscence. Old age, pulmonary disease, surgical site infection, and emergency surgery have been identified to be independent risk factors [9–12].

Patients who are prone to develop incisional hernia are also those who undergo open aortic abdominal aneurysms repair (AAA). This is often explained by the fact that these patients suffer from underlying connective tissue disorders [9]. The quality of connective tissue is mainly determined by the amount and ratio of collagen type I and type III, which is the central protein of extra cellular matrix. Collagen type I, which is larger in diameter than collagen type III, is responsible for maintaining tensile strength. Collagen type III, which is an immature collagen, is found in early wound healing. A reduced type I/III collagen ratio indicates reduced mechanical stability of connective tissue, and it is associated with impaired wound healing [14–17]. An impaired scarring process can lead to decreased scar tissue quality and altered collagen synthesis. Other reported risk factors for incisional hernia include diabetes, pulmonary disease, malignancy, smoking, steroid use, surgical site infection, malnutrition, and midline abdominal incisions [10–13].

Assessment of risks of burst abdomen, incisional hernia, recurrence, or mortality can be used for patient counseling. It can also be used for preoperative patient optimization and selection of appropriate surgical technique and mesh choice. Veljkovic et al. developed a risk model for incisional hernia after identification of four variables with predictive value for development of incisional hernia: a suture length to wound length ratio <4.2, deep or organ/space surgical site infection, time to suture removal or complete epithelialization over 16 days, and body mass index over 24.4 kg/m^2 [14]. A study on data from the Danish Ventral Hernia Database reported risk factors for readmission, reoperation, and recurrence.

*Contributed equally to this chapter

A. Jairam, M.D. • J.F. Lange, M.D., Ph.D.
Erasmus University Medical Center,
Rotterdam, The Netherlands

G.H. van Ramshorst, M.D., Ph.D. (✉)
VU Medical Center, Amsterdam, The Netherlands
e-mail: g.vanramshorst@vumc.nl

© Springer International Publishing Switzerland 2016
Y.W. Novitsky (ed.), *Hernia Surgery*, DOI 10.1007/978-3-319-27470-6_5

A previous vertical incision and large defect size were independent risk factors for readmission.

Considering all the risk associated with fascial dehiscence and incisional hernia, prevention remains of primary interest. Consequently, several methods of wound closure and hernia prevention strategies have been investigated. These include different suture techniques and suture materials, as well as preventive mesh repair. These various methods will be outlined in this chapter.

Surgical Risk Factors

In many studies midline incisions have been evaluated and compared to transverse incisions. In the majority of high-quality studies, including the Cochrane Review by Brown et al., the midline incision was identified as a risk factor for incisional hernia compared to the transverse incision [15–19]. It has previously been suggested that midline incisions should be reserved for emergency surgery and other surgical procedures for which the entire abdominal cavity should be accessible [3]. Due to the relatively low incidence of abdominal wound dehiscence, few studies were adequately designed to detect a statistically significant risk associated with type of incision [7, 15, 20–24]. In conclusion, it appears it might be preferable to avoid midline incisions when possible to lower the incidence of postoperative hernia.

Suture Materials

Suture materials can be compared based on various characteristics such as method of production (monofilament vs. multifilament) and duration of resorption (slowly vs. rapidly absorbable and non-absorbable). Various suture materials and techniques were compared for incidence of postoperative hernia in randomized trials performed in the 1980s and 1990s. Van't Riet et al. published a meta-analysis which demonstrated that slowly absorbable and non-absorbable suture materials resulted in fewer incisional hernias

than quickly absorbable suture material. Non-absorbable suture materials, however, were associated with increased wound pain and sinus formation [25].

Suture Technique

One of the other technical factors that may influence the development of an incisional hernia is the suture technique used. The technique of an optimal wound closure is most important, since the technique can strengthen the wound and, thereby, prevent incisional hernia [26]. Ideally, tensile strength should be maintained during the healing process of the wound. The method of suture application (mass closure vs. layered closure; continuous vs. interrupted sutures) and amount of suture material used for fascia closure (suture length to wound length ratio) are of clinical importance with regard to formation of postoperative hernia.

Mass Closure vs. Layered Closure

Layered closure of the rectus sheath has been compared with mass closure, which comprises closure of all abdominal layers except the skin, in a number of studies. It has been shown in meta-analyses that layered closure results into higher hernia and dehiscence rates [27, 28]. Therefore, mass closure is preferred over layered closure.

Continuous vs. Interrupted Sutures

In a multicenter randomized trial by Wissing et al., interrupted and continuous closure with quickly absorbable and non-absorbable suture materials were compared. Although no statistically significant differences were found for wound dehiscence, the incidence of incisional hernia was significantly lower in the group with continuously used nylon compared to continuous polyglactin 910 (10.3% vs. 20.6%) [29]. These effects could not be reproduced in some other studies [30, 31]. However, the continuous method is preferred based on the fact that this method is faster, easier, and can, thus, save operating time [25, 32, 33].

Suture Length to Wound Length Ratio

The suture length to wound length ratio has been an underestimated variable of abdominal wall closure. It comprises the length of the suture material in relation to the length of the wound and it relates the size of the stitches and the interval between them [34]. In general, many surgeons have been trained to use large stitches (tissue bites) for abdominal wall closure. Large stitches have been described as sutures placed at 10 mm distance from the wound edge and at intervals of 10 mm. Small stitches, on the other hand, are placed at 5–8 mm distance from the wound edge and stitch intervals of less than 5 mm [34].

It has been shown in several animal experiments that high suture tension is associated with impaired collagen synthesis, wound weakness, and increased tissue necrosis and infec-tion. There is strong evidence that a suture length to wound length ratio of at least 4:1 should be used for closure of the abdominal wall to minimize the risk of incisional hernia [34, 35]. A suture to wound length ratio of less than 4:1 has been associated with a threefold increased risk of developing incisional hernia [35]. Millbourn et al. also described that a lin-ear correlation exists between the stitch length and the risk of developing wound infection. In order to achieve a suture length to wound length ratio of at least 4:1, it has been recommended to measure and document the achieved ratio for each patient [36].

This ratio can be achieved by placing many bites at close intervals, or by placing fewer bites at greater intervals. As a simple rule, the length between stitches must not exceed the distance between the fascia edge and the stitch (Fig. 5.1). An experimental study in animals by Cengiz et al. showed higher wound tensile strength after 4 days when small stitches were used [37]. Other clinical studies performed on this topic by Israelsson, Millbourn, and the STITCH study group also supported that wound closure should

Fig. 5.1 Examples of small bites and large bites techniques

a

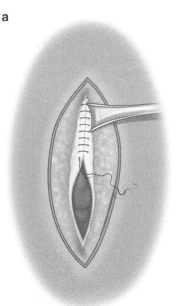

b

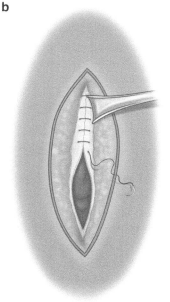

Small Stitches
Stitches placed at 5 to 8 mm
distance from the wound edge,
stitch intervals less than 5 mm.

Large Stitches
Stitches placed at 10 mm
distance from the wound edge,
stitch intervals 10 mm.

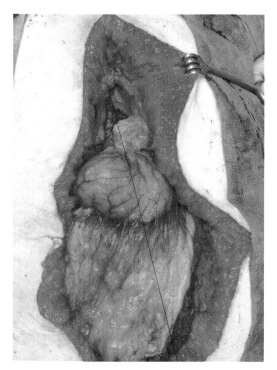

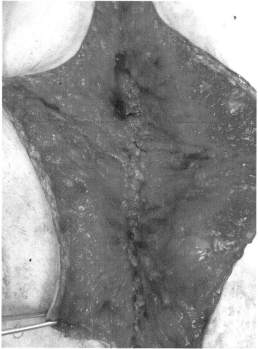

Fig. 5.2 Median laparotomy wound in obese patient, closure of aponeurosis with small stitches using PDS® Plus antibacterial (polydioxanone) 2-0 suture (Courtesy of Dr. A.G. Menon, surgeon, Havenziekenhuis Rotterdam, Rotterdam, the Netherlands)

Fig. 5.3 Result after closure of median laparotomy wound with small bites; a SL:WL ratio of 6:1 was achieved (Courtesy of Dr. A.G. Menon, surgeon, Havenziekenhuis Rotterdam, Rotterdam, the Netherlands)

be performed with small stitches [34, 35, 38, 39]. A clinical example of the small stitches technique is shown in Figs. 5.2 and 5.3. Small stitches have been associated with a decreased risk of incisional hernia and surgical site infections. In the Swedish randomized trial by Millbourn et al., incisional hernia was found in 49/272 patients (18.0%) in the large stitch group and in 14/250 patients (5.6%) in the small stitch group ($p < 0.001$). Also, 1/381 patients with large bites developed abdominal wound dehiscence compared to none of the 356 allocated to the small bites technique (0.3% vs. 0%, $p > 0.99$) [34].

The STITCH trial (Suture Techniques to reduce the Incidence of The incisional Hernia) was a randomized controlled trial, in which the large bites technique was compared with the small bites technique. In the large bite technique the bite width was 1.5 cm and the intersuture space 1 cm. In the small bites technique, bite widths and inter suture spacing of 0.5 cm were applied. The primary endpoint of the study was incisional hernia after 1 year postoperatively. The study showed that the incidence of incisional hernia at 1 year was statistically significantly lower (13% vs. 21%) in the small bites group. In addition, 2/284 patients in the large bites group developed abdominal wound dehiscence vs. 4/276 patients in the small bites group (0.7% vs. 1.4%, $p = 0.392$) [38]. In the Swedish study, multivariate analysis showed that patients treated with large stitches were exposed to a relative risk of 2 for infection and 4 for incisional hernia. In the STITCH trial, small stitches were not associated with decreased rate of surgical site infection and neither study was adequately powered for detection of a statistically significant difference in the incidence of abdominal wound dehiscence. However, the STITCH trial confirmed that the small bites technique is superior compared to the large bites technique in the prevention of incisional hernia after closure of abdominal midline wounds.

The positive effects of small stitches on wound healing can be explained as follows: the aponeurosis has limited possibilities for regeneration and cannot bridge over a large defect [6]. With a large stitch, not only aponeurosis tissue is included, but also fat and muscle. In combination with increased intra-abdominal pressure, soft tissue can be compressed and damaged. This can result into slackening and separation of wound edges, tissue devitalization, and infection. A separation of wound edges of more than 12 mm during the first postoperative period has been strongly associated with development of incisional hernia [3]. Closing patients with the use of small stitches has been associated with longer operation time of 4–5 min [34, 36]. However, if the reduced incidence of incisional hernia (repairs) is taken into account, using small stitches should be considered a safe, easy, and cost-effective method [39]. In conclusion, the ideal suture technique for closing of the fascia should be with performed with a continuous mass technique, using slowly absorbable suture material and suture to wound length ratio of 4 to 1 [40].

Preventive Abdominal Binders

Prevention of abdominal wound dehiscence and/or incisional hernia by using preventive abdominal binders is highly surgeon-dependent. In some countries, abdominal binders and/or corsets are widely used in spite of the fact that the effects of these medical aids have been disputed [41]. The prescription of these binders is motivated by the conception that externally applied pressure may help in diminishing chances of developing postoperative seroma and dehiscence of fascial edges, thereby preventing abdominal wound dehiscence and incisional hernia. In midline laparotomy, fascial edges are tended toward separation instead of approximation by the forces exerted by contractions of the oblique and transverse abdominal muscles. In theory, it seems unlikely that lateral forces separating fascia edges will be diminished by externally applied forces exercised by abdominal binders. Clinical studies on the use of abdominal binders are scarce, but in one study patients reported to have abandoned wearing supportive corsets and/or binders due to perceived discomfort, whereas another study reported increased patient comfort [42, 43]. Moreover, it is imaginable that diminished elasticity of the abdominal wall could result in lower abdominal—and thereby, thoracic volume, with less possibility for lung expansion. The use of abdominal binders should, therefore, be considered carefully and weighed against potential risks of lung atelectasis and possible pneumonia.

Primary Mesh Augmentation

Placement of mesh to prevent incisional hernia has been investigated in several studies since the mid-1990s of the previous century. Its use has primarily been investigated in high-risk patient groups, such as patients with abdominal aortic aneurysms and obesity. In these patient groups, incidences of incisional hernia of up to 38% and 50% have been found, respectively [2, 9, 12, 44, 45]. Different mesh positions are possible in primary mesh augmentation. In the onlay position, mesh is placed on the anterior rectus fascia. The sublay technique comprises the positioning of the mesh on the posterior rectus fascia and peritoneum (Figs. 5.4, 5.5 and 5.6). In the preperitoneal technique, mesh is placed directly on the peritoneum.

Bhangu et al. published a systematic review in which randomized controlled trials and prospective cohort studies were included [46]. Recently, Timmermans et al. conducted a meta-analysis which included randomized controlled trials only [47]. All studies featured in the review by Bhangu et al. were high-risk patients for incisional hernia, such as patients with connective tissue disorders (including abdominal aortic aneurysm), obesity, or other relevant comorbidity. Bhangu et al. concluded that the rate of incisional hernia was significantly reduced (OR 0.15, $p < 0.001$) after primary mesh placement (3.9%, 9/238), compared with primary suture repair (22%, 67/305). There was, however, an increased rate of postoperative

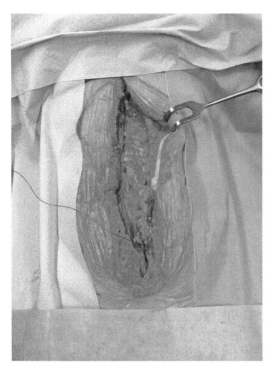

Fig. 5.4 Preparation of closure of median laparotomy with prophylactic mesh: continuously sutured posterior rectus fascia using PDS® (polydiaxonone) 0 suture (Courtesy of Dr. I. Dawson, surgeon, Ijsselland Ziekenhuis, Capelle aan den Ijssel, the Netherlands)

seroma formation in the mesh group (12.9%, 26/201 vs. 6.9%, 18/262 in the suture group), with a borderline significant p-value of 0.050. With a random effect model, no significant increase in seroma rate was found (OR 1.86, $p = 0.210$). Incidences of surgical site infections and hematomas were comparable for both groups. There was an increased rate in chronic pain for the mesh group, although this increase was non-significant [46].

In the meta-analysis by Timmermans et al., five randomized controlled trials were included. In one of these trials, primary (polypropylene) mesh augmentation was compared to primary suture repair. The outcome data were pooled, and the authors also concluded that incisional hernia occurred significantly less in the group with primary mesh augmentation (RR 0.25, 95% CI 0.12–0.52, $p < 0.001$). There were no statistically significant differences between the groups of primary mesh augmentation and primary suture repair with regard to wound infection, seroma formation, and chronic pain. However, a trend was found of more chronic pain in the primary mesh augmentation group. Some important outcome measurements, such as hematoma, operation

Fig. 5.5 Prophylactic Progrip™ mesh in retrorectus position. The mesh is fixated using interrupted polyglactin 910 3-0 sutures (Courtesy of Dr. I. Dawson, surgeon, Ijsselland Ziekenhuis, Capelle aan den Ijssel, the Netherlands)

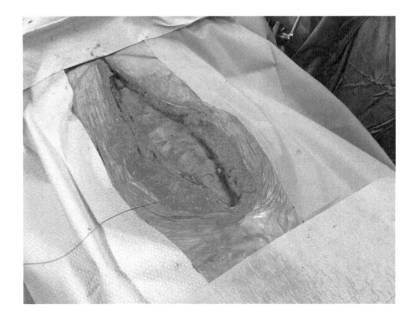

Fig. 5.6 Closure of anterior rectus fascia over Progrip™ mesh in retrorectus position using PDS® (polydiaxonone) 0 suture (Courtesy of Dr. I. Dawson, surgeon, Ijsselland Ziekenhuis, Capelle aan den Ijssel, the Netherlands)

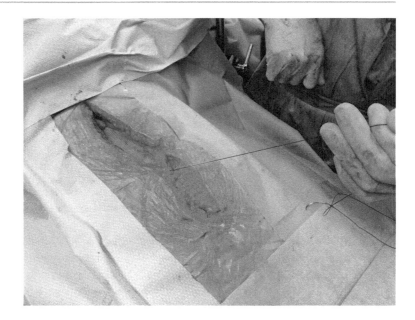

time, quality of life, and cost-effectiveness, were not reported in all of the included studies [47].

Not included in the aforementioned meta-analyses was a randomized clinical study by Caro Tarrago et al. This study included (mainly) oncological patients with elective midline laparotomies. In this RCT, published in March 2014, it was shown that placement of prophylactic mesh in supra-aponeurotic position was associated with a reduction of incisional hernia. The likelihood of incisional hernia at 12 months for patients with mesh placement was 1.5%, compared to 35.9% in the group without mesh ($p < 0.0001$) [12]. Significantly, more seromas were found in the mesh group (29% vs. 11%, $p < 0.01$).

There are no studies available in which different mesh types have been compared. In one study, biological mesh was used (Alloderm, Lifecell, Branchburg, NJ, USA), whereas in all other studies polypropylene mesh was used. In the study by Caro-Tarrago et al., a large pore/lightweight polypropylene mesh was used (Biomesh Light, Cousin), but in all other studies small pore, heavyweight meshes were used. Different meth-

ods of mesh position and mesh fixation were used. In none of the studies different mesh positioning techniques were compared. The onlay technique is, in general, the easiest and quickest way, but has been associated with increased seroma formation and wound infections.

With regard to primary mesh augmentation, limited data are available concerning secondary outcomes such as quality of life or cost-effectiveness of mesh placement. Placement of a preventive mesh could potentially lead to complications or re-operations with adverse effects on quality of life. Long-term follow-up results of these studies will provide the surgical community with more evidence regarding the possible benefits of primary mesh augmentation in selected patient groups.

Future Perspectives

Several trials are currently in progress, and the results of these studies are expected to influence daily practice in hernia surgery. The Dutch PRIMA trial will be the first trial to be published comparing different mesh positioning techniques: primary mesh augmentation in onlay or sublay position, compared to primary suture. Other upcoming trials include the PRIMAAT trial from Belgium, the results of which are expected shortly as well. The ProphMesh group from Switzerland compares Dynamesh IPOM with primary suture in high-risk patients. The Austrian Hernia Study group set up another RCT, comparing onlay mesh with primary suture, and the findings of this study are expected in 2016.

The use of preventive mesh with abdominal wound dehiscence as primary end point has not been studied extensively. The methods reported in older literature include intraperitoneal polyglactin 910 mesh compared to either polyamide mesh glued to the skin or extraperitoneal retention sutures. Three studies published on this topic were of poor quality, including small or incomparable patient groups or had non-randomized designs [48–50]. Recently, an international multicenter study was ended prematurely mainly due to low patient enrollment. Patients with fascial dehiscence were randomized between Strattice® Reconstructive Tissue Matrix (Lifecell) placed either as an intraperitoneal underlay or as retro-rectus sublay, or standard repair by re-approximating wound edges using sutures with or without absorbable (polyglactin) mesh. The endpoints of the study were occurrence of incisional hernia, fascial redehiscence, and other adverse events. Eventually, 18 patients were treated with Strattice® and 19 patients with standard repair. The incidence of fascial redehiscence was significantly lower after Strattice® repair (5.6% vs. 36.8%, $p = 0.015$), whereas no increase in adverse events was found. In spite of low patient numbers, the results of this study plead for use of biological mesh in patients with fascial dehiscence, in spite of the implicated high costs (Jeekel J, presented at congress of European Hernia Society 2014 in Edinburgh).

Personal Thought on Patient, Technique and Mesh Selections

On principle, minimally invasive techniques should be considered in every patient undergoing abdominal surgery. If minimally invasive techniques cannot be used, a transverse or paramedian incision should be considered. If a midline laparotomy is chosen, the abdominal fascia should be closed in a continuous fashion using slowly absorbably suture material with small bites and a suture length to wound length ratio of 4:1. In high-risk patients, such as patients with abdominal aortic aneurysms or obesity, primary mesh augmentation should be considered. Polypropylene mesh in sublay position might be preferred over onlay position based on a lower risk of wound morbidity. Figure 5.7 shows a flow chart which can be followed for patients undergoing abdominal surgery.

Personal Tips and Tricks: Small Bites and Prophylactic Mesh Placement

All patients diagnosed with an aneurysm of the abdominal aorta, undergoing a midline laparotomy, should receive a mesh to prevent an incisional hernia. For the small bites technique, a slowly absorbable 2–0 single suture with a 36-mm needle should be chosen. It should be recommended to have sterile rulers included in all laparotomy instrument sets to facilitate sterile measuring of the wound length and length of suture remnants. Standard measurement and documentation of the achieved suture length to wound length ratio could contribute to shortening of the learning curve and to the process of quality monitoring.

Fig. 5.7 Flowchart for patients undergoing abdominal surgery

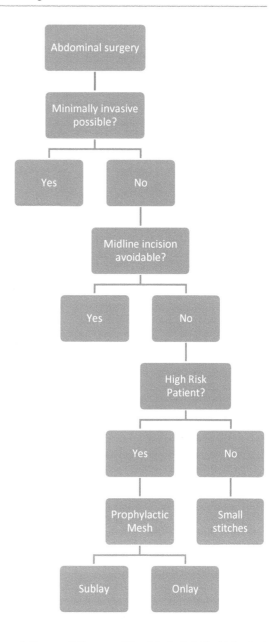

References

1. Timmermans L, Eker HH, Steyerberg EW, Jairam A, de Jong D, Pierik EG, et al. Short-term results of a randomized controlled trial comparing primary suture with primary glued mesh augmentation to prevent incisional hernia. Ann Surg. 2014;261(2):276–81.
2. Strzelczyk JM, Szymanski D, Nowicki ME, Wilczynski W, Gaszynski T, Czupryniak L. Randomized clinical trial of postoperative hernia prophylaxis in open bariatric surgery. Br J Surg. 2006;93(11):1347–50.
3. Burger JW, van't Riet M, Jeekel J. Abdominal incisions: techniques and postoperative complications. Scand J Surg. 2002;91(4):315–21.
4. Dubay DA, Franz MG. Acute wound healing: the biology of acute wound failure. Surg Clin North Am. 2003;83(3):463–81.
5. Van't Riet M, De Vos Van Steenwijk PJ, Bonjer HJ, Steyerberg EW, Jeekel J. Incisional hernia after repair of wound dehiscence: incidence and risk factors. Am Surg. 2004;70(4):281–6.
6. Carlson MA. Acute wound failure. Surg Clin North Am. 1997;77(3):607–36.

7. Gislason H, Gronbech JE, Soreide O. Burst abdomen and incisional hernia after major gastrointestinal operations—comparison of three closure techniques. Eur J Surg. 1995;161(5):349–54.

8. Gislason H, Viste A. Closure of burst abdomen after major gastrointestinal operations—comparison of different surgical techniques and later development of incisional hernia. Eur J Surg. 1999;165(10):958–61.

9. Bevis PM, Windhaber RA, Lear PA, Poskitt KR, Earnshaw JJ, Mitchell DC. Randomized clinical trial of mesh versus sutured wound closure after open abdominal aortic aneurysm surgery. Br J Surg. 2010;97(10):1497–502.

10. Hidalgo MP, Ferrero EH, Ortiz MA, Castillo JM, Hidalgo AG. Incisional hernia in patients at risk: can it be prevented? Hernia. 2011;15(4):371–5.

11. El-Khadrawy OH, Moussa G, Mansour O, Hashish MS. Prophylactic prosthetic reinforcement of midline abdominal incisions in high-risk patients. Hernia. 2009;13(3):267–74.

12. Caro-Tarrago A, Olona Casas C, Jimenez Salido A, Duque Guilera E, Moreno Fernandez F, Vicente GV. Prevention of incisional hernia in midline laparotomy with an onlay mesh: a randomized clinical trial. World J Surg. 2014;38(9):2223–30.

13. Llaguna OH, Avgerinos DV, Nagda P, Elfant D, Leitman IM, Goodman E. Does prophylactic biologic mesh placement protect against the development of incisional hernia in high-risk patients? World J Surg. 2011;35(7):1651–5.

14. Veljkovic R, Protic M, Gluhovic A, Potic Z, Milosevic Z, Stojadinov A. Prospective clinical trial of factors predicting the early development of incisional hernia after midline laparotomy. J Am Coll Surg. 2010; 210(2):210–9.

15. Brown SR, Goodfellow PB. Transverse verses midline incisions for abdominal surgery. Cochrane Database Syst Rev. 2005;(4):CD005199.

16. Halm JA, Lip H, Schmitz PI, Jeekel J. Incisional hernia after upper abdominal surgery: a randomised controlled trial of midline versus transverse incision. Hernia. 2009;13(3):275–80.

17. Seiler CM, Deckert A, Diener MK, Knaebel HP, Weigand MA, Victor N, et al. Midline versus transverse incision in major abdominal surgery: a randomized, double-blind equivalence trial (POVATI: ISRCTN60734227). Ann Surg. 2009;249(6):913–20.

18. Fassiadis N, Roidl M, Hennig M, South LM, Andrews SM. Randomized clinical trial of vertical or transverse laparotomy for abdominal aortic aneurysm repair. Br J Surg. 2005;92(10):1208–11.

19. Grantcharov TP, Rosenberg J. Vertical compared with transverse incisions in abdominal surgery. Eur J Surg. 2001;167(4):260–7.

20. Proske JM, Zieren J, Muller JM. Transverse versus midline incision for upper abdominal surgery. Surg Today. 2005;35(2):117–21.

21. Armstrong CP, Dixon JM, Duffy SW, Elton RA, Davies GC. Wound healing in obstructive jaundice. Br J Surg. 1984;71(4):267–70.

22. Stone HH, Hoefling SJ, Strom PR, Dunlop WE, Fabian TC. Abdominal incisions: transverse vs vertical placement and continuous vs interrupted closure. South Med J. 1983;76(9):1106–8.

23. Greenall MJ, Evans M, Pollock AV. Midline or transverse laparotomy? A random controlled clinical trial. Part I: influence on healing. Br J Surg. 1980;67(3): 188–90.

24. Riou JP, Cohen JR, Johnson Jr H. Factors influencing wound dehiscence. Am J Surg. 1992;163(3): 324–30.

25. van't Riet M, Steyerberg EW, Nellensteyn J, Bonjer HJ, Jeekel J. Meta-analysis of techniques for closure of midline abdominal incisions. Br J Surg. 2002; 89(11):1350–6.

26. Niggebrugge AH, Trimbos JB, Hermans J, Steup WH, Van De Velde CJ. Influence of abdominal-wound closure technique on complications after surgery: a randomised study. Lancet. 1999;353(9164):1563–7.

27. Weiland DE, Bay RC, Del Sordi S. Choosing the best abdominal closure by meta-analysis. Am J Surg. 1998;176(6):666–70.

28. Berretta R, Rolla M, Patrelli TS, Piantelli G, Merisio C, Melpignano M, et al. Randomised prospective study of abdominal wall closure in patients with gynaecological cancer. Aust N Z J Obstet Gynaecol. 2010;50(4):391–6.

29. Wissing J, van Vroonhoven TJ, Schattenkerk ME, Veen HF, Ponsen RJ, Jeekel J. Fascia closure after midline laparotomy: results of a randomized trial. Br J Surg. 1987;74(8):738–41.

30. Gupta H, Srivastava A, Menon GR, Agrawal CS, Chumber S, Kumar S. Comparison of interrupted versus continuous closure in abdominal wound repair: a meta-analysis of 23 trials. Asian J Surg. 2008;31(3): 104–14.

31. Seiler CM, Bruckner T, Diener MK, Papyan A, Golcher H, Seidlmayer C, et al. Interrupted or continuous slowly absorbable sutures for closure of primary elective midline abdominal incisions: a multicenter randomized trial (INSECT: ISRCTN24023541). Ann Surg. 2009;249(4):576–82.

32. Diener MK, Voss S, Jensen K, Buchler MW, Seiler CM. Elective midline laparotomy closure: the INLINE systematic review and meta-analysis. Ann Surg. 2010;251(5):843–56.

33. Hoer J, Stumpf M, Rosch R, Klinge U, Schumpelick V. Prevention of incisional hernia. Chirurg. 2002; 73(9):881–7.

34. Millbourn D, Cengiz Y, Israelsson LA. Effect of stitch length on wound complications after closure of midline incisions: a randomized controlled trial. Arch Surg. 2009;144(11):1056–9.

35. Israelsson LA, Jonsson T. Suture length to wound length ratio and healing of midline laparotomy incisions. Br J Surg. 1993;80(10):1284–6.

36. van Ramshorst GH, Klop B, Hop WC, Israelsson LA, Lange JF. Closure of midline laparotomies by means of small stitches: practical aspects of a new technique. Surg Technol Int. 2013;23:34–8.

37. Cengiz Y, Blomquist P, Israelsson LA. Small tissue bites and wound strength: an experimental study. Arch Surg. 2001;136(3):272–5.
38. Deerenberg EB, Harlaar JJ, Steyerberg EW, Lont HE, Van Doorn HC, Heisterkamp J, Wijnhoven BP, Schouten WR, Cense HA, Stockmann HB, Berends FJ, Dijkhuizen FP, Dwarkasing RS, Jairam AP, van Ramshorst GH, Kleinrensink GJ, Jeekel J, Lange JF. Small bites versus large bites for closure of abdominal midline incisions (STITCH): a double-blind, multi-centre, randomised controlled trial. Lancet. 2015;386: 1254–60.
39. Millbourn D, Wimo A, Israelsson LA. Cost analysis of the use of small stitches when closing midline abdominal incisions. Hernia. 2013;18(6):775–80.
40. Muysoms FE, Antoniou SA, Bury K, Campanelli G, Conze J, Cuccurullo D, et al. European Hernia Society guidelines on the closure of abdominal wall incisions. Hernia. 2015;19(1):1–24.
41. Bouvier A, Rat P, Drissi-Chbihi F, Bonnetain F, Lacaine F, Mariette C, et al. Abdominal binders after laparotomy: review of the literature and French survey of policies. Hernia. 2014;18(4):501–6.
42. van Ramshorst GH, Eker HH, van der Voet JA, Jeekel J, Lange JF. Long-term outcome study in patients with abdominal wound dehiscence: a comparative study on quality of life, body image, and incisional hernia. J Gastrointest Surg. 2013;17(8):1477–84.
43. Christoffersen MW, Olsen BH, Rosenberg J, Bisgaard T. Randomized Clinical Trial on the postoperative use of an abdominal binder after laparoscopic umbilical and epigastric hernia repair. Hernia. 2014;19(1): 147–53.
44. Nachiappan S, Markar S, Karthikesalingam A, Ziprin P, Faiz O. Prophylactic mesh placement in high-risk patients undergoing elective laparotomy: a systematic review. World J Surg. 2013;37(8):1861–71.
45. Strzelczyk J, Czupryniak L. Polypropylene mesh in prevention of postoperative hernia in bariatric surgery. Ann Surg. 2005;241(1):196. author reply-7.
46. Bhangu A, Fitzgerald JE, Singh P, Battersby N, Marriott P, Pinkney T. Systematic review and meta-analysis of prophylactic mesh placement for prevention of incisional hernia following midline laparotomy. Hernia. 2013;17(4):445–55.
47. Timmermans L, de Goede B, Eker HH, van Kempen BJ, Jeekel J, Lange JF. Meta-analysis of primary mesh augmentation as prophylactic measure to prevent incisional hernia. Dig Surg. 2013;30(4–6):401–9.
48. Paye F, Rongere C, Gendreau D, Lenriot JP. Intra-peritoneal resorbable mesh in the prevention of postoperative wound dehiscence. A comparative study. Ann Chir. 1992;46(6):518–22.
49. Gainant A, Boudinet F, Cubertafond P. Prevention of postoperative wound dehiscence in high risk patients. A randomized comparison of internally applied resorbable polyglactin 910 mesh and externally applied polyamide fiber mesh. Int Surg. 1989;74(1): 55–7.
50. Tohme C, Brechet E, Bernard A, Arnaud R, Viard H. Prevention of postoperative wound dehiscence. Comparative study of polyglactin 910 mesh and total reinforced extraperitoneal sutures. Ann Chir. 1991; 45(6):513–6.
51. Webster C, Neumayer L, Smout R, Horn S, Daley J, Henderson W, et al. Prognostic models of abdominal wound dehiscence after laparotomy. J Surg Res. 2003; 109(2):130–7.
52. Gomez Diaz CJ, Rebasa Cladera P, Navarro Soto S, Hidalgo Rosas JM, Luna Aufroy A, Montmany Vioque S, et al. Validation of abdominal wound dehiscence's risk model. Cir Esp. 2014;92(2):114–9.
53. van Ramshorst GH, Nieuwenhuizen J, Hop WC, Arends P, Boom J, Jeekel J, et al. Abdominal wound dehiscence in adults: development and validation of a risk model. World J Surg. 2010;34(1):20–7.
54. Kenig J, Richter P, Lasek A, Zbierska K, Zurawska S. The efficacy of risk scores for predicting abdominal wound dehiscence: a case-controlled validation study. BMC Surg. 2014;14:65.
55. Junge K, Klinge U, Rosch R, Mertens PR, Kirch J, Klosterhalfen B, et al. Decreased collagen type I/III ratio in patients with recurring hernia after implantation of alloplastic prostheses. Langenbecks Arch Surg. 2004;389(1):17–22.
56. Klinge U, Si ZY, Zheng H, Schumpelick V, Bhardwaj RS, Klosterhalfen B. Abnormal collagen I to III distribution in the skin of patients with incisional hernia. Eur Surg Res. 2000;32(1):43–8.
57. Peeters E, De Hertogh G, Junge K, Klinge U, Miserez M. Skin as marker for collagen type I/III ratio in abdominal wall fascia. Hernia. 2014;18(4):519–25.
58. Rosch R, Junge K, Knops M, Lynen P, Klinge U, Schumpelick V. Analysis of collagen-interacting proteins in patients with incisional hernias. Langenbecks Arch Surg. 2003;387(11–12):427–32.
59. van Ramshorst GH, Eker HH, Hop WC, Jeekel J, Lange JF. Impact of incisional hernia on health-related quality of life and body image: a prospective cohort study. Am J Surg. 2012;204(2):144–50.
60. Helgstrand F, Rosenberg J, Kehlet H, Bisgaard T. Outcomes after emergency versus elective ventral hernia repair: a prospective nationwide study. World J Surg. 2013;37(10):2273–9.
61. Martinez-Serrano MA, Pereira JA, Sancho JJ, Lopez-Cano M, Bombuy E, Hidalgo J, et al. Risk of death after emergency repair of abdominal wall hernias. Still waiting for improvement. Langenbecks Arch Surg. 2010;395(5):551–6.
62. Halasz NA. Dehiscence of laparotomy wounds. Am J Surg. 1968;116(2):210–4.
63. Keill RH, Keitzer WF, Nichols WK, Henzel J, DeWeese MS. Abdominal wound dehiscence. Arch Surg. 1973;106(4):573–7.
64. Waldhausen JH, Davies L. Pediatric postoperative abdominal wound dehiscence: transverse versus vertical incisions. J Am Coll Surg. 2000;190(6): 688–91.

65. Campbell DP, Swenson O. Wound dehiscence in infants and children. J Pediatr Surg. 1972;7(2): 123–6.

66. van Ramshorst GH, Salu NE, Bax NM, Hop WC, van Heurn E, Aronson DC, et al. Risk factors for abdominal wound dehiscence in children: a case-control study. World J Surg. 2009;33(7): 1509–13.

67. Albertsmeier M, Seiler CM, Fischer L, Baumann P, Husing J, Seidlmayer C, et al. Evaluation of the safety and efficacy of MonoMax(R) suture material for abdominal wall closure after primary midline laparotomy-a controlled prospective multicentre trial: ISSAAC [NCT005725079]. Langenbecks Arch Surg. 2012;397(3):363–71.

68. Penninckx FM, Poelmans SV, Kerremans RP, Beckers JP. Abdominal wound dehiscence in gastroenterological surgery. Ann Surg. 1979;189(3):345–52.

69. Khorgami Z, Shoar S, Laghaie B, Aminian A, Hosseini Araghi N, Soroush A. Prophylactic retention sutures in midline laparotomy in high-risk patients for wound dehiscence: a randomized controlled trial. J Surg Res. 2013;180(2):238–43.

70. Israelsson LA, Millbourn D. Closing midline abdominal incisions. Langenbecks Arch Surg. 2012;397(8): 1201–7.

Synthetic Mesh: Making Educated Choices

Issa Mirmehdi and Bruce Ramshaw

Background

In 1951, Benjamin Pease filed a patent titled, "Nonmetallic Mesh Surgical Insert for Hernia Repair." The patent was awarded in 1954 (Fig. 6.1). In 1958, Usher described the use of this patented material in the form of polypropylene mesh for hernia repair [1]. It was later popularized by the technique outlined by Lichtenstein et al. in 1989 [2]. Today, a mesh hernia repair is the most common technique to repair inguinal and ventral hernias, although there are many technique and mesh variations to choose from. Several studies have demonstrated lower recurrence rates for mesh repair of abdominal wall defects. A meta-analysis of 13 randomized trials comparing open hernia repair with mesh versus without mesh showed a significantly lower incidence of recurrent hernia when mesh was used [3]. The EU Hernia Trialist Collaboration looked at 58 randomized controlled trials and found the use of synthetic mesh was superior with respect to recurrence in

both open and laparoscopic hernia operations [4, 5]. Mesh, therefore, potentially results in a more durable hernia repair. At first, the thought process employed by surgeons was that a heavyweight polypropylene material that can withstand maximum intra-abdominal pressure of 170–200 mmHg and that induced significant fibrosis and scar tissue formation was best to buttress a weakened fascia. However, the use of such a mesh and the subsequent fibrotic reaction were later found to be associated with chronic post-hernia repair neuralgia, mesh migration and contraction as well as potential functional restrictions for some patients. The next step in the evolution of polypropylene synthetic mesh was the introduction of mid and lightweight material that had less density of material and wider pores which potentially led to less fibrotic reaction while still providing enough tensile strength to withstand maximum intra-abdominal pressures [6]. Despite the advantage of a less aggressive foreign body response, these newer mesh products continued to have various complications including loss of tensile integrity, erosion, intra-abdominal adhesions, bowel obstruction, and fistula/abscess formation in some patients. Consequently, various medical device companies have joined the quest for the development of the single "ideal" mesh. Other material such as polyester, polytetrafluoroethylene (PTFE), absorbable compounds, and biological meshes have been introduced. While numerous patients have ben-

I. Mirmehdi
General Surgery, Halifax Health, Daytona Beach, FL, USA

B. Ramshaw (✉)
Department of Surgery, The University of Tennessee Knoxville Graduate School of Medicine, Knoxville, TN, USA
e-mail: BRamshaw@utmck.edu

© Springer International Publishing Switzerland 2016
Y.W. Novitsky (ed.), *Hernia Surgery*, DOI 10.1007/978-3-319-27470-6_6

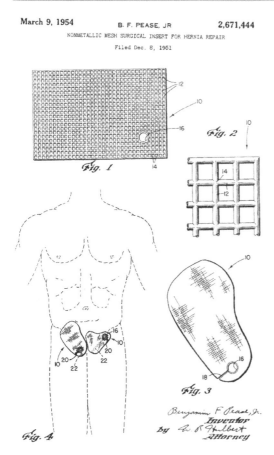

Fig. 6.1 The original plastic hernia mesh patent

all types of hernias in all hernia repair techniques all the time. Today, there are hundreds of different meshes manufactured with the above materials. Each addresses some of the concerns related to biocompatibility of synthetic prostheses while posing potential disadvantages. This has created a challenge for many surgeons, particularly in the setting of increasing complexity of hernias seen in everyday practice. Selecting the right mesh for the right patient requires the surgeon to have a relatively thorough understanding of the potential benefits and deficiencies for all types of hernia mesh and the requirements for each specific clinical scenario. With that knowledge, the surgeon is still left with numerous choices and uncertainty in predicting the outcomes for each patient.

Defining Hernia Mesh

Table 6.1 describes types of hernia mesh available in the US market by the plastic polymer used and divided be those which are macroporous (not used in the abdominal cavity) and those that have microporous surfaces (potentially used in the abdominal cavity).

Polypropylene (Figs. 6.2, 6.3, 6.4, 6.5, and 6.6) is synthesized from the monomer propylene via addition reaction. It is a hydrophobic compound and theoretically resistant to many chemical

efitted from each of these materials, none has yielded a superior outcome for all patients with

Table 6.1 Description of available hernia meshes based on type of polymer, pore size and location for use

Basic polymer	Macroporous (used in abdominal wall)	Microporous (potential for use in abdominal cavity)
Polypropylene	Lightweight Mid-weight Heavyweight Coated polypropylene	Polypropylene with absorbable microporous barrier Polypropylene with permanent microporous barrier Microporous PTFE and Polypropylene composite
Polyester	Multifilamented polyester Monofilamented polyester	Polyester with absorbable microporous barrier
PTFE	Macroporous PTFE	Microporous PTFE Dual-sided PTFE (smooth and textured) Microporous PTFE and Polypropylene composite
Absorbable synthetic	Macroporous absorbable synthetic	Microporous absorbable synthetic

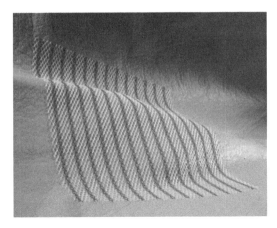

Fig. 6.2 Lightweight Polypropylene (macroporous)

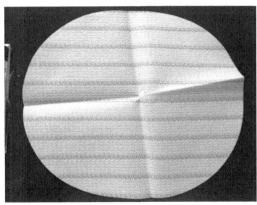

Fig. 6.5 Polypropylene with a microporous absorbable cellulose surface

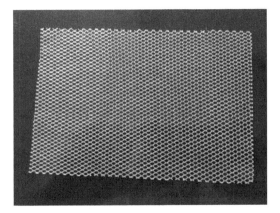

Fig.   6.3 Polyurethane-coated   polypropylene (macroporous)

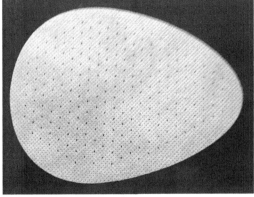

Fig. 6.6 Non-woven polypropylene

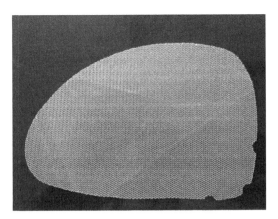

Fig. 6.4 Omega-3 fatty acid-coated polypropylene (macroporous)

solvents, bases, and acids. It is, however, thermo-plastic and can be remelted and reformed. Hernia mesh is made with semicrystalline polypropylene fibers extruded and then woven into monofilament or multifilament structures. Recently, non-woven and coated polypropylene fibers have also been made available to the growing list of hernia mesh choices. In vivo, polypropylene mesh has been shown to degrade by undergoing oxidation. It occurs when C–H bonds are compromised, creating free radicals that will bind oxygen. If chain scission or cross-linking occurs, the mesh may change its property and become stiff and/or contract. Heavy-weight polypropylene mesh, defined as having greater than 90 g/m^2 area of material and pore size <3–5 mm, has been shown, in some patients and animal studies, to induce an intense foreign body reaction. Examples of polypropylene mesh are in Figs. 6.2, 6.3, 6.4, 6.5, and 6.6.

Polyethylene Terephthalate (PET) is a member of the polyester family (Figs. 6.7 and 6.8). It is synthesized from the monomer bis-β-hydroxyterephthalate via condensation reaction by either esterification (water as a by-product) or transesterification (methanol as a by-product). It is less hydrophobic than polypropylene. Yet its thermoplastic property is similar to polypropylene. The degradation mechanism of concern is hydrolysis. The physiochemical changes that occur during degradation of PET include discoloration, chain scissions resulting in reduced molecular weight, formation of acetaldehyde, and formation of cross-links. Because of its macroporous design, a significant inflammatory reaction with tissue ingrowth occurs that results in variable degree of scar formation. Polyester mesh can be constructed in monofilament or multifilament forms. Recent data, however, suggest that monofilament polyester may be too fragile with resultant frequent central mesh failures.

Polytetrafluoroethylene (PTFE) (Fig. 6.9) is a fluorocarbon-based polymer that is synthesized via a free-radical polymerization of tetrafluoroethylene. PTFE is highly crystalline, significantly hydrophobic, and one of the most chemically inert polymers in the market. The high strength of the fluoro-carbon bind is mostly responsible for the inertness of this polymer. Expanded PTFE (ePTFE), commonly used in hernia mesh, is produced when PTFE is heated and then stretched, creating micropores. The hydrophobic, microporous nature of this material can lead to fibrous encapsulation and mesh contraction in some patients. There have also been rare reports of chronic, active seromas. This material was used in one of the first meshes designed for placement against the viscera (primarily using a laparoscopic approach for ventral/incisional hernia repair). In this type of PTFE product, one side of the material is rough to induce tissue ingrowth, while the other side is smooth to reduce tissue ingrowth from the viscera. Monofilament PTFE mesh with an open macroporous design is another PTFE-based product that may allow better tissue integration.

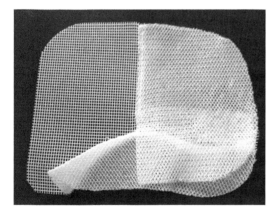

Fig. 6.7 Multifilamented polyester (macroporous)

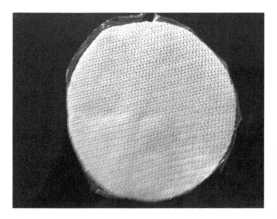

Fig. 6.8 Multifilamented polyester with a microporous absorbable collagen barrier

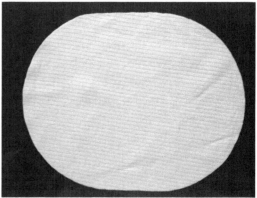

Fig. 6.9 Dual-sided PTFE mesh (microporous)

Mesh design is an important factor that needs to be taken into consideration before selecting a mesh. Unfortunately, despite recent advances, all meshes incite variable degrees of foreign body response. In order to improve this response, the mesh design could be better optimized. The parameters influencing the mesh design are weight, pore size, and the weave. Heavy-weight meshes with small pores were initially thought to be the best to withstand maximum intra-abdominal pressure of 170–200 mmHg. However, they were later found to be over-engineered for most people. In addition, they formed a rigid scar plate and granuloma bridging in many patients due to their small pores. The introduction of mid and lightweight meshes with larger pores (>1 mm) reduced the foreign body response and granuloma bridging [7] Despite this reduction, the foreign body response has not been eliminated and lower ratio of type I/III collagen continues to occur, highlighting the need for additional research. The weave design will dictate the overall mechanical properties, pore size, and the foreign body response. Isotropic and anisotropic qualities of the mesh are also determined by the weave design. Isotropic mesh design displays equal mechanical properties in any direction of applied force, while anisotropic mesh exhibits different mechanical properties depending on the direction of the force.

abdominal visceral organs and is designed to prevent ingrowth. (More recent mesh options include non-woven microfibers of polypropylene.)

The use of synthetic hernia mesh in a *contaminated or potentially contaminated field* has been controversial. Contamination has long been regarded as a relative contraindication to the use of permanent synthetic mesh. As a result, in such a setting, a multi-stage operation with delayed definitive hernia repair has been advocated [8, 9] More recently, a single-stage repair with the use of biologic mesh has become widely popular in the USA. Despite its relatively safe profile, higher wound complications and higher 3-year recur-

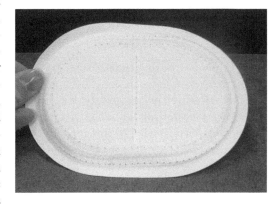

Fig. 6.10 Microporous PTFE and macroporous Polypropylene composite mesh

Hernia Mesh for Specific Clinical Scenarios

Direct *viscus exposure* to the synthetic hernia mesh can lead to adhesions or the ingrowth of bowel and other visceral organs causing erosion, fistula, abscess, and/or obstruction. A variety of mesh options for intra-abdominal placement have been designed to address this issue. A solid permanent (PTFE or silicone) or absorbable (many types) barrier is used on a variety of polypropylene or polyester meshes. This combination is referred to as "composite" mesh (Fig. 6.10). There are also PTFE meshes with a rough surface that is intended to promote ingrowth into the abdominal wall and a smooth surface that faces the intra-

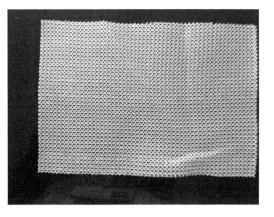

Fig. 6.11 Macroporous long-term resorbable synthetic mesh

rence (about 50%) have been associated with this technique [10]. Furthermore, a systematic review of 32 studies comparing the use of biologic mesh to synthetic non-absorbable mesh in contaminated fields during single-stage repairs did not find any advantage favoring the use of biologic material. While wound infection rates were similar, the recurrent hernia rate was significantly higher with biologic mesh [11]. The value of biologic mesh and other options will need to be measured. The use of long-term absorbable synthetic material has also been documented for both multi-staged and single-stage hernia repairs in contaminated fields (Fig. 6.11).

New Concepts in Improving Mesh Biocompatibility

Animal studies have demonstrated that *randomly generated fibers*, or non-woven material, such as non-woven polypropylene, may be beneficial for biocompatibility when compared to woven or knitted fibers [12]. Based on this principle, hernia meshes made with non-woven fibers have been introduced. Long-term outcomes have yet to be demonstrated.

Another relatively new concept in mesh design, aimed at minimizing fibrotic tissue, ingrowth, and/or scar tissue formation, are *coated polypropylene or polyester prostheses*. Most coated products are designed to prevent ingrowth to the viscera by coating the visceral side of the mesh with a microporous coating. Different types of coatings that are currently available in the market for this purpose include collagen, omega 3 fatty acid, hyaluronic acid, and other degradable polymers. Coatings can also be applied to individual mesh fibers to mask the bodies' foreign body response to polypropylene. Coatings available for this purpose include titanium and polyurethane. Because these mesh products are macroporous, they are not designed to prevent ingrowth and may not be the best choice for placement against the viscera. However, they may be beneficial in decreasing the foreign body response.

The Medical and Legal Aspects of Synthetic Mesh Manufacturing and Marketing

Most hernia meshes fall in the class II medical device category of FDA and enter the market with a 510K application process. Class II devices are subject to general controls and special controls. Special controls include safety measures such as postmarket surveillance and premarket data requirements. However, no clinical study or premarket approval is generally necessary as long as a predicate device is identified. Therefore, biocompatibility defined as "the ability of a material to perform with an appropriate host response in a specific application" [13] is not typically tested in humans prior to use in patients. With respect to postmarket surveillance, there are currently two mechanisms in place. The Safe medical Devices Act of 1990 requires user facilities to report device-related deaths to the FDA and the manufacturer and report serious injuries to the manufacturer, who then reports to the FDA. This law does not address whether or not the device responsible for death or serious injury needs to be returned to the manufacturer and/or studied [14]. The second mechanism for postmarket surveillance is a voluntary web-based program known as MedWatch. This program allows health care professionals and consumers to report adverse events directly to the FDA [15].

Is There an "Ideal" Mesh?

Since the introduction of the synthetic material to the hernia world, there has been a quest to find the "ideal" mesh. Various attempts have been made to either manufacture or describe the qualities of an "ideal" prosthesis. Clinical studies have not yet found a single hernia mesh that has ideal tensile strength which also behaves as the most biocompatible in all patients with all types of hernias all the time. While the "ideal" mesh may not exist when looking at the hernia patient population as a whole, there are individuals whose hernias have been repaired with what they would consider "ideal" mesh for that particular patient, or a sub-population of patients. Unfortunately, traditional clinical research tools, such as prospective randomized controlled trials, are inadequate to help us identify those individuals and sub-populations. Identifying sub-populations of patients that would do best, or worst, with various mesh options is a future challenge for hernia researchers.

Shared Decision-Making Process

The general public awareness about hernia mesh is on the rise. Whether it is due to increased conversation on social media or the negative advertisements by various legal firms, or both, more and more patients today expect to play an active role in the technique and mesh selection process. Surgeons are often able to narrow down the options based on the understanding of the potential benefits and deficiencies of different hernia mesh choices and their application to any specific clinical scenario. But, for a growing number of patients, a shared-decision process for the choice of mesh and technique for hernia repair is preferred.

Applying Complexity Science and Nonlinear Data Analytics: A Novel Approach

As mentioned earlier, traditional research methodologies are insufficient to best identify the sub-population of patients who may benefit from or be harmed by a certain type of mesh. This is due to the fact that hernia disease (as with other medical phenomenon) is a complex entity while traditional clinical research tools are designed for simple (or isolated) systems. Recently, the principles of complexity science have been introduced into the health care. Complexity science tools can potentially categorize patients into subpopulations that are more likely to demonstrate biocompatibility with one type of hernia mesh

versus others. One tool that can be used to better determine appropriate mesh choice is the use of clinical quality improvement (CQI) principles. CQI includes defining a dynamic care process, preferably based on the entire cycle of care, for patients with hernia disease. It also involves defining outcome measures that ultimately determine the value of care. The data can be gathered from multiple sources during real patient care, including from the patient. Many institutions that have begun CQI projects have also introduced disease-specific multidisciplinary teams. These teams tend to maintain a better contact with the patient throughout the entire cycle of care and, therefore, collect a great deal of information pertaining to the process and outcome measures. As more data are collected, certain patterns begin to emerge. These patterns can potentially be quantified using nonlinear data analytics. Identifying the factors (variables) that matter in determining outcomes can generate predictive algorithms that can assist surgeons and patients in determining the appropriate mesh (and technique) choice for each patient group [16]. Although the application of complexity science to patient care is in its infancy, the potential to improve outcomes through predictive analytics using data generated by real-world patient care is significant.

Summary

Mesh selection for patients undergoing hernia repair can be a challenging process. Due to the complexity of the hernia patient population and the vast choices of hernia mesh, traditional research mechanisms to determine the best, and worst, mesh for each technique, patient, and patient sub-populations are inadequate. Currently, a shared decision process allows the surgeon and patient to make choices that include each perspective. In the future, the use of complexity science tools such as CQI will facilitate predictive analytics that will allow for more informed choices that will benefit both the surgeon and the patient.

References

1. Usher FC, Ochsner J, Tuttle Jr LLD. Use of Marlex mesh in the repair of incisional hernias. Am Surg. 1958;24:969.
2. Lichtenstein IL, Shulman AG, Amid PK, et al. The tension free hernioplasty. Am J Surg. 1989;157:188–93.
3. Scott NW, McCormack K, Graham P, et al. Open mesh versus non-mesh for repair of femoral and inguinal hernia. Cochrane Database Syst Rev. 2002; CD002197.
4. EU Hernia Trialists Collaboration. Repair of groin hernia with synthetic mesh: meta-analysis of randomized controlled trials. Ann Surg. 2002;235:322–32.
5. EU Hernia Trialists Collaboration. Mesh compared with non-mesh methods of open groin hernia repair: systematic review of randomized controlled trials. Br J Surg. 2000;87:854–9.
6. Brown CN, Finch JG. Which mesh for hernia repair? Ann R Coll Surg Engl. 2010;92:272–8.
7. Klinge U, Binnebosel M, Mertens PR. Are collagens the culprits in the development of incisional and inguinal hernia disease? Hernia. 2006;10(6):472–7.
8. Fabian TC, Croce MA, Pritchard FE, et al. Planned ventral hernia. Stagedmanagement for acute abdominal wall defects. Ann Surg. 1994;219:643–50. discussion 651–653.
9. Jernigan TW, Fabian TC, Croce MA, et al. Staged management of giant abdominal wall defect: acute and long-term results. Ann Surg. 2003;238:349–55. discussion 355-357.
10. Rosen MJ, Krpata DM, Ermlich B, Blatnik JA. A 5-year clinical experience with single-staged repairs of infected and contaminated abdominal wall defects utilizing biologic mesh. Ann Surg. 2013;257(6):991–6.
11. Lee L, Mata J, Landry T, Khwaja KA, Vassiliou MC, Fried GM, Feldman LS. A systematic review of synthetic and biologic materials for abdominal wall reinforcement in contaminated fields. Surg Endosc. 2014;28:2531–46.
12. Raptis DA, Vichova B, Breza J, Skipworth J, Barker S. A comparison of woven versus nonwoven polypropylene (PP) and expanded versus condensed polytetrafluoroethylene (PTFE) on their intraperitoneal incorporation and adhesion formation. J Surg Res. 2011;169(1):1–6.
13. Ratner BD, Hoffman AS, Schoen FJ, Lemons JE, editors. Biomaterials science: an introduction to materials in medicine. 2nd ed. London: Elsevier; 2004.
14. Lowe NS, W.L. Medical device reporting for user facilities. Center for devices and radiological health. 1996.
15. Medwatch. http://www.fda.gov/medwatch/.
16. Siegel E. Predictive analytics: the power to predict who will click, buy, lie, or die. Hoboken: Wiley; 2013.

Biologic Mesh: Classification and Evidence-Based Critical Appraisal

Corey R. Deeken

Current State of the Art

At least thirty types of biologic meshes exist for soft tissue repair applications such as hernia repair/abdominal wall reconstruction, breast reconstruction, wound healing, urogenital/pelvic floor reconstruction, and musculoskeletal reconstruction [1–6]. Of these, fifteen are commonly utilized for hernia repair applications and are fully described in Table 7.1. Biologic meshes are touted to possess many advantages over permanent synthetic meshes. Since biologic meshes are derived from biological tissues, these materials are eventually degraded and remodeled by the host, providing the benefit of a temporary scaffold at the repair site with low risk of long-term inflammation and fibrosis. In addition, biologic meshes can be utilized in clean-contaminated or contaminated settings where synthetic meshes may be contraindicated. It is believed that revascularization of these materials during the remodeling process effectively clears pathogens from the mesh. Despite these potential advantages, there are also some disadvantages associated with biologic mesh use, namely the high cost of these materials compared to synthetic meshes, variability in biologic mesh properties due to donor characteristics, and production of these materials in limited sizes and geometries. Furthermore, biologic meshes may be problematic for patients with religious or ethical concerns surrounding the use of human or animal tissue-derived products [7].

In the future, biologic mesh designs may expand to include antibacterial coatings to reduce or inhibit microbial colonization. This could be particularly useful in clean-contaminated or contaminated settings. One such mesh, XenMatrix™ AB Surgical Graft (C.R. Bard/Davol, Inc., Warwick, RI), has recently received 510 k approval from the FDA. This mesh is comprised of acellular porcine dermis, coated with a resorbable polymer (L-tyrosine succinate) that serves as a carrier for two antimicrobial agents, derivatives of rifamycinB and tetracycline (180 µg/cm^2 each). According to the Instructions for Use (IFU), preclinical studies have demonstrated that these antimicrobial agents reduce or inhibit microbial colonization of the mesh when compared to a control mesh. However, data have not yet been acquired in human subjects.

Classification of Biologic Mesh

Biologic meshes are typically classified according to three major categories as shown in Table 7.1: (1) species of origin, (2) tissue type, and (3) processing conditions. These materials are derived from a variety of species (i.e., human, bovine, porcine, and equine) and tissue types

C.R. Deeken, Ph.D. (✉)
Covalent Bio, LLC, Eureka, MO, USA
e-mail: deekenc@wudosis.wustl.edu

© Springer International Publishing Switzerland 2016
Y.W. Novitsky (ed.), *Hernia Surgery*, DOI 10.1007/978-3-319-27470-6_7

Table 7.1 Modern Inventory of Biologic Meshes

Trade name	Manufacturer	Species	Tissue type	Intentionally crosslinked	Sterilization method
AlloDerm, X-Thick	LifeCell Corp., Branchburg, NJ	Human	Dermis	No	Not terminally sterilized
AlloMax	C.R. Bard/Davol, Inc., Warwick, RI	Human	Dermis	No	Low-dose gamma
CollaMend	C.R. Bard/Davol, Inc., Warwick, RI	Porcine	Dermis	YES 1-ethyl-(3-dimethylaminopropyl)-carbodiimide hydro-chloride (EDC)	Ethylene oxide
CollaMend FM	C.R. Bard/Davol, Inc., Warwick, RI	Porcine	Dermis (fenestrated)	YES (EDC)	Ethylene oxide
FlexHD	Ethicon, Inc., Somerville, NJ	Human	Dermis	No	Decontamination with ethanol and peracetic acid (not terminally sterilized)
Fortiva	RTI Biologics, Inc., Alachua, FL	Porcine	Dermis	No	RTI's Tutoplast® Tissue Sterilization Process with low dose gamma irradiation
GraftJacket	Wright Medical Technology, Inc., Arlington, TN	Human	Dermis	No	Not terminally sterilized
OrthAdapt	Synovis Orthopedic & Woundcare, Irvine, CA	Equine	Pericardium	Yes (Proprietary)	Proprietary
PeriGuard	Synovis Surgical Innovations, St. Paul, MN	Bovine	Pericardium	YES (glutaraldehyde)	Ethanol and propylene oxide
Permacol	Covidien, Norwalk, CT	Porcine	Dermis	YES (hexamethylene diisocyanate)	Gamma irradiation
Strattice, Firm	LifeCell Corp., Branchburg, NJ	Porcine	Dermis	No	E-Beam
SurgiMend	TEI Biosciences, Inc., Boston, MA	Bovine (fetal)	Dermis	No	Ethylene oxide
Surgisis, Biodesign	Cook Medical, Bloomington, IN	Porcine	Small intestine submucosa	No	Ethylene oxide
Veritas	Synovis Surgical Innovations, St. Paul, MN	Bovine	Pericardium	No	E-beam
XenMatrix	C.R. Bard/Davol, Inc., Warwick, RI	Porcine	Dermis	No	E-Beam

(i.e., dermis, pericardium, and small intestine submucosa). The species and type of tissue from which a biologic mesh is derived determine the structure, composition, and mechanical properties of the resulting biologic mesh and can have important implications when implanted in human subjects. However, more attention has historically been paid to the method by which the original tissue is processed to become a biologic mesh, particularly the crosslinking process.

At a minimum, all biologic meshes undergo a decellularization process to remove cells and cellular debris, leaving behind the extracellular matrix (ECM) component of the original. This is an extremely important aspect of biologic mesh development since the recipient's immune response is directly influenced by the efficacy of the decellularization process. Residual cellular debris can lead to an inflammatory response and should be eliminated to the extent possible without damaging the structure or composition of the ECM. Numerous decellularization techniques exist such as treatments with enzymes [8, 9], solvents [10–12], acids/bases, detergents [11–13], hypertonic/hypotonic solutions [14, 15], chelating agents [16, 17], and toxins [4]. The decellularization technique must be optimized for the species and tissue type from which the mesh is derived, and the details of the decellularization process are often withheld by the manufacturer as proprietary.

In addition to decellularization, some biologic meshes are also *intentionally* crosslinked through chemical treatments or dehydration. Crosslinking is typically done to improve the strength of the mesh and/or to prevent rapid degradation of the mesh in vivo. Crosslinking can be accomplished through a variety of chemicals such as carbodiimides [18–21], glutaraldehyde [22–24], or hexamethylene diisocyanate [22]. Variables such as crosslinking agent, concentration, temperature, pH, and exposure time all contribute to the number and type of new bonds that are introduced into the tissue [18, 22, 25].

Xenogeneic meshes are terminally sterilized using gamma irradiation, ethylene oxide, or e-beam treatments, while allogeneic meshes are subjected only to a final disinfection process such as ethanol or peracetic acid treatment. Inadvertent crosslinking may occur during the sterilization process, which can have unfavorable consequences, such as reducing cellular infiltration and scaffold degradation.

Preservation of the tissue for long-term packaging and storage is the final step in the processing of biologic meshes. Some are dehydrated, while others are stored in a hydrated state or even submerged in a preservation fluid. These conditions can lead to unintended disruption of the structure and composition of the ECM, which may influence the remodeling process in vivo.

In summary, there are a tremendous number of variables due to the number of species, tissue types, and processing conditions involved in the production of biologic mesh materials. Furthermore, the details of many of the processing techniques are withheld by the manufacturers as proprietary, making it even more challenging to directly compare biologic mesh products and scientifically determine the effect of a single variable. Human tissue-derived biologic meshes are also plagued by the added variables of donor age, sex, comorbidities, and anatomical location from which the tissue is procured.

Evidence-Based Critical Appraisal

Characterization of Biologic Meshes

The physical, thermal, and mechanical characteristics of twelve biologic meshes were evaluated in a recent study via laser micrometry, differential scanning calorimetry, suture retention strength testing, tear resistance testing, and ball burst testing [26]. The results were compared based on species, tissue type, and processing conditions, namely crosslinking. These tests were designed to fully characterize the pre-implantation properties of biologic meshes and to test the hypothesis that *crosslinked materials possess greater pre-implantation strength than non-crosslinked materials.*

The results of this study revealed a wide variety of pre-implantation characteristics between different types of biologic meshes. In contrast to the hypothesis, crosslinked meshes exhibited lower mechanical strengths than non-crosslinked meshes in all three mechanical tests performed (i.e., suture retention strength testing, tear resistance testing, and ball burst testing). This was especially true of the porcine dermis-derived meshes. The bovine pericardium-derived meshes exhibited similar mechanical strengths between the crosslinked and non-crosslinked meshes, indicating little effect of crosslinking on the mechanical characteristics of bovine pericardium tissue. It was expected that the human dermis-derived meshes would exhibit similar mechanical strengths since all are derived from the same species/type of tissue and none are crosslinked. However, the three human dermis-derived meshes exhibited a wide range of mechanical strengths. These results indicate that other factors such as donor variables (i.e., age, sex, tissue procurement site, comorbidities, etc.) or conditions during the decellularization and decontamination processes significantly influenced the resulting properties of the human dermis-derived meshes.

Repetitive Loading

A subset of biologic meshes was further evaluated in another study involving repetitive loading experiments [27]. Nine types of biologic meshes were subjected to cycles of uniaxial tensile loading, and series of 10, 100, and 1000 cycles were completed for each mesh type. It was hypothesized that *crosslinked materials resist damage during repetitive loading and maintain baseline strength while non-crosslinked materials sustain damage during repetitive loading and exhibit a significant reduction in strength.*

Consistent with this hypothesis, one of the crosslinked porcine dermis meshes (Permacol™) was significantly stronger than the non-crosslinked porcine dermis meshes (Strattice™ and XenMatrix™) at baseline and after 10, 100, or 1000 cycles of loading. However, the other crosslinked porcine dermis mesh (CollaMend™)

exhibited similar results as the non-crosslinked porcine dermis meshes at baseline and after 10, 100, or 1000 cycles, indicating that the particular crosslinking agent or conditions utilized to achieve decellularization, crosslinking, and/or sterilization significantly influenced the properties of this material. Additionally, both crosslinked porcine dermis meshes (Permacol™ and CollaMend™) and one of the non-crosslinked porcine dermis meshes (XenMatrix™) maintained their baseline tensile strength even after exposure to repetitive loading conditions, while the other non-crosslinked porcine dermis (Strattice™) exhibited a significant decrease in tensile strength with increasing number of cycles. As expected, the crosslinked bovine pericardium mesh (PeriGuard®) was significantly stronger than the non-crosslinked bovine pericardium mesh (Veritas®) at baseline and after 10, 100, or 1000 cycles of loading. However, both bovine pericardium meshes maintained their baseline tensile strength even after 1000 cycles of loading, regardless of the presence of crosslinking. These results contrast those of porcine dermis-derived meshes, indicating that variables such as species, tissue type, and processing conditions may all play a role in determining the final properties of these materials. As in the previous study, wide variation was observed between the human dermis-derived meshes, pointing to donor variables, in addition to processing conditions, as particularly problematic for human tissue-derived meshes.

In general, crosslinked meshes resisted damage during repetitive loading and maintained baseline tensile strength, while non-crosslinked meshes sustained damage during repetitive loading and exhibited significant reduction in tensile strength. However, widespread generalizations should not be made, as this study demonstrated exceptions, particularly for porcine-dermis-derived products.

Resistance to Enzymatic Degradation

In another study, the same subset of biologic meshes was also exposed to collagenase enzymes in vitro in order to assess the impact of enzymatic degradation on the uniaxial tensile strength of these materials [28]. It was hypothesized that *crosslinked materials resist enzymatic degradation and maintain baseline strength while non-crosslinked materials undergo enzymatic degradation and exhibit a significant reduction in strength.*

Nine types of biologic mesh materials were exposed to collagenase solution at 37 °C. After 30 hours of exposure, both crosslinked and non-crosslinked porcine dermis meshes exhibited significantly reduced tensile strength compared to their respective baseline tensile strengths, indicating significant enzymatic degradation. This result was observed regardless of crosslinking. Even so, one of the crosslinked porcine dermis meshes (Permacol™) maintained significantly greater tensile strength than the two non-crosslinked porcine dermis meshes (Strattice™ and XenMatrix™) and the other crosslinked porcine dermis mesh (CollaMend™) throughout the exposure period. On the other hand, one of the non-crosslinked porcine dermis meshes (XenMatrix™) was so significantly degraded that it was difficult to measure the tensile strength of the specimens beyond 12 hours of exposure to collagenase solution.

Similarly, the non-crosslinked bovine pericardium mesh (Veritas®) exhibited significantly reduced tensile strength compared to its baseline tensile strength after just 6 hours of exposure to collagenase solution, indicating significant and rapid in vitro degradation of this particular material. However, the crosslinked bovine pericardium mesh (PeriGuard®) maintained its baseline tensile strength and did not show any evidence of degradation even after 30 hours of exposure to collagenase. The crosslinked bovine pericardium mesh (PeriGuard®) also maintained significantly greater tensile strength than its non-crosslinked counterpart (Veritas®) throughout the exposure period, as expected.

The human dermis-derived meshes displayed wide variation in baseline properties and in their ability to resist enzymatic degradation. Although the baseline tensile strength of FlexHD® was lower than that of AlloMax™, FlexHD® resisted enzymatic degradation more effectively. AlloMax™ was so significantly degraded after just 12 hours of exposure that tensile strength could not be reliably measured beyond that point.

The results of this study demonstrated that in general, crosslinking did not improve the resistance of porcine dermis-derived meshes to enzymatic degradation. However, crosslinking did significantly improve the resistance of bovine pericardium-derived meshes to enzymatic degradation. These results suggest that the effects of crosslinking may be species/tissue dependent or related to the specific chemical compounds utilized to achieve crosslinking and the number of additional bonds ultimately introduced into these tissues. Additionally, differences were observed between non-crosslinked materials, suggesting that widespread generalizations of all non-crosslinked materials should not be made. Differences due to species, tissue type, and other processing conditions appear to be extremely influential.

Porcine Model of Ventral Hernia Repair

The mechanical strength of a hernia repair site and the host tissue response to six types of biologic meshes were evaluated in several recent studies using a well-established porcine model of ventral hernia repair [29–31]. This model was designed to fully characterize the post-implantation properties of biologic meshes and to test the hypotheses that (1) *crosslinked materials augment the strength of native tissue, leading to a stronger hernia repair and that* (2) *crosslinked materials resist degradation, thereby reducing cellular infiltration and overall tissue remodeling compared to non-crosslinked materials.*

In this study, a total of four hernia defects (5 cm each) were surgically created in each animal, one in each abdominal quadrant. The musculature and fascia of the abdominal wall were incised and left open, creating the abdominal wall defects. The subcutaneous fat, areolar tissue, and skin were closed in separate layers to prevent wound dehiscence. The defects were allowed to mature for 21 days and were then repaired with biologic mesh positioned in the retromuscular/preperitoneal space. Animals were subsequently survived for 1, 6, or 12 months. Mesh-tissue composites were procured at the end of the survival period and subjected to uniaxial tensile testing to provide a measure of the biomechanics of the repair site. Specimens were also stained with hematoxylin and eosin (H&E) and semi-quantitatively assessed for six characteristics of tissue response: cellular infiltration, cell types, scaffold degradation, ECM deposition, neovascularization, and fibrosis. Possible scores in each category ranged from 0 to 3, with higher scores representing more favorable characteristics of tissue response. A composite score was also generated from the mean of the six component scores and was utilized as an overall measure of tissue remodeling.

Mechanical testing of the mesh-tissue composites revealed that all repair sites exhibited similar tensile strengths at all time points regardless of biologic mesh type or presence/absence of crosslinking. Furthermore, the strength of the native tissue of the porcine abdominal wall was not significantly augmented by any of the biologic meshes, including crosslinked materials.

Histological analysis revealed that in the short-term, crosslinking of biologic meshes impacted characteristics of tissue remodeling such as cellular infiltration and neovascularization. As shown in Fig. 7.1, non-crosslinked meshes exhibited higher scores at earlier time points than crosslinked meshes. However, at later time points, scores for crosslinked materials tended to reach levels similar to non-crosslinked materials. Thus, crosslinking did not appear to significantly influence cellular infiltration over the long-term as anticipated. Other processing conditions such as differences in decellularization and sterilization techniques may have impacted tissue remodeling characteristics more substantially and should be evaluated in future studies.

Biologic Meshes Explanted from Human Subjects

The remodeling characteristics of biologic meshes after implantation in human subjects for abdominal wall reconstruction are not well understood. Thus, two recent studies have evaluated biopsies of biologic meshes procured from human subjects during abdominal re-exploration [32, 33].

In the study by Cavallo et al., biopsies were obtained from forty human subjects [32]. Mesh type was identified in 37 out of 40 biopsies and included 23 human dermis-derived biologic meshes, 11 porcine dermis-derived biologic meshes, and 3 bovine dermis-derived biologic meshes. After procurement, the specimens were stained with hematoxylin and eosin (H&E) and semi-quantitatively assessed for six characteristics of tissue response: cellular infiltration, cell types, scaffold degradation, ECM deposition, neovascularization, and fibrosis. Possible scores in each category ranged from 0 to 3, with higher scores representing more favorable characteristics of tissue response. A composite score was also generated from the mean of the six component scores and was utilized as an overall measure of tissue remodeling.

Cellular infiltration, ECM deposition, and neovascularization scores were 2 for 80%, 64%, and 64% of the specimens, respectively, indicating that the majority of cells, host ECM deposition, and vasculature infiltrated beyond the periphery and began to penetrate deeper into the mesh, even reaching the center of the biopsy in some cases. Cell types scores were <3 in 57% of the specimens, indicating that the majority of meshes showed evidence of inflammatory infiltrate. Only 43% of the specimens scored ≥3 for cell types, indicating the presence of fibroblasts only without any inflammatory cells. Scaffold degradation and fibrosis scores were ≥2 in 56% and 70% of cases, respectively, indicating that the majority of the meshes were significantly degraded with mild fibrous encapsulation of less than 25% of the mesh periphery. In general, the biologic mesh biopsies indicated favorable host remodeling scores with cells (primarily fibroblasts), host ECM deposition, and new vasculature beginning to reach the center of the biopsies, which were almost fully degraded with minimal inflammatory or fibrous reaction.

When the meshes were subdivided by mesh type, it was revealed that human dermis-derived

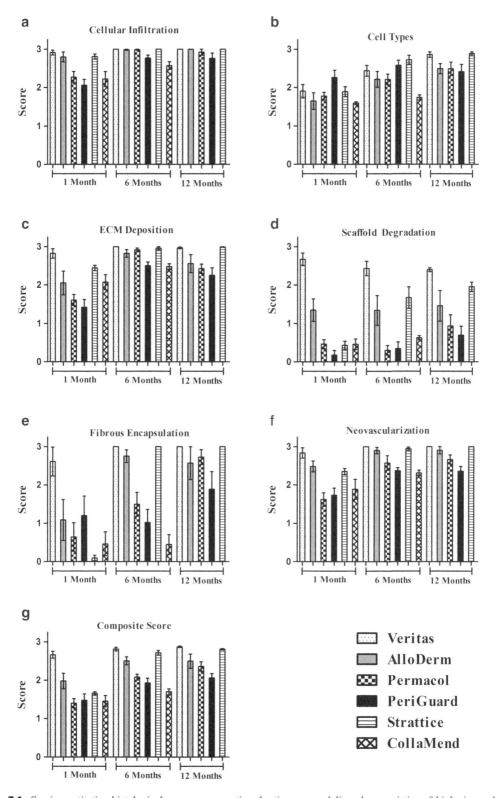

Fig. 7.1 Semi-quantitative histological scores representing the tissue remodeling characteristics of biologic meshes explanted from a porcine hernia model (H&E stained slides)

meshes exhibited significantly improved cellular infiltration, ECM deposition, scaffold degradation, and neovascularization scores compared to porcine dermis-derived meshes and trended toward improved scores compared to bovine dermis-derived meshes. Thus, the species of origin appears to significantly impact remodeling of biologic meshes when implanted in human subjects.

In the study by De Silva et al., biopsies were obtained from fourteen ($n = 14$) human subjects who underwent biologic mesh repairs placed as an intraperitoneal underlay [33]. Mesh type was identified in all biopsies with $n = 7$ crosslinked porcine dermis (Permacol™) and $n = 7$ non-crosslinked porcine dermis (Strattice™). After procurement, the specimens were stained with hematoxylin and eosin (H&E) and Masson's trichrome and evaluated for acute and chronic inflammatory response, foreign body reaction, fibrous capsule formation, cellular infiltration, neovascularization, and degradation/remodeling. Possible scores in each category were 0 (none), 1 (minimal), 2 (mild), 3 (moderate), or 4 (extensive).

The crosslinked porcine dermis specimens exhibited mild foreign body reaction, moderate fibrous capsule formation, no neovascularization, no cellular infiltration, and no quantifiable new collagen deposition. The non-crosslinked porcine dermis specimens exhibited similar characteristics with mild to moderate foreign body reaction, mild to moderate fibrous encapsulation, no neovascularization. However, non-crosslinked grafts did demonstrate some neo-cellularization at the periphery of the mesh, albeit without any quantifiable new collagen deposition. Regardless of crosslinking, the porcine dermis-based biopsies showed no evidence of significant remodeling at the time of explantation. Although the findings of the study questioned the concept of biologic mesh remodeling, this finding might be a factor of the underlay mesh positioning.

Conclusions

A large number of biologic meshes are currently available. Those meshes are touted to possess many advantages over permanent synthetic meshes. It is believed that revascularization of these materials during the remodeling process effectively clears pathogens from the mesh. Mesh remodeling has proven to be inconsistent. Crosslinking is not the only factor that determines the properties or performance of biologic meshes. Other aspects of the tissue treatment process (i.e., decellularization method, crosslinking technique, extent of crosslinking, sterilization process, and packaging conditions) or species/tissue from which these meshes are derived all contribute and should be explored in more detail in future studies. Overall, biologic mesh use appears to have peaked several years ago and recent disappointing clinical data and high cost have begun to limit its utilization.

References

1. Cornwell KG, Landsman A, James KS. Extracellular matrix biomaterials for soft tissue repair. Clin Podiatr Med Surg. 2009;26:507–23.
2. Badylak SF. Xenogeneic extracellular matrix as a scaffold for tissue reconstruction. Transpl Immunol. 2004;12:367–77.
3. Badylak SF. The extracellular matrix as a biologic scaffold material. Biomaterials. 2007;28:3587–93.
4. Badylak SF. Decellularized allogeneic and xenogeneic tissue as a bioscaffold for regenerative medicine: factors that influence the host response. Ann Biomed Eng. 2014;42:1517–27.
5. Zienowicz RJ, Karacaoglu E. Implant-based breast reconstruction with allograft. Plast Reconstr Surg. 2007;120:373–81.
6. Cook JL, Fox DB, Kuroki K, Jayo M, De Deyne PG. In vitro and in vivo comparison of five biomaterials used for orthopedic soft tissue augmentation. Am J Vet Res. 2008;69:148–56.
7. Jenkins ED, Yip M, Melman L, Frisella MM, Matthews BD. Informed consent: cultural and religious issues associated with the use of allogeneic and xenogeneic mesh products. J Am Coll Surg. 2010;210:402–10.
8. Meyer SR, Chiu B, Churchill TA, Zhu L, Lakey JR, Ross DB. Comparison of aortic valve allograft decellularization techniques in the rat. J Biomed Mater Res Part A. 2006;79:254–62.
9. Lynch AP, Ahearne M. Strategies for developing decellularized corneal scaffolds. Exp Eye Res. 2013;108:42–7.
10. Horowitz B, Bonomo R, Prince AM, Chin SN, Brotman B, Shulman RW. Solvent/detergent-treated plasma: a virus-inactivated substitute for fresh frozen plasma. Blood. 1992;79:826–31.

11. Cartmell JS, Dunn MG. Effect of chemical treatments on tendon cellularity and mechanical properties. J Biomed Mater Res. 2000;49:134–40.
12. Woods T, Gratzer PF. Effectiveness of three extraction techniques in the development of a decellularized bone-anterior cruciate ligament-bone graft. Biomaterials. 2005;26:7339–49.
13. Deeken CR, White AK, Bachman SL, Ramshaw BJ, Cleveland DS, Loy TS, et al. Method of preparing a decellularized porcine tendon using tributyl phosphate. J Biomed Mater Res B Appl Biomater. 2011;96:199–206.
14. Gillies AR, Smith LR, Lieber RL, Varghese S. Method for decellularizing skeletal muscle without detergents or proteolytic enzymes. Tissue Eng Part C Methods. 2011;17:383–9.
15. Gratzer PF, Harrison RD, Woods T. Matrix alteration and not residual sodium dodecyl sulfate cytotoxicity affects the cellular repopulation of a decellularized matrix. Tissue Eng. 2006;12:2975–83.
16. Zhang AY, Bates SJ, Morrow E, Pham H, Pham B, Chang J. Tissue-engineered intrasynovial tendons: optimization of acellularization and seeding. J Rehabil Res Dev. 2009;46:489–98.
17. Rieder E, Kasimir MT, Silberhumer G, Seebacher G, Wolner E, Simon P, et al. Decellularization protocols of porcine heart valves differ importantly in efficiency of cell removal and susceptibility of the matrix to recellularization with human vascular cells. J Thorac Cardiovasc Surg. 2004;127:399–405.
18. Damink LHHO, Dijkstra PJ, vanLuyn MJA, vanWachem PB, Nieuwenhuis P, Feijen J. Cross-linking of dermal sheep collagen using a water-soluble carbodiimide. Biomaterials. 1996;17:765–73.
19. Abraham GA, Murray J, Billiar K, Sullivan SJ. Evaluation of the porcine intestinal collagen layer as a biomaterial. J Biomed Mater Res. 2000;51:442–52.
20. Billiar K, Murray J, Laude D, Abraham G, Bachrach N. Effects of carbodiimide crosslinking conditions on the physical properties of laminated intestinal submucosa. J Biomed Mater Res. 2001;56:101–8.
21. Olde Damink LH, Dijkstra PJ, van Luyn MJ, van Wachem PB, Nieuwenhuis P, Feijen J. In vitro degradation of dermal sheep collagen cross-linked using a water-soluble carbodiimide. Biomaterials. 1996;17:679–84.
22. Khor E. Methods for the treatment of collagenous tissues for bioprostheses. Biomaterials. 1997;18:95–105.
23. Courtman DW, Errett BF, Wilson GJ. The role of crosslinking in modification of the immune response elicited against xenogenic vascular acellular matrices. J Biomed Mater Res. 2001;55:576–86.
24. HardinYoung J, Carr RM, Downing GJ, Condon KD, Termin PL. Modification of native collagen reduces antigenicity but preserves cell compatibility. Biotechnol Bioeng. 1996;49:675–82.
25. Gratzer PF, Lee JM. Control of pH alters the type of cross-linking produced by 1-ethyl-3-(3-dimethylaminopropyl)-carbodiimide (EDC) treatment of acellular matrix vascular grafts. J Biomed Mater Res. 2001;58:172–9.
26. Deeken CR, Eliason BJ, Pichert MD, Grant SA, Frisella MM, Matthews BD. Differentiation of biologic scaffold materials through physiomechanical, thermal, and enzymatic degradation techniques. Ann Surg. 2012;255:595.
27. Pui CL, Tang ME, Annor AH, Ebersole GC, Frisella MM, Matthews BD, et al. Effect of repetitive loading on the mechanical properties of biological scaffold materials. J Am Coll Surg. 2012;215:216–28.
28. Annor AH, Tang ME, Pui CL, Ebersole GC, Frisella MM, Matthews BD, et al. Effect of enzymatic degradation on the mechanical properties of biological scaffold materials. Surg Endosc. 2012;26:2767–78.
29. Deeken CR, Melman L, Jenkins ED, Greco SC, Frisella MM, Matthews BD. Histologic and biomechanical evaluation of crosslinked and non-crosslinked biologic meshes in a porcine model of ventral incisional hernia repair. J Am Coll Surg. 2011;212:880–8.
30. Jenkins ED, Melman L, Deeken CR, Greco SC, Frisella MM, Matthews BD. Biomechanical and histologic evaluation of fenestrated and nonfenestrated biologic mesh in a porcine model of ventral hernia repair. J Am Coll Surg. 2011;212:327–39.
31. Cavallo JA, Greco SC, Liu J, Frisella MM, Deeken CR, Matthews BD. Remodeling characteristics and biomechanical properties of a crosslinked versus a non-crosslinked porcine dermis scaffolds in a porcine model of ventral hernia repair. Hernia. 2013;19(2):207–18.
32. Cavallo JA, Roma AA, Jasielec MS, Ousley J, Creamer J, Pichert MD, et al. Remodeling characteristics and collagen distribution in biological scaffold materials explanted from human subjects after abdominal soft tissue reconstruction: an analysis of scaffold remodeling characteristics by patient risk factors and surgical site classifications. Ann Surg. 2013.
33. De Silva GS, Krpata DM, Gao Y, Criss CN, Anderson JM, Soltanian HT, et al. Lack of identifiable biologic behavior in a series of porcine mesh explants. Surgery. 2014;156:183–9.

Biodegradable Meshes in Abdominal Wall Surgery

Garth Jacobsen and Christopher DuCoin

Introduction

Tension-free hernia repair with reinforcement by synthetic, nonresorbable mesh has led to a drastic reduction in the rate of hernia recurrence. However, these permanent foreign materials have been implicated in causing the development of chronic inflammation and fibrosis, which have been attributed to post-operative issues such as chronic pain and abdominal wall stiffness [1–3]. Most surgeons fear their use in contaminated environments due to the high risk of mesh infection and subsequent required explant [4]. Thus acellular, biological meshes of both human and animal origin have been suggested as the alternative to the synthetics in contaminated fields [5, 6]. However, the high cost of biological meshes, at roughly $25–30 per cm^2, has been shown to result in a median net financial loss of $8370 per hospital admission for large abdominal wall hernias [7]. Recently, the use of reduced-weight polypropylene synthetic mesh in clean-contaminated and contaminated fields was studied and found to have both similar surgical site occurrences and mesh removal rates when compared to biologics [8]. However, no mesh to this point has been FDA approved for the use in contaminated

surgical fields. This leaves us in a state of confusion. The dogma remains that synthetic mesh provides radically lower rates of hernia recurrence and that biologics are supreme when used in dirty surgical fields. There may be more lure to these assumptions than evidence based understanding, and thus these teachings should no longer be taken as definitive rule. So where does this leave us, is there a happy medium between synthetic and biologic? Yes, the benefits of both synthetics and biologics can be found in the synthetic bioabsorbable meshes.

Types of Bioabsorbables

Bioabsorbables are composed of synthetic resorbable monofilament polymers, either in a single or double layer that is gradually degraded over time. Yet, as the mesh is being degraded it is also providing the structural framework for the host tissue to incorporate with, and allows for the remodeling of the abdominal wall with native tissue. The end result is that the abdominal wall strength is provided by the host's own tissue. Thus, as there is no permanent foreign body, the likelihood of infection is drastically reduced. Currently there are four major types of bioabsorbable mesh. These meshes include Ethicon Vicryl Mesh (Ethicon Inc., Somerville, NJ), Phasix Mesh (C. R. Bard, Inc./Davol Inc., Warwick, RI), Tigr Matrix (Novus Scientific, Uppsala, Sweden), and Gore Bio-A (W.L. Gore

G. Jacobsen, M.D. (✉) • C. DuCoin, M.D., M.P.H.
Department of Surgery, University of California,
San Diego, 9500 Gilman Drive, MC 0740 l,
La Jolla, CA 92093-0740, USA
e-mail: gjacobsen@ucsd.edu; cducoin@ucsd.edu

© Springer International Publishing Switzerland 2016
Y.W. Novitsky (ed.), *Hernia Surgery*, DOI 10.1007/978-3-319-27470-6_8

Table 8.1 Inventory of Bioabsorbable meshes

	Collagen deposit	Majority of strength lost	Full resorption (months)	Studies
VICYRL	Low	75% of strength lost in 14 days	2–3	Animal
				Human
PHASIX	Not reported	4–8 months	12–18	Animal
TIGR	Mixed ratio over 36 months	8–9 months	36	Animal
				Human
BIO-A	100% Type 1 at 30 days	3–4 months	6	Animal
				Human

Electron Microscopy of Synthetic Bioabsorbable Mesh

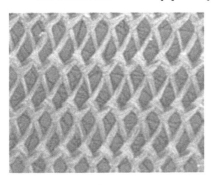

Vicryl™ Mesh
SEM photo, 20x

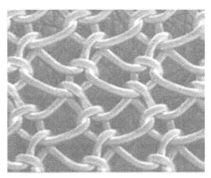

Phasix™ Mesh
SEM photo, 20x

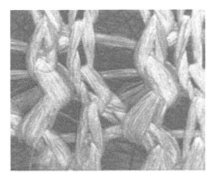

TIGR® Matrix
SEM photo, 20x

Bio-A®Mesh
SEM photo, 20x

Fig. 8.1 Electron microscopy of synthetic bioabsorbable mesh at twenty times magnification. The images delineate the intricate woven matrix styles and size, along with the caliber of porosity. Vicryl mesh is a tightly woven single layer mesh with a symmetrical pattern. Phasix mesh has a greater caliber matrix with more porosity. TIGR Matrix is composed to two polymers that are degraded at different rates, with differed caliber size and vast porosity. Bio-A mesh is also composed of copolymers but possesses a unique non-woven matrix

and Associates, Inc., Flagstaff, AZ) which will be reviewed in greater detail (Table 8.1). Fundamentally these meshes have very different structural patterns as can be seen with electron-microscopy (Fig. 8.1).

Vicryl (polyglactin 910) woven mesh is prepared from a synthetic absorbable co-polymer of glycolide and lactide. This tightly woven mesh is prepared from uncoated, undyed fiber identical in composition to that used in Vicryl synthetic absorbable suture. This material has been found to be inert, nonantigenic, nonpyrogenic and to elicit only a mild tissue reaction during absorption. Vicryl woven mesh is intended for use as a buttress to provide temporary support during the healing process. However, Vicryl loses 77% of its strength in the first 14 days (0.5 month) in rat models, and it is fully resorbed in approximately 60–90 days (2–3 months). Thus, Vicryl mesh is absorbed the fastest of all the synthetic bioabsorbables. Vicryl degrades in vivo through hydrolysis and is known to decrease the pH in the local tissues [9]. When compared to other biologics, Vicryl was found to have lower collagen deposition and neovascularization, which has been attributed to this decrease in pH [9, 10]. There is also an increase in inflammation at the wound site as Vicryl mesh degrades [9, 10]. Overall, Vicryl mesh is resorbed quickly, losing its mechanical strength too fast, making it less than ideal for hernia repair [11]. A mesh that provides greater structural support of the hernia site for a longer period of time will be required to allow for adequate completion of tissue remodeling [11].

Thus, more recent absorbable scaffold designs have been developed which utilize long lasting polymers that degrade slower. Bard's Phasix Mesh is constructed of monofilament poly-4-hydroxybutyrate (P4HB), a resorbable polymer. P4HB is a naturally derived, fully absorbable polymer produced by *Escherichia coli* K12 bacteria via transgenic fermentation techniques [12]. P4HB degrades in vivo through both hydrolysis and a hydrolytic enzymatic digestive process and is fully resorbed in approximately 365–545 days (12–18 months) [12]. The resulting by-products (carbon dioxide and water) are metabolized quickly via the Krebs Cycle and beta-oxidation, with minimal effect on the local wound environment [12]. Unlike absorbable scaffolds such as Vicryl, whose by-products decrease the local pH, degradation of P4HB is not as acidic, which may reduce the inflammatory response associated with these materials [12]. An animal study evaluated Phasix Mesh and P4HB Plug repair sites over a 52 week period and showed a significantly greater burst strength and relative stiffness with the mesh when compared to the native abdominal wall at all-time intervals [11]. In addition, histological assessment revealed a comparable and mild inflammatory response, and mild to moderate granulation tissue/vascularization associated with the P4HB material regardless of its configuration as a mesh or a plug [11]. Studies thus far have all been completed in animal models and additional human models will hopefully show the same benefits.

Tigr Matrix is knitted from two fibers having different resorption rates. The first fiber makes up approximately 40% of the overall mesh by weight and is a copolymer of polyglycolide, polylactide, and polytrimethylene carbonate. This fiber degrades in vivo through hydrolysis, loses substantial mechanical strength in the first 14 days (0.5 month), and is fully resorbed in approximately 120 days (4 months). The second fiber makes up approximately 60% of the overall mesh by weight and is a copolymer of polylactide and polytrimethylene carbonate. This fiber also degrades in vivo through hydrolysis, but it retains its mechanical strength longer than the first fiber. It begins to demonstrate loss of mechanical strength after approximately 270 days (9 months) and is fully resorbed in approximately 1095 days (36 months). Tigr Matrix has been evaluated in a long-term animal model, and a clinical trial is currently underway. In the animal study, Tigr Matrix was compared to permanent polypropylene mesh in sheep with full thickness abdominal wall defects over the course of 4, 9, 15, 24, and 36 months [13]. The results showed the typical long-term inflammatory response found with the permanent polypropylene mesh. However, Tigr Matrix demonstrated a medium-term inflammatory response similar to that of polypropylene, with the important difference being that inflammation declined after 24 months and was practically absent after 36 months once the mesh had been completely resorbed [13]. Tigr Matrix also exhibited collagen deposition at the repair site that increased over time and eventually resembled native connective tissue [13]. In the study no defect recurrences were noted in either the test or control group. Since Tigr Matrix loses the bulk of its mechanical strength after 6 months, it can be assumed that the restored tissue is evidently strong enough to carry the abdominal loads found in these sheep models [13]. In the clinical trial, 40 subjects were enrolled and followed for 1 year after placement of Tigr Matrix to repair a primary inguinal hernia [14]. Pain and recurrence were evaluated at 0.5, 1, 3, 6, and 12 months, and pain scores were reduced from an average of 17.4 before surgery to 0.3 after just 6 months post operatively [14]. In conclusion, Tigr Matrix is fully resorbed in 3 years, shows an inflammatory response that reduces over time, and is associated with a reduction in post-operative pain.

Gore Bio-A is a copolymer composed of polyglycolic acid and trimethylene carbonate (PGA-TMC) that degrades in vivo through both hydrolytic and enzymatic mechanisms. Bio-A is fully resorbed within approximately 180 days (6 months). Published studies to date are mainly in animal models with an international multi-center human clinical trial having just been completed. In an animal study, Bio-A showed higher degree of cellular and vascular ingrowth, and collagen deposition than three commonly used biologic meshes in a sterile field [15]. In regard to vascular ingrowth, Bio-A showed a statistically significant increase in blood vessel ingrowth when compared to biologics ($p < 0.0001$) [15]. The vascular ingrowth for Bio-A was greatest between days 7–14, while the biologics had no significant change after 7 days [15]. Samples of Bio-A demonstrated that at 30 days the collagen was 100% Type 1 [15]. This is significantly earlier than the biologics ($p = 0.006$) [15]. Bio-A also exhibited the least inflammatory infiltrate over time [15]. The outcomes thus far have been promising with low rates of recurrence, infection, and pain.

A recently completed international multi-center prospective human study evaluated Bio-A in clean contaminated and contaminated ventral hernia repairs with outcome measures of hernia recurrence, surgical site events (SSE), and quality of life. Of the 104 patients enrolled the mean follow-up time was 16 months. Findings at that time of evaluation showed a hernia recurrence rate of 14% and a SSE rate of 28%, with a surgical site infection rate (SSI) of 18% ($n = 21$). When the group analyzed the risk factors for hernia recurrence

they found that body mass index (BMI), previous infected mesh, position of mesh, and post-operative SSI were statistically significant contributors to risk of recurrence. It was also found that the average BMI for no midline recurrence was 27 kg/m^2 while the BMI for recurrence of midline hernia was 34 kg/m^2 (p-value 0.004), and that previous mesh infection had a p-value of 0.031. Position of mesh was also important in that there was a significantly lower recurrence rate when the mesh was placed into the retro-rectus position. When the mesh was placed in an intrapertioneal position the recurrence rate was 30%, yet when placed retro-rectus the recurrence rate dropped to 5% (p-value 0.028). Also, with a post-operative SSI the recurrence rate was 21% while in those without post-operative SSI the recurrence rate was 5% (p-value 0.035). In regard to SSI, 18% had infections post-operatively, but since all Bio-A mesh was placed into contaminated fields in this study, it can be argued that 82% of patients were cured of their previous infection. Of the SSI's, nine were superficial and responded to antibiotic treatment only, while ten were deep requiring drain placement with antibiotics. However, no mesh required explant. When looking at risk factors for SSI, diabetes mellitus ($p = 0.042$), fistula take down ($p = 0.001$), and previous mesh ($p = 0.019$) were found to be significant risk factors. When evaluating for quality of life scores, the data showed an initial drop. However, over time there was a significant improvement. The authors concluded that the hernia recurrence rate was acceptable and improved with retro-rectus placement, that mesh infection could be managed conservatively, and patients benefited from an improved quality of life.

Placement into Infected Surgical Fields

The infected surgical field remains the most challenging area of mesh placement as mesh infection can be a catastrophic and mortal event to the patient. As mentioned above, synthetic bioabsorbable mesh has been used successfully in this setting. The study above showed that Bio-A used

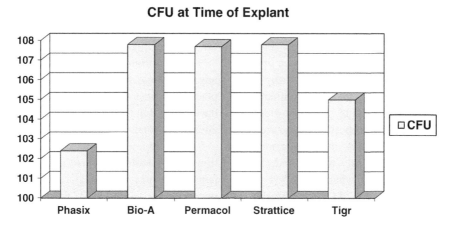

Fig. 8.2 Bacterial clearance

in clean contaminated and contaminated ventral hernia repairs had a post operative surgical site infection rate (SSI) of 18%. The astonishing finding in this study is that no mesh required removal and that all infections, both superficial and deep, could be treated with conservative measures. An animal study found that Bio-A was safe to use in a contaminated surgical field [16]. In a rat model, that used methicillin resistant *Staphylococcus aureus* (MRSA) as contaminate, bacteria were cleared from the Bio-A mesh more effectively than either Vicryl or Tigr Matrix at an inoculum greater than 106 [16]. However, at an inoculum of 104 or less, all three scaffolds performed equally. All three of the scaffolds exhibited reduced tensile strength and increased rate of mesh failure regardless of composition if there was any inoculum present [16]. A similar study recently completed by Dr. Voeller et al. compared Phasix Mesh to various other mesh types. In this study, a rabbit dorsal model using one of the mesh types was inoculated with MRSA 1×10^8 colony forming unites (CFU)/mL. On post operative day number seven the mesh was explanted then examined for number of CFU/mL. All mesh types showed a decrease in CFU/mL, however Phasix and Tigr Mesh showed the greatest reduction (Fig. 8.2). As the data of these two studies can be somewhat confusing, each

study showing a different mesh with better bacterial clearance, it is still evident that synthetic bioabsorbable mesh can not only tolerate placement into an infected field, but can also clear the bacteria present.

Another animal study examined the infection rates when the mesh was impregnated with antibiotics, specifically cefazolin [17]. In this study 90 white rats were divided into four groups where Bio-A was placed in an intraperitoneal position. Group 1 consisted of mesh only (control group), in group 2 the mesh was infected at 1 week post operative with 1×10^8 CFU of *S. aureus*, in group 3 antibiotic-impregnated mesh used and then infected at 1 week's time, and in group 4 the antibiotic quantity was double that of group 3 and subsequently infected at 1 weeks time. The groups were then examined at 1 week post infection, or post-op week 2 for bacterial colonization. Evident decrease of bacterial colonization was observed in groups 3 and 4, the ones impregnated with cefazolin, in comparison with the group 2, infected without previous antibiotic impregnation, with statistically significant results ($p < 0.001$). Thus, the authors suggest that impregnation of an absorbable hydrophilic prosthesis, such as Bio-A, with cefazolin will help reduce the rate of mesh infection when placed in a contaminated field.

Which Mesh to Use and When to Use It and Where to Put It

It has been our practice to base the type of mesh selection on a case-by-case basis, as truly every patient is unique in regard to abdominal wall reconstruction. When using synthetic mesh we prefer lightweight macro-porous mesh. We have moved away from the classic biologic mesh as empirically little benefit was found at an extremely elevated cost when compared to the synthetic bioabsorbables. Synthetic bioabsorbable mesh is roughly 1/3–1/10 the cost of a matched piece of biologic mesh. Over the last 5 years when treating complex abdominal wall hernias with the possibility of either a clean-contaminated or contaminated field we have opted to use a bioabsorbable mesh. Our outcomes have been so positive that we no longer stock biologic mesh at our center.

When looking at our data in regard to bioabsorbable mesh for complex abdominal wall hernias we found that over the last 5 years 147 patients have been treated with either Bio-A or Tigr Matrix. These hernia defects have consisted of extremely large areas with the average hernia defect being 130.8 cm². Of these 147 patients, 52 of them (35.4%) presented with a recurrent hernia that had undergone previous attempted repair, with a cumulative of 83 previous attempted hernia repairs. A CDC wound classification was found to be Class II or greater in 41 patients (27.9%). The average follow-up duration for this study population was 582 days. There was a total number of 27 (18.3%) wound complications, consisting of seroma ($N=13$), wound infection ($N=7$), retro-rectus hematoma ($N=4$), and flap necrosis ($N=3$). In the study population there were four recurrences (2.7%), and a single explant. Though the average follow-up for this study group is less than 2 years, we feel the wound complication rate and the drastically lower recurrence rate when compared to biologic mesh warrants the use of synthetic bioabsorbables in large complex abdominal wall hernia reconstruction where there is risk of contamination.

In regard to placement of mesh, we use a very straight forward algorithm (Fig. 8.3). Our goal is to always place the mesh in a sublay fashion, in an attempt to reduce wound complications and infections, in the belief that it is a more appropriate physiological placement. For any defect less than 25 cm² we will attempt to place our mesh in a retro-rectus position. We have found that for defects larger than 25 cm² an alternate fascial release is required. In determining which type of release to use, we use resection of panniculectomy as the determinant. If a panniculectomy is to be performed usually the morbidity of creating skin flaps has already taken place. Thus, we will use a standard component separation with an onlay mesh placement that is sutured to the lateral edge of the released external oblique fascia under moderate tension. If a panniculectomy is not part of the abdominal wall hernia repair, then we will continue with our retro-rectus dissection and extend it to a Transversus abdominis muscle release (TAR), detailed in Chapter 13. In this fashion the midline can be brought back together and the mesh placed behind the transversus abdominis and the rectus muscles, cut to fit and not affixed. Multiple drains are placed to combat seroma formation and allow for good tissue approximation and mesh ingrowth.

Conclusion

Synthetic bioabsorbable meshes provide the initial rigidity found in synthetic mesh while degrading over time, much like a biologic, reducing the risk of infection and need for mesh removal. Our data supports that they have a lower recurrence rate when compared to biologics while maintaining the same complication risk when used in contaminated fields. They do this at a drastically reduced cost. Excluding Vicryl mesh, bioabsorbable meshes have been shown to have collagen deposition that resembles native connective tissue. When compared to synthetics they have a lower inflammatory response which facilitates greater tissue ingrowth. Thus, in large complex abdominal wall hernias where there is a possibility of clean contaminated or contaminated wounds, we have chosen synthetic

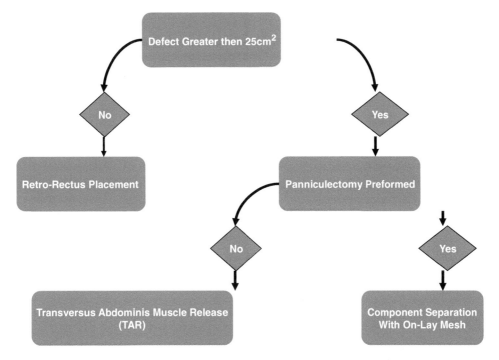

Fig. 8.3 The UCSD algorithm for mesh placement. It is our institutional preference to perform mesh placement in an underlay fashion. We have found that if the defect is less than 25 cm² the mesh can be placed into the retro-rectus space without tension. However, if the defect is larger than 25 cm² a greater facial release will be required. We prefer the Transversus Abdominis Muscle Release (TAR). However, if a panniculectomy is performed simultaneously with the hernia repair and the morbidity of the skin flaps has already been created, then we perform the standard components separation with an onlay mesh

bioabsorbable mesh over biologics. Both, a large multi-center international study along with our data supports this decision, that there is a lower hernia recurrence rate with similar wound complications when compared to biologics at a reduced cost.

References

1. Kingsnorth A, LeBlanc K. Hernias: inguinal and incisional. Lancet. 2003;362:1561.
2. Binnebose M, Von Trotha KT, Jansen PL, Conze J, Neumann UP, Junge K. Biocompatibility of prosthetic meshes in abdominal surgery. Semin Immunopathol. 2011;33:235.
3. Peeters E, Barneveld K, Schreinemacher M, Hertogh G, Ozog Y, Bouvy N, Miserez M. One-year outcome of biological and synthetic bioabsorbable meshes for augmentation of large abdominal wall defects in a rabbit model. J Surg Res. 2013;180(2):274–83.
4. Engelsman AF, Van Der Mei HC, Ploeg RJ, et al. The phenomenon of infection with abdominal wall reconstruction. Biomaterials. 2007;28:2314–24.
5. Badylak SF. The extracellular matrix as a biologic scaffold material. Biomaterials. 2007;28:3587.
6. Cavallaro A, Lo Menzo E, Di Vita M, et al. Use of biological meshes for abdominal wall reconstruction in highly contaminated fields. World J Gastroenterol. 2010;16(15):1928–33.
7. Reynolds D, Davenport DL, Korosec RL, Roth JS. Financial implications of ventral hernia repair: a hospital cost analysis. J Gastrointest Surg. 2013;17(1):159–66.
8. Carbonell AM, Criss CN, Cobb WS, Novisky YW, Rosen MJ. Outcomes of synthetic mesh in contaminated ventral hernia repairs. J Am Coll Surg. 2013;217(6):991–8.
9. Rice RD, Ayubi FS, Shaub ZJ, Parker DM, Armstrong PJ, Tsai JW. Comparison of surgisis, AlloDerm, and Vicryl Woven Mesh grafts for abdominal wall defect repair in an animal model. Aesthetic Plast Surg. 2010;34(3):290–6.
10. Laschke MW, Häufel JM, Scheuer C, Menger MD. Angiogenic and inflammatory host response to surgical meshes of different mesh architecture and polymer composition. J Biomed Mater Res B. 2009;91(2):497–507.
11. Deeken CR, Matthews BD. Characterization of the mechanical strength, resorption properties, and histologic characteristics of a fully absorbable material

(poly-4-hydroxybutyrate—PHASIX mesh) in a porcine model of hernia repair. ISRN Surg. 2013;2013:238–67.

12. Martin DP, Williams SF. Medical applications of poly-4-hydroxybutyrate: a strong flexible absorbable biomaterial. Biochem Eng J. 2003;16(2):97–105.

13. Hjort H, Mathisen T, Alves A, Clermont G, Boutrand JP. Three-year results from a preclinical implantation study of a long-term resorbable surgical mesh with time-dependent mechanical characteristics. Hernia. 2012;16:191.

14. Ruizjasbon F. Norrby six months results of first-in-man trial of a new synthetic long-term resorbable mesh for inguinal hernia repair. Istanbul: European Hernia Society; 2010.

15. Zemlyak AY, Colavita PD, Tsirline VB, Belyansky I, El-Djouzi S, Norton HJ, Lincourt AE, Heniford BT. Absorbable glycolic acid/trimethylene carbonate synthetic mesh demonstrates superior in-growth and collagen deposition. Abdominal Wall Reconstruction Conference, June 13–16, 2012, Washington, DC.

16. Blatnik JA, Krpata DM, Jacobs MR, Novitsky YW, Rosen MJ. Effect of wound contamination on modern absorbable synthetic mesh. Abdominal Wall Reconstruction, June 2011.

17. Suarez JM, Conde SM, Galan VG, Cartes JA, Durantez FD, Ruiz FJ. Antibiotic embedded absorbable prosthesis for prevention of surgical mesh infection: experimental study in rats. Hernia. 2012;19(2):187–94.

Abdominal Wall Spaces for Mesh Placement: Onlay, Sublay, Underlay

Gina L. Adrales

Introduction

Ventral hernia remains a vexing problem for the surgeon and the public alike. Laparotomy is associated with an incisional hernia rate of 3–23% [1, 2]. Despite contemporary efforts to understand and implement best practice techniques in fascial closure, the rate of ventral herniorrhaphy continues to rise. In the United States, where this health problem is compounded by an obesity epidemic, 384,000 ventral hernia repairs were performed in 2006 at a staggering cost of 3.2 billion dollars [3]. Hernia recurrence rates also remain unacceptably high, particularly considering the healthcare and societal costs. Mesh repair has decreased the longterm rate of recurrence from 63% for primary repair to 32% [4], but questions remain as to the optimal positioning of the prosthetic for reduction in hernia recurrence and other complications (Fig. 9.1).

Herein, onlay, sublay, and underlay mesh placement are explored and an algorithm based on the available evidence is proposed. Uniformity in the definition of the positions of mesh is imperative and the European proposed guideline is employed [5]. Inlay (interposition) mesh placement by which the mesh fills the defect and is attached to the fascial edges of the defect is discouraged due to the prohibitive risk of hernia recurrence and is not discussed further [6–8].

Technique

Onlay Mesh Placement

Onlay repair involves placement of the mesh on the anterior rectus fascia below the subcutaneous layer after approximation of the anterior rectus fascia. The advantage of this technique is its ease of application. Depending on the degree of bowel adhesions and the chronicity and thickness of the hernia sac, limited subfascial and intraabdominal dissection may be possible. For small hernias where the fascia is more easily approximated, this is an attractive option. Onlay mesh placement is associated with a shorter operative time compared to sublay positioning [9]. Additionally, the mesh is not directly in contact with the intraabdominal contents limiting the risk for bowel adherence and erosion. In contrast, there is at least a theoretical increased risk for infection from skin flora related to contact of the mesh with the skin during placement or potential for dissemination of infection from a superficial site infection to this anteriorly placed mesh. Because this technique involves subcutaneous dissection to develop the space for mesh placement, it is suspected that the risk for seroma is elevated compared to deeper mesh placement. However,

G.L. Adrales, M.D., M.P.H. (✉)
Division of Minimally Invasive Surgery,
The Johns Hopkins University School of Medicine,
Baltimore, MD, USA
e-mail: gadrale1@jhmi.edu

© Springer International Publishing Switzerland 2016
Y.W. Novitsky (ed.), *Hernia Surgery*, DOI 10.1007/978-3-319-27470-6_9

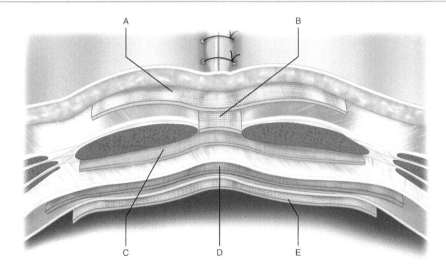

Fig. 9.1 Diagram of ventral hernia and mesh positioning (**a**) Onlay mesh (**b**) Inlay mesh (**c**) Retrorectus sublay mesh (**d**) Underlay preperitoneal (**e**) Underlay intraperitoneal

the clinical significance of sterile seroma formation is questionable.

In onlay repair, the hernia sac is dissected free and reduced. The hernia sac may be left intact though the necessity of inspection of the herniated contents may warrant opening of the sac. The anterior, subcutaneous space is developed through blunt and sharp dissection typically aided by cautery just above the anterior fascia. The anterior fascia is reapproximated in the midline. When this is not possible due to tension on the closure, components separation is employed. The optimal mesh size for this technique relative to the hernia size is not well established. The mesh is affixed widely with transfascial sutures. Self-adhering mesh or fixation with adhesives are alternative options. Drain placement, with careful handling and prompt removal as permitted, is recommended to address the expected seroma in the dissected subcutaneous space.

Sublay Mesh Placement

Sublay repair refers to placement of the prosthetic in the retromuscular space posterior to the rectus abdominis and anterior to the posterior rectus fascia. The retrorectus repair, popularized by Rives and later Stoppa and Wantz, revolutionized hernia repair by offering a robust treatment of complicated incisional hernias with a low recurrence rate [10, 11]. Contemporary series of the Rives-Stoppa repair have reaffirmed the value of the repair with reports of a low hernia recurrence rate of 5% while demonstrating an improved wound infection rate of 4% [12].

The retrorectus repair addresses the attenuation and lateralization of the rectus abdominis muscles and recreates the natural tension of the lateral obliques on the abdominal wall. The retrorectus space is well vascularized offering a favorable environment for tissue incorporation of the mesh. As with the onlay repair, the mesh is not in direct contact with the viscera if the posterior fascial closure is complete; however, the dissection associated with the retrorectus repair is decidedly more challenging than the onlay repair, particularly for recurrent hernias.

In the retrorectus Rives-Stoppa repair (Chapter 12), the midline skin is opened and the hernia sac is exposed and dissected free from the fascial edges as with the onlay repair. The sac may be adherent to overlying thin and sometimes ulcerated skin and may require excision of both. After opening of the sac, the bowel in inspected and adhesiolysis is performed to free the intestinal loops from the abdominal wall. The abdominal wall is inspected for additional fascial defects. After completion of the intraabdominal dissection and irrigation, the posterior rectus fascia is opened at its medial edge on each side sharply with or without cautery and the space between the posterior rectus sheath and the rectus abdominis is developed in this avascular plane primarily with blunt dissection. The dissection is continued laterally to the margin of the rectus muscle where the landmark of the neurovascular bundles marks the extent of the dissection. Of note, below the arcuate line, the dissection is performed in the preperitoneal space of Retzius and of Bogros laterally, and thus the prosthetic mesh will only be separated from the peritoneal cavity by the peritoneum inferior to the arcuate line. The posterior layers are reapproximated in the midline and the mesh is placed in the retrorectus space. The anterior fascia is then reapproximated in the midline. For large defects where midline fascial approximation is not possible, separation of components may be needed either with external oblique release or transversus abdominis muscle release. Drains are placed at the surgeon's discretion. While frequently placed in the subcutaneous space, drain placement in the retrorectus space adjacent to the mesh should be done only after weighing the benefit of tissue apposition versus the risk of infection. An advantage of the retrorectus repair, compared to the onlay approach, is that the subcutaneous dissection is limited, made possible by the suture passing devices for the lateral transfascial mesh fixation sutures.

Underlay Mesh Placement

Underlay mesh placement describes mesh positioning in the preperitoneal subfascial space or the intraperitoneal space deep to the fascia and peritoneum. The intraperitoneal repair may be performed with either an open or laparoscopic approach, the latter associated with a lower infection risk [13, 14]. Compared to suture repair, both laparoscopic and open underlay mesh placement decreased recurrence risk without increasing the risk of serious mesh infection or fistula formation [7]. Underlay repair spares the perforating vessels compared to a wide onlay repair and avoids skin and musculofascial flaps potentially lessening the risk for ischemia and wound complications. In contrast to overlay repair, underlay may be more difficult and lengthy but more straightforward than sublay mesh positioning. Underlay mesh repair for incisional hernias may require extensive dissection and adhesiolysis to allow a clear space for a widely overlapping mesh repair. Additionally, if the overlying fascia cannot be reapproximated, a bridging mesh repair will not restore the midline. For some active patients, the functionality of such a repair is not optimal. Careful selection of the prosthetic mesh is critical to the longterm success of intraperitoneal underlay repair due to the exposure of the intestines to the mesh and potential for adhesions or erosion.

Similar to the other described techniques, underlay mesh placement involves freeing the hernia sac from the fascial edges and adhesiolysis of any adherent bowel or omentum. For preperitoneal underlay repair, the hernia sac is left intact if possible and the preperitoneal space is widely developed to allow adequate overlap of the mesh repair. Because preservation of the peritoneum can be difficult due to its thin nature, this technique is utilized primarily for smaller ventral defects such as umbilical or epigastric hernia repairs. These preperitoneal repairs are typically performed with open technique though laparoscopic repair has been reported [15].

Open intraperitoneal mesh placement is conducted in similar fashion but extensive adhesiolysis may be needed to identify all ventral hernia defects and to clear a wide berth for placement of the prosthetic with wide overlap of the hernia(s). Close abdominal wall inspection is essential for avoidance of the early hernia recurrence which may actually be a missed hernia defect. The intestine must be protected from the synthetic mesh with use of an adhesion-barrier coated polyester or polypropylene mesh or an expanded polytetrafluoroethylene mesh. Alternatively, in cases of contamination, biologic mesh is favored although its longterm durability is limited due to eventual eventration and reherniation, especially in cases of where the overlying fascia cannot be closed. [16] The mesh is secured with transfascial mattress sutures and may be supplemented by absorbable or permanent tacks in between sutures to reduce the risk of bowel slippage anterior to the mesh in between the transabdominal sutures. Another common example of an intraperitoneal underlay mesh use is the Laparoscopic ventral hernia repair [17], described in detail in Chapters 21–22.

Evidence-based Surgery: The Best Position for Mesh Placement in Ventral Hernia Repair

Review of the available evidence does not yield a superior positioning technique for all aspects of ventral hernia repair. Much of the published literature is restricted to single-center retrospective series. However, some themes have emerged from the literature and are highlighted.

Mesh Position, Recurrence, and Seroma

Laparoscopic intraperitoneal repairs and retrorectus sublay repairs have the lowest reported hernia recurrence rates. A 2013 systematic review of 62 articles of ventral hernia repair and mesh positioning and over 5800 patients determined that the rate of hernia recurrence was highest for onlay (17%) or interposition (17%) compared to retrorectus (5%) or underlay mesh implantation (7.5%) [18]. In this systematic review, bridging interposition mesh repair was associated with the highest rate of overall complications, such as seromas. Of note, there were many more underlay repairs ($N=3641$) than retrorectus repairs ($N=743$) in this review. Additionally, the underlay group was heterogeneous in that it included both open and laparoscopic repairs and intraperitoneal and subfascial repairs.

The retrorectus repair may be the safest option in contaminated hernia cases. Rosen et al evaluated the surgical outcomes for biologic mesh repairs in contaminated fields [19]. In this post hoc analysis of a retrospective multicenter trial with short term follow up (1 year), the recurrence risk favored retrorectus repair despite larger defects in the intraperitoneal mesh repairs. A multicenter group also reported a low recurrence rate of 7% in contaminated ventral hernia repairs with macroporous lightweight polypropylene, with over half of the recurrences involving recurrent parastomal hernias [20]. The repairs in this study were heterogeneous but mesh was placed in the retrorectus space in 94% of the patients.

Laparoscopic repair compares favorably with open mesh repair in uncontrolled series. Helgstrand reported that laparoscopic repair decreased the risk of recurrence compared to open (15 versus 21%) [21]. Open repair, hernia defects larger than 7 cm, and open repair with onlay or intraperitoneal mesh were found to be risk factors for poor late outcomes. In another study, 50 unselected laparoscopic repair patients were compared to those with Rives-Stoppa herniorraphy [22]. The laparoscopic group had larger hernia defects, shorter hospital stay, fewer complications (24% versus 30%) and a lower rate of hernia recurrence (2% versus 10%) over a mean follow up of almost 21 months.

In contrast, a Cochrane review highlighted the limited conclusions that can be drawn from available randomized trials due to the short-term follow-up [23]. This review included ten randomized control trials with 880 patients and found that the hernia recurrence rate was the same for laparoscopic and open repair of various mesh positioning but half of the trials had less than two-year follow up. An earlier Cochrane review of eight trials concluded that open repair was superior to suture repair in terms of recurrence but insufficient evidence as to which mesh position or type was best [24]. Another metaanalysis of eight randomized controlled trials comparing laparoscopic and open incisional or ventral hernia repair found no difference in recurrence [14].

Mesh Position and Subsequent Surgery

The positioning of the mesh in ventral herniorraphy holds implications for future surgery. The best operative repair should be performed for the problem at hand without undue influence of the mere possibility of future surgery. However, there are subgroups of patients, such has Crohn's patients who have required prior surgery, for whom the possibility of future intraabdominal surgery and implications of intraperitoneal mesh should enter into the preoperative discussion with the patient while considering the options for repair and prosthetic type. Abdominal surgery after ventral hernia repair is not uncommon. In the United States, the Veterans Affairs National Surgical Quality Improvement Program data demonstrated that 25% of patients required subsequent abdominal surgery after ventral incisional hernia repair, with almost two-thirds of these involving recurrent repair [25]. Underlay or inlay polypropylene mesh repair was associated with increased operative time in subsequent abdominal surgery but without increased risk of inadvertent enterotomy.

In the Netherlands, Halm et al found that intraperitoneal polypropylene mesh repair complicated subsequent laparotomy in 76% compared to 29% with preperitoneal mesh and led to small bowel resection in 26% compared to 4% [26]. This learned group of European hernia experts recommended that intraperitoneal polypropylene mesh should be avoided.

Infection

Laparoscopic repair appears to be favored in terms of surgical site infection. While the systematic review by Albino et al concluded that surgical site infection was lowest for sublay ret-rorectus repair at 4%, the underlay group was heterogeneous including both open and laparoscopic repairs [18]. Another metaanalysis of 15 observational studies found that laparoscopic repair resulted in shorter length of stay, operative time, and a significant reduction in wound abscess and superficial site infection with a trend towards reduced hernia recurrence rate [13]. Systematic reviews of randomized controlled trials comparing laparoscopic and open ventral hernia repairs supported a decreased risk of wound infection in the laparoscopic group with a relative risk of 0.22–0.26 [14, 23].

Summary

The lack of a definitive solution to ventral herniorraphy in terms of the ideal mesh positioning underscores the complexity of this problem. No hernia patient or hernia defect is the same. Additional evidence is needed. Collaborative evaluation of the outcomes of various repairs and prosthetics is imperative. On an individual basis, the types of repairs within a given surgeon's armamentarium should be matched to the goals of the patient tempered by the characteristics of the hernia defect and the co-morbidities of the patient which might affect the surgical outcome. The shortcomings and benefits of the myriad of mesh products, both biologic and permanent synthetic, must be considered. This is an ever-changing environment in which the hernia surgeon must be vigilant and knowledgeable. The author's personal algorithm is outlined in the accompanying table and flowchart (Table 9.1 and Fig. 9.2). While such algorithms are based on available evidence, the decision ultimately is made between the patient and surgeon through thoughtful discussion and examination of the value of hernia repair for that individual patient.

Table 9.1 Author's approach to ventral hernia repair and mesh placement

Concern	Author's preferred approach based on available evidence	Author's reasoning
Contaminated ventral hernia repair	Open retrorectus repair with biologic graft or bioabsorbable synthetic mesh. Bridging or partially bridging repair may be needed depending on hernia defect size	While there are published reports of use of lightweight polypropylene mesh in the setting of contamination, the lower risk of hernia recurrence associated with the permanent prosthetic must be weighed against the risk of chronic infection and need for subsequent procedures particularly with combined colon surgery. If a recurrence occurs (higher risk with a bridging repair), recurrent hernia repair could then be performed laparoscopically or open with presumably less bioburden of infection
Chronically infected mesh with recurrent hernia with wide defect	Open repair and removal of foreign body with retrorectus or underlay biologic or bioabsorbable mesh reinforcement +/- components separation if midline closure or partial fascial closure can be achieved. Otherwise bridging underlay repair reserving definitive treatment after infection is cleared	Addresses chronic infection which is likely the main complaint. Thorough preoperative discussion and education is vital to patient satisfaction especially if staged repair beginning with bridging biologic mesh repair is indicated. Components separation can be performed but if it is apparent that midline closure is not achievable, this should be reserved for later definitive repair
Chronically infected mesh with recurrent small defect	Open repair and removal of foreign body with retrorectus or underlay biologic or bioabsorbable mesh +/- components separation	Addresses chronic infection which is likely the main complaint. Of the open repair options, rectorectus repair appears favorable in terms of infection risk
Obesity	Preoperative risk modification (weight loss) and laparoscopic underlay intraperitoneal mesh repair with primary closure of smaller defects	Lower risk of wound infection compared to open repair and allows for wide overlapping mesh repair
Healthy active patient with ventral hernia and main complaint of laxity	Open retrorectus repair with permanent synthetic mesh	Addresses laxity issue and functionality through reconstruction of the midline with a lower risk of hernia recurrence and skin complications compared to onlay or underlay mesh placement
Ventral incisional hernia without infection with undesired redundant skin and wide scar	Open retrorectus repair with permanent synthetic mesh with or without components separation depending on defect size combined with plastic surgery	Addresses patient priorities of repair of symptomatic hernia and scar revision/panniculectomy with lowest infection risk for open repair
Recurrent ventral hernia after failed open repair	Laparoscopic repair if failed open repair (onlay repair, components separation with/without mesh, or primary repair)	Avoids prior operative field and repair associated with equivalent recurrence risk but lower infection risk. Caution should be exercised with adhesiolysis after prior intraperitoneal mesh
Ventral incisional hernia with expectation of subsequent laparotomy (e.g., Crohn's disease)	Open retrorectus repair with permanent synthetic mesh (lightweight macroporous polypropylene mesh)	Intraperitoneal mesh may complicate future surgery and could become the site of infection with subsequent bowel surgery. Lightweight polypropylene mesh may be salvageable after surgical site infection

Concern	Author's preferred approach based on available evidence	Author's reasoning
Atypically located ventral hernia (high epigastric, suprapubic, lateral or flank)	Laparoscopic repair with bony mesh fixation for suprapubic and lateral or flank hernias	Allows wide mesh overlap even under rib margin and bony/ligamentous fixation
Morbid obesity bariatric surgery candidate with non-obstructed ventral hernia	Bariatric surgery first (laparoscopic sleeve gastrectomy if bowel herniation or extensive adhesions); If hernia does not need to be addressed (e.g., herniated omentum) then the defect is left unrepaired. If the defect is disturbed (contents reduced), it is repaired with underlay bridging biologic mesh deferring definitive repair until after weight loss	Addresses underlying problem and patient prioritized problem of morbid obesity while allowing the most effective hernia repair optimally performed after weight loss

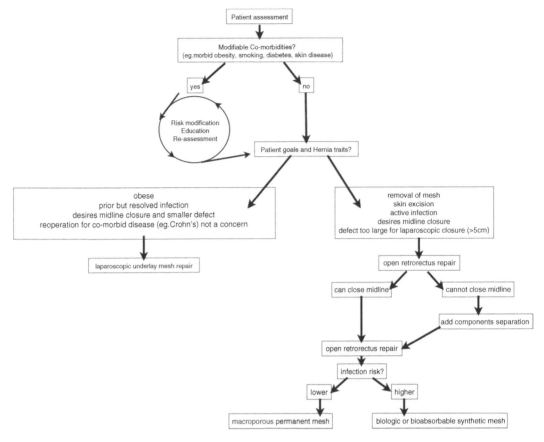

Fig. 9.2 Algorithm for technique/mesh selection

References

1. Burger JWA, Halm JA, Wisjmuller AR, ten Raa S, Jeekel J. Evaluation of new prosthetic meshes for ventral hernia repair. Surg Endosc. 2006;20:1320–5.
2. Cassar K, Munro A. Surgical treatment of incisional hernia. Br J Surg. 2002;89:534–45.
3. Poulose BK, Shelton J, Phillips S, Moore D, Nealon W, Penson D, Beck W, Holzman MD. Epidemiology and cost of ventral hernia repair: making the case for hernia research. Hernia. 2012;16(2):179–83.
4. Burger JW, Luijendijk RW, Hop WC, Halm JA, Verdaasdonk EG, Jeekel J. Long-term follow-up of a randomized controlled trial of suture versus mesh repair of incisional hernia. Ann Surg. 2004;240(4):578–83.
5. Muysoms F, Campanelli G, Champault GG, DeBeaux AC, Dietz UA, Jeekel J, Klinge U, Köckerling F, Mandala V, Montgomery A, Morales Conde S, Puppe F, Simmermacher RK, Śmietański M, Miserez M. EuraHS: the development of an international online platform for registration and outcome mea-

surement of ventral abdominal wall hernia repair. Hernia. 2012;16(3):239–50.
6. Ventral Hernia Working Group, Breuing K, Butler CE, Ferzoco S, Franz M, Hultman CS, Kilbridge JF, Rosen M, Silverman RP, Vargo D. Incisional ventral hernias: review of the literature and recommendations regarding the grading and technique of repair. Surgery. 2010;148(3):544–58.
7. Hawn MT, Snyder CW, Graham LA, Gray SH, Finan KR, Vick CC. Long-term follow-up of technical outcomes for incisional hernia repair. J Am Coll Surg. 2010;210(5):648–55.
8. de Vries Reilingh TS, van Geldere D, Langenhorst B, de Jong D, van der Wilt GJ, van Goor H, Bleichrodt RP. Repair of large midline incisional hernias with polypropylene mesh: comparison of three operative techniques. Hernia. 2004;8(1):56–9.
9. Timmermans L, de Goede B, van Dijk SM, Kleinrensink GJ, Jeekel J, Lange JF. Meta-analysis of sublay versus onlay mesh repair in incisional hernia surgery. Am J Surg. 2014;207(6):980–8.
10. Rives J, Lardennois B, Pire JC, Hibon J. Large incisional hernias. The importance of flail abdomen and

of subsequent respiratory disorders. Chirurgie. 1973;99(8):547–63.

11. Stoppa RE. The treatment of complicated groin and incisional hernias. World J Surg. 1989;13(5):545–54.

12. Iqbal CW, Pham TH, Joseph A, Mai J, Thompson GB, Sarr MG. Long-term outcome of 254 complex incisional hernia repairs using the modified Rives-Stoppa technique. World J Surg. 2007;31(12):2398–404.

13. Salvilla SA, Thusu S, Panesar SS. Analysing the benefits of laparoscopic hernia repair compared to open repair: a meta-analysis of observational studies. J Minim Access Surg. 2012;8(4):111–7.

14. Forbes SS, Eskicioglu C, McLeod RS, Okrainec A. Meta-analysis of randomized controlled trials comparing open and laparoscopic ventral and incisional hernia repair with mesh. Br J Surg. 2009;96(8):851–8.

15. Hilling DE, Koppert LB, Keijzer R, Stassen LP, Oei IH. Laparoscopic correction of umbilical hernias using a transabdominal preperitoneal approach: results of a pilot study. Surg Endosc. 2009;23(8):1740–4.

16. Blatnik J, Jin J, Rosen M. Abdominal hernia repair with bridging acellular dermal matrix—an expensive hernia sac. Am J Surg. 2008;196(1):47–50.

17. Heniford BT, Park A, Ramshaw BJ, Voeller G. Laparoscopic repair of ventral hernias: nine years' experience with 850 consecutive hernias. Ann Surg. 2003;238(3):391–9.

18. Albino FP, Patel KM, Nahabedian MY, Sosin M, Attinger CE, Bhanot P. Does mesh location matter in abdominal wall reconstruction? A systematic review of the literature and a summary of recommendations. Plast Reconstr Surg. 2013;132(5):1295–304.

19. Rosen MJ, Denoto G, Itani KM, Butler C, Vargo D, Smiell J, Rutan R. Evaluation of surgical outcomes of retro-rectus versus intraperitoneal reinforcement with bio-prosthetic mesh in the repair of contaminated ventral hernias. Hernia. 2013;17(1):31–5.

20. Carbonell AM, Criss CN, Cobb WS, Novitsky YW, Rosen MJ. Outcomes of synthetic mesh in contaminated ventral hernia repairs. J Am Coll Surg. 2013;217(6):991–8.

21. Helgstrand F, Rosenberg J, Kehlet H, Jorgensen LN, Bisgaard T. Nationwide prospective study of outcomes after elective incisional hernia repair. J Am Coll Surg. 2013;216(2):217–28.

22. Lomanto D, Iyer SG, Shabbir A, Cheah WK. Laparoscopic versus open ventral hernia mesh repair: a prospective study. Surg Endosc. 2006;20(7):1030–5.

23. Sauerland S, Walgenbach M, Habermalz B, Seiler CM, Miserez M. Laparoscopic versus open surgical techniques for ventral or incisional hernia repair. Cochrane Database Syst Rev. 2011;3, CD007781.

24. den Hartog D, Dur AHM, Tuinebreijer WE, Kreis RW. Open surgical procedures for incisional hernias. Cochrane Database Syst Rev. 2008;3, CD006438.

25. Snyder CW, Graham LA, Gray SH, Vick CC, Hawn MT. Effect of mesh type and position on subsequent abdominal operations after incisional hernia repair. J Am Coll Surg. 2011;212(4):496–502.

26. Halm JA, de Wall LL, Steyerberg EW, Jeekel J, Lange JF. Intraperitoneal polypropylene mesh hernia repair complicates subsequent abdominal surgery. World J Surg. 2007;31(2):423–9.

Parag Bhanot and Ryan Ter Louw

Introduction

Ventral hernias represent an incredibly varied clinical entity with a wide spectrum of disease. It is important for the surgeon to be comfortable with several techniques as specific interventions may prove more or less favorable for a given hernia. Consequently, the reconstructive options for hernia repair are diverse and must be tailored to a given clinical situation. Patient comorbidities, hernia characteristics, and skin/soft tissue factors will each impact the technique chosen for the repair. In addition, intra-operative findings should guide the reconstructive approach to optimize outcomes. It is critical to perform the first hernia repair with the proper approach, technique, and mesh selection to avoid even higher failure rates with subsequent repairs [1]. This chapter will outline the authors' approach and management of the common small fascial defects encountered in umbilical, epigastric, and small incisional hernias.

Patient Selection

Results following AWR are variable. Differences in surgical outcomes are partially attributed to differences in patient demographic. Age, gender, obesity, smoking, and medical comorbidities each independently impact outcomes following ventral hernia repair. (Table 10.1) Age is an independent risk factor for hernia recurrence, 30-day major morbidity, and mortality.

Postoperative morbidity following VHR is increased for each decade after 50 (OR 1.63), preoperative (partial or total) functional dependence (2.34), presence of ascites (9.71), pulmonary compromise (2.47), acute renal failure (11.45), and hyponatremia (3.34). The risk of hernia recurrence increases proportionately with the number of prior failed repairs; patients presenting for an initial hernia repair are much less likely to develop a postoperative complication. The success of surgical repair is inversely related to the number of prior surgical attempts at VHR. Functional status is another critical element to consider as patients who are not functionally independent are significantly more likely to develop complications following hernia repair. Inactive and sedentary patients may not require surgical repair if there is no involvement of bowel

P. Bhanot, M.D., F.A.C.S. (✉)
Department of Surgery, Medstar Georgetown University Hospital, 3800 Reservoir Road, PHC Building, 4th Floor, Washington, DC 20007, USA
e-mail: Parag.Bhanot@medstar.net

R. Ter Louw, M.D.
Department of Plastic Surgery, Medstar Georgetown University Hospital, 3800 Reservoir Road, Washington, DC 20007, USA
e-mail: rpt2@gunet.georgetown.edu

© Springer International Publishing Switzerland 2016
Y.W. Novitsky (ed.), *Hernia Surgery*, DOI 10.1007/978-3-319-27470-6_10

Table 10.1 Demographic variables associated with inferior surgical outcomes (30-day major morbidity, 30-day mortality, and/or hernia recurrence)

Age	Ascites	Coronary artery disease
Functional dependence	Pulmonary compromise	Hypoalbuminemia
Obesity	Acute renal failure	Chronic steroid dependence
Nicotine consumption	Hyponatremia	Immunosupression
COPD	Anemia	Reactive airway disease

within the hernia sac. It is critical to optimize the medical management of patient's comorbid conditions prior to surgery through a multi-disciplinary approach for preoperative risk reduction, select patients for hernia repair with a baseline functional capacity warranting surgery, and determine the safest surgical procedure to ensure a successful repair [2].

Approach (Open or Laparoscopic)

In addition to patient demographics, hernia morphology affects outcomes and should also dictate treatment. It is critical that the surgeon personally review the imaging study, if available, to determine the extent of the structural involvement to formulate the surgical plan. However, the authors do not advocate the routine use of imaging for small noncomplicated hernias. The factors that need to be considered include: (1) defect size (2) number of defects, and (3) location of the defect(s).

In general, repairs can be classified as static or functional (Fig. 10.1). Open repairs that do not re-approximate muscle and fascia and most laparoscopic repairs are considered static repairs because they do not restore the inherit anatomy of the abdominal wall. Small defects may be amenable to closure with a laparoscopic approach as well and possibly offer additional advantage over traditional repair.

The following represents the authors' algorithm based on personal clinical experience and a review of the literature. A primary, single defect <3 cm in a non-obese patient may be repaired with suture repair alone (Fig. 10.2). This situation represents a compromise between a slightly

higher recurrence rate and the avoidance of mesh related complications. It is critical to assess the quality of the fascia if mesh is excluded from the repair. The approximation of poor quality tissue, regardless of the fascia defect size, will lead to an unacceptable recurrence rate. In addition, a rectus diastasis should be addressed as well [3].

All other patients, in the optimal setting, should have a mesh reinforcement of the repair. The decision to proceed with a laparoscopic versus open approach is dependent not only on the size of the defect, but also on the quality of the skin and soft tissue coverage (Fig. 10.3).

Adequate Skin/Soft Tissue Coverage

In these patients, the decision to proceed with a laparoscopic or open approach is dependent on the size of the defect. Recurrent hernias, single defects between 3–10 cm, several midline defects ("swiss-cheese type"), or primary defects less than 3 cm in a morbidly obese individual are ideal for a laparoscopic approach with synthetic mesh (Fig. 10.4). The presence of a significant rectus diastasis may prompt an open approach.

Inadequate Skin/Soft Tissue Coverage

Regardless of the size of the defect, if there is a potential for exposure of the synthetic mesh or the repair is performed in the setting of contamination, we would favor the open approach with the use of a biological mesh. There is currently no data to support the use of a biological product via a laparoscopic approach.

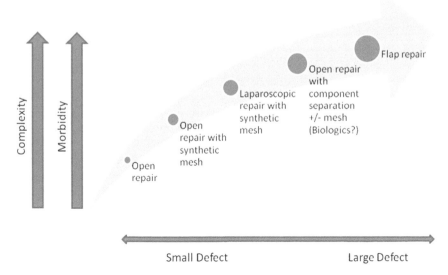

Fig. 10.1 There are a myriad of techniques available for AWR. Small defects are amenable to both an open and laparoscopic approach. Larger defects may require a more complex operation for adequate repair. With increasing complexity of technique, the surgeon should expect a higher morbidity rate

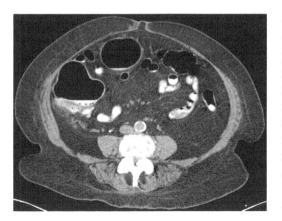

Fig. 10.2 CT scan image of small fascial defect (<3 cm)

Location of Mesh Placement

After selecting the ideal mesh product to reinforce a given VHR, the material may be placed in a number of different locations within the abdominal wall for reinforcement [4]. Mesh may be sutured superficial to the primarily closed fascia (onlay), directly to the fascial edges as a bridged repair (interposition), posterior to the rectus abdominis muscle (sublay), or deep to the peritoneum (underlay). Each of these has distinct advantages given a particular clinical situation. In general, underlay or retrorectus mesh placement results in the lowest complication rates including less infection, seroma, and hernia recurrence as compared to onlay or interposition mesh placement. Within the context of biologic mesh, interposition mesh placement when primary fascial approximation is not feasible will result in the highest rate of hernia recurrence, approaching 100%.

Specific Hernias

Umbilical Hernias

Hernias involving the umbilicus can be congenital or occur spontaneously. Many congenital umbilical hernias will spontaneously close by 2–3 years of age. The repair of the pediatric hernia is not the focus of the following discussion. In adults, multiparity, obesity, ascites, as well as any other pathology that elevates intra-abdominal pressure, increase the risk of a fascial defect. Though umbilical hernias are common, the differential diagnosis should include soft tissue tumors and urachal cysts. The contents of an

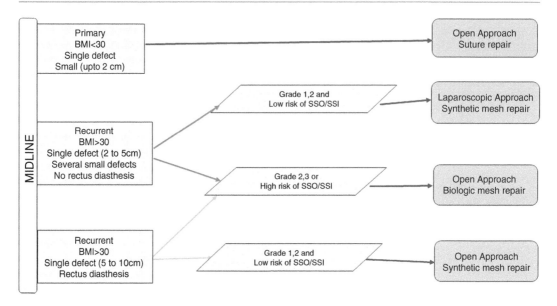

Fig. 10.3 Algorithm for AWR for small to moderate size defects

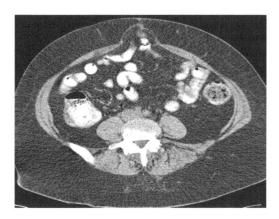

Fig. 10.4 CT scan image of moderate fascial defect (3–8 cm)

umbilical hernia may include pre-peritoneal fat, mesenteric fat, and/or bowel.

As discussed, the size of the defect, comorbidities, and the skin factors should be considered in the choice of surgical technique. With our established algorithm, most of the umbilical hernias repaired in our practice in the non-obese population are a primary suture repair without mesh reinforcement. This does represent a compromise between recurrence rates and mesh related complications. A randomized study by Arroyo et al. showed that umbilical hernia repair with prosthetic mesh had a recurrence rate of 1%

at 64 months compared to 11% with direct suture repair alone. Complications in both groups were similar [5].

Given the same small defect size in an obese individual, mesh reinforcement is necessary. The protocol for synthetic versus biological mesh has been previously discussed. In the setting of appropriate skin coverage, a laparoscopic approach is recommended with synthetic mesh [6]. Typically, these cases are short and can be performed as a same day operation. With less than ideal skin coverage, absent or attenuated skin, a laparoscopic approach is not recommended. An open repair with reduced-weight polypropylene mesh or biological mesh is appropriate.

Epigastric Hernias

Epigastric hernias are another common fascial defect encountered by general surgeons and may be present in up to 2% of the population. They mostly occur spontaneously as a function of the anatomy of the linea alba which becomes thinner and wider cephalad from the umbilicus. These hernias have a male prevalence and can have multiple defects in upto 20% of patients. Given the small defect size which often has a small piece of incarcerated preperitoneal fat, the level of discomfort can be more than expected. The diagnosis is usually made with the clinical exam confirming a palpable bulge. Imaging is not necessary, but can be obtained if the exam is equivocal.

The algorithm for repair has been described in the preceding section [7]. As with umbilical hernias, the authors recommend repair of any associated rectus diastasis to minimize recurrence or development of metachronous defects.

Incisional Hernias

Incisional hernias develop in up to 20% of patients. The associated pathology is quite variable and thus so is the technique utilized for repair. A recent Cochrane database review of open surgical techniques for incisional hernias has shown that even in small defects, the use of suture repair was associated with less surgical site infection and seroma but an increased rate of recurrence [8]. Therefore, mesh reinforcement is advocated for in all incisional hernias, regardless of defect size [9].

There are multiple randomized controlled trials evaluating laparoscopic versus open repair of abdominal wall hernias. The laparoscopic approach provides for lower overall complication rates, decreased wound complications, decreased length of stay, and decreased recurrence rates.

However, there is a higher rate of bowel injury with inexperienced surgeons [10].

Technique for Open Repair With/ Without Mesh Reinforcement

1. An incision is made over the fascial defect to provide proper exposure in either a vertical or horizon fashion. For umbilical hernias, the umbilical stalk is dissected free from the hernia sac. It is important not to button-hole the skin.
2. The hernia sac/contents are dissected away from the edges of the fascia. Without the involvement of omentum or bowel, violation of the peritoneal cavity should be avoided. Especially important are individuals with the presence of ascites.
3.
   (a) The fascial edges are clearly delineated. With a less than 2 cm defect, a primary repair is carried out using absorbable suture such as 0-PDS figure of eight sutures transversely. We typically place our corner sutures beyond the defect (Fig. 10.5a, b).
   (b) With a defect larger than 2 cm and/or accounting for patient risk factors, mesh can be utilized. The authors recommend underlay mesh (intraperitoneal or sublay) rather than an onlay technique. The size of the mesh should allow for at least 3–4 cm support circumferential.

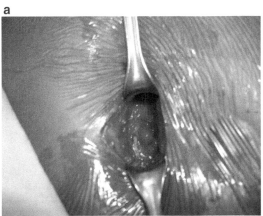 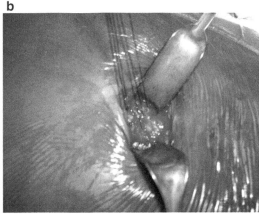

Fig. 10.5 (a) The small defect size is clearly delineated after the fascial edge is cleared circumferentially. (b) A primary suture repair is performed in a transverse fashion with figure-of-8 PDS sutures starting beyond the actual defect

The mesh is secured with at least 0-PDS sutures transfascial. The fascia is then re-approximated over the mesh. (Fig. 10.6a–c).

4. Closure of the incision. For umbilical hernias, the umbilicus is tacked back down to the linea alba with absorbable suture.

Technique for Laparoscopic Repair with Mesh Reinforcement

1. The authors prefer to gain access to the peritoneal cavity via a Veress needle at the anterior axillary line, but is based on surgical history.

2. Trocar placement is based upon surgical history. 3 (5 mm) and 1 (12 mm) trocars are required. It is important to place the trocars at ample distance from the actual defect to allow appropriate overlap with the mesh.

3. A lysis of adhesions is usually not required in the absence of previous surgery. However, we prefer to take down the falciform ligament from the posterior sheath with ultrasonic shears to allow adequate penetration by tacking device (Fig. 10.7a–f).

4. The hernia contents should be fully reduced. If possible, the hernia sac can be excised.

5. The fascial defect is measured by a standard technique previously described using a spinal needle. It is up to the surgeon's preference whether to close the small defect or not.

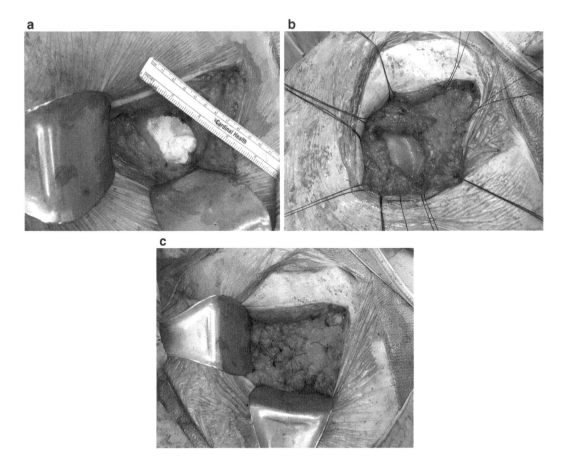

Fig. 10.6 (a) A 5 cm fascial defect is exposed at site of prior incision. (b) Mesh reinforcement is utilized given the defect size and association with prior incision. Location is intraperitoneal. The mesh is parachuted in after placement of #1-PDS sutures transfascial. (c) After securing the mesh, the fascia is then re-approximated with additional #1-PDS sutures, providing autologous tissue coverage

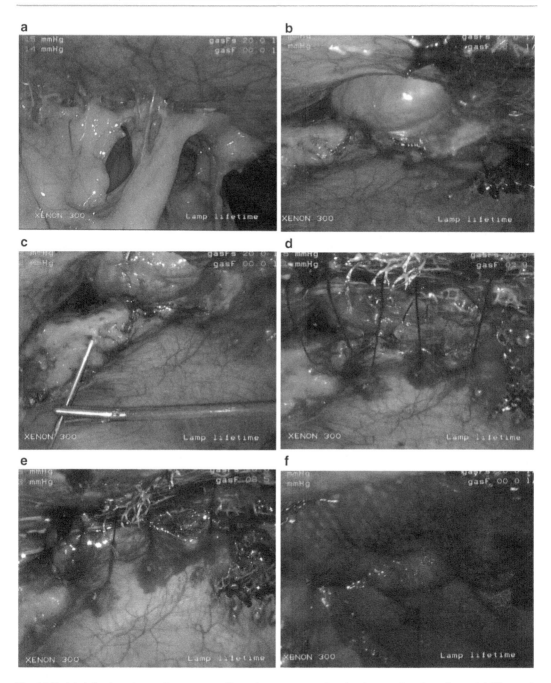

Fig. 10.7 (**a**) Adhesions from prior surgery will need to be addressed to expose the small fascial defect. (**b**) A single small fascial defect is visualized measuring 5×5cm. (**c**) Given the small defect size and compliance of the abdominal wall, closure of the defect is performed prior to mesh placement. A suture passer device is utilized to place several figure-of-8 sutures. (**d**) Depicted are the sutures placed prior to tying them down. (**e**) The small defect has been re-approximated without exceeding physiological tension. (**f**) The mesh is then placed in a standard laparoscopic fashion. With the small defect re-approximated, less mesh material is needed to provide the proper overlap

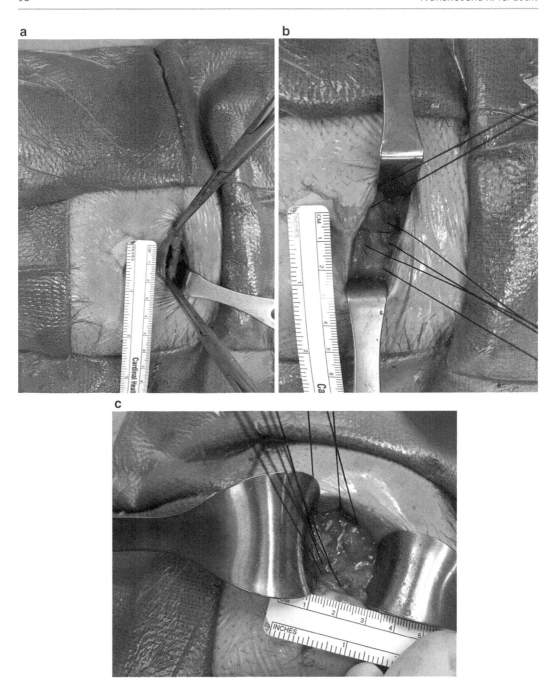

Fig. 10.8 (**a**) A 2 cm fascial defect is isolated after reduction of omentum. The fascia is attenuated with a 3 cm wide thin linea alba. (**b**) The defect is closed in a transverse fashion with figure-of-8 0-PDS sutures. Mesh is not utilized given the defect size. (**c**) An additional suture line is placed in a vertical fashion to plicate the rectus muscles over the first suture line to provide additional support

6. The mesh is selected and measured to allow for at least 5 cm overlap.
7. The mesh is fixated with both transfascial sutures as well as circumferential tacks. The authors prefer an absorbable tacker given the intraperitoneal location of the mesh.

Technique for Repair of Rectus Diastasis

1. The incision is a vertical midline incision to provide proper exposure from the xiphoid process infra-umbilical. The small fascial defect is repaired as described above with or without mesh reinforcement (Fig. 10.8a–c).
2. The extent of the diastasis is delineated to allow for maximal plication.
3. Either a single or double row of sutures can be utilized depending upon surgeon preference. The authors prefer either a single row of figure-of-8 #1-PDS sutures or a double row consisting of figure-of-8 0-PDS sutures followed by running #1-PDS. Additional onlay mesh reinforcement is not necessary.

Summary

Reconstructive options for AWR are vast and should start with optimizing patient selection. It is important to note that not all patients require repair and the decision to offer surgery should be based on reasonable expectations. The surgeon should have within his/her armamentarium a myriad of options to perform the optimal surgery. An algorithm should be incorporated into clinical practice based on high level data that will allow the surgeon to define which approach, technique, and mesh reinforcement should be utilized for each individual patient. The ultimate goals of ventral hernia repair are (1) prevent complications from the hernia, (2) restore functional abdominal wall, (3) improve cosmesis, and (4) minimize future complications including recurrence.

References

1. Flum DR, Horvath K, Koepsell T. Have outcomes of incisional hernia repair improved with time? A population-based analysis. Ann Surg. 2003;237:129–35.
2. Breuing K, Butler CE, Ferzoco S, et al. Incisional ventral hernias: review of the literature and recommendations regarding the grading and technique of repair. Surgery. 2010;148(3):544–58.
3. Köhler G, Luketina RR, Emmanuel K. Sutured repair of primary small umbilicaland epigastric hernias: concomitant rectus diastasis is a significant risk factor for recurrence. World J Surg. 2015;39(1):121–6.
4. Albino FP, Patel KM, Nahabedian MY, et al. Does mesh location matter in abdominal wall reconstruction? A systematic review of the literature and a summary of recommendations. Plast Reconstr Surg. 2013;132(5):1295–304.
5. Arroyo A, García P, Pérez F, et al. Randomized clinical trial comparing suture and mesh repair of umbilical hernia in adults. Br J Surg. 2001;88(10):1321–3.
6. Sauerland S, Walgenbach M, Habermalz B, et al. Laparoscopic versus open surgical techniques for ventral or incisional hernia repair. Cochrane Database Syst Rev. 2011; 3.
7. Christoffersen MW, Helgstrand F, Rosenberg J, et al. Lower reoperation rate for recurrence after mesh versus sutured elective repair in small umbilical and epigastric hernias. A nationwide register study. World J Surg. 2013;37(11):2548–52.
8. den Hartog D, Dur AH, Tuinebreijer WE, et al. Open surgical procedures for incisional hernias. Cochrane Database Syst Rev. 2008;3.
9. Nguyen MT, Berger RL, Hicks SC, et al. Comparison of outcomes of synthetic mesh vs suture repair of elective primary ventral herniorrhaphy: a systematic review and meta-analysis. JAMA Surg. 2014;149(5):415–21.
10. Pierce RA, Spitler JA, Frisella MM, et al. Pooled data analysis of laparoscopic vs. open ventral hernia repair: 14 years of patient data accrual. Surg Endosc. 2007;21(3):378–86.

Onlay Ventral Hernia Repair

11

Nathaniel Stoikes, David Webb, and Guy Voeller

11.1 Introduction

There are many ways to approach the repair of a ventral or incisional hernia (VIH). Varying techniques are based on where the mesh is placed in relation to the abdominal wall. Furthermore, there is a relationship between the repairs and their histories. Options include intraperitoneal placement of mesh, retrorectus or retromuscular placement (Rives 1973) and premuscular or onlay mesh placement (Chevrel 1979). The two major techniques described by Rives and Chevrel occurred in the 1970s and essentially run parallel to each other. In their time, both techniques maintained popularity and had similar outcomes. However, during the past 20 years retromuscular mesh placement as described by Rives has become the standard of care for ventral hernias while Chevrel's onlay technique was forgotten. The lack of popularity of the onlay repair in the USA has a historical basis. The Rives retrorectus repair was brought to the United

Electronic supplementary material: The online version of this chapter (doi:10.1007/978-3-319-27470-6_11) contains supplementary material, which is available to authorized users.

N. Stoikes, M.D. (✉) • G. Voeller, M.D.
Department of Surgery, University of Tennessee Health Science Center, Germantown, TN, USA
e-mail: nstoikes@uthsc.edu

D. Webb, M.D.
Baptist Memphis and Methodist Germantown, Memphis, TN, USA

States in the 1980s by George Wantz, who was a hernia surgeon from New York. Dr Wantz travelled to France to learn many of their hernia repair methods. One of our mentors, Eugene Mangiante, brought Dr. Wantz to our institution in the early 1980s and taught the senior author the Rives' sublay repair. This repair became our repair of choice and is taught to our residents to this day. As we developed our laparoscopic repair we realized that suture fixation would be critical to long term success and we used pictures in the hernia atlas produced by Dr. Wantz of the Rives repair to show how the two repairs were similar. The main difference is that the mesh is behind the rectus muscles in the Rives repair and intraperitoneal in the laparoscopic. The first laparoscopic ventral hernia repair course ever taught was in Memphis, TN in the mid 1990s; at this course and many others that followed, American surgeons were introduced to the open Rives repair as the basis for laparoscopic ventral hernia repair. At this time, most V/I hernia repairs in the USA were done as an inlay with the mesh being sewed to the edges of the hernia defect. As more surgeons learned the laparoscopic repair and were exposed to the Rives open repair, the Rives repair became the standard for most herniologists in the USA. In the process, Chevrel's onlay technique, which was not known in the USA had been more or less forgotten except by its practitioners in France. In 2003 we began using fibrin glue for mesh fixation for our TEP inguinal hernia repairs and this stimulated our interest in Chevrel's onlay method for V/I hernia repair.

11.2 Chevrel's Logic

In the classic Chevrel repair, the primary goal is to recreate the linea alba. Chevrel based this on biomechanical studies which he and Rath conducted to identify the strongest and weakest portions of the abdominal wall. In these studies, they evaluated the abdominal wall above and below the arcuate line of Douglas as well as the anterior and posterior sheaths. When looking at breaking strain and deformability, the anterior sheaths and posterior sheaths were similar above and below the arcuate line. However, differences were found in bursting strength. The strongest area was the supraarcuate anterior sheath, which was significantly stronger than the infraarcuate anterior sheath. The supraarcuate posterior sheath was stronger than the infraarcuate posterior sheath but was not statistically significant. In all, the supraarcuate anterior sheath was stronger than the posterior sheath at all levels [1].

Chevrel also studied the linea alba and found that the infraumbilical linea alba was stronger (linear traction) than the supraumbilical linea alba. He then compared this to the rectus sheath and found the anterior rectus sheath to have the most comparable values. The results of the posterior sheath values are the most compelling in that the posterior sheath is weaker on all levels than the linea alba but especially the infraumbilical posterior sheath ($P < 0.01$) [2].

These studies form Chevrel's logic for a premuscular prosthesis. First, the anterior rectus sheath is the strongest and best tissue to use for recreation of the linea alba. Second, a premuscular prosthesis placement is favorable to the retrorectus location due to the weakness of the posterior sheath. In reference to retrorectus prosthesis placement, Chevrel stated "The posterior sheath then becomes the layer which separates the prosthesis from the peritoneum and the viscera, and the first to sustain the action of the intraabdominal pressure." He goes on to conclude: "this layer is thus weaker than the underlying prosthesis and will give way under an increase in intraabdominal pressure, risking exposing the viscera to the prosthesis." Chevrel also felt infections were easier to treat in a premuscular than a retromuscular prosthesis and the retromuscular mesh may have to be removed while that is rarely necessary when the mesh is premuscular [3]. In our clinical experience with onlay ventral hernia repair, we have found the management of wound infections to be straight forward with salvage of mesh in all cases.

11.3 Chevrel's Technique

As previously stated, the goal of Chevrel's technique is to reconstruct the linea alba. After making skin flaps, this is accomplished by creating a four layer reconstruction that includes three tissue layers and a premuscular prosthesis. The three tissue layers are accomplished by first closing the midline fascia. Chevrel used Gibson or Clotteau-Premont type relaxing incisions if required to get the midline closed. Vertical incisions are then made along the rectus muscles bilaterally 2 cm from their medial borders and these flaps are folded over each other and sutured. The lateral edges of each flap of rectus sheath are rolled toward the midline and sutured with two rows of interrupted "u" stitches. These flaps create the second and third tissue layers. The prosthesis in the onlay position is the fourth layer (Fig. 11.1). The periphery of the mesh is fixated with running absorbable suture and the middle portion of the mesh is molded to the midline closure by spraying 2 mL of fibrin glue. Chevrel did this to fix the mesh to the midline closure which took tension off of the midline closure immediately until granulation tissue served that function. Two to four closed suction drains are then placed and the skin is closed in two layers. Chevrel left his drains until there was no drainage for 48 hours and he maintained an abdominal truss day and night for 2 months. He felt it took this long for adequate granulation tissue to grow through the mesh [3].

11.4 Clinical Data

Looking at Chevrel's original series, it is important to note that he compiled other techniques with the technique just described and treated 426 incisional hernias from 1979 to 1998. He used

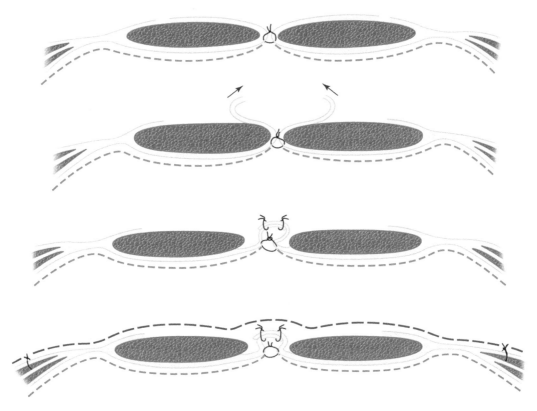

Fig. 11.1 Chevrel's technique for recreation of the linea alba

the fibrin glue technique in 143 repairs and they followed up 93% of them for between 1 and 20 years. His recurrence rate was 4.9% and no prosthesis was lost to mesh infection. He also found that seroma formation was greater when larger amounts of fibrin glue were used [3].

Kingsnorth in 2007 published a series of ventral hernia repairs using mesh onlay, components separation, and suture and fibrin glue. The technique included midline closure and selective use of Ramirez type component separation. The mesh was fixated with running sutures on the periphery of the mesh. With regard to fibrin glue use, it was directed for treatment of the skin flaps instead of mesh fixation. The study population included 116 patients with a median follow up of 15.2 months. Seroma rate was 9.5% and skin infection rate was 8.6%. There were no mesh infections. The recurrence rate was 3.4% over the follow up period [4].

Stoikes et al. published their initial series of 50 patients of an onlay technique using fibrin glue alone for mesh fixation. Our technique differs from the classic Chevrel in that it utilizes an onlay of the mesh prosthesis, however, it is positioned initially with skin staples and then fixated to the entire anterior fascia with fibrin glue alone. The senior author noticed when he first did this that there was immediate strong fixation of the mesh over the entire abdominal wall and stress was immediately taken off of the midline suture closure. The technique includes tension free primary closure of the midline with selective use of myofascial advancement flaps when required. Mean follow up was 19.5 months with no known recurrences identified. The seroma rate was 16% and skin infection rate was 6%. There were no mesh infections [5]. An update to the data is in process and now numbers over 100 patients. New data includes use of the technique in clean-contaminated and contaminated scenarios with no associated infectious complications or reoperations. Overall skin infection rate is 4 with

100% salvage of mesh in all situations with infection. BMI is the only risk factor linked to infection and reoperation.

11.5 Logic and Technique for Onlay Ventral Hernia Repair with Fibrin Glue Fixation

The key to a successful onlay ventral hernia repair is a tension free primary midline closure. Accomplishing this requires the use of advancement flaps in the form of external oblique releases and posterior rectus fascia releases in a selective manner as described by Ramirez. Independently, the mesh should be viewed as a buttress that integrates into the abdominal wall for long-term strength and recurrence prevention. The addition of fibrin glue to fixate the mesh is what provides immediate fixation to all surfaces thereby allowing immediate load sharing and reduced tension on the midline in the short-term.

Understanding the principles, one should select patients with defect sizes where the surgeon believes that the midline can be recreated with acceptable tension on the primary midline closure. This means that good quality fascia can be brought together or overlapped with acceptable tension. In our practice, this generally applies to patients with defect widths of 15 cm or less. Other applications for onlay include off-midline hernias such as flank hernias or paramedian defects where there may be insufficient space for appropriate sublay of mesh or fixation of mesh.

11.5.1 Technique Description

After a reduction of the hernia and lysis of adhesions, the hernia defect is delineated and skin flaps are made generally out past the semilunar line. Since the onlay technique requires creation of skin and subcutaneous flaps, it should not be done in patients who have had the collateral circulation to the skin compromised, i.e., those that have had aortic surgery where the lumbar collaterals have been sacrificed. In addition, we do not

operate on smokers unless they stop for 2 months and this is especially true for the onlay method where the skin flaps will be compromised. We also try to avoid operating on the morbidly obese hernia patient until they lose weight since these flaps can be compromised. Generally speaking, we would like patient BMI to be optimized to 35 or less, but in some cases that is not possible given the characteristics of the hernia or symptoms. Regardless, we exhaust all avenues for weight loss including diet, exercise, and bariatric referral coupled with office follow up for weight monitoring. Unfortunately, there are cases where patients are noncompliant in which case they only receive a hernia repair in the emergency setting. At each step of medialization of the fascial edges, the defect edges should be assessed for tension as they are brought together. While tension free midline advancement is important, any component release principally weakens the native abdominal wall in another region, so it should not be done dogmatically. Ramirez described a stepwise approach for myofascial advancement beginning with skin flap creation. If this is not enough, then the posterior rectus fascia is incised on one side, making sure to release each inscription (one sees a "pop" of the fascia when these are cut). If necessary the other rectus fascia is released and then if required the external releases are done one at a time. Generally this will address elliptical defects up to 15 cm wide. A running or interrupted primary closure of #1 nonabsorble suture is then used to close the midline (Fig. 11.2).

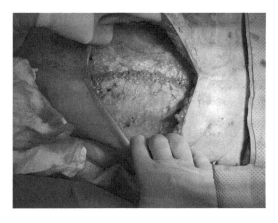

Fig. 11.2 Closure of the midline after myofascial advancement

A macroporous, light weight (or microporous, heavier mesh if necessary) polypropylene mesh is then placed in the onlay position such that it covers the entire area of exposed fascia and any external releases. Overlap of the midline closure should be a minimum of 8 cm. A simple skin stapler is used as a placeholder for proper positioning of the mesh. Fibrin glue is then applied first to the midline. The glue typically has a dual nozzle with an attachable common spout. We prefer to allow the glue to be applied through the dual nozzle and use our hands to mix and massage the glue components into the mesh and abdominal wall. In this way, the mesh is first molded to the midline closure as Chevrel originally described. The remaining mesh is then completely covered with the fibrin glue to fixate all aspects

(Fig. 11.3a–d). Staples are used at the periphery as well as the central area of the mesh. If external oblique releases have been done we use a running absorbable suture to sew the mesh to the lateral edge of the release on each side (Fig. 11.4). Two to four large bore drains are placed in the subcutaneous space and secured with nylon sutures. The skin and remaining hernia sack is then debrided and subsequently closed in two layers. Absorbable 3-0 sutures are used to close the dermal layer and then a running absorbable 4-0 suture is used to close the skin or a combination of nylon sutures and skin staples. We use a BioPatch (Ethicon, Cincinnati, OH) around each drain with a Tegaderm (3M, St. Paul, MN) and change these weekly. Patients are sent home on minocycline as long as the drains are in place.

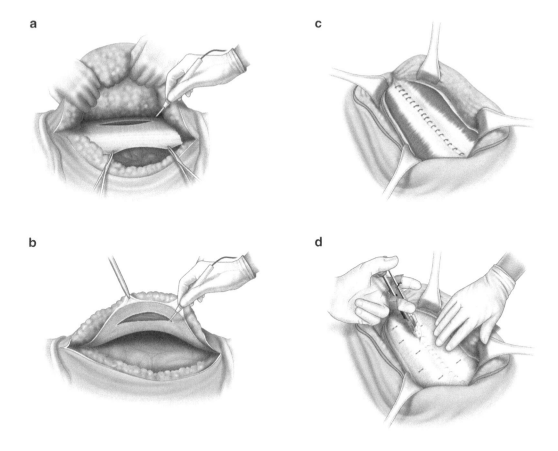

Fig. 11.3 (**a**)–(**d**) Onlay ventral hernia repair with fibrin glue fixation of mesh

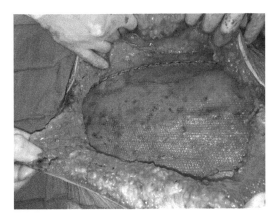

Fig. 11.4 Onlay mesh placement fixated with skin staples, fibrin glue, and running absorbable suture along the external oblique release

Post-operatively the patients are kept NPO until bowel function resumes and the patient wears an abdominal binder at all times. We have no strict numbers as to when drains are removed. Since seromas are more common with skin flap creation we leave drains in until almost nothing is coming out from the drains. This will help limit seroma formation. As a general rule, drains should be kept in for 10–14 days at minimum.

11.6 Discussion

When thinking about mesh fixation in ventral hernias, one must keep in mind that risks factors and inherent genetics contribute to hernia formation. Whether a sublay or onlay is used, mesh has to be anchored and typically by mechanical fixation. The problem with mechanical fixation is that one relies on inherent tissue strength to support the mechanical anchoring that is being done, which in a way perpetuates the problem of recurrence in a patient who is already prone to hernia formation. This line of thought led our group to the use of adhesives, which has been shown by multiple investigators to be an excellent fixation method for inguinal hernia repairs.

To better understand adhesive fixation, Stoikes et al. compared fibrin glue fixation of mesh to suture fixation with an onlay model in Mongrel pigs. At 24 hours, 7 days, and 14 days, the two groups were evaluated with biomechanical shear testing and histology. Biomechanically, shear strengths were stronger at 24 hours for the sutured group but by 7 days the groups were equal. Specifically, by 7 days the lightweight macroporous mesh was so integrated into the abdominal wall that the mesh/fascia interface was found to be stronger than the mesh or fascia itself. Coupled with similar histologies and no mesh migrations with glue, it was concluded that fibrin glue fixation has excellent fixation properties. Another interesting point studied was that the contraction rate of mesh was less with the glue group, though it did not reach statistical significance. It was speculated that this was due to the advantage of having all surfaces of the mesh fixated as opposed to point fixation with sutures, which allows for mesh to ripple and fold as it scars into the abdominal wall [6].

Understanding the principles and application of adhesives for mesh fixation allows for a different perspective on ventral hernia repair: *suture fixation is a function of suture strength and tissue strength; whereas adhesive fixation is a function of surface area alone*. One can see how adhesive use coupled with a broad premuscular prosthesis could have distinct advantages for ventral hernia repair. We have been impressed at the immediate strength one sees of the repair when the mesh is fixated with fibrin glue. We have had cases where the muscle relaxant has worn off intraoperatively after the mesh has been glued, the patient "bucks" on the endotracheal tube and generates tremendous intraabdominal pressure. The mesh will not budge and the suture closure of the midline shows no stress. There is no need to wait for tissue ingrowth for stress to be removed from the midline suture closure and this is the key in our method of onlay repair.

Future directions of the adhesive advantage could include prevention of mesh contraction as it relates to chronic pain. An article recently published by Bendavid et al. discussed mesh contraction and fixation as a cause of chronic pain in inguinal hernia repairs. While the article focuses on inguinal hernia, the discoveries about mesh and how it potentially causes chronic pain, directly translates to ventral hernia as well.

Bendavid concluded that part of the problem was deformation and contraction of mesh, which created pockets and warped surface areas for potential nerve impingement or ingrowth [7]. Such findings are consistent with point fixation of mesh. Because adhesive fixation results in complete fixation of all portions of the mesh, contraction and deformation may be preventable and needs further evaluation.

Clinically, we have observed anecdotal evidence that patients have significantly less postoperative pain and less narcotic requirement compared with intraperitoneal or retrorectus repairs. Intuitively, it makes sense for several reasons including that there is no muscle and fascia penetration by sutures that strangulate tissues and entrap nerves. In addition, complete fixation creates a better load sharing environment compared to point fixation which may cause a patient to experience pulling and tugging at the various fixated locations.

Another advantage of onlay ventral hernia repair is that mesh is not located intraabdominally or separated from the viscera by the weakest layer of the abdominal wall where viscera and mesh can come into contact with one another as in the Rives repair. Reoperations for other pathologies are less technically demanding and also the risks of mesh complications are less. Most importantly, in situations of post-operative infection or intraoperative contamination we have had a 100% salvage rate of the mesh and clearance of infection. The combination of the onlay location of mesh and selection of a macroporous configuration allows for quick integration of the mesh with vacuum wound systems.

References

1. Rath A, Zhang J, Chevrel J. The sheath of the rectus abdominis muscle: an anatomical and biomechanical study. Hernia. 1997;1:139–42.
2. Rath A, Attali P, Dumas J, et al. The abdominal linea alba: an anatomo-radiologic and biomechanical study. Surg Radiol Anat. 1996;18:281–8.
3. Chevrel J, Rath A. The use of fibrin glues in the surgical treatment of incisional hernias. Hernia. 1997;1:9–14.
4. Kingsnorth A, Shahid M, Valliattu A, et al. Open onlay mesh repair for major abdominal wall hernias with selective use of components separation and fibrin sealant. World J Surg. 2008;32:26–30.
5. Stoikes N, Webb D, Voeller G, et al. Preliminary report of a sutureless onlay technique for incisional hernia repair using fibrin glue alone for mesh fixation. Am Surg. 2013;79:1177–80.
6. Stoikes N, Sharpe J, Voeller G, et al. Biomechanical evaluation of fixation properties of fibrin glue for ventral incisional hernia repair. Hernia. 2015;19(1):161–6.
7. Bendavid R, Lou W, Koch A, et al. Mesh related SIN syndrome. A surreptitious irreversible neuralgia and its morphologic background in the etiology of post-herniorraphy pain. Int J Clin Med. 2014;5:799–810.

Alfredo M. Carbonell II

Introduction

When Jean Rives and Rene Stoppa independently embarked on the development of the retromuscular and preperitoneal repair of incisional hernias, neither could have predicted the impact their eponymous operations would have on future generations of hernia surgeons. This sublay mesh technique is increasingly becoming the world's standard approach to the complex repair of ventral hernias, due to its durability and long term outcomes in addition to the fact that mesh is excluded from the visceral contents and thus does not pose a problem for future abdominal surgery.

History

In 1965, Rene Stoppa, a native of French Algiers, began to develop the preperitoneal space to place a large 16×24 cm sheet of polyester mesh for the repair of complex and multiply recurrent bilateral inguinal hernias. He called this operation the Giant Preperitoneal Prosthesis Repair (GPPR) [1]. The thought was that the intraabdominal pressure, acting through Pascal's principles of hydrostatics, would instantly splint the prosthesis between the peritoneum and the abdominal wall. The mesh would then become incorporated into the surrounding tissue. The basis of his technique; the same stresses which act to form hernias are now harnessed to protect against recurrences.

Jean Rives, another French Algierian, and a friend of Rene Stoppa is credited with having introduced polyester mesh to France. In 1966, he revolutionized the technique of repairing incisional hernias by placing the mesh directly behind the rectus muscle with the posterior rectus sheath dorsal to the mesh in an effort to protect the mesh from visceral exposure. Below the arcuate line, the transversalis fascia and peritoneum formed the protective layer over the visceral sac below [2]. This retromuscular, prefascial repair quickly became the preferred approach, and minor modifications were made by Stoppa [3] who began to utilize this natural extension of his GPPR technique, more cranial, to repair incisional hernias.

George Wantz, who practiced at New York Hospital as Clinical Professor of Surgery at Cornell University Medical Center, developed his own version of Stoppa's GPPR, but for unilateral hernias, termed the Giant Prosthetic Reinforcement of the Visceral Sac (GPRVS). He is also credited with popularizing the retromuscular prefascial repair of incisional hernias in the United States [4, 5].

A.M. Carbonell II, D.O., F.A.C.S., F.A.C.O.S. (✉)
Division of Minimal Access and Bariatric Surgery,
Hernia Center, Greenville Health System, University
of South Carolina School of Medicine Greenville,
701 Grove Road, Greenville, SC 29605, USA
e-mail: acarbonell@ghs.org

© Springer International Publishing Switzerland 2016
Y.W. Novitsky (ed.), *Hernia Surgery*, DOI 10.1007/978-3-319-27470-6_12

Biomechanical Principles of Repair

It is unlikely that Rives, by completing the retrorectus dissection, was actually setting out to perform a myofascial release of the rectus muscle; however, this is exactly what occurred. Opening the rectus sheath and dissecting the posterior lamina away from the rectus muscle serves to liberate the rectus muscle from its very encasement in the sheath. This release allows the rectus muscle to widen and further medializes the linea alba, offsetting the tension at the suture line during midline abdominal wall reconstruction.

Oscar Ramirez beautifully demonstrated this concept, albeit by happenstance. In the landmark paper describing his components separation technique, Ramirez performed an anatomic study on ten fresh cadavers. He found that each rectus muscle with the overlying rectus sheath could be advanced 3, 5, and 3 cm (Fig. 12.1), respectively, in the upper, middle, and lower thirds of the abdomen once the rectus muscle was removed from its encasement in the rectus sheath (essentially, the Rives dissection). This one maneuver, which is integral to the Ramirez components separation, is often neglected when surgeons attempt to replicate it. Nevertheless it demonstrates how developing the retrorectus plane alone, serves as a myofascial release and allows for the reapproximation of defects up to 10 cm wide at the mid abdomen.

The retrorectus space serves as a well-vascularized position where mesh prostheses become incorporated. This sublay mesh position has benefits both at a molecular level, as well as a pure mechanical level. In an animal model, mesh placed in the retrorectus position is associated with a perifilamentous collagen deposition with a much higher type I/III ratio compared to mesh in the onlay or premuscular condition [6]. The higher degree of type I, or mature collagen, results in a higher tensile strength of the wound. This was demonstrated clinically in a study of human mesh explants, where the highest ratio of type I/III collagen was found in meshes explanted from the retrorectus space. Interestingly, in the patients in whom the mesh was explanted for recurrence, the ratio was much lower than those in whom the mesh was explanted for chronic pain [7]. This confirms the importance of a high collagen type I/III ratio for wound healing and mesh stabilization, however, it is not the only piece of the puzzle.

The mechanical advantage of the retrorectus space has been demonstrated utilizing a novel in vitro incisional hernia simulation. In this study, the onlay mesh position resulted in decreased stability of the mesh and increased extrudability compared to the sublay position [8]. This was borne out clinically in studies demonstrating a higher recurrence rate for onlay repairs compared to sublay. A large Swedish national database study by Israelsson et al. [9] demonstrated a recurrence rate of 19.3% with onlay and 7.3% with sublay repairs. Similarly, a nationwide study of the Danish Ventral Hernia Database demonstrated the lowest cumulative risk of reoperation for recurrence in the sublay group (12.1%) versus the onlay (16.1%) and intraperitoneal (21.2%) mesh groups ($p = 0.03$) [10].

Operative Steps

The operation typically begins with a midline incision with or without excision of the prior scar. Alternatively, the retrorectus repair may be performed at the same time as dermolipectomy. Once the skin flap has been raised of the abdominal wall and hernia sac, the operation may commence.

Hernia Sac

It is recommended that the hernia sac be preserved since it can be later used to make up for any deficiency in either the posterior rectus sheath to reconstruct and close the visceral sac or the anterior sheath, so as to exclude the mesh from the subcutaneous tissues [11]. The hernia sac should thus be divided in the midline and the

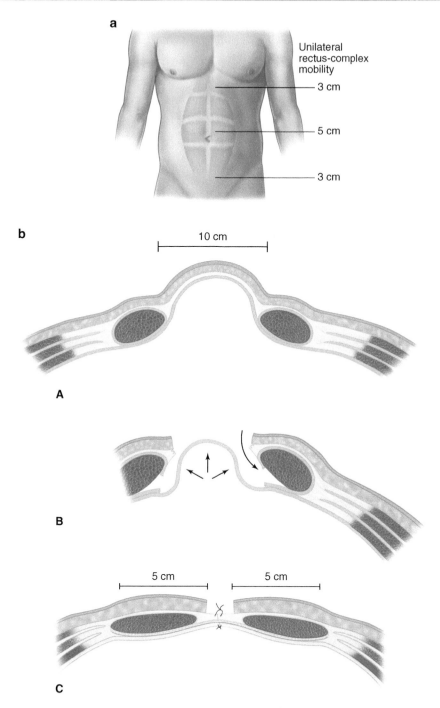

Fig. 12.1 (**a**) Distance of unilateral advancement of the rectus muscle to the midline after dissection of the retromuscular plane. (**b**) Axial illustration demonstrating the widening of the rectus muscle after dissection

peritoneum is entered. This allows for a full exploration of the visceral contents and any concomitant operations can be performed. A full lysis of adhesions from the anterior abdominal wall is recommended, as it will help with the mobility of closing the posterior rectus sheath and peritoneum in the midline.

Posterior Rectus Sheath Dissection

One side of the hernia sac is preserved and the dissection proceeds ventral to the hernia sac until the medial edge of the rectus sheath is encountered on the one side. Next, the rectus sheath is incised along the entire vertical length of the incision (Fig. 12.2). On the contralateral side, the hernia sac may be left attached anteriorly, and the incision of the posterior rectus sheath can be made immediately lateral to the medial most edge of the hernia defect on that side.

The dissection of the posterior rectus sheath is then continued cranial and caudal to the her-

nia defect for a minimum distance of 5–8 cm. This will provide ample space for mesh overlap across the vertical dimension of the hernia. The posterior rectus sheath is fused to the linea alba at its lateral most aspect. The linea alba may be of variable width. To create a space for mesh placement which crosses the midline behind the rectus muscles above and below the hernia defect, the posterior sheath must be divided off of the linea alba. Great care is taken in dividing the posterior sheath off of the lateral most portion of the linea alba on both sides of the abdomen. This ensures preservation of the linea alba as it will be the midline thrust bearing portion of the abdominal wall ventral to the mesh in the areas both above and below the hernia. If possible, the layer of peritoneum dorsal to the linea alba can be preserved and dissected posteriorly, serving as a bridge between the cut edges of the posterior rectus sheaths above and below the hernia (Fig. 12.3).

The dissection of the posterior sheath off of the overlying rectus muscle proceeds laterally, towards the edge of the rectus sheath envelope.

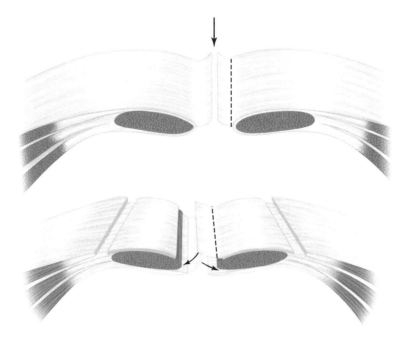

Fig. 12.2 With the hernia sac preserved, the edge of the rectus sheath is penetrated to begin the retromuscular dissection

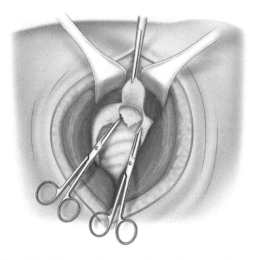

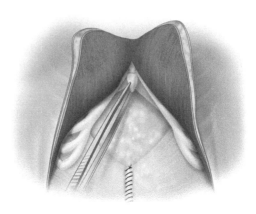

Fig. 12.4 The posterior sheath divided off the xiphoid process and the retroxophoid preperitoneal fatty plane is exposed

Fig. 12.3 The posterior rectus sheath has been disconnected from the linea alba, bilaterally, while preserving the peritoneum which was mobilized off the linea alba

The dissection can be performed bluntly with finger or sponge dissection or with cautery. During this retrorectus dissection, care should be taken to preserve the inferior epigastric vessels as well as the segmental innervation of the rectus muscle emanating from the lateral most edge of the rectus sheath and coursing anteriorly towards the rectus muscle.

Should the hernia defect extend into the upper abdomen, the surgeon may need to extend the dissection up to the costal margin and behind the xiphoid process. The posterior rectus sheath is attached to the dorsal aspect of the xiphoid process. The posterior sheath can be divided off of the xiphoid process and dropped posteriorly and the dissection carried out in the preperitoneal plane dorsal to the xiphoid (Fig. 12.4).

Below the arcuate line, the posterior rectus sheath ceases to exist and only transversalis fascia, preperitoneal fat and peritoneum remain. For hernias extending below the umbilicus, the surgeon will need to maintain these structures so as to have tissue to close the visceral sac. The dissection may extend into the preperitoneal spaces of Retzius and Bogros, exposing the pubic bone, Cooper's ligaments, and the iliac vessels on both sides.

Visceral Sac Closure

Once the dissection is complete, the posterior rectus sheath is approximated in the midline in a continuous fashion with a size 2-0, absorbable, polydioxanone suture. Closure of this layer should be aided by having preserved at least some portion of the hernia sac, which is still attached. Despite the relatively weak nature of the transversalis fascia/peritoneal layer below the arcuate line, its elasticity easily allows for approximation and visceral sac closure. If the sutures appear to be tearing utilizing the standard running technique, the suture bites may be oriented in a horizontal mattress fashion, incorporating more tissue, thus adding strength. It is critical that the posterior sheath be closed completely, so as to prevent any bowel from slipping in between the mesh and the posterior sheath, which could result in a bowel obstruction. Additionally, visceral sac closure ensures the mesh will not come in contact with the viscera. Should there be difficulty reapproximating the posterior sheaths in the midline due to excessive tension, two options arise. The fascial edges of the posterior sheaths can be sutured directly to the omentum, effectively closing the visceral sac. Alternatively, an absorbable mesh can be sewn as an interpositional graft to make up for any defect in the posterior sheath.

Mesh Fixation

The width of each rectus muscle and thus the entire retrorectus space is quite variable between patients. Ideally, the mesh should occupy this entire retrorectus space; ultimately the mesh width may vary from 10 cm to over 20 cm. The space may be measured and the mesh trimmed to size. Alternatively, the uncut mesh can be placed into the space and trimmed as it is being fixated. The mesh should be fixated circumferentially with spaced, full-thickness slowly absorbable sutures through the abdominal wall utilizing the Reverdin needle. If the mesh extends to the costal margin, the mesh may be placed below the ribs and suture fixated to the costal cartilage. I have not found this fixation to be fraught with the problems suggested by others. For hernias extending into the low abdomen, the mesh is fixated to the symphysis pubis and Cooper's ligaments bilaterally, here with a permanent monofilament suture. The mesh should lay taut in this space taking into consideration the fact that the space will become even smaller once the rectus muscle is reapproximated overtop the mesh (Fig. 12.5). Ideally, the surgeon should avoid introducing wrinkles into the mesh as it decreases mesh-tissue area interface.

There is no real consensus on the need for mesh fixation in this retromuscular plane. Rives et al. [2] originally described permanent sutures, placed abundantly along the mesh perimeter. As the focus of hernia repair outcomes shifted from recurrence to postoperative pain and function, many groups modified their fixation approach. I have progressively been decreasing the amount of sutures that I place and use size 2-0, absorbable polydioxanone suture. Others have been using absorbable fixation devices, and even fibrin sealants. For years, many Europeans have been fixating the mesh with permanent suture directly to the posterior rectus sheath, albeit with the risk of intestinal injury with this blind suture technique. Although there has not been a clinical trial to assess fixation methods in the retrorectus space, one animal study demonstrated no difference in fixation strength between permanent and absorbable sutures, fibrin sealant, and no fixation [12]. Fixation will remain a personal choice.

Midline Abdominal Wall Reconstruction

At the conclusion of mesh placement, two closed suction drains are placed, through separate stab incisions, into the retromuscular space. The drains will rest directly on top of the mesh. The midline abdomen is now reconstructed by suture reapproximating the edges of the linea alba in a continuous fashion with a size 0, absorbable, polydioxanone suture. Reconstructing the midline serves three purposes. First, it restores the central tendon of the abdomen, thus producing a functional anatomic repair. Secondly, it provides an increased area of mesh/tissue interface, and a reliable backstop for the mesh to resist the pressure of the abdominal cavity. Thirdly, closure of the fascia overtop the mesh has been demonstrated to reduce the incidence of prosthetic mesh infection [13].

Special Considerations

Assessing Anterior Tension

At the time of midline closure, the surgeon should decide whether the bilateral rectus myofascial release performed will be sufficient

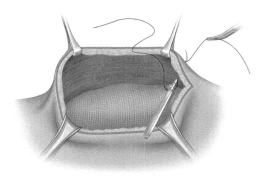

Fig. 12.5 The mesh is being deployed in the retromuscular plane. The Reverdin needle facilitates suture passage

enough to allow the anterior rectus sheaths to be approximated in the midline. This is done by placing clamps on the fascial edges and pulling in opposite directions. If the tension is minimal, then the surgeon may proceed with anterior fascial closure. Should the tension be excessive, a decision should be made regarding the next step. Options are numerous, and include leaving the fascia open. The surgeon may perform the Ramirez component separation [14], which will allow further medialization of the rectus muscles. A newer approach is to perform a posterior component separation where a myofascial release is effected by dissecting between the oblique muscle layers, lateral to the rectus sheath. From superficial to deep, Mathes et al. [15] described the space between the external and internal oblique muscle. Carbonell et al. [16] demonstrated the space between the internal oblique and transversus abdominis muscle. Novitsky described the transversus abdominis release (TAR) [17] where this muscle is divided, thus gaining access to the preperitoneal/pre-transversalis plane lateral to the rectus muscle. Each of these myofascial releases affords further medialization of the rectus muscles and obviates the need for any subcutaneous flap elevation, which is required for the Ramirez, or anterior component separation. My preference is now the TAR for its ease and reproducibility. Of all the posterior releases, it allows the most medialization of the posterior rectus sheath as it is attached to the highly expansile peritoneum laterally.

Lateral Defect

Concomitant lateral defects such as a former stoma site hernia can be addressed at the same time as the Rives-Stoppa repair. These defects can be within the rectus muscle itself, but often lie at the semilunar line, or worse yet, within the oblique musculature. To extend the retrorectus dissection lateral enough to these defects, the surgeon will need to perform a posterior component separation as previously described. This will allow a wide dissection lateral to the off-midline defect. Once the dissection is complete, the

defect within the posterior rectus sheath will need to be closed, as well as the defect anteriorly within the rectus muscle or oblique complex.

Parastomal Hernia

Similarly, when there is a current parastomal hernia of the colon, ileum, or urinary conduit, in addition to the midline defect being repaired, a posterior component separation will also be required. Options include, leaving the stoma in place, which will require working circumferentially around the stoma. In this scenario, the mesh will need to be keyhole split from one edge towards its mid-aspect. The mesh is then placed around the stoma, fixated properly, and then the keyhole slit is reconstructed with a permanent suture. Alternatively, the stoma can be completely dismantled and re-sited through a circular trephination created in the mesh.

Limitations

Since the Rives-Stoppa repair is a technique described for midline hernias, it should not be used for defects that are solely lateral, without a midline component. Lateral defects can be best approached directly over the defect and the pre-peritoneal space developed for mesh placement. Developing the retrorectus space will be exceedingly difficult, if not untenable in patients who have undergone resection of one or both of the rectus muscles such as women who have undergone a transverse rectus abdominis myocutaneous (TRAM) reconstruction of the breast. These patients may be better suited for an intraperitoneal or onlay placement of mesh.

Postoperative Care

Postoperatively, closed suction drains are left in position until they are draining less than 30 mL in a 24 hour period. I routinely discharge patients home with drains and do not prescribe antibiotics during this period. An abdominal binder is placed for comfort and support during the convalescent period.

It is not uncommon for patient to develop postoperative ileus due to entering the peritoneal cavity, particularly if an extensive lysis of adhesions was performed. I do not routinely leave a nasogastric tube in position after the operation; rather reserve its placement should the patient become increasingly symptomatic postoperatively.

The most common complications postoperatively are wound complications. Patients with multiple cicatrices of the abdomen may have disrupted the normal vascular supply to the skin of the abdomen. These patients are best evaluated by a plastic surgeon preoperatively to determine the ideal placement of the incision for hernia repair. Wound complications include skin ischemia, skin dehiscence, seroma, hematoma, and surgical site infection.

The incidence of surgical site infection is directly proportional to the degree of bacterial contamination or wound classification during the hernia repair. Mesh in the retromuscular space is quite resistant to infection, particularly the newer varieties of wide-pore meshes. Multiple investigators have shown that they can often be easily salvaged with negative pressure wound therapy, should a deep space surgical site infection occur [18–20].

A particularly under reported complication is that of a postoperative interparietal hernia. This can manifest as a small bowel obstruction due to the small bowel becoming trapped within the space between the posterior rectus sheath and the mesh. This occurs only if there is a breakdown in the posterior fascial closure, which likely occurs more than we believe. A high-index of suspicion for this entity should arise if a patient fails to progress postoperatively as expected. A computed tomographic exam will demonstrate the defect in the posterior sheath closure with bowel in the interparietal space [21].

Overall, the recurrence rate of the Rives-Stoppa incisional hernia repair has been shown, in multiple large series, to be less than 10% [9, 10, 13, 22–25].

In summary, the Rives-Stoppa technique for the repair of incisional hernias continues to stand the test of time since its inception close to 50 years ago. It should be the standard by which all other techniques are compared.

References

1. Stoppa R, Petit J, Abourachid H, Henry X, Duclaye C, Monchaux G, et al. Original procedure of groin hernia repair: interposition without fixation of Dacron tulle prosthesis by subperitoneal median approach. Chirurgie. 1973;99(2):119–23.
2. Rives J, Lardennois B, Pire JC, Hibon J. Large incisional hernias. The importance of flail abdomen and of subsequent respiratory disorders. Chirurgie. 1973;99(8):547–63.
3. Stoppa RE. The treatment of complicated groin and incisional hernias. World J Surg. 1989;13(5):545–54.
4. Wantz GE. Giant prosthetic reinforcement of the visceral sac. Surg Gynecol Obstet. 1989;169(5):408–17.
5. Wantz GE. Incisional hernioplasty with Mersilene. Surg Gynecol Obstet. 1991;172(2):129–37.
6. Binnebösel M, Klink CD, Otto J, Conze J, Jansen PL, Anurov M, et al. Impact of mesh positioning on foreign body reaction and collagenous ingrowth in a rabbit model of open incisional hernia repair. Hernia. 2010;14(1):71–7.
7. Junge K, Klinge U, Rosch R, Mertens PR, Kirch J, Klosterhalfen B, et al. Decreased collagen type I/III ratio in patients with recurring hernia after implantation of alloplastic prostheses. Langenbecks Arch Surg. 2004;389(1):17–22.
8. Binnebösel M, Rosch R, Junge K, Flanagan TC, Schwab R, Schumpelick V, et al. Biomechanical analyses of overlap and mesh dislocation in an incisional hernia model in vitro. Surgery. 2007;142(3):365–71.
9. Israelsson LA, Smedberg S, Montgomery A, Nordin P, Spangen L. Incisional hernia repair in Sweden 2002. Hernia. 2006;10(3):258–61.
10. Helgstrand F, Rosenberg J, Kehlet H, Jorgensen LN, Bisgaard T. Nationwide prospective study of outcomes after elective incisional hernia repair. J Am Coll Surg. 2013;216(2):217–28.
11. Picazo-Yeste J, Morandeira-Rivas A, Moreno-Sanz C. Multilayer myofascial-mesh repair for giant midline incisional hernias: a novel advantageous combination of old and new techniques. J Gastrointest Surg. 2013;17(9):1665–72.
12. Grommes J, Binnebösel M, Klink CD, Trotha KT, Junge K, Conze J. Different methods of mesh fixation in open retromuscular incisional hernia repair: a comparative study in pigs. Hernia. 2010;14(6):623–7.
13. Petersen S, Henke G, Zimmermann L, Aumann G, Hellmich G, Ludwig K. Ventral rectus fascia closure on top of mesh hernia repair in the sublay technique. Plast Reconstr Surg. 2004;114(7):1754–60.
14. Ramirez OM, Ruas E, Dellon AL. "Components separation" method for closure of abdominal-wall defects: an anatomic and clinical study. Plast Reconstr Surg. 1990;86(3):519–26.
15. Mathes SJ, Steinwald PM, Foster RD, Hoffman WY, Anthony JP. Complex abdominal wall reconstruction: a comparison of flap and mesh closure. Ann Surg. 2000;232(4):586–96.

16. Carbonell A, Cobb W, Chen S. Posterior components separation during retromuscular hernia repair. Hernia. 2008;12(4):359–62.

17. Novitsky YW, Elliott HL, Orenstein SB, Rosen MJ. Transversus abdominis muscle release: a novel approach to posterior component separation during complex abdominal wall reconstruction. Am J Surg. 2012;204(5):709–16.

18. Rueda Perez JM, Cano Maldonado AJ, Romera Barba E, Navarro Garcia I, Espinosa Lopez FJ, Galvez Pastor S, et al. Manejo conservador de la infección de la herida quirúrgica asociada a material protésico, con terapia de presión negativa. Revista Hispanoamericana de Hernia. 2013;1(2):81–5.

19. Meagher H, Clarke Moloney M, Grace PA. Conservative management of mesh-site infection in hernia repair surgery: a case series. Hernia. 2015;19(2):231–7.

20. Berrevoet F, Vanlander A, Sainz-Barriga M, Rogiers X, Troisi R. Infected large pore meshes may be salvaged by topical negative pressure therapy. Hernia. 2013;17(1):67–73.

21. Carbonell AM. Interparietal hernias after open retromuscular hernia repair. Hernia. 2008;12(6):663–6.

22. McLanahan D, King LT, Weems C, Novotney M, Gibson K. Retrorectus prosthetic mesh repair of midline abdominal hernia. Am J Surg. 1997;173(5):445–9.

23. Martín-Duce A, Noguerales F, Villeta R, Hernández P, Lozano O, Keller J, et al. Modifications to Rives technique for midline incisional hernia repair. Hernia. 2001;5(2):70–2.

24. Flament JB, Palot JP, Lubrano D, Levy-Chazal N, Concé JP, Marcus C. Retromuscular prosthetic repair: experience from France. Der Chirurg; Zeitschrift für alle Gebiete der operativen Medizen. 2002;73(10):1053–8.

25. Novitsky YW, Porter JR, Rucho ZC, Getz SB, Pratt BL, Kercher KW, et al. Open preperitoneal retrofascial mesh repair for multiply recurrent ventral incisional hernias. J Am Coll Surg. 2006;203(3):283–9.

Posterior Component Separation Via Transversus Abdominis Muscle Release: The TAR Procedure

13

Yuri W. Novitsky

Introduction

Evolution of hernia surgery has led to popularization of reconstructive techniques. I believe that the goal of most, if not all, herniorrhaphies should be restoration of a functional abdominal wall with autologous tissue repair strengthened by mesh reinforcement. Anterior component separation techniques described in Chapters 14–16 typically involve release of the external oblique muscle and fascia. The traditional approach described by Ramirez involves creation of large skin flaps and associated significant wound morbidity in up to 63% of cases [1–3]. Minimally invasive modifications are known to reduce skin flaps and wound complications, but limit mesh placement to intraperitoneal underlay in the vast majority of cases. In an effort to reduce wound morbidity, I prefer to utilize retromuscular sublay techniques. For moderate-sized defects, classic Rives-Stoppa retrorectus repairs, described in Chapter 12, provide durable outcomes with low morbidity [4–7]. However, the major limitations of the classic retrorectus repair

include limited medial myofascial advancement and lack of sufficient sublay space for wide overlap of the visceral sac in many hernias. Although techniques to overcome the limitations of the rectus sheath by utilizing pre-peritoneal or intra-muscular repairs have been described [7, 8], both are fraught with disadvantages of limited myofascial medialization and/or neurovascular bundle damage.

To address the shortfalls of the traditional retromuscular repairs, I have recently developed another novel technique of posterior component separation using transversus abdominis muscle release (TAR) [9]. This modification allows for significant posterior rectus fascia advancement, wide lateral dissection, preservation of the neurovascular supply of the rectus abdominis muscle, and provides a large space for mesh sublay. Most importantly, this technique allows for medialization of the abdominal wall components without raising lipocutaneous flaps. In this chapter, I will describe the history of this technique, its anatomic and physiologic basis, indications/limitations, detailed technical considerations of TAR as well as a variety of clinical outcomes.

Electronic supplementary material: The online version of this chapter (doi:10.1007/978-3-319-27470-6_13) contains supplementary material, which is available to authorized users.

Y.W. Novitsky, M.D., F.A.C.S. (✉)
Department of Surgery, Case Comprehensive Hernia Center, University Hospitals Case Medical Center, 11100 Euclid Avenue, Cleveland, OH 44106, USA
e-mail: yuri.novitsky@uhhospitals.org;
ynovit@gmail.com

History of TAR

The first TAR was performed in the late 2006. Prior to that, an aforementioned Rives-Stoppa with the pre-peritoneal extension was my procedure of choice. As I happened to be involved in the cadaveric dissections during normal anatomy classes, I serendipitously noted a significant medial extension of the transversus abdominis muscle (TA) past linea semilunaris as well as its dorsal relationship with the costal margin (Fig. 13.1). The initial series of my TAR patients was first presented at the 2009 World Hernia Congress and received mixed reviews, with skepticism about its efficacy, reproducibility, and potential deleterious effects of TA transection on the stability of the abdominal wall. However, following publication of the technical details [10] of the first 42 patients with longer follow-up and further evidence of safety and efficacy of this approach, there has been a steady increase in the acceptance and utilization of TAR by the surgical community worldwide.

Anatomic and Physiologic Basis of TAR

As mentioned above and described in detail in Chapter 1, the anatomy of the TA muscle makes it the ideal target for posterior component separation. In the upper third of the abdomen, it extends medially far beyond the semilunar line (and the lateral edge of the rectus muscle) (Fig. 13.1) and ultimately inserts into the edge of the costal margin (costal cartilages of 7–12th ribs) and xiphoid process. It also interdigitates with the diaphragm at its cephalad aspect. The medial extent of the TA muscle diminishes as one moves caudally. At the level of the umbilicus and below, only the transversus abdominis aponeurosis and almost no TA muscle fibers are present. In addition, the orientation of the TA muscle fibers is in the direction of the desired (horizontal) advancement of the rectus complex, as opposed to the external and internal oblique muscles. This largely contributes to successful medialization of all abdominal components during TAR.

The physiologic function of TA is another key factor for its targeting during posterior component separation. It is one of the principal muscles in the maintenance of the intra-abdominal pressure and together with the internal oblique, but not external oblique, it provides hoop tension throughout the entire thoracolumbar fascia. In fact, it is widely viewed as the "corset" of the abdomen. Its release and subsequent mobiliza-

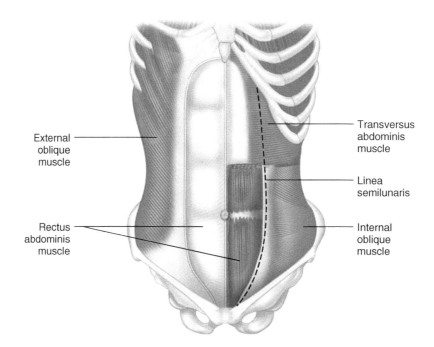

Fig. 13.1 Muscles of the abdominal wall. Notably, the transversus abdominis muscle extends medial to the semilunar line in the upper abdomen

tion off the underlying fascia removes the muscle's contribution to the "tone" of the lateral abdominal wall. Logically, this leads to the largest expansion of the abdominal girth and medial advancement of the entire rectus complex. These physiologic functions are central in the ability of TAR to provide medialization of not only posterior, but also anterior components of the abdominal wall, especially in cases of wide abdominal defects.

Indications and Patient Selection

My personal algorithm for procedure selection for a given patient begins with considering the suitability of the laparoscopic approach. Patients who have small to medium defects (<8 cm wide), without previous intraperitoneal mesh or skin changes/skin grafts/wound healed by secondary intention are generally approached laparoscopically. The remaining patients I will approach via an open technique. While some of the patients undergoing open repairs may be effectively treated using a traditional Rives-Stoppa, most of those patients in my practice would have undergone a laparoscopic repair. Thus, I utilize TAR for the vast majority of my open repairs. Posterior component separation is particularly important for those patients who need myofascial release for their abdominal wall reconstruction, but are not candidates for the anterior component separations. Those may include patients with subcostal/Chevron incision hernias, patients with old appendectomy incisions, and those with a history of abdominoplasty and previous anterior releases, among others. Furthermore, patients with large subxiphoid, parailiac, and suprapubic hernias do not usually enjoy the benefits of anterior component release, and therefore may be best suited for posterior release and TAR. Finally, in my practice, most patients with parastomal herniations are also considered to be good candidates for reconstructions with TAR.

While there are no absolute contraindications to TAR, relative contraindications include previously pre-peritoneal and/or retromuscular repairs,

need for panniculectomy/abdominoplasty, and history of severe necrotizing pancreatitis (given resultant scarring of the retroperitoneum). It is also important to point out that TAR should not be combined with the anterior component release. This practice would likely result in significant lateral laxity or lateral hernia formation from creating the environment where internal oblique muscle is a sole provider of lateral abdominal wall integrity. However, in patients who present with recurrences following anterior release, the TAR approach is useful and possibly the "last resort" approach, despite associated risks of lateral bulging in those challenging patients. We have recently reported our experience in those challenging patients, with good short-term outcomes [11]. Of note, in this unique cohort, I advocate the use of a heavy-weight polypropylene mesh to allow for more durable prosthetic reinforcement.

Pre-operative Planning

Careful pre-operative imaging is paramount to a successful ventral hernia repair, especially when any degree of complexity is anticipated. I recommend routine abdominal/pelvic CT imaging. No oral or intravenous contrast is generally necessary. CT delineates all abdominal wall defects: this is of particular importance in obese patients where physical examination carries significant limitations. Furthermore, in addition to uncovering occult intra-abdominal pathology contributing to patient's symptoms, abdominal CT allows for detection of previous synthetic meshes and/or latent infections. I also mandate a screening colonoscopy in appropriate patients prior to undertaking any major abdominal wall reconstructions.

Pre-operative optimization is one of the most important steps to maximize surgical outcomes. General principles of patient optimizations are already covered in Chapter 4. Our hernia center provides nutritional evaluation and counseling for all obese patients contemplating hernia repair. For those with non-obstructive symptoms, major abdominal wall reconstructions are delayed until commonly agreed weight loss criteria are reached. Admittedly, I do not have established BMI criteria that preclude repairs and generally consider multiple factors to decide on appropriate timing of the repair. It is important to point out that a fairly large proportion of obese patients with symptomatic hernias will progress to require urgent and emergent operations, which are significantly more difficult and morbid. To assist with weight loss goals, our bariatric team evaluates patients to select appropriate candidates for weight-loss surgery. Unfortunately, insurance limitations often preclude pre-operative weight-loss surgery for hernia patients. While concomitant bariatric/abdominal wall repairs may become routine in the future, their utility remains investigational at the present time. We also emphasize strict blood glucose control and postpone any elective repairs until HgA1C is less than 8. Smoking cessation is mandatory prior to any elective repairs.

Operative Technique

Patient Positioning

The patient is placed in the supine position. The abdomen should be prepped from the nipples to mid-thigh. Laterally, the prepped field is extended to the posterior axillary lines. I routinely use an Ioban drape (3M, St. Paul, MN) to minimize the risks of mesh infection.

Step 1: Incision/Adhesiolysis

A generous midline laparotomy is performed in the majority of cases. Elliptical or "tear-drop" incisions are used to incorporate previous scars as well as all attenuated or ulcerated skin. For most patients, and especially the morbidly obese with large midline hernias, I recommend routine excision of the umbilicus to minimize post-operative wound morbidity. While some surgeons prefer to remain extra-peritoneal, I advocate a complete lysis of all intestinal adhesions to the anterior abdominal wall. This is essential for several important reasons. First, undivided adhesions may contribute to peritoneal/posterior sheath tears during myofascial release/advancement. Second, the

adhered viscera may be vulnerable to inadvertent (and likely unrecognized) visceral injury during tissue releases. Lastly, dense intra-peritoneal adhesions to the anterior abdominal wall may impede medialization of the posterior components. I typically abstain from lysing inter-loop adhesions unless there are pre-operative obstructive symptoms or any intestinal resections are undertaken. Following adhesiolysis, a countable towel is placed on top of the viscera with its edges "tucked" into the gutters, pelvis, above the liver, and toward the esophageal hiatus. This helps to protect the viscera during subsequent myofascial releases.

Step 2: Rectus Sheath Release/Retro-Rectus Dissection

Following adhesiolysis, the posterior rectus sheath is incised. The precise location of this initial incision might be difficult, especially in patients with large defects where the rectus muscles are retracted laterally (Fig. 13.2). It is important to identify the junction of the rectus muscle and hernia sac. Only after that is done, the rectus sheath is incised about 0.5–1 cm from its medial edge (Fig. 13.3a, b). It is critical that the fibers of rectus abdominis are clearly visualized (Fig. 13.4). If this is not done, one may erroneously divide the hernia sac and enter the subcutaneous plane. I typically aim to initiate this step either above or below the hernia neck, in order to access the retrorectus plane where the muscle is not lateralized. Another useful maneuver is to palpate the rectus muscle to facilitate identification of its medial extent. The retromuscular plane is then developed toward the linea semilunaris. For this plane, I utilize bovie electrocautery to control/divide the fine areolar tissue and small perforating branches of the epigastric artery. In addition, blunt instrument or finger dissection could be utilized. An important aspect of this dissection is the constant traction/counter-traction applied by Richardson retractors under the rectus muscles and multiple Allis clamps placed on the medial edge of the incised posterior rectus sheath (Fig. 13.5). The lateral extent of this dissection is the perforators to the rectus muscle, which are the branches of the thoraco-abdominal nerves, penetrating the lateral edge of the posterior rectus sheath just medial to linea semilunaris

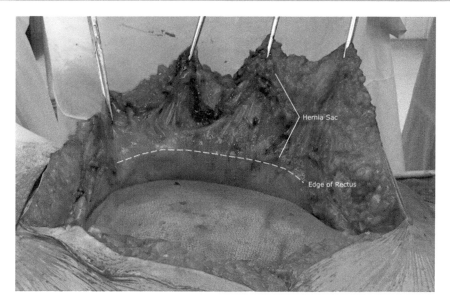

Fig. 13.2 Countable towel covers the entire visceral sac and rectus muscle edge is defined

(Fig. 13.6). The plane is extended cephalad toward the costal margin. Importantly, the attachments of the falciform ligament to the undersurface of the right posterior rectus sheath need to be preserved during the cranial dissection of the right retro-rectus space (Fig. 13.7). The cranial extent of this dissection depends on the extent of the hernia defect and may extend to the epigastric area or all the way to and above the xiphoid process (discussed below). The transition from the retromuscular plane within the rectus sheath into the pelvis involves the division of the medial attachments of the arcuate line of Douglas to the linea alba. Following that, it is imperative to enter and develop the pre-peritoneal plane. The inferior deep epigastric vessels, which run ventral to the transversalis fascia and along the posterolateral surface of the rectus abdominis muscles need to be identified and preserved. Dissection in the pre-transversalis plane may lead to vascular injuries. Caudally, I typically will proceed to dissect into the space of Retzius, exposing the pubis symphysis and Cooper's ligaments (Fig. 13.8).

Step 3: Exposure and Division of the Transversus Abdominis Muscle

Once the retromuscular plane is developed to the linea semilunaris, the limit of the traditional

Rives-Stoppa approach has been reached. Posterior component separation and TAR, if necessary, is then undertaken. Starting in the upper third of the abdomen (or at the cephalad-most part of the retro-rectus dissection), the posterior rectus sheath is incised again and the underlying fibers of the transversus abdominis muscle are identified (Fig. 13.9a, b). It is important to make the incision just medial to the perforating neurovascular bundles to minimize their damage and subsequent chance of denervating the rectus muscle (Fig. 13.10). As mentioned above (Fig. 13.1), the medial extension of TA is significantly medial to the linea semilunaris, the key anatomic feature that allows the TAR procedure. If this incision is undertaken too medially, the muscle fibers may be difficult to visualize and peritoneum may be cut. Similarly, if this step is undertaken in the mid or lower abdomen, the muscular portion of the TA is more lateral in those areas and, as a result, more difficult to identify properly. In fact, at the level of the umbilicus, almost no muscle fibers of TA extend to linea semilunaris. Further caudally, only the transversus abdominis aponeurosis persists. The posterior rectus sheath is then incised in the cranial-caudal direction. The lateral aspect of the arcuate line is divided at its junction with the semilunar line (Fig. 13.11).

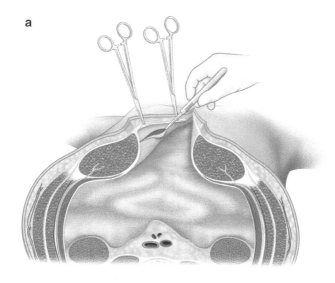

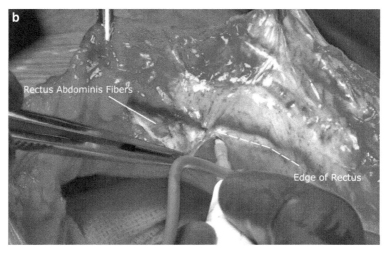

Fig. 13.3 Incision of the posterior sheath just lateral to the linea alba (**a**) is a drawing and (**b**) is an intra-op pic demonstaring the same concept

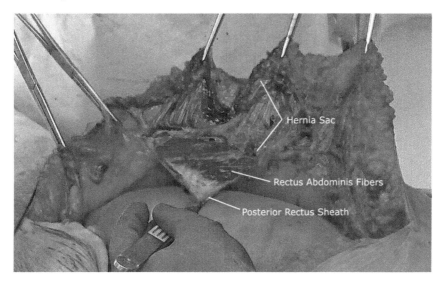

Fig. 13.4 The fibers of the rectus muscle must be visualized to ensure the correct location of the initial incision in the posterior rectus sheath, just lateral to the edge of the hernia sac

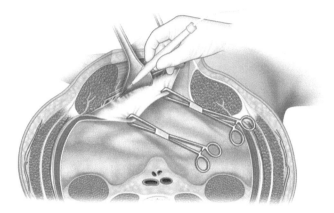

Fig. 13.5 Retro-rectus dissection toward the linea semilunaris

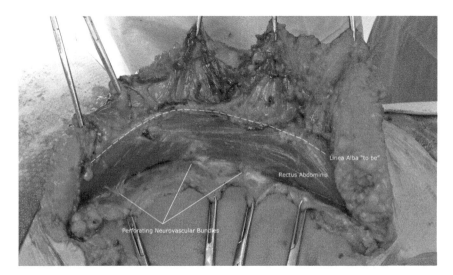

Fig. 13.6 Completed retro-rectus dissection. Note that neurovascular bundles to the rectus muscles that perforate the posterior sheath just medial to the linea semilunaris are preserved

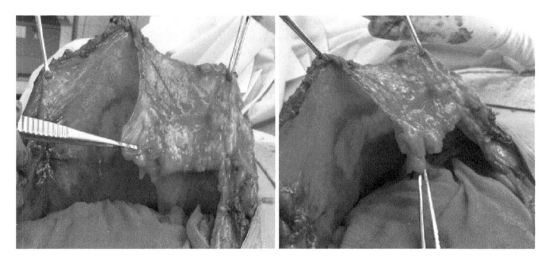

Fig. 13.7 Falciform ligament is kept attached to the right posterior rectus sheath

I then turn my attention to the TA muscle itself. One must avoid dissecting in the plane ventral to the muscle, as this would lead to the intramuscular plane and damage the previously identified perforating nerves. The TA muscle is divided along its entire medial edge using electrocautery. This step is initiated in the upper third of the abdomen where medial fibers of the transversus abdominis muscle are easiest to identify and separate from the underlying fascia (Fig. 13.12a, b). The use of right-angled dissector significantly facilitates this release and minimizes injury to the underlying transversalis fascia and peritoneum. Muscle release allows entrance to the space between the transversalis fascia and the divided transversus abdominis muscle. This is my preferred plane in the upper abdomen. Furthermore, I prefer to perform a limited finger dissection just underneath the costal margin to verify the correct plane of dissection dorsal to the ribs. Being ventral to the costal margin is incorrect; lateral progression should be stopped, TA muscle should be re-identified and divided properly. It is important to understand that the only path from the rectus sheath into the pre-peritoneal plane cranial to the costal margin is via the described division of the TA fibers.

Step 4: Lateral/Retroperitoneal Dissection

Once the TA muscle is divided, the plane deep to it is developed in the medial to lateral direction. To minimize tears of the posterior layers, careful blunt dissection is necessary. I place a right-angled dissector on the cut edge of the TA to provide anterior retraction. The Kittner dissector is then used for blunt dissection between the muscle and underlying transversalis fascia (Fig. 13.13). The Allis clamps on the cut edge of the posterior rectus sheath are used to provide counter-traction. This plane is bloodless and any difficulties/bleeding at this point should alert to the possibility of erroneous entry into the intramuscular plane. Occasionally, the transversalis fascia is difficult to distinguish and it is divided creating entry into the pre-peritoneal plane. One must be careful not to damage the very thin peritoneal layer. If fenestrations do occur, they can be sutured primarily. I

utilize running or figure-of-eight 2-0 Vicryl sutures to close those fenestrations in the transverse (but not vertical) direction, in order to minimize tension on this suture line.

The pre-transversalis/pre-peritoneal plane is contiguous with the retroperitoneum and the transition to it is often marked with retroperitoneal fatty tissue. Subsequent blunt dissection will expose the lateral edge of the psoas muscle, if necessary. The lateral edge of the psoas is my "safety" landmark and I use it to guide me during my caudal dissection toward the space of Bogros and myopectineal orifice. At the completion of this step, significant medialization of the posterior rectus fascia and extensive retromuscular pocket is developed (Fig. 13.14).

Step 5: Inferior Dissection

After exposing both Cooper's ligaments and the pubis (described above), the dissection is extended laterally across the entire myopectineal orifice. It is important to follow the direction of the iliopubic tract in order to avoid inadvertent neurovascular injuries. In women, the round ligament is divided routinely. In men, the spermatic cord is identified and carefully de-parietalized (similarly to cord dissection during laparoscopic inguinal hernia repair). All direct and indirect inguinal hernia should be reduced. In fact, if inguinal/femoral hernias are a major concern pre-operatively, this dissection is extended to expose at least 5 cm of the distal psoas muscle with subsequent mesh placement overlapping the inferior edge of the myopectineal orifice, similar to laparoscopic inguinal hernia repairs. The urinary bladder may be filled with saline to facilitate its identification and dissection. This is particularly prudent in patients with previous history of pelvic surgery, such as prostatectomy, cystectomy, etc.

Alternatively, this plane could be dissected from the lateral to medial direction. Starting cranially, after the TA release and dissection into the retroperitoneum is performed (discussed above), one can move caudally along the lateral edge of the psoas muscle to approach the inferior-lateral edge of the myopectineal orifice. At that point, one can begin to bluntly sweep medially to get

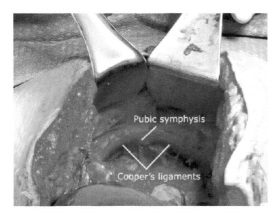

Fig 13.8 Dissection of the space of Retzius and Cooper's ligaments

dorsal to the transversus aponeurosis (but ventral to the peritoneum) and transition to the space of Retzius. I prefer to dissect both myopectineal orifices and Cooper's ligaments prior to connecting the planes underneath the intact caudal portion of the linea alba.

Step 6: Superior Dissection

Depending on the location of the hernia, the superior dissection may extend to the upper epigastrium or above the xiphoid process to the retrosternal space. The maneuvers utilized for each of those scenarios are different and will be described in detail separately.

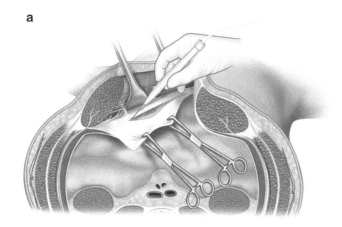

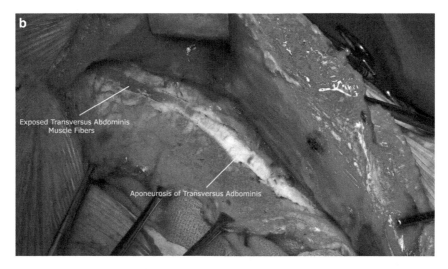

Fig. 13.9 Incision of the lateral aspect of the posterior rectus sheath. This step is best started as cephalad in the rectus sheath as possible (**a**) is a drawing and (**b**) is an intra-op picture demonstaring the same concept

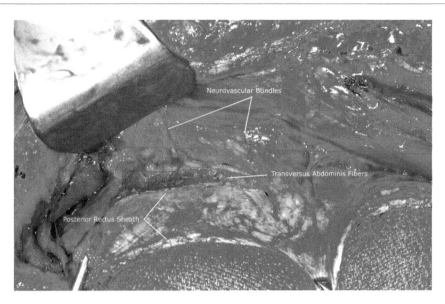

Fig. 13.10 Lateral (second) incision of the posterior rectus sheath just medial to the preserved neurovascular perforating bundles to the rectus muscles

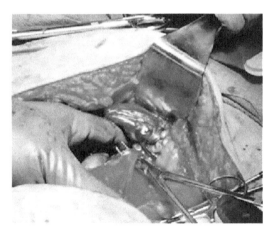

Fig. 13.11 Division of the lateral aspect of the arcuate line, as it joins linea semilunaris

(a) *Transition in the epigastrium*

For midline hernias with cephalad extension at least 6–8 cm below the xiphoid process, a plane needs to be established to connect bilateral retro–rectus spaces across the midline. Typically, the linea alba prevents the continuity of those two planes. To prevent recurrent herniations off the superior edge of the dissection/mesh, the linea alba is maintained in continuity ventral to the mesh for at least 5 cm by dividing the insertion of the posterior rectus sheaths into the linea alba

(Fig. 13.15). This is accomplished by cutting the insertion of each posterior sheath in the cranial direction about 0.5 cm lateral to the linea alba on the respective sides. The posterior sheaths will subsequently be reconnected, and the mesh will be placed dorsal to the intact linea alba. To facilitate this step, I usually delay this transition until the rest of the dissection/releases are accomplished on both sides.

(b) *Transition at or cranial to xiphoid process*

For the vast majority of mid and upper abdominal defects, I believe cephalad dissection to the retrosternal space is critical to minimize superior/subxiphoid recurrences. First, the linea alba is divided to the xiphoid process. Then, posterior insertion of the posterior rectus sheath into the xiphoid process is incised as well. This provides access to a fatty triangle that is extended cephalad in a substernal plane. Finally, the continuity of this space with the retromuscular dissection is created. The incision line at the lateral aspect of the posterior rectus sheath is extended to and slightly above the costal margin. This is then followed by complete division of the uppermost fibers of the transversus abdominis muscle just off the lateral edge of the xiphoid.

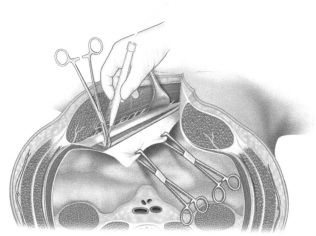

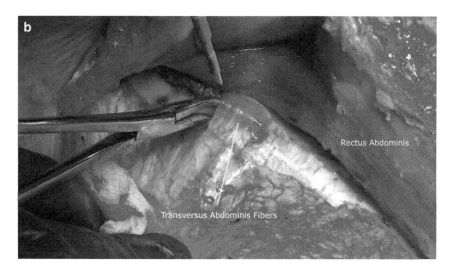

Fig. 13.12 Incision of the transversus abdominis muscle (**a**) is a drawing and (**b**) is an intra-op pic demonstaring the same concept

Care must be taken not to transect the fibers of the anterior diaphragm that are interdigitated with the transversus abdominis in its cranial-medial aspect. Failure to do so may result in an iatrogenic Morgagni hernia. The retromuscular dissection plane can be extended dorsal to the sternum by sweeping the peritoneum/transversalis fascia off of the diaphragm laterally. For the hernia defects in the upper abdomen, further retrosternal dissection to expose the upper aspect of the central tendon of the diaphragm (Fig. 13.16) is necessary for adequate mesh overlap. Once

again, this is best accomplished as the last step, once both retromuscular planes have been completely established.

Step 7: Closure of the Posterior Layers

Once similar release is performed on both sides (as is often needed in most complex repairs), the posterior rectus sheaths are re-approximated in the midline with a running 2-0 Vicryl or PDS suture (Fig. 13.17a, b). In rare instances when posterior fascial edges cannot be brought together the gap(s) in that layer are buttressed with native tissue (i.e., omentum), patched with polyglycolic

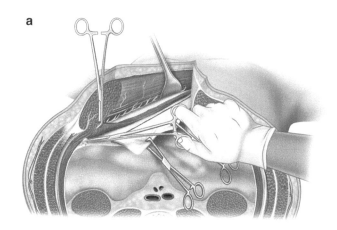

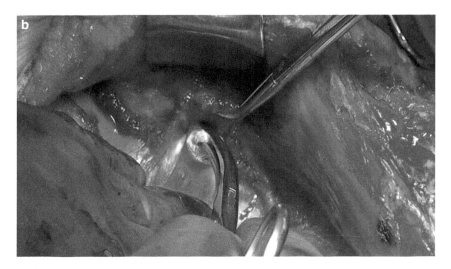

Fig. 13.13 Posterior component separation by dissecting deep to the divided transversus abdominis muscle

Fig. 13.14 Medialization of
the posterior layers and
retromuscular dissection into
the lateral retroperitoneum

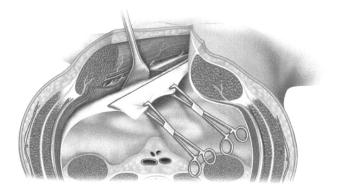

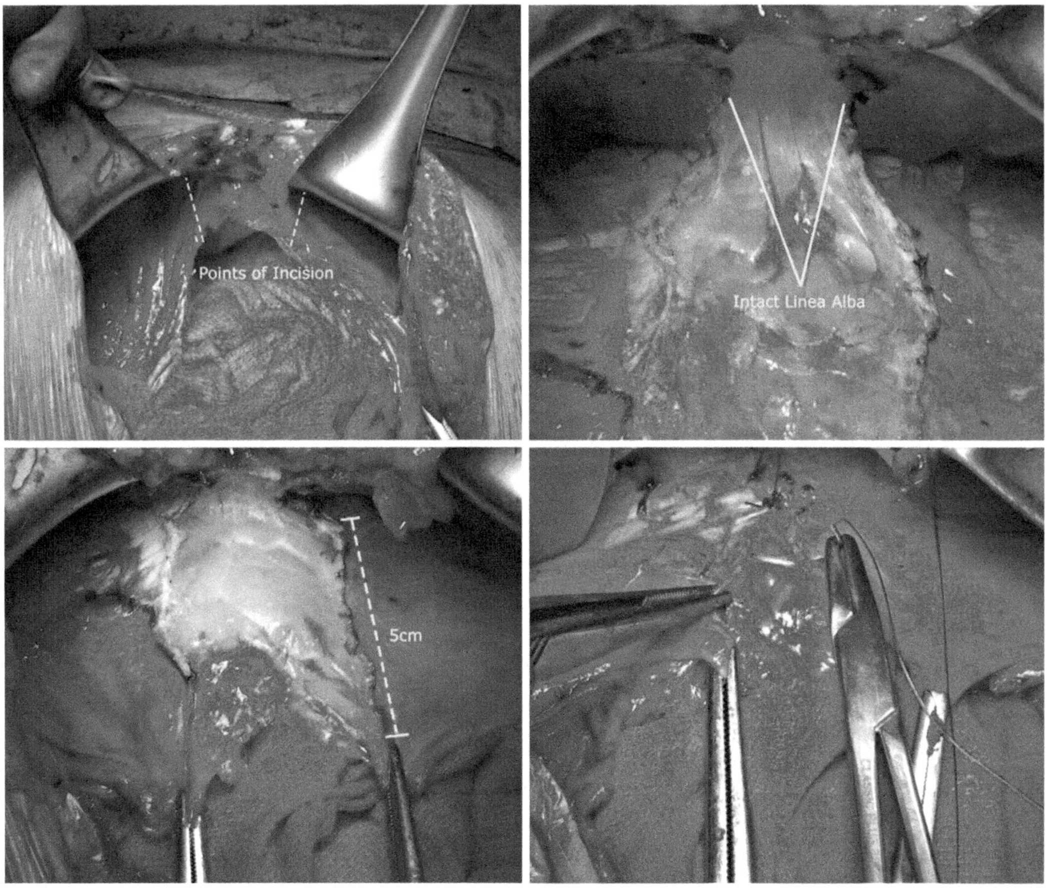

Fig. 13.15 Connecting dissection planes in the epigastric region. The retro-rectus dissection extends for at least 5-cm cranial to the intact linea alba. The advanced posterior rectus sheaths are then reconnected, allowing for sufficient mesh overlap below the intact linea alba, minimizing risks of recurrence of the cranial edge of the mesh

Fig. 13.16 Connecting dissection planes in the subxiphoid/retro-sternal region. The plane may be extended to expose the central tendon of the diaphragm

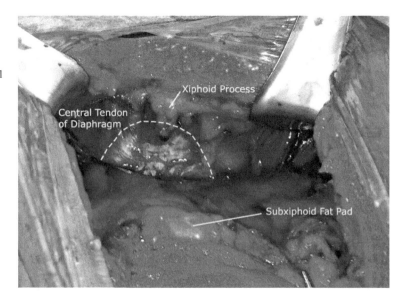

acid (Vicryl) mesh (Fig. 13.18a), or biologic mesh (Fig. 13.18b). There are several reasons why closure of the posterior sheaths is needed: first, it avoids herniation of the intra-abdominal viscera between the mesh and the abdominal wall layers. Second, it negates the need for costly composite meshes, since there is no exposure of the abdominal viscera to mesh that is placed pre-peritoneally. Finally, I believe this step might provide some minor additional strength to the reconstruction of the abdominal wall.

Step 8: Irrigation of the Extraperitoneal Space and TAP Block

Once the posterior layers are reconnected, a completely extraperitoneal pocket has been created. In clean contaminated and contaminated cases, I use antibiotic pressurized pulse lavage of the space prior to mesh placement. We have discovered that this strategy results in a significant reduction of the bioburden of contaminated wounds. Following the lavage, a transversus abdominis plane bock can be performed. Since the intramuscular plane that contains the nerves can be easily visualized, I place 80–100 cm³ of dilute liposomal bupivacaine in both TA planes under direct vision (Fig. 13.19).

Step 9: Mesh Placement/Fixation

The mesh is placed as a sublay in the retromuscular space. Adhering to the principle of "giant prosthetic reinforcement of the visceral sac" is critical to ensure durability of the repair. I aim to place the mesh to at least the anterior axillary line in the vast majority of my TAR cases. Choosing the size of the mesh is not proportional to the size of the original defect, as is commonly done in other type of repairs. This strategy essentially eliminates possibilities of lateral recurrences. For defects that extend to the umbilicus, I dissect the entire space of Retzius and extend/fixate the mesh to the Cooper's ligaments. I typically first place two interrupted sutures, one in each of the Cooper's ligament, (Fig. 13.20a) and then pass the tail through the mesh so that the knots will be tied at the dorsal surface of the mesh (Fig. 13.20b). This strategy not only facilitates mesh placement, but

allows us to ensure mesh overlap in the retropubic space. One must be careful to pass the suture tails from each stitch at a distance similar to the distance between the stitches in the Cooper's ligaments. Inferior fixation is essential to counteract the vectors of the intra-abdominal forces that are directed inferiorly, so as to reduce the odds of the suprapubic recurrences. Superiorly, the mesh extends to the epigastric area or to the retrosternal plane (as described above).

Mesh fixation is accomplished by placing a #1 absorbable monofilament suture into the mesh and then pass the tails of the mesh (about 1 cm apart through the abdominal wall) out of the same skin incision using a Carter-Thomason suture passer (Cooper Surgical, Trumbull, CT, USA) (Fig. 13.21). In the past, I have used 10–14 of such full-thickness, trans-abdominal points of fixation. Over the years, however, I found that this was not necessary, especially laterally. If I am able to achieve a desired overlap of the visceral sac and I am able to reconstruct the linea alba in the midline without undue tension, I have evolved to minimize or almost completely forego lateral mesh fixation. However, I still almost uniformly employ inferior fixation to both Cooper's ligament using two interrupted monofilament sutures (as shown above). Superiorly, the mesh could be positioned cephalad to the costal margin and in the retro-xiphoid space. It is secured with interrupted sutures around the xiphoid process. Those sutures are placed 4–5 cm off the edge of the mesh to allow for large overlap, especially for upper abdominal defects.

Mesh selection remains to be a controversial topic. My preferred material is a macroporous mid-weight polypropylene. In patients where linea alba reconstruction is impossible or under excessive tension, a heavy-weight polypropylene mesh is used. In addition, patients with flank defects and those after previous failed anterior component separation are best treated with a heavier weight polypropylene material. I am strongly against utilization of polyester-based meshes during major open abdominal wall reconstructions. The role of bioabsorbable and newer biologic meshes for retro-muscular repairs is evolving.

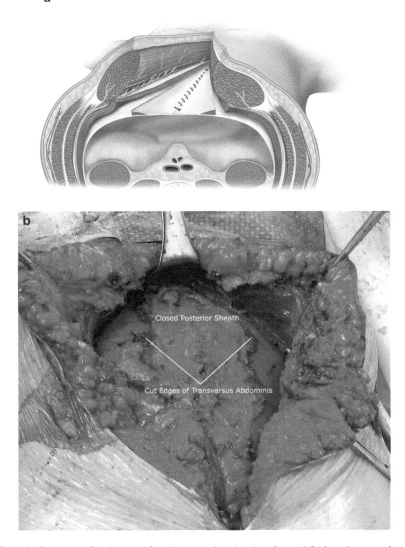

Fig. 13.17 Posterior layers are closed; visceral sac is restored (**a**) is a drawing and (**b**) is an intra-op picture demonstaring the same concept

Step 10: Anterior Fascia and Skin Closure

Large closed suction drains are placed on top of the mesh. Given the medial advancement of both rectus muscles, the linea alba is then reconstructed with a running monofilament suture ventral to the mesh (Fig. 13.22). Occasionally, interrupted figure-of-8 stitches can be placed, especially when restoration of the entire linea alba is uncertain or difficult. The soft tissue is closed in layers. All redundant and attenuated skin and soft tissue should be excised to minimize wound complications. If subcutaneous pockets cannot be eliminated, additional subcutaneous drain(s) are utilized. The skin is closed with a running suture or staples. Areas of tension are reinforced with vertical mattress 000 Nylon sutures.

Post-operative Care

Intra-operative hemodynamics and airway pressures affect post-operative care. Pulmonary plateau pressure has become my most important guide. In patients undergoing complex abdominal

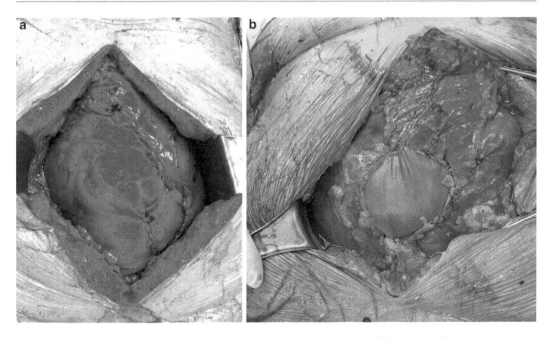

Fig. 13.18 Posterior layer/visceral sac may be patched with an absorbable (**a**) or biologic mesh (**b**)

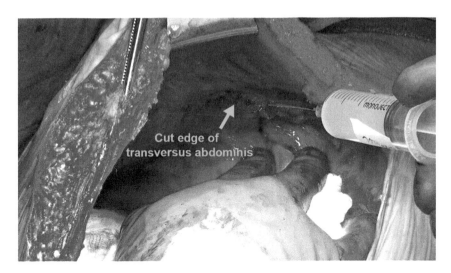

Fig. 13.19 Transversus abdominis plane (TAP) block

wall reconstructions, increase of pulmonary plateau pressure above 6 mmHg necessitates keeping the patient intubated, at least overnight. Provided that myofascial releases are performed, abdominal compliance improves within 12–24 hours post-operatively and pulmonary physiology returns to baseline allowing for safe extubation. In addition, those patients with increase in plateau airway pressures >11 mmHg are kept paralyzed

for 24 hours post-operatively [12]. Please note, we have found that bladder pressure measurements are not as useful in this setting. The closed suction drains are kept in place until the output is <30–50 cm^3 per day. However, for patients with synthetic mesh repairs, I usually remove the drains prior to discharge, even in the setting of higher drain output. This is due to fears of introducing mesh infection (via a drain's direct contact

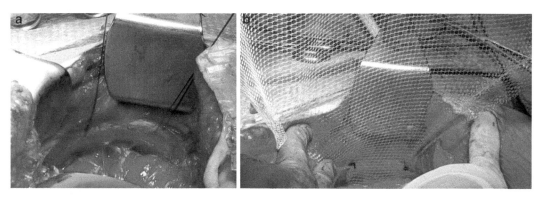

Fig. 13.20 Inferior mesh fixation to Cooper's ligaments. An interrupted monofilament stitch is placed in each of the Cooper's ligaments (**a**) and the tails are passed through the mesh so that the knots are on the dorsal aspect of the mesh (**b**), facilitating mesh overlap in the retro-pubic space

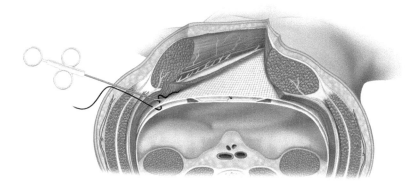

Fig. 13.21 Lateral mesh fixation utilizing a suture-passer. The knots are tied in the subcutaneous space

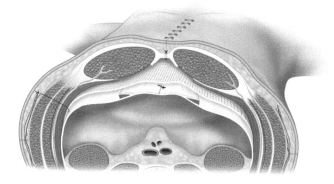

Fig. 13.22 Linea alba is reconstructed ventral to the mesh

Table 13.1 Our validated ventral hernia repair phone survey (VHR-PS)

1.	Do you feel that your hernia is back?
2.	Has any physician told you that your hernia is back?
3.	Do you have a bulge/lump where your hernia used to be?
4.	Do you have any painful areas on your abdominal wall?

with mesh) in the outpatient setting. Alternatively, when a biologic graft is used, the drains are left in place for at least 2 weeks, regardless of the output. The drains are kept longer in the setting of biologics because I found that with increased ambulation after discharge, the drain output increases. Antibiotics are continued for up to 24 hours, unless otherwise indicated. Aggressive deep vein thrombosis prophylaxis is mandatory. I do not use systemic anticoagulation and/or caval filters, unless specifically indicated. Aggressive ambulation is avoided until the second post-operative day. Abdominal binders are used in the early postoperative period. Beyond the first week, their use is liberalized at the patients' discretion. Routine nasogastric tube decompression is avoided. Diet advancement is per our Enhanced Recovery after Surgery (ERAS) protocol [13].

Typical post-operative follow-up consists of a physical exam at 3–4 weeks, 3 months, 6 months, 1 year, and then annually. Abdominal Computed Tomography (CT) scans are obtained routinely at 1 year or earlier to investigate any abdominal discomfort. In addition, we have developed a telephone survey, which is administered to those who miss or are unable to come for a follow-up visit (Table 13.1). We have internally validated this survey to be 100% sensitive, in that no one has ever had a documented recurrence in the setting of all negative responses. Alternatively, any *positive* answer is considered a recurrence until proven otherwise by a physical exam and/or imaging.

Outcomes

The most effective operative approach to complex ventral hernia repairs remains debatable. The TAR procedure allows for safe and reliable medial fascia/rectus muscle advancement and large retromuscular space dissection in patients undergoing major abdominal wall reconstruction. In 2012, I published my first series of 42 patients with massive ventral defects undergoing posterior component release using TAR [9]. Ten (23.8%) patients developed wound complications; requiring re-operation/debridement in three patients. At a median follow up of 26 months, there have been only two (4.7%) recurrences [9]. My recent data on over 400 patients undergoing TAR with synthetic mesh reinforcement revealed 3.7% rate of recurrence at a mean follow up of over 30 months.

The potential deleterious effects of TAR on the lateral abdominal wall and spine stabilization were a matter of early skepticism and concern. However, our recent investigations have alleviated some of those fears. First, we demonstrated rectus muscle hypertrophy following linea alba restoration as well as, very importantly, a compensatory hypertrophy of the external and internal oblique muscles [14]. Furthermore, a dynamometry study revealed an improvement in core abdominal wall functionality post-TAR reconstruction [15]. While the power of the aforementioned results about improvements of the abdominal wall hypertrophy and functionality is insufficient to claim any superiority of TAR, the data clearly support the safety of the division of the transversus abdominis muscle during abdominal wall reconstructions.

Conclusion

Transversus abdominis release is rapidly becoming one of the common approaches to major abdominal wall reconstructions. There are three main advantages to this approach. First, transversus abdominis muscle release results in significant medial mobilization of the posterior rectus sheath and creation of the extraperitoneal pocket. Second, it allows for extensive lateral dissection between the transversus muscle and the underlying transversalis fascia/peritoneum that allows for sublay placement of mesh, reinforcing the entire visceral sac. Finally, it provides for medialization of rectus muscles and linea alba reconstruction in vast majority of complex hernia patients. We found its usefulness in complex scenarios including parastomal, flank, and subxiphoid defects. Furthermore, TAR might be the only reliable approach for patients with failures after open component separation. Overall, the TAR procedure allows not only for a relatively tension-free repair with a large sublay mesh, but also myofascial reconstruction ventral to the mesh, thus markedly minimizing risks of prosthetic infections. Finally, this reconstruction not only provides for a durable repair, but may also facilitate restoration of physiologic properties of the repaired abdominal wall.

References

1. Korenkov M, Sauerland S, Arndt M, Bograd L, Neugebauer EAM, Troidl H. Randomized clinical trial of suture repair, polypropylene mesh or autodermal hernioplasty for incisional hernia. Br J Surg. 2002;89(1):50–6.
2. de Vries Reilingh TS, van Goor H, Charbon JA, Rosman C, Hesselink EJ, van der Wilt GJ, et al. Repair of giant midline abdominal wall hernias: "Components Separation Technique" versus prosthetic repair. World J Surg. 2007;31(4):756–63.
3. Flum DR, Horvath K, Koepsell T. Have outcomes of incisional hernia repair improved with time? A population-based analysis. Ann Surg. 2003;237(1): 129–35.
4. Novitsky YW, Porter JR, Rucho ZC, Getz SB, Pratt BL, Kercher KW, et al. Open preperitoneal retrofascial mesh repair for multiply recurrent ventral incisional hernias. J Am Coll Surg. 2006;203(3):283–9.
5. Stoppa R, Petit J, Abourachid H, Henry X, Duclaye C, Monchaux G, et al. Original procedure of groin hernia repair: interposition without fixation of Dacron tulle prosthesis by subperitoneal median approach. Chirurgie. 1973;99(2):119–23.
6. Mehrabi M, Jangjoo A, Tavoosi H, Kahrom M, Kahrom H. Long-term outcome of Rives-Stoppa technique in complex ventral incisional hernia repair. World J Surg. 2010;34(7):1696–701.
7. Iqbal CW, Pham TH, Joseph A, Mai J, Thompson GB, Sarr MG. Long-term outcome of 254 complex incisional hernia repairs using the modified Rives-Stoppa technique. World J Surg. 2007;31(12): 2398–404.
8. Carbonell AM, Cobb WS, Chen SM. Posterior components separation during retromuscular hernia repair. Hernia. 2008;12(4):359–62.
9. Novitsky YW, Elliott HL, Orenstein SB, Rosen MJ. Transversus abdominis muscle release: a novel approach to posterior component separation during complex abdominal wall reconstruction. Am J Surg. 2012;204(5):709–16.
10. Krpata DM, Blatnik JA, Novitsky YW, Rosen MJ. Posterior and open anterior components separations: a comparative analysis. Am J Surg. 2012;203(3): 318–22.
11. Pauli EM, Wang J, Petro CC, Juza RM, Novitsky YW, Rosen MJ. Posterior component separation with transversus abdominis release successfully addresses recurrent ventral hernias following anterior component separation. Hernia. 2015;19(2):285–91.
12. Petro CC, Raigani S, Fayezizadeh M, Novitsky YW, Rosen MJ. Permissive abdominal hypertension following open incisional hernia repair: a novel concept. Plast Reconstr Surg. 2015;136(4):868–81.
13. Fayezizadeh M, Petro CC, Rosen MJ, Novitsky YW. Enhanced recovery after surgery pathway for abdominal wall reconstruction: pilot study and preliminary outcomes. Plast Reconstr Surg. 2014;134(4 Suppl 2):151S–9S.
14. De Silva GS, Krpata DM, Hicks CW, Criss CN, Gao Y, Rosen MJ, et al. Comparative radiographic analysis of changes in the abdominal wall musculature morphology after open posterior component separation or bridging laparoscopic ventral hernia repair. J Am Coll Surg. 2014;218(3):353–7.
15. Criss CN, Petro CC, Krpata DM, Seafler CM, Lai N, Fiutem J, et al. Functional abdominal wall reconstruction improves core physiology and quality-of-life. Surgery. 2014;156(1):176–82.

Open Anterior Component Separation

Peter Thompson and Albert Losken

Introduction

The method of anterior "components separation" was first described by Ramirez et al. in 1990 [1]. In this elegant anatomic study, the authors described a technique whereby the muscular layers of the anterior abdominal wall could be separated and then medially mobilized in order to achieve closure of large ventral defects, restoring the anatomic relationship of the rectus muscles at the midline.

Though the use of external oblique relaxing incisions was originally described as early as 1916 [2], Ramirez and colleagues are credited with important technical refinements and development of the surgery in common use today. In dissections of ten cadavers, Ramirez et al. described development of the avascular plane between the external and internal oblique muscular layers through relaxing incisions lateral to the rectus sheath. Combined with freeing the rectus from its attachments to the posterior sheath, this technique created myofascial advancement flaps with potential for significant medialization: 5 cm at the epigastrium, 10 cm at the waist, and 3 cm in the suprapubic region per side, allowing clo-

sure of defects up to 20 cm in diameter at the waist. They went on to describe a series of eleven patients with abdominal wall hernias of various etiologies including trauma, infected prostheses, and TRAM defects.

Prior to popularization of component separation and the availability of acellular dermal matrix, ventral defects which could not be closed by en bloc mobilization of the abdominal wall required placement of bridging synthetic mesh to prevent loss of abdominal domain, a technique which exposed patients to the potential of mesh infection, extrusion, fistulization, and high hernia recurrence rates [3–5]. Defects with inadequate fascial or soft tissue coverage were addressed with the inventive use of autologous tissue transfers such as the free or pedicled tensor fascia lata flap [6, 7], also with significant associated morbidity and hernia recurrence. The development of component separation therefore represented an important advance with major implications for the care of patients with this difficult surgical problem.

The goal of component separation in abdominal wall reconstruction is a tension-free re-approximation of the linea alba, thereby restoring the normal anatomic relationship of the abdominal wall muscles and off-loading the constant lateral pull of the oblique and transverse muscular system. Anterior component separation is indicated for the repair of large abdominal wall defects of any etiology; two of the most common indications include the multiply recurrent ventral hernia resulting in a hostile abdomen in which

P. Thompson, M.D. (✉) • A. Losken, M.D.
Emory Division of Plastic and Reconstructive Surgery, Emory University,
3200 Downwood Circle, Suite 640-A, Atlanta, GA 30327, USA
e-mail: pwthomp@emory.edu; alosken@emory.edu

© Springer International Publishing Switzerland 2016
Y.W. Novitsky (ed.), *Hernia Surgery*, DOI 10.1007/978-3-319-27470-6_14

laparoscopic repair would be contraindicated, and abdominal trauma managed with damage control laparotomy resulting in "planned" ventral hernia. Both etiologies may be complicated by loss of abdominal domain and often occur in the setting of a contaminated field (such as infection of previously placed mesh or enterocutaneous fistula). In such situations, component separation is an indispensible tool to restore normal abdominal wall physiology and provide a durable repair.

Outcomes

Despite widespread acceptance and application of the technique, anterior component separation remains an operation plagued by high surgical morbidity. This is likely a function of both the surgery itself and the general poor state of health of many of the candidates for abdominal wall reconstruction. Common complications are the logical sequelae of large myofascial and subcutaneous flap elevation and include seroma, hematoma, infection, skin edge necrosis, wound breakdown, and hernia recurrence. Recurrence rates following anterior components separation range from 5 to 32% in major series; rates of wound complications range from 7.5 to 48%. These outcomes are summarized in Table 14.1.

Current Trends

Since the original description by Ramirez et al., various modifications of the components separation technique have been proposed in order to reduce surgical morbidity. Several of these innovations, including the type and position of mesh to be used in reinforcement of repair and the use of minimally invasive techniques for component release, continue to be topics of discussion and debate.

Minimal Dissection Technique

As originally described by Ramirez, separation of the abdominal wall components involves significant subcutaneous undermining from the midline to the level of the semilunar line in order to achieve exposure of the external oblique. The large potential space created after raising this flap predisposes to postoperative fluid collection, with rates up to 11.6% for hematoma [8] and 10% for seroma [9]. In addition, undermining of the skin and subcutaneous tissues necessitates division of lipocutaneous perforators, particularly in the periumbilical region, resulting in a relatively devascularized flap. This can increase the rate of skin necrosis and ischemia, which can complicate up to 20% of anterior component separation repairs [9]. Modifications of the traditional open anterior components separation have been suggested which provide exposure of the external oblique without the need for aggressive subcutaneous undermining. These include use of either longitudinal [10] or transverse [11] paramedian incisions to access the external oblique aponeurosis lateral to the semilunar line. Endoscopic-assisted minimally invasive release of the external oblique has also been described [12]. Despite differences in technique, the common goal of each of these modifications is preservation of the periumbilical perforators, an important blood supply to the midline abdominal skin. Periumbilical perforator-sparing techniques have been associated with decreased rates of wound healing complications, including skin necrosis and infection [13]. While minimal undermining and skin flap dissection may be preferable, there are clearly clinical scenarios in which preservation of periumbilical perforators is not possible. In very large hernias with loss of abdominal domain, retracted skin edges may tether the abdominal wall, and fascial approximation at the midline may not be possible without full release of the skin and subcutaneous tissue from the underlying layers. Also, in the setting of multiple previous abdominal operations, previous mesh onlay or previous component release, periumbilical perforators may have already been divided or no clear dissection plane may exist.

Type of Mesh: Synthetic vs. Biologic

In the original description of the components separation technique by Ramirez et al., fascial layers were reapproximated primarily in the mid-

Table 14.1 Outcomes following anterior component separation

Author (year)	Number of patients undergoing ACS	Mean follow-up (months)	Number of recurrences (%)	Number of wound complications (%)	Comments
Girotto et al. (1999) [8]	37	21	2 (6.1)	11 (30)	ACS without mesh
Saulis et al. (2002) [9]	66	12	5 (7.6)	9 (14)	ACS with or without PUP-sparing
DeVries Reilingh et al. (2003) [10]	43	15.6	12 (32)	15 (35)	ACS without mesh
Girotto et al. (2003) [11]	96	26	22 (23)	25 (26)	ACS with mesh onlay "when necessary"
Jernigan et al. (2003) [12]	73	24	4 (5.5)	–	ACS after open abdomen, most without mesh
Lowe et al. (2003) [13]	30	9.5	3 (10)	35 (?)	ACS mostly without mesh
Gonzales et al. (2005) [14]	42	16	3 (7)	14 (33)	LR vs. ACS; with and without mesh
Espinosa-de-los-Monteros et al. (2007) [15]	37	13	2 (5)	10 (26)	ACS with ADM onlay
Ko et al. (2009) [16]	200	10.3	43 (21)	38–86 (19–43)	ACS via lateral access incisions; no mesh, ADM or soft synthetic mesh as underlay
Sailes et al. (2010) [17]	545	–	100 (18)	41 (7.5)	ACS with various mesh types over 10 years
Ghazi et al. (2011) [18]	75	34	10 (13)	9 (12)	ACS with and without mesh
Krpata et al. (2012) [19]	56	9.1	8 (14)	27 (48)	PCS vs. ACS with mesh underlay

ACS anterior component separation, *PUP* periumbilical perforator, *LR* laparoscopic repair, *ADM* acellular dermal matrix, *PCS* posterior component separation

line without mesh reinforcement. This resulted in a hernia recurrence rate of up to 53% at 7 months [14]. In agreement with widely accepted principles for repair of incisional hernias [15, 16], mesh reinforcement of components separation appears to decrease hernia recurrence to as low as 5% [17]. Various types of synthetic and biologic mesh have been used as adjuncts to component separation, each with distinct advantages and disadvantages. Synthetic materials such as polypropylene have been available for use for decades. While the strength of this material may provide long-lasting protection from recurrence compared to biologic materials [11, 18], synthetic permanent mesh is often contraindicated in the contaminated field. It creates a dense inflammatory reaction that can predispose to infection, adhesion formation, and enterocutaneous fistula formation [3]. In contrast, biologic materials such as human or porcine acellular dermal matrix are generally considered safe to use in the contaminated field. These materials incorporate, revascularize, and remodel with host tissue after implantation, with minimal host inflammatory response. Biologics have been used in situations where permanent synthetic mesh is contraindicated but appears to have a tendency to stretch over time [19], resulting in recurrence rates that in some series were higher than that observed with no mesh at all [11]. The type of mesh selected for reinforcement of a components separation repair depends on numerous variables including patient comorbidities, the presence of contamination, or infection in the surgical field and the size of the hernia defect. When used correctly, the biologic mesh can provide the benefits of synthetic mesh closure through reinforcement and tension reduction, without the infection risks often associated with synthetic mesh.

Mesh Position

The position for mesh placement is also a source of debate. Investigators have described reinforcement of component separation-based abdominal wall reconstructions using mesh placed in onlay [20], underlay [11], bridging [9], or sublay (retrorectus) [21] positions. Other authors have described using a combination of these approaches for a so-called "sandwich" repair [21]. There are clearly advantages and disadvantages to each technique. For example, by placing a layer of tissue between bowel and mesh, the onlay technique theoretically decreases risk of bowel-to-mesh adhesion and enteric fistula formation. This technique also avoids the need for more extensive intraperitoneal dissection and adhesiolysis, making it a preferable option in the setting of the hostile abdomen. However, a recent review of the available literature regarding mesh position suggests that compared to the underlay position, mesh placed in the onlay position had a higher incidence of overall complications and hernia recurrence regardless of the type of mesh used [22].

Personal Algorithms and Technique

Preoperative Evaluation

Patients with large abdominal wall defects often experience significant deformity, pain, and decreased energy due to loss of normal abdomi-

nal wall mechanics, severely impacting their quality of life; however, it is important to remember that abdominal wall reconstruction is always an elective procedure, and one with potential for significant morbidity. Therefore, candidates should be chosen based on their overall likelihood of a successful repair balanced against their risk of surgical or medical complication. Patient selection for abdominal wall reconstruction with components separation begins with a thorough history and physical exam.

Careful attention should be paid to patients' medical comorbidities, in particular diabetes, smoking, and morbid obesity, all of which increase the risk of wound complications and hernia recurrence. The importance of preoperative counseling cannot be over-stressed, and patients should be encouraged to correct modifiable risk factors with tight blood glucose control, smoking cessation and weight loss as possible. For an elective surgery which will usually require considerable operative risk, complicated postoperative care and considerable use of hospital resources, it is reasonable to request that patients make an effort to stack the odds in their favor by losing weight and stopping smoking prior to being scheduled for surgery. Preexisting cardiac and pulmonary comorbidities necessitate preoperative consultation with the appropriate specialist in order to ensure medical optimization and fitness to undergo major surgery. Malnutrition is an equally prevalent problem in patients who may be chronically debilitated from multiple previous operations and prolonged hospital stays. Every effort should be made to optimize nutritional status as determined by trends in weight and laboratory markers such as albumin, prealbumin, and transferrin.

Likewise, a detailed knowledge of the patient's surgical history is essential for success. For patients with multiply recurrent ventral hernias, careful attention to the number and technique of previous hernia repairs, the location and type of any previously placed mesh, and the location of any scars on the anterior abdominal wall will help shape the intraoperative plan and guide technique and mesh selection (Fig. 14.1).

Preoperative imaging with CT or MRI of the abdomen can provide essential information about

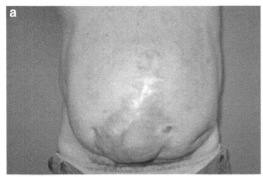
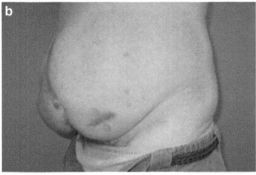
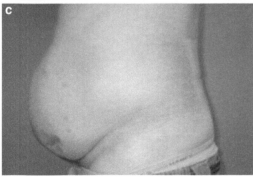

Fig. 14.1 (**a**) Anterior (**b**) oblique and (**c**) lateral preoperative photos of a patient scheduled for component separation. This middle-aged male had a history of multiple previous failed hernia repairs secondary to mesh infections, resulting in a large ventral hernia with relative loss of domain

the anatomy of the anterior abdominal musculature, position of previously placed mesh, and location of any stomas or enterocutaneous fistulas (Fig. 14.2). Most importantly for large midline defects, preoperative imaging can precisely measure the distance between the true fascial edges. In general, a full separation of anterior components can be expected to produce a unilateral rectus sheath advancement of 10–15 cm at the waistline; therefore, fascial approximation of midline defects

up to 30 cm can be obtained with a full bilateral release. Less advancement is expected in the epigastric and suprapubic regions, around 5–8 cm and 3–6 cm respectively per side. The presence of a stoma, history of previous component release, or large defects in the upper or lower thirds of the abdomen may therefore preclude repair with anterior components separation alone. Preoperative imaging can help make this important determination before entering the operating room. In our practice, all patients being considered for abdominal wall reconstruction undergo some form of preoperative cross-sectional imaging. Other preoperative evaluation includes laboratory assessment of hematologic indices, serum chemistry, and nutritional markers as well as EKG and plain film chest X-ray for high-risk patients.

Timing of abdominal wall reconstruction is critical. As mentioned previously, the most common indications for components separation repair at our institution include the open abdomen after trauma with loss of abdominal domain and the multiply recurrent incisional hernia. Both of these conditions often occur in association with enterocutaneous fistulae, infected mesh, or an otherwise contaminated field. The posttraumatic open abdomen is often managed at our institution using a staged approach as previously described [23]; patients become candidates for definitive abdominal wall reconstruction 6–12 months after creation of the "planned" hernia defect by placement of split thickness skin graft on top of exposed viscera. After this period of time, inflammation and dense adhesions generally resolve and the skin graft can usually be dissected easily from the underlying bowel. A simple test to determine a patient's readiness for definitive reconstruction is the "pinch test." If the grafted skin can be easily picked up with the thumb and index finger and pinched with no intervening bowel, then surgery may safely proceed. Similarly, in the setting of recurrent ventral incisional hernias, a waiting period of at least 6 months is advisable following the most recent attempt at hernia repair; component separation or any other definitive reconstruction attempted in the setting of acute inflammation will be more likely to fail secondary to poor tissue strength.

Fig. 14.2 Preoperative cross-sectional imaging with computed tomography (CT) demonstrating (**a**) thin, attenuated fascia over previously placed mesh (*yellow arrow*) and (**b**) significant rectus muscle diastasis/hernia recurrence (*yellow arrows*)

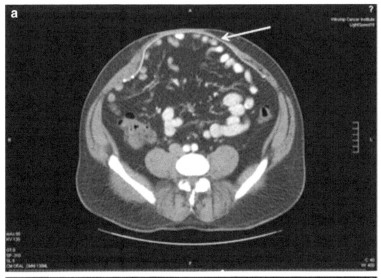

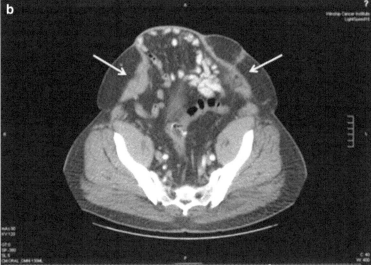

Surgical Technique

At our institution, most abdominal wall reconstructions are performed in careful coordination with a general surgery team. Patients are maintained NPO after midnight on the eve of surgery. Bowel preparation is performed at the discretion of the general surgeon. In the operative suite, patients are positioned supine with arms out. Appropriate monitoring devices are placed by the anesthesia team. Hair is removed from the operative site with clippers and the skin is prepped with chlorhexidene solution. The field is widely prepped and draped from nipples to upper thigh and to the level of the bed over each flank. Thin strips of Ioban (3M; St. Paul, MN) are often useful to secure drapes in place during these long procedures. Thromboembolic prophylaxis with sequential compression devices on the lower extremities is essential.

The operation begins usually with a full midline laparotomy followed by extensive lysis of adhesions performed by the general surgery team. The general surgery portion of the procedure also includes excision of any previously placed or infected prosthetic material, take down and repair of enterocutaneous fistulae, and bowel resections as indicated.

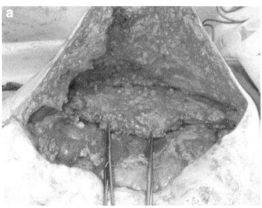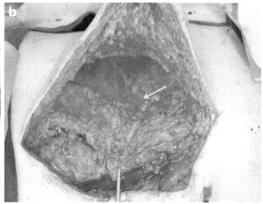

Fig. 14.3 Intraoperative photos. (**a**) After lysis of adhesions, the fascial edges are grasped with Kocher clamps and a lipocutaneous flap raised. (**b**) The external oblique aponeurosis is then incised lateral to the rectus muscle bundle. The medial cut edge of external oblique aponeurosis is designated by the *yellow arrow*

The plastic surgery team begins the reconstructive portion of the procedure with assessment of the resultant defect. The edges of the rectus sheath are grasped with Kocher clamps and pulled bilaterally toward the midline in order to determine how much advancement is necessary to recreate the linea alba (Fig. 14.3a). Identification of the true fascial edge is often difficult in the presence of dense scar, and careful dissection is often needed to locate the rectus sheath. This is an essential step as misidentification and subsequent approximation of scar tissue instead of fascia will almost certainly result in hernia recurrence.

The next step is determined by the size of the defect to be reconstructed. Often, after lysis of adhesions and freeing attachments of viscera to the overlying abdominal wall, primary approximation of fascial edges may be possible without any component release. In this instance, a mesh-reinforced primary repair is performed, with a components release added if needed to reduce midline tension. Most commonly for defects 10–30 cm in width, recreation of the linea alba will not be possible without component release. An anterior component separation is performed in the following fashion, originally described by Ramirez [1]. The fascial edge of the side to be released is grasped with a Kocher and retracted toward the midline. Counter-traction is applied by the assistant who retracts the skin edge with either a toothed forcep or handheld retractor.

Dissection proceeds in a subcutaneous plane just above the rectus fascia to a point 1–2 cm lateral to the linea semilunaris, from the costal margin superiorly to the anterior superior iliac spine (ASIS) inferiorly. The external oblique aponeurosis is incised at this lateral point along the entire length of the dissection (Fig. 14.3b). Confirmation of position lateral to the linea semilunaris can be obtained by manually palpating the rectus muscle or by making a small nick in the fascia and examining the orientation of the underlying muscle fibers. Obliquely oriented fibers of the internal oblique muscle should be visible. Dissection then proceeds in the avascular plane between the internal and external oblique laterally to the mid-axillary line. Following completion of unilateral release, the bilateral fascial edges are again grasped and pulled together to check midline approximation. If a tension-free recreation of the linea alba is now possible, contralateral component release is not necessary. Avoiding contralateral dissection preserves this plane for future reconstructive procedures in the event of recurrence, and decreases the likelihood of abdominal wall necrosis, seroma formation and a lateral bulge. If tension-free approximation is not possible with unilateral external oblique release, a bilateral release is performed. If following bilateral external oblique release approximation is still inadequate, a posterior rectus sheath relaxing incision may be made as described by Ramirez

[1], however in our experience this maneuver will add only 1–2 cm of advancement at most.

Our experience [24] and that of others [17, 25] has demonstrated that an abdominal components separation repair reinforced with mesh has a lower rate of recurrence than a non-reinforced repair; for this reason, we consider mesh reinforcement an essential step in an anterior component separation repair. Our preference in clean and some clean-contaminated situations such as bowel resection or presence of a stoma is to use synthetic mesh such as lightweight polypropylene (Prolene®, Ethicon) or a composite mesh of polyester and non-adherent collagen film (Parietex™, Covidien) given superior strength and lower risk of recurrence of synthetics. In contaminated cases, such as removal of infected mesh or gross spillage of enteric contents, our preference is to use a porcine acellular dermal matrix. Whenever possible, mesh is placed in an intraperitoneal underlay position in order to decrease the risk of mesh contamination and seroma. It is our feeling that an underlay provides a stronger repair than mesh placed in an onlay position. The mesh is fashioned into the shape of a diamond and secured in position with transfascial U-stitches of #1 Prolene (Fig. 14.4a). The first stitches are placed at the four corners of the diamond, left untied and secured with hemostats in order to set the appropriate tension on the mesh. Additional stitches are then placed at intervals of 2–3 cm around one lateral border of the mesh (Fig. 14.4b). All sutures are controlled with hemostats and tied after all are in place, taking care that no viscera are entrapped during tying. The repair should then be probed with a finger to ensure that no gaps remain between sutures through which a loop of bowel might slip. Additional sutures are placed as needed to fill in these gaps. This process is repeated on the contralateral border of the mesh. The mesh should overlap the rectus to the external oblique for a distance of at least 4 cm and should tension the myofascial flaps in such a way as to offload the midline approximation. When the mesh is in place, the medial edges of the rectus sheath may be sutured together over the mesh using a #1 PDS in an interrupted or running fashion (Fig. 14.4c).

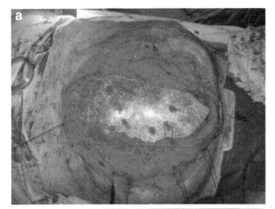
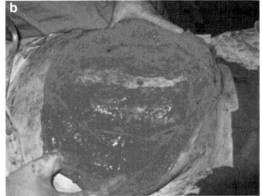
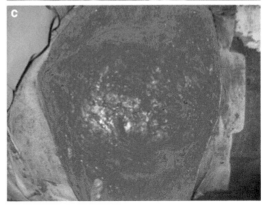

Fig. 14.4 A mesh underlay is performed with a large piece of acellular dermal matrix. (**a**) Widely spaced, interrupted #1 Prolene transfascial sutures are used to set the appropriate mesh tension. (**b**) The mesh is then secured circumferentially with additional transfascial sutures. (**c**) The overlying fascia is primarily reapproximated in the midline and sutured with interrupted or running #1 PDS suture

Subcutaneous closed suction drains are placed and brought out through the inferior skin lateral to the laparotomy incision. The skin is closed with staples.

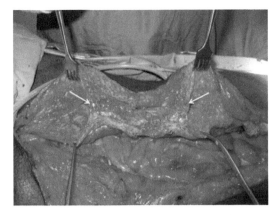

Fig. 14.5 Important perforators supplying the abdominal wall skin may be spared during anterior component separation by avoiding dissection in the periumbilical region (between *yellow arrows*). A tunnel can be created lateral to these perforators through which the external oblique relaxing incision can be made

Several unique situations deserve mention. As described previously, several authors have endorsed a periumbilical perforator-sparing approach during elevation of skin flaps [13] in order to decrease rates of seroma, skin edge necrosis, and subsequent wound healing complications. This technique is particularly useful in patients at risk for poor soft tissue perfusion such as those with peripheral vascular disease, smoking history, diabetes, and the super-obese. In our practice, we attempt to preserve perfusion of the abdominal wall in this population as much as possible through use of minimal skin flap elevation and avoidance of dissection in the periumbilical region (Fig. 14.5); however, there are two situations in which this approach is less useful. In the patient with multiple previous hernia repairs or a previous component release, the periumbilical blood supply may have already been divided. In addition, some patients (i.e., the skin-grafted trauma patient) may not have adequate skin coverage of fascia without full elevation of the skin laterally to the anterior axillary line, creating an additional sliding flap of soft tissue that can then be approximated at the midline. Other options if soft tissue coverage is inadequate include pedicled flaps such as a tensor fascia lata (TFL) or anterolateral thigh (ALT) flap, or if inadequate skin is suspected preoperatively abdominal wall tissue expanders may be used.

Postoperative Management

Postoperatively, patients are often left intubated and monitored in the ICU. Drains are placed to wall suction for anywhere from 24 hours to 5 days postoperatively depending on the extent of dissection and the surgeon's preference, and then placed to bulb suction. Perioperative antibiotics are continued for 24 hours after surgery. Some surgeons prefer continuation of antibiotics throughout the recovery period for as long as drains are in place. Postoperative imaging is often obtained at the surgeon's discretion to provide a baseline for future follow-up (Fig. 14.6).

Conclusion

Separation of abdominal components has become an essential and powerful weapon in the armamentarium of surgeons across specialties, gaining widespread popularity for the closure of abdominal wall defects resulting from trauma, infection, and previous surgery. This technique has been utilized for a variety of problems with reproducible, consistent outcomes. Further refinements by surgical innovators continue to reduce morbidity and hernia recurrence.

References

1. Ramirez OM, Ruas E, Dellon AL. "Components separation" method for closure of abdominal-wall defects: an anatomic and clinical study. Plast Reconstr Surg. 1990;86(3):519–26.
2. Gibson CL. Post-operative intestinal obstruction. Ann Surg. 1916;63(4):442–51.
3. Leber GE, Garb JL, Alexander AI, Reed WP. Long-term complications associated with prosthetic repair of incisional hernias. Arch Surg. 1998;133(4):378–82.
4. de Vries Reilingh TS, van Geldere D, Langenhorst B, de Jong D, van der Wilt GJ, van Goor H, et al. Repair of large midline incisional hernias with polypropylene mesh: comparison of three operative techniques. Hernia. 2004;8(1):56–9.
5. Lichtenstein IL, Shore JM. Repair of recurrent ventral hernias by an internal "binder". Am J Surg. 1976;132(1):121–5.
6. Williams JK, Carlson GW, deChalain T, Howell R, Coleman JJ. Role of tensor fasciae latae in abdominal wall reconstruction. Plast Reconstr Surg. 1998;101(3):713–8.

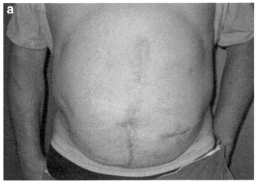

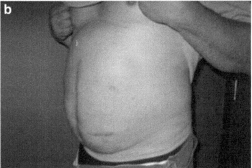

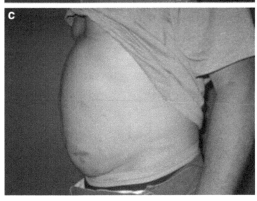

Fig. 14.6 (**a**) Anterior (**b**) oblique and (**c**) lateral postoperative photos following anterior component separation with mesh underlay

7. Williams JK, Carlson GW, Howell RL, Wagner JD, Nahai F, Coleman JJ. The tensor fascia lata free flap in abdominal-wall reconstruction. J Reconstr Microsurg. 1997;13(2):83–90. discussion 90-81.

8. de Vries Reilingh TS, van Goor H, Rosman C, Bemelmans MH, de Jong D, van Nieuwenhoven EJ, et al. "Components separation technique" for the repair of large abdominal wall hernias. J Am Coll Surg. 2003;196(1):32–7.

9. Lowe III JB, Lowe JB, Baty JD, Garza JR. Risks associated with "components separation" for closure of complex abdominal wall defects. Plast Reconstr Surg. 2003;111(3):1276–83. quiz 1284-1275; discussion 1286-1278.

10. Maas SM, van Engeland M, Leeksma NG, Bleichrodt RP. A modification of the "components separation" technique for closure of abdominal wall defects in the presence of an enterostomy. J Am Coll Surg. 1999;189(1):138–40.

11. Ko JH, Wang EC, Salvay DM, Paul BC, Dumanian GA. Abdominal wall reconstruction: lessons learned from 200 "components separation" procedures. Arch Surg. 2009;144(11):1047–55.

12. Lowe JB, Garza JR, Bowman JL, Rohrich RJ, Strodel WE. Endoscopically assisted "components separation" for closure of abdominal wall defects. Plast Reconstr Surg. 2000;105(2):720–9. quiz 730.

13. Saulis AS, Dumanian GA. Periumbilical rectus abdominis perforator preservation significantly reduces superficial wound complications in "separation of parts" hernia repairs. Plast Reconstr Surg. 2002;109(7):2275–80. discussion 2281-2272.

14. de Vries Reilingh TS, van Goor H, Charbon JA, Rosman C, Hesselink EJ, van der Wilt GJ, et al. Repair of giant midline abdominal wall hernias: "components separation technique" versus prosthetic repair: interim analysis of a randomized controlled trial. World J Surg. 2007;31(4):756–63.

15. Burger JW, Luijendijk RW, Hop WC, Halm JA, Verdaasdonk EG, Jeekel J. Long-term follow-up of a randomized controlled trial of suture versus mesh repair of incisional hernia. Ann Surg. 2004;240(4):578–83. discussion 583-575.

16. den Hartog D, Dur AH, Tuinebreijer WE, Kreis RW. Open surgical procedures for incisional hernias. Cochrane Database Syst Rev. 2008;(3):CD006438.

17. Espinosa-de-los-Monteros A, de la Torre JI, Marrero I, Andrades P, Davis MR, Vasconez LO. Utilization of human cadaveric acellular dermis for abdominal hernia reconstruction. Ann Plast Surg. 2007;58(3):264–7.

18. Ko JH, Salvay DM, Paul BC, Wang EC, Dumanian GA. Soft polypropylene mesh, but not cadaveric dermis, significantly improves outcomes in midline hernia repairs using the components separation technique. Plast Reconstr Surg. 2009;124(3):836–47.

19. Schuster R, Singh J, Safadi BY, Wren SM. The use of acellular dermal matrix for contaminated abdominal wall defects: wound status predicts success. Am J Surg. 2006;192(5):594–7.

20. Sailes FC, Walls J, Guelig D, Mirzabeigi M, Long WD, Crawford A, et al. Synthetic and biological mesh in component separation: a 10-year single institution review. Ann Plast Surg. 2010;64(5):696–8.

21. Pauli EM, Rosen MJ. Open ventral hernia repair with component separation. Surg Clin North Am. 2013;93(5):1111–33.

22. Albino FP, Patel KM, Nahabedian MY, Sosin M, Attinger CE, Bhanot P. Does mesh location matter in abdominal wall reconstruction? A systematic review of the literature and a summary of recommendations. Plast Reconstr Surg. 2013;132(5):1295–304.

23. Jernigan TW, Fabian TC, Croce MA, Moore N, Pritchard FE, Minard G, et al. Staged management of giant abdominal wall defects: acute and long-term

results. Ann Surg. 2003;238(3):349–55. discussion 355-347.

24. Ghazi B, Deigni O, Yezhelyev M, Losken A. Current options in the management of complex abdominal wall defects. Ann Plast Surg. 2011;66(5):488–92.

25. Holton III LH, Kim D, Silverman RP, Rodriguez ED, Singh N, Goldberg NH. Human acellular dermal matrix for repair of abdominal wall defects: review of clinical experience and experimental data. J Long Term Eff Med Implants. 2005;15(5):547–58.

Endoscopic Anterior Component Separation

15

David Earle

Introduction

The term component separation has no single meaning. It currently refers to some sort of tissue rearrangement of the trunk for the purposes of restoration of linea alba, usually for hernia repair. In this chapter, I will discuss the separation of the internal and external oblique muscles, and the separation, or division, of the insertion of the external oblique along its aponeurosis lateral to the rectus muscle. This was first described for hernia repair by Dr. Young in 1961, but without the separation of the oblique muscles [1]. It wasn't until 1990 when Dr. Ramirez described the modern day technique that also separated the oblique muscles [2]. They coined the term "component separation" to describe their technique. Finally, in 2000, Dr. Lowe and colleagues described an endoscopi-

cally assisted technique for the external oblique separation, which dramatically reduced wound complications [3].

Indications

The purpose of component separation is usually aimed at medialization of the rectus muscles and reduction of the intra-operative tension on the closure of midline hernia defects. To this day, this rationale for performing this technique is consistently discussed. The determination of intra-operative tension, however, is subjective, typically determined by the surgeon pulling the medial borders of the rectus muscles toward the midline, and making a tension estimate. In my opinion, the appropriate tension estimated by the surgeon in the operating room with the patient supine, and under general anesthesia, is inaccurate as it does not take into account postoperative tension. In my practice, endoscopic component separation (ECS) technique is used for patients who have midline larger midline hernias, with the goal of hernia repair *and* restoration of a normal abdominal wall contour. Distance between the rectus muscles should be at least 5 cm in width. For defect widths in the 5–10 cm, there will be significant variability in abdominal wall contour abnormalities and goals of repair; thus, the component separation technique is used less frequently than it would be for defects greater than 10 cm in width [4].

Electronic supplementary material: The online version of this chapter (doi:10.1007/978-3-319-27470-6_15) contains supplementary material, which is available to authorized users.

D. Earle, M.D., F.A.C.S. (✉)
Tufts University School of Medicine,
Springfield, MA, USA
e-mail: davidearle59@gmail.com

Technique

The decision about whether or not to perform an ECS is made preoperatively, based on patient goals, history, abdominal wall contour, midline location, and the distance between rectus muscles.

Patient Position

The patient is positioned supine, with the arms tucked at the sides. Occasionally, we will simply swing the arm boards to the patient's side, then swing it back out for the open portion of the procedure. This is more helpful with obese patients. All appropriate precautions should be taken to avoid inadvertent injury to the upper extremity.

Access and Muscle Separation

We usually perform the ECS as the first part of the procedure to reduce the time the laparotomy incision is open. If there is a transverse/oblique incision, or ostomy on one side, we will do the side without incisions first. The initial 2–4 cm incision is made transversely, near the costal margin, near the tip of the 11th rib. This is more lateral than you would anticipate, and we often tilt the table away from us to improve exposure and ergonomics. The monopolar pencil with a protected electrode is used to divide the subcutaneous fascia, and three "S" shaped retractors are used. The external oblique muscle fibers (not aponeurosis) are then positively identified, and bluntly separated until the most posterior fibers are sliding free from the underlying internal oblique. The internal oblique fascia will appear white, although it is quite thin (Fig 15.1a, b). While it is possible to start on the external oblique aponeurosis, this area carries a higher risk to divide all the way through common junction of the oblique muscles, and is more difficult to use as an effective port site because it is near the insertion of the external oblique, which is divided as part of the release. We also start on the muscle belly when performing open external oblique release.

Once the space between the oblique muscles has been accessed, one of the "S" shaped retractors is placed under the external oblique to lift it off the internal oblique. A round balloon dissector (Covidien; North Haven, CT; USA) is introduced and pushed blindly toward the ipsilateral groin along a trajectory that takes it 2–3 cm medial of the anterior superior iliac spine. It is important to note that while the balloon is being pushed toward the inguinal ligament, the tip should be angled anteriorly to avoid going through the internal oblique. Once the tip of the balloon is near the inguinal ligament, it is inflated and deflated 3–4 times, beginning distally and moving proximally. While there is no specific amount of air introduced, or number of pumps of the inflator, there is both visual inspection and palpation of the size of the balloon as it is being distended. If there is any doubt, under distention is better than over distention, which can tear the muscle fibers of the internal oblique (Fig. 15.2a, b). The balloon is then removed, the introducer reinserted, and after elevating the external oblique with an "S" retractor, is redirected above the costal margin. I initially use the uninflated balloon in a back-and-forth motion above the costal margin before inflation, and inflate the balloon less than inferiorly. Usually, only one to two inflation sequences are required here (Fig. 15.3a, b).

Port Placement

After separating the oblique muscles with balloon dissector, I place a 12 mm blunt-tipped AirSeal™ port (Surgiquest; Orange, CT; USA) through the incision, and insufflate to 12 mmHg with CO_2. I used to use a round balloon-tipped port (Covidien; North Haven, CT; USA), but the balloon often impeded the view of the external oblique insertion, and is easily damaged by energy sources. With the AirSeal™ port and insufflation system, impedance of the external oblique insertion, smoke evacuation, or loss of insufflation with a gas leak are rare. Once the space is insufflated, visual inspection confirms whether the correct plane was dissected, and whether or not there has been any injury to the muscle belly of the internal oblique. We then place two 5 mm ports under direct visualization—one medial, and inferior to the anterior superior iliac spine, and

a

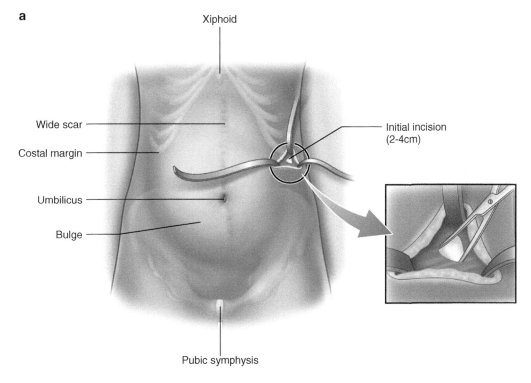

b

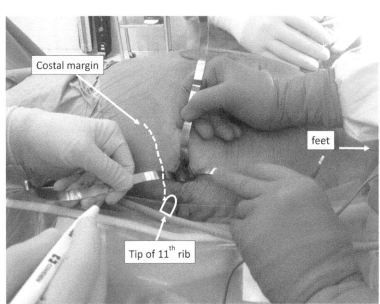

Fig. 15.1 The location of the initial incision is near the tip of the 11th rib, and its size will be dependent on the amount of subcutaneous fat (2–4 cm). The blunt tipped clamp will spread the external oblique fibers and allow visualization of the whitish fascia over the internal oblique. The "S" retractor can be used to start the dissection between the obliques and lift the external oblique to allow introduction of the dissection balloon. (**a**) Access is illustrated in the *left upper quadrant*. (**b**) Photo depicts access in the *right upper quadrant*

Fig. 15.2 Lift the external oblique anteriorly and insert the balloon dissector toward the inguinal ligament, passing just medial to the anterior superior iliac spine (ASIS). It is important to keep the tip pressure anteriorly and lateral to avoid inadvertent penetration through the internal oblique or common junction. The tip should be inserted all the way to, but not through the inguinal ligament. The balloon is then serially inflated and deflated beginning distally and moving proximally to the area under the initial insertion site. Then remove the dissector and reassemble. There is no specific amount that the balloon should be distended; however, under-inflation is generally less risky than over-inflation. (**a**) Placing the balloon dissector on the *left side*. (**b**) Placing the balloon dissector on *right side*

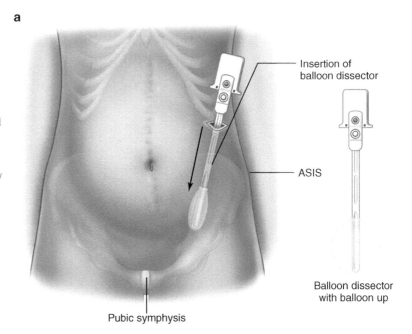

Insertion of balloon dissector

ASIS

Balloon dissector with balloon up

Pubic symphysis

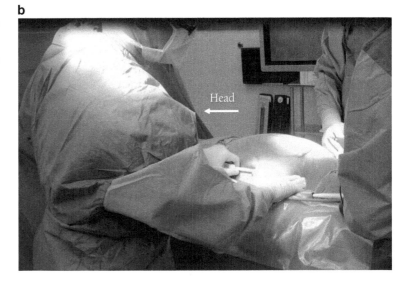

Head

one in between, at the same lateral margin as the 12 mm port. The superior and inferior ports are for the scope, and the middle port is used for the instruments used to divide the external oblique insertion (Fig. 15.4a, b).

Troubleshooting

If the initial inspection reveals an injury to the internal oblique muscle, an assessment must be made about the severity. If just the fascia is torn,

Fig. 15.3 After beginning the superior dissection over the costal margin with the index finger, the balloon dissector is then reinserted superiorly, also over the costal margin, again keeping the pressure on the tip anterior and slightly lateral. It generally only takes one to two inflation-deflation sequences with less distention than inferiorly. Generally, under-inflation is less risky than over-inflation. (**a**) Placing balloon dissector on *left side*. (**b**) Placing the balloon dissector on *right side*. (**c**) Inflating the balloon dissector on the *right side*

a

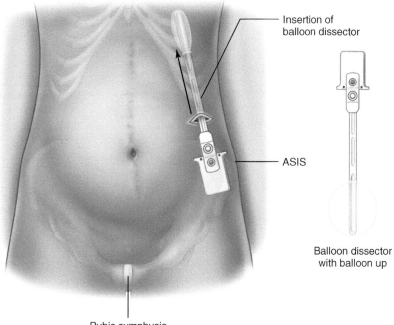

Insertion of
balloon dissector

ASIS

Balloon dissector
with balloon up

Pubic symphysis

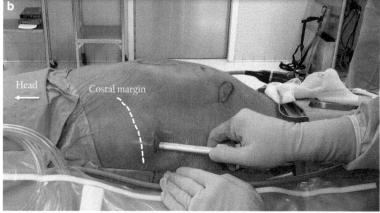

Head

Costal margin

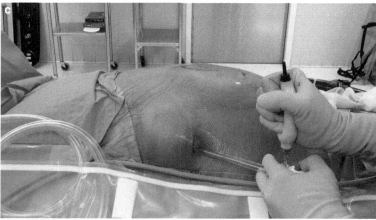

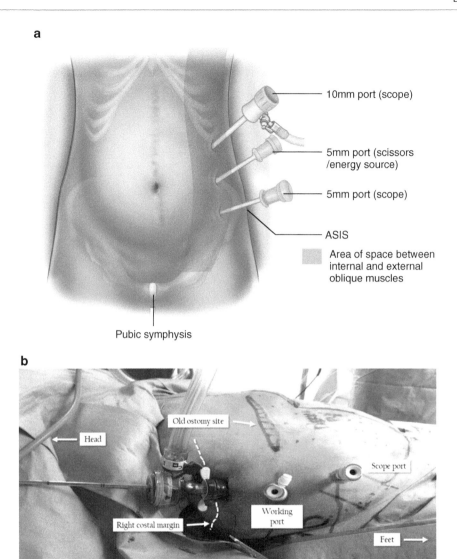

Fig. 15.4 The ports are all placed laterally, with the superior and inferior ports being used for the scope and the middle port used for the dissection and cutting instruments. With no specimen extraction, all 5 mm ports could be used. We use a 10–12 mm port superiorly to take advantage of a unique AirSeal™ insufflation system or blunt, balloon tipped port. As smaller ports with these features become available, the size could be scaled down. (**a**) *Left sided* port set-up. (**b**) *Right sided* port set-up. Note the slight medial placement of the inferior port. This allows for less interference of the field of view by the instrument in the working port. An angled rigid or flexible tip scope can also help avoid this

but the muscle belly is largely intact, nothing needs to be done. If there is significant disruption of the muscle belly, it should be repaired with long acting absorbable suture, and consideration for covering the defect with a prosthetic in this space, or as part of the hernia repair should be undertaken. If there is an injury to the external oblique, nothing needs to be done as this muscle is being divided anyway. If there is an injury to the common junction medially, either during the balloon dissection or during the division of the external oblique, this must be repaired. We repair these with long acting absorbable, barbed suture material. Placement of a prosthetic of any type should be done if there is doubt that the suture repair was adequate. The prosthetic can be placed in this space, or as part of the hernia repair if an intra-peritoneal mesh is being used. It is also possible to place the balloon dissector too superficially and dissect the subcutaneous space rather than the space between the oblique muscles. This requires nothing be done other than acknowledging the correct plane, and reinserting the balloon between the oblique muscles while holding the space open with an "S" shaped retractor, thus insuring the balloon enters the correct plane.

External Oblique and Subcutaneous Fascial Division

Once the muscles have been separated, the space insufflated with CO_2, and the ports have been placed, you will see the initial view of the space between the oblique muscles (Fig. 15.5). Now it's time to divide the external oblique insertion. With the scope in the upper (12 mm) port and the scissors in the middle (5 mm) port, any remaining fibro-areolar connective tissue not separated by the balloon is divided to complete the separation. A small opening is then made directly perpendicular to the port and lateral to the common

junction. You should see yellow, subcutaneous fat (Fig. 15.6a). If you see muscle fibers, you are in the wrong plane, and need to reassess the anatomy. This may require restarting more laterally. This can be done by extending the initial incision, and rotating the table away from the surgeon. Once the initial incision is made, and subcutaneous fat is seen, the jaws of the scissors can be opened, and one blade inserted above the fascia. The shaft can then be slightly rotated downward, and this will help avoid cutting into the subcutaneous tissue too deeply, which has a risk of excess bleeding. This incision is then carried down to just above the inguinal ligament. When dividing the external oblique insertion, it is important to stay parallel and lateral to the common junction of the oblique muscle complex and the lateral border of the rectus muscle. This can be difficult with the small working space, oblique instrument angles that change as you move along, and a visual horizon that may rotate (Fig. 15.6b). Once the insertion has been divided along the majority of its length, the subcutaneous fascia is divided, which gives the majority of the medial mobilization that can easily be seen as the fascia is released. An energy device is very helpful here to control bleeding. When dividing the subcutaneous fascia, it is important to stay in a line perpendicular to the external oblique division, and avoid straying too medial (Fig. 15.6c). If this part of the dissection deviates too medial, there can be

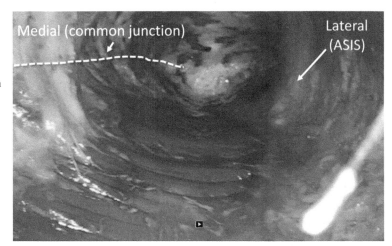

Fig. 15.5 Initial view of the *right side* (looking distally) after creating the space between the oblique muscles. Note the fascia of the internal oblique has been stripped from the muscle belly by the initial insertion of the balloon dissector or slight over distension of the balloon. Because there is no defect in the muscle, no repair is required. The common junction is marked by the white dashed line, and the anterior superior iliac spine (ASIS) is seen laterally

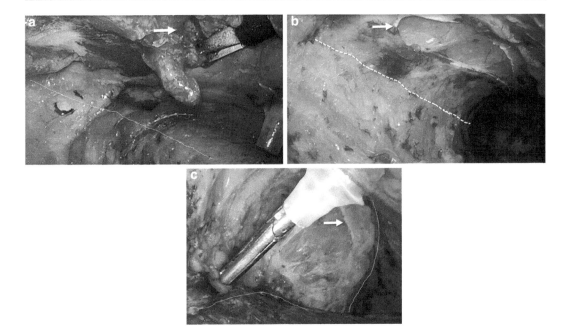

Fig. 15.6 (**a**) Initial division of external oblique (*View*: right side, looking distally). The scope is currently in the most superior port. The initial incision (*arrow*) in the external oblique is made medial to the common junction (*dashed line*) and perpendicular to the middle port through which the scissors have been placed. Note the subcutaneous fat, confirming complete division of the external oblique aponeurosis. (**b**) Distal external oblique division. (*View*: right side, looking distally) The incision (*arrow*) is made medial and parallel to the common junction (*dashed line*) all the way to, but not including the inguinal liga-ment. Note the narrowing where an old ostomy site was. (**c**) Subcutaneous tissue division. (*View*: right side, look-ing distally) Staying parallel to the common junction, the subcutaneous fascia is divided with an energy source. We utilize an ultrasonic device, but many utilize a monopolar device. The cut edges of the external oblique (*dashed line*) can be seen, and are much further apart after division of the subcutaneous tissue. Note the aponeurotic portion of Scarpa's fascia (*arrow*) superficially. This is inconsis-tently seen. The grasper can be used to estimate the amount of separation

an injury to the hernia sac or bowel. Additionally, if there is an ostomy present, subcutaneous redundancy of the bowel is common, and the viscera are at increased risk of injury during this portion of the procedure.

After the inferior portion of the external oblique insertion and subcutaneous fascia has been divided, the scope position is changed to the inferior (5 mm) port. The superior portion is then accomplished in the same way. Near the costal margin, however, the external oblique insertion will become more muscular, and is usually divided with an energy source only. It will remain this way the entire distance above the costal margin (Fig. 15.7).

Limits of Dissection

The limits of the muscle separation are the inguinal ligament, the common junction of the oblique muscle complex and rectus muscle, the superior attachment of the external oblique about 5–7 cm above the costal margin, and the lateral neurovascular bundles between the internal and external oblique muscles. For more inferior defects, the superior portion is less important and vice versa. For smaller defects, the lateral separation is less important. The limits of the external oblique division are typically just above the inguinal ligament to about 5–7 cm above the costal margin. As with the muscle separation, these limits can

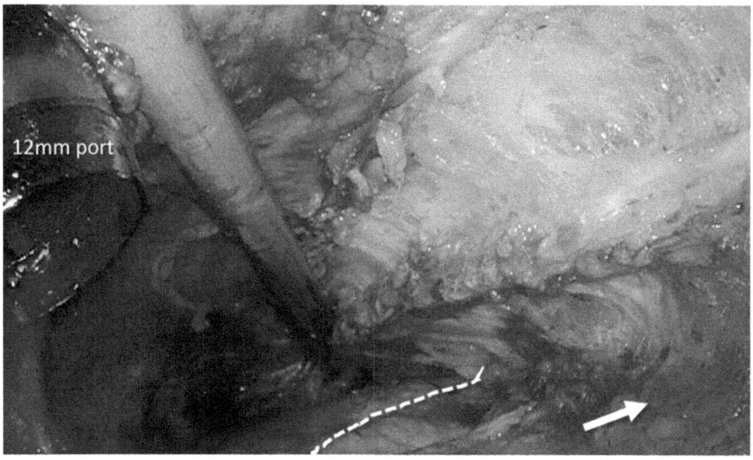

Fig. 15.7 Proximal division of external oblique. (*View*: right side, looking proximally). Although there is no common junction of the oblique muscles above the costal margin (*dashed line*), the line of division of the external oblique and subcutaneous tissue remains parallel to the common junction (*arrow*). Note the aponeurosis does not extend above the costal margin at this position, and the muscle belly of the exter-nal oblique can be seen near the costal margin. We utilize an ultrasonic device, but an alternative energy source can be used. It is also important to note the lateral placement of the 12 mm port in the right upper quadrant. If this is placed too medially, it may impede instrument manipulation. Also, if a balloon-tipped port is used here, care must be taken to avoid contact with the balloon with the energy source

be adjusted depending on the size and location of the defect. This is the same for the limits of the subcutaneous dissection.

Troubleshooting

If the initial incision through the perceived external oblique aponeurosis reveals muscle fibers, the wrong plane has been entered. You will need to reassess the anatomy by critically analyzing the direction of the muscle fibers and fascia to confirm that you are in the space between the internal and external oblique muscles. If you are not in the right plane, or can't tell, then start over by identifying the external oblique muscles fibers, not aponeurosis. This may require extending the initial incision laterally. If you are in the right plane, it's possible that you are too far laterally on the external oblique. If this is the case, it is acceptable to continue by dividing these muscle fibers parallel to the common junction. You may however be working too close to the ports, and can thus carry the incision line slightly more medial. If the muscle fibers are oriented in the craniocaudal plane, it is probably the rectus mus-cle, and you will need to start over by positively identifying the external oblique fibers, which will require lateral extension of the initial incision.

When dividing the subcutaneous tissue, it is possible to enter the hernia sac. If this happens, make sure to open the sac enough to assess for evidence of a bowel injury, as any part of the GI tract can be densely adherent to the sac from adhesions. If this is not possible, the area must be assessed during the hernia repair phase of the operation. If planning on this, Consider marking the area with a suture to positively identify the area later. If there is an ostomy present, it is common for redundant bowel to be present in the subcutaneous space, or for there it be a parastomal hernia containing adjacent loops of bowel. A slower and more meticulous subcutaneous dissection is warranted in this situation. If a bowel injury occurs, appropriate action for repair is in order.

Exiting the Space

Like any laparoscopic procedure, the ports are all removed under direct vision, and the CO_2 is allowed to escape. We do not place drains in this space, except when management of the overlying soft tissue envelope requires excision of excess tissue and opens this space. The drains are then placed in an open fashion. If drains are placed, we prefer drains with metal spikes that are placed from the inside, as we believe it creates a better seal at the skin. The fascia of the external oblique at the port sites obviously does not need to be closed, and the skin is closed according to surgeon's preference.

Completing the Hernia Repair

We then typically perform an open scar excision and retro-rectus sublay with a variety of prosthetics and fixation methods depending on the clinical situation and goals of the operation. I utilize long-acting absorbable, barbed suture material with a short stitch technique for both the posterior and anterior sheath closure. During the anterior sheath closure, the fascial edges are freed of excess scar tissue, hernia sac, and fat. Care is taken to avoid cutting too far back where the anterior sheath is thin. We also take significant precautions to avoid suturing any muscle fibers.

Limitations

Use of an endoscopic approach to external oblique release is primarily for midline hernia defects only. Its use is limited for hernias that extend beyond the semilunar line, such as flank and subcostal hernias. If there is an associated parastomal or incisional hernia at an old stoma site, these can usually be repaired transversely with long acting absorbable suture and covered with the sublay mesh. One example where an open perforator sparing technique may be more appropriate is during a concomitant panniculectomy for a lower midline hernia. A long, low transverse incision will expose the lateral abdominal wall, and tunneling cephalad to avoid the perforators will give ample operative exposure to the external oblique for a release.

Complications and Outcomes

Complications of ECS are few and infrequent, but can be serious. This is particularly true of if the common junction of the oblique muscle complex and rectus muscles are inadvertently divided. The sublay mesh placed over the rectus sheath will not cover the iatrogenic defect laterally, and a postoperative flank hernia will develop. We have had one case early on in our series where this occurred, and a laparoscopic hernia repair was successfully performed utilizing a barrier coated, intra-peritoneal prosthetic. Additionally, long-term seromas requiring operative drainage procedures occur about 5% of the time in our patients. Reoperation is performed if the seroma has been persistent for more than 6 months, and is accomplished with local/sedation or general anesthesia. The old port sites are used, and the seroma is drained and the majority of the lining excised endoscopically. A drain is placed and removed when the output is less than 30 cm^3 per 24 hours for at least two consecutive days. Short-term seromas in the ECS site occur in about 30% of our patients and are evenly distributed between unilateral and bilateral.

References

1. Young D. Repair of epigastric incisional hernia. Br J Surg. 1961;48(211):514–6.
2. Ramirez OM, Ruas E, Dellon AL. "Components separation" method for closure of abdominal-wall defects: an anatomic and clinical study. Plast Reconstr Surg. 1990;86(3):519–26.
3. Lowe JB, Garza JR, Bowman JL, Rohrich RJ, Strodel WE. Endoscopically assisted "components separation" for closure of abdominal wall defects. Plast Reconstr Surg. 2000;105(2):720–30.
4. Rohrich RJ, Lowe JB, Hackney FL, Bowman JL, Hobar PC. An algorithm for abdominal wall reconstruction. Plast Reconstr Surg. 2000;105(1):202–16.

Open Anterior Component Separation with Perforator Preservation

Gregory A. Dumanian

Introduction

As surgeons, we can all agree that blood flow to tissues is associated with healing, while ischemia is associated with tissue loss and complications. In regard to hernia repair, a technique called "perforator preservation" serves to maintain pulsatile skin blood flow while still performing a components separation hernia repair by avoiding the undermining of skin flaps. This style of ventral hernia repair is more than simply avoiding the division of blood vessels to the skin; it also requires an understanding of abdominal skin blood flow, an appreciation of the forces at the suture/tissue interface (STI), a means to achieve primary fascial closure with mesh using concepts of force distribution, and excision of redundant midline skin. In the following chapter, a brief introduction of laminar versus pulsatile blood flow and the angiosome theory of perfusion will be presented. The history of perforator preservation as an adjunct to the components separation technique will be recounted. The value of compo-

nents separation as a means to reduce suture pull-through will then be introduced. The technique of perforator preservation at the time of components separation and use of a narrow mesh will be presented in a video demonstrating this repair in a 76 year old gentleman with heart disease, a one pack per day current smoker, four previous attempts at repair including prior mesh, and with a 16 cm in transverse dimension hernia by CT.

Laminar Versus Pulsatile Blood Flow/Blood Flow of the Abdominal Wall

Vascular surgeons have extensive studies correlating the quality of tissue perfusion with the healing of surgical incisions. In the early 1970s, lower extremity blood flow was analyzed using a combination of pulse-volume recordings and blood pressures [1]. A tiny blood pressure cuff placed on a toe or across the instep of the foot would have a small incremental change in pressure due to the stroke volume of blood introduced into the aorta by the heart during systole. Normal blood flow is pulsatile, correlating to each heartbeat. Laminar flow, in contradistinction, does not experience the repeated episodic increases in pressure. Laminar flow is associated with numerous conditions familiar to surgeons including prior scar, radiation, proximal vascular obstruction, and division of native vascularity. It has been shown experimentally and clinically that primary healing

Electronic supplementary material: The online version of this chapter (doi:10.1007/978-3-319-27470-6_16) contains supplementary material, which is available to authorized users.

G.A. Dumanian, M.D. (✉)
Northwestern Feinberg School of Medicine,
Northwestern Memorial Hospital, Chicago, IL, USA
e-mail: gdumania@nm.org

occurs more predictably when tissue is vascularized with pulsatile blood flow [2–4].

An angiosome is defined as a three-dimensional block of tissue supplied by a single named blood vessel. The size of a particular angiosome varies depending on the flow in the vessel and has patterns based on locations in the body. At the borders of the angiosome exist choke vessels that are normally without flow, but that can open and provide flow when a border area becomes ischemic. Over time, choke vessels can reestablish pulsatile blood flow in an area that has lost its original vascularity. The opening of choke vessels occurs more slowly with advancing age, when the adjacent angiosome is itself not well perfused, when the tissues have been radiated, and in smokers. In a typical patient, choke vessels between skin angiosomes do not open robustly for 2–3 weeks.

The blood flow of the abdominal wall comes from numerous sources. The central tissue is predominantly supplied from *periumbilical perforators* traveling through the rectus abdominis muscle from the deep inferior and the superior epigastric arteries. The tendinous inscription of the rectus muscles that exists typically 1 cm above the umbilicus is the inexact boundary between these two arterial territories. Inferolaterally, perfusion is from the superficial inferior epigastrics, commonly coagulated during inguinal hernia repair. The superficial and deep inferior epigastrics have overlapping territories for the abdominal skin, with one vessel being able to supply the other's territory when necessary. Congenitally large deep systems usually coexist with small superficial systems, and vice versa. Superiorly and laterally, the segmental intercostal vessels and lumbar arteries give off perforators through the external oblique muscle at the level of the mid-axillary line. Connections exist between the periumbilical perforators and these lateral segmental vessels in imaginary dermatomal lines traveling between the umbilicus and the tip of the scapula.

Plastic surgery and flaps require a basic understanding of the limits of tissue undermining. In general, tissue elevation during the creation of skin flaps requires that an adjacent angiosome supply the newly elevated skin. Rather than having pulsatile blood flow, the newly elevated skin is maintained with laminar blood flow, and healing may be somewhat compromised. Common skin flap elevations where history and experience teaches that the quality of laminar blood flow is sufficient for healing include the standard abdominoplasty skin elevation from the symphysis pubis to the xiphoid, and the oblique rectus abdominis myocutaneous flap (ORAM) [5]. As these flaps require the immediate opening of choke vessels to allow perfusion, these flaps are not performed when perpendicular scars are present, or in smokers. Judgment is involved in what can be elevated safely and what would be considered unreliable. The importance of what lies underneath the skin is also critical. In an abdominoplasty, there is intact well-vascularized abdominal wall, while in a spanning mesh hernia repair; there would be exposed prosthetic mesh if the skin were to become nonviable. While in the former, one may rely on skin with a large laminar component, a spanning prosthetic mesh would almost demand skin with pulsatile flow to increase the odds for healing.

History of Perforator Preservation

The concept of perforator preservation [6] can be traced to a morbidity and mortality conference at the University of Pittsburgh in 1994. Advances in treatment of the abdominal wall came from this institution, both due to the huge demands placed on the abdominal wall for liver transplantation, and due to the fact that Dr. Oscar Ramirez had been a plastic surgery resident at the University of Pittsburgh soon after performing his cadaveric abdominal wall muscle dissections in Baltimore, MD. The morbidity and mortality conference presented a patient who had undergone a components release hernia repair for a massive hernia that developed after placement of a tube graft for an abdominal aortic aneurysm. Large skin flaps were elevated as was the standard, dividing the periumbilical perforators in order to access the semilunar lines for division of the external oblique muscle and fascia. The skin lost its primary blood flow with division of the periumbilical perforators, and the adjacent angiosomes fed by the lumbar perforators were unable to compensate due to a prior division of segmental vessels off of the aorta at the time of the tube graft. This patient, therefore, had a near total loss of blood flow to the skin, and therefore lost all of the skin of the abdominal wall that had been elevated. Dr. Kenneth Shestak, during the discussion, questioned if it would be possible to go around the periumbilical perforators and still perform a components release. Dr. Jaime Garza was the chief resident sitting next to me during this conference and later he took a position at the University of Texas in Austen. There, he helped to perform seven components separation hernia repairs where a laparoscope was used to access the semilunar lines. These patients were presented at a regional meeting in 1997, and Dr. Garza published the account in 2000 [7]. Across the Atlantic nearly simultaneously, Maas in 1999 used a lateral incision to perform an external oblique release in four patients to avoid an enterostomy [8]. At Northwestern several years later, I was having an unacceptable wound complication rate after components separation hernia repairs with standard skin undermining. Remembering Dr. Shestak's comments, I started to go around the periumbilical perforators either through subcutaneous tunnels or later through lateral incisions. Our report in 2002 was the first to directly compare wound complication rates in components procedures with and without perforator preservation [9]. An addtitional publication directly comparing the hernia repairs complications of standard open components with perforator preservation was written by Butler in 2011 [10].

Decrease Forces at the STI with Components Releases

A central question is why are releases of the abdominal wall musculature beneficial during the performance of ventral hernia repairs. It is well established that suture repairs of abdominal wall hernias fail at alarming rates. Even the laparoscopy incision closure in some patient groups will develop hernias over 30% of the time [11]. The central question remains as to why divided tissues approximated by sutures go on to fail and not demonstrate a lasting union. There are three types of suture failures. Acute failure, as in catastrophic evisceration after a laparotomy, results from tearing of sutures through intact tissue [12–14]. Subacute failures of laparotomy suture lines were demonstrated by Pollock [15, 16] and later confirmed by Burger [17]. Early separation of metal clips placed on either side of a laparotomy closure can be seen radiographically within the first month after surgery in patients who will later develop an incisional hernia. The gapping of newly opposed tissues sewn under tension has recently been shown in laboratory animals [18]. Chronic failures are represented by hernia formation late after laparotomy [19] and occur when scar contained within the suture loop remodels and thins over time [20]. Surgeons refer to this chronic remodeling of scar tissue as "cheesewiring", and it is the result of chronic suture migration through tissue. A problem central to sutures is that the forces required to achieve tissue apposition can cause local damage at the STI from pressure-induced ischemia and overtightening [21]. The greater the force, such as in laparotomy closure, the greater the potential for tissue damage. After laparotomy closure, episodic waves of force directed at the new suture line from coughs, movement, lifting, and stairs further stress the STI. A stiff abdominal wall will transmit those energy waves more than would compliant musculature. While many surgeons view components releases as moving the rectus muscles to the midline, I view components releases as a means to improve lateral abdominal wall compliance and to protect the new suture line from tearing. A second means to ensure lower forces at the STI is to better distribute the forces with mesh, as will be discussed. The trick is to have a means to fixate the mesh while at the same time performing a components release and to maintain skin pulsatile blood flow. This surgical problem is addressed by using a narrow mesh to minimize the necessary skin elevation, and lateral incisions to avoid devascularization of the skin for the components release.

Patient Preoperative Evaluation

The evaluation of a patient with a midline ventral hernia is rather straightforward, as many old operative reports are collected as possible. A CT scan both delineates the transverse separation of the rectus muscles and rules out unexpected intra-abdominal pathology. An assessment needs to be made as to abdominal wall compliance. The patient should be placed flat for examination, and pressure is applied onto the abdominal wall to assess compliance. Weight loss, a history of large pregnancies, and a history of treated ascites all favorably influence compliance. Being at one's maximum weight, prior lateral incisions, a history of intra-abdominal sepsis, COPD, and multiple prior abdominal wall procedures negatively influence compliance. The amount of bowel found within the hernia sac is important in terms of concepts of loss of domain, but this only rises in importance in a patient with low muscle compliance.

The wider the separation of the rectus muscles in a transverse plane, and the less compliant the abdominal wall, the more a components release will be necessary to prevent tearing at the midline suture line. For patients with normal compliance, rectus separations of 6 cm or less rarely need a components release. Over 10 cm, separations are almost always required. Patients in the middle ground have an intra-operative decision as to the need for a release or not.

Weight loss for patients prior to surgery is beneficial and is encouraged but is not a requirement for the majority of patients with body mass indices under 35. Cessation of tobacco is clearly supported in the medical and hernia literature, but has not been overly problematic for the procedure to be described. Immunosuppression (in the absence of steroids) for transplantation has not been an issue with healing, and likewise for a diabetic in reasonable control. The patient is cleared for surgery for major cardiopulmonary issues, and a bowel prep of clear liquids, a half bottle of magnesium citrate, and two dulcolax tablets suffice to clear the majority of particulate matter within the bowel. The bowel preparation is performed to minimize the controllable intra-abdominal volume to minimize the forces at the STI.

Surgery Technique

This procedure as well as mesh choice has remained essentially unchanged for the last decade. The goals of the procedure are to approximate the rectus complexes in the midline, to fix a narrow mesh flat and tight with numerous sutures coursing through the rectus muscles to distribute the forces across the repair, and to maintain pulsatile blood flow for closure.

1. The patient is prepped and draped widely under general anesthesia. The room should be kept warm during induction to maintain patient normothermia.
2. The midline incision is widely opened. In general, the length of the incision will be *far longer* than the length of the hernia because above and below the actual hernia rectus diastasis exists that will also need to be repaired. Repair of the rectus diastasis will actually take tension off of the repair at its widest point by "working out the dog ear" [22].
3. The posterior aspect of the hernia sac and the posterior aspect of the abdominal wall are cleared of any attachments to the viscera so that eventual medial movement of the rectus muscles will not pull bowel with it. The procedure is kept as two-dimensional as possible, and so individual bowel loops are not separated. The preoperative CT scan suffices to rule out bowel pathology. If facile, the omentum is mobilized for eventual coverage of the bowel in the midline.
4. The anterior rectus fascia is cleared of soft tissue for 4 cm along its width for the length of the muscle to be repaired. *Perforator preservation, therefore, is of the perforators more than 4 cm from the medial edge of the rectus.*
5. Tension is applied to the rectus muscles to see if their medial aspects can be brought together to the midline. In general, if this can be achieved with finger tension only, a components release does not need to be performed.

6. A decision at this point is made if the mesh will be placed intra-abdominally or in the retro-rectus position. Both are acceptable with advantages and disadvantages. As mesh incorporation will occur from both sides when in the retro-rectus position, this is preferred. The widest hernia defects are repaired with the mesh intra-abdominally placed.

7. In the video supplement, the retro-rectus space is created with care taken to maintain the patency of the inferior epigastric arteries.

8. Through a 6-cm transverse incision at the inferior aspect of the rib cage (Fig. 16.1), dissection is performed through Scarpa's fascia to reach the abdominal wall. With spreading, the semilunar line is reached, and the anterior-most fibers of the external oblique are visualized. A small perforator often requires coagulation. Spreading with a Mayo scissor or equivalent vertically along the semilunar line begins the visualization of the semilunar line, and the exposure is completed using a 1 in. Deaver retractor bluntly aimed superiorly and a bit medially. The external oblique muscle is held and elevated with forceps to confirm it is not the anterior rectus fascia, and then it is incised under direct vision with a cautery. Yellow fat is typically seen immediately deep to the external oblique fascia. A dissecting finger sweeps laterally to confirm the space between the external and internal oblique muscles, and this dissecting finger continues to sweep the space now on top of the ribs. With the external oblique extension into the anterior rectus fascia completely visualized on top of the rib cage, cautery divides the external muscle and fascia. A fascia layer deep to the external oblique but still above the internal oblique needs to be identified and divided for best movement. The Deaver retractor is now replaced to aim toward the anterior superior iliac spine, and again blunt force opens the tissues without bleeding or excessive force. The same dissecting finger between the external and internal obliques now develops the plane inferiorly to be divided by cautery.

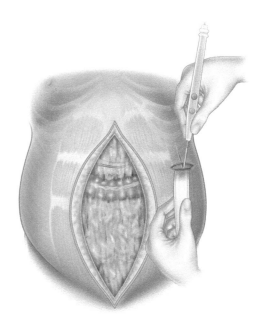

Fig. 16.1 Semilunar lines exposed through 6 cm transverse incisions located at the inferior aspect of the rib cage

One trick is required to complete the division of the external oblique toward the symphysis pubis. From the midline incision and low on the abdominal wall, a tunnel is created from the midline to the lateral semilunar line dissection (Fig. 16.2). The end of the divided external oblique muscle is captured by feeling for the cut end of the fascia, and it feels like the inner vertex of the letter "V". This fascia is pulled into the midline wound where cautery serves to complete the release. Alternatively, especially for very obese patients where the lower midline tissue is not incised, the completion of the external oblique release can be performed through a second transverse skin incision located near the ASIS.

Finally, the space between the external and internal oblique muscles is widely undermined with digital pressure from the upper transverse incision. The entire external oblique release can be performed while still maintaining pulsatile blood flow to the skin and takes 4–5 min to perform without special lighting or equipment.

9. A 7.5 cm wide mesh is cut that will extend the length of the hernia and any associated

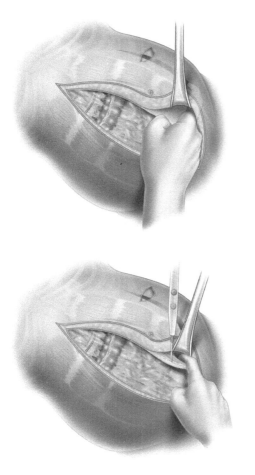

Fig. 16.2 The inferior aspect of the divided external oblique is captured by the index finger through a suprapubic tunnel to effect the completion of the release

rectus diastasis. The mesh is quilted to the undersurface of the rectus muscles with through-and-through full-thickness bites of 0-polypropylene suture introduced through the anterior rectus fascia, through the muscle, grabbing a small bite of mesh, and back through muscle and fascia. When two rows of sutures are placed 4 cm from the medial aspect of the rectus muscles and with a 7.5 cm wide mesh, the medial aspect of the rectus muscles will be brought together in the midline when the sutures are tied. By geometry, the mesh will be flat and tight, and the tension on the mesh will fight wrinkles. Chronic pain has not been an issue for these

patients, as the segmental nerves of the rectus muscles are relatively small so close to the midline. The medial aspect of the rectus muscles is approximated over the mesh to achieve a direct supported repair (Fig. 16.3). Sutures are located 2–3 cm from each other to distribute the forces, and approximately 40 sutures are used for the three vertical lines for a full midline repair. Done in this manner, while the total tension on the midline may initially seem too tight, the tension experienced by each suture is below the point for suture pull-through. The added compliance achieved with the lateral releases will also be protective of the repair.

10. Medialization of the rectus muscles and the attached overlying skin produces redundant skin in the midline. Excess skin is excised in the midline as a vertical panniculectomy—an important issue both to remove the most undermined skin and to leave a smaller potential space where fluid collections can exist. Two or three subcutaneous drains are used for the time in the hospital. On occasion, "pumpkin-teeth" skin flaps are fashioned to create a neo-umbilicus. Not only cosmetically important, these skin flaps can be tacked down to the abdominal wall for improved soft tissue healing. Figures 16.4, 16.5, and 16.6 demonstrate an older gentleman who smokes with a large 16 cm hernia treated with this technique.

Outcomes

Components separation hernia repairs are associated with increased numbers of wound complications, and perforator preservation is one technical modification to decrease the rate of these problems. In Dumanian's 2002 series of 66 patients, wound complications dropped from 20% down to 2% when skin vascularity was maintained. Performing this procedure with lateral incisions for 12 years, there has been uniform acceptance of the transverse scars, and they heal quite well being located along the natural crease lines of the abdominal wall. Butler's 2012 series of 107

Fig. 16.3 Geometry of narrow mesh placement with three rows of sutures in this direct supported repair

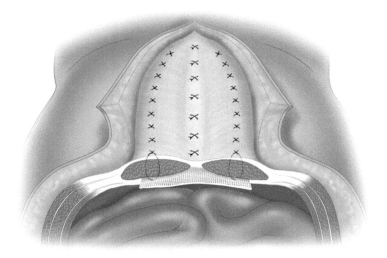

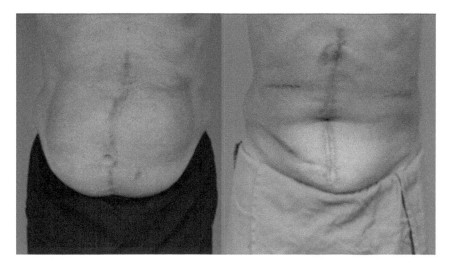

Fig. 16.4 Preoperative and postoperative anterior views of an older gentleman with a large midline hernia

patients mirrored these results when comparing open vs perforator preserving techniques during components separation. Despite a more challenging patient population in the perforator-sparing group, all wound-healing complications dropped from 32% down to 14%. In both series, the incidence of long-term hernia recurrences was the same or lower with perforator preservation. The soft tissue complication rates with these perforator sparing procedures are similar to that reported in a recent meta-analysis of laparoscopic releases of the external oblique [23].

Discussion

Hernia repairs are a balancing act, and the goal of the procedure is to approximate the abdominal wall under tension without the sutures tearing the tissue. It is clear that neither sutures alone [24] nor sutures with components alone [25] suffice to completely avoid the development of hernias. Therefore, a midweight macroporous uncoated polypropylene mesh is added to the procedure to distribute forces, but then fixation of the mesh becomes an issue. What may be unique to the

Fig. 16.5 Separation of the
rectus muscles is 16 cm by CT
scan

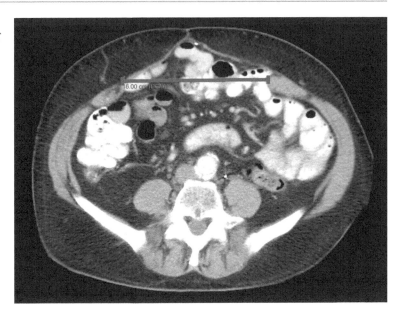

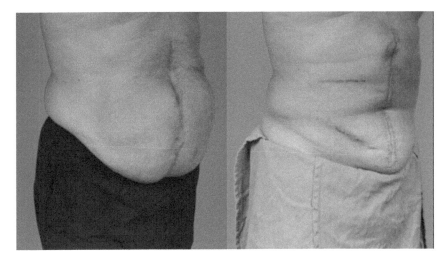

Fig. 16.6 Preoperative and postoperative oblique views. Final closure achieved after placement of a narrow well fixed
retrorectus mesh, vertical panniculectomy, and umbilicus recreation

hernia repair described in this chapter is the use
of a narrow mesh firmly fixed to the rectus complex. It is a plastic surgery principle that a well-
fixed implant does not become infected. A recent
series of mesh placed in this fashion documented
no mesh infections, a surgical site infection incidence rate of 3%, and a surgical site occurrence
rate of 10% in 100 consecutive cases [26]. The
few complications were sporadic and were not
predicted by the Ventral Hernia Working Group

classification scheme. Chronic pain is not an
issue with this procedure as the nerves are smaller
closer to the midline. The narrow mesh requires
less skin elevation from the anterior rectus sheath
for placement of the sutures. Mesh placed in this
fashion can be loaded with a fair degree of tension to avoid bridging. I believe it is the combination of a narrow mesh, achievement of a direct
supported repair, and lateral incisions/perforator
preservation to perform the external oblique

releases, that is the optimal balance between a secure closure and minimizing abdominal wall dissection. These procedures are routinely now performed in under 2½ hours.

In comparison, larger meshes require greater elevation of tissue planes, more foreign material, and greater difficulty with fixation. Surgeons who advocate no suture fixation with giant meshes open large tissue planes permitting fluid to collect, and large meshes may have wrinkling at the outer edges when trying to fit a flat mesh to a curved surface. The large mesh and soft tissue dissection probably can cause uncomfortable stiffening in the lateral abdominal wall compliance over time that the patient may notice. A middle ground with large (not giant) meshes and transcutaneous fixation risks the capturing of larger segmental nerves. It may not be surprising that Rives-Stoppa hernia repairs with large meshes have a 27% chronic pain rate [27].

Perforator preservation alone is not a magic bullet to avoid all complications in components separation hernia repairs. In combination with a focus of the forces at the STI, force distribution with a narrow mesh, long repairs that address rectus diastasis, and excess vertical skin excision, wide hernia repairs in these components patients can be performed safely and with low morbidity.

References

1. Raines JK, Jaffrin MY, Rao S. A non-invasive pressure-pulse recorder: development and rationale. Med Instrum. 1973;7:245.
2. Gibbons GW, Wheelock FC, Hoar CC, et al. Predicting success of forefoot amputations in diabetics by noninvasive testing. Arch Surg. 1979;114:1034.
3. Chang N, Mathes SJ. Comparison of the effect of bacterial inoculation on musculocutaneous and random pattern flaps. Plast Reconstr Surg. 1982;70:1.
4. Feng LF, Price D, Hohn D, Mathes SJ. Blood flow changes and leukocyte mobilization in infection: a comparison between ischemia and well-perfused skin. Surg Forum. 1983;34:603.
5. Abbott DE, Halverson AL, Wayne JD, Kim JY, Talamonti MS, Dumanian GA. The oblique rectus abdominis myocutaneous flap for complex pelvic wound reconstruction. Dis Colon Rectum. 2008; 51:1237–41.
6. Dumanian GA. Discussion: minimally invasive component separation with inlay bioprosthetic mesh (MICSIB) for complex abdominal wall reconstruction. Plast Reconstr Surg. 2011;128:710–2.
7. Lowe JB, Garza JR, Bowman JL, Rohrich RJ, Strodel WE. Endoscopically assisted "components separation" for closure of abdominal wall defects. Plast Reconstr Surg. 2000;105:720–9.
8. Maas SM, van Engeland M, Leeksma NG, Bleichrodt RP. A modification of the "components separation" technique for closure of abdominal wall defects in the presence of an enterostomy. J Am Coll Surg. 1999;189:138–40.
9. Saulis A, Dumanian GA. Periumbilical rectus abdominis perforator preservation significantly reduces superficial wound complications in "Separation of Parts" hernia repairs. Plast Reconstr Surg. 2002; 109:2275.
10. Ghali S, Turza K, Baumann DP, Butler CE. Minimally invasive component separation results in fewer wound-healing complications than open component separation for large ventral hernia repairs. J Am Coll Surg. 2012;214:981–9.
11. Armananzas L, Ruiz-Tovar J, Arroyo A, et al. Prophylactic mesh vs suture in the closure of the umbilical trocar site after laparoscopic cholecystectomy in high-risk patients for incisional hernia: a randomized clinical trial. J Am Coll Surg. 2014; 218:960–8.
12. Alexander CH, Prudden JF. The causes of abdominal wound disruption. SGO. 1966;122:1223–9.
13. Rodeheaver GT, Nesbit WS, Edlich RF. Novafil, a dynamic suture for wound closure. Ann Surg. 1986;204:193–9.
14. Israelsson LA, Millbourn D. Closing midline abdominal incisions. Langenbecks Arch Surg. 2012; 397:1201–7.
15. Playforth MJ, Sauven PD, Evans M, Pollock AV. The prediction of incisional hernias by radio-opaque markers. Ann Royal Col Surg Eng. 1986;68:82–4.
16. Pollock AV, Evans M. Early prediction of late incisional hernias. Br J Surg. 1989;76:953–4.
17. Burger JW, Lange JF, Halm JA, Kleinrensink G-J, Jeekel H. Incisional hernia: early complication of abdominal surgery. World J Surg. 2005;29:1608–13.
18. Xing L, Culbertson EJ, Wen Y, Franz MG. Early laparotomy wound failure as the mechanism for incisional hernia formation. J Surg Res. 2013;182:e35–42.
19. Ellis H, Gajraj H, George CD. Incisional hernias: when do they occur? Br J Surg. 1983;70:290–1.
20. Hoes J, Fischer L, Schachtrupp A. Laparotomy closure and incisional hernia prevention—what are the surgical requirements. Zentralbl Chir. 2011;136:42–9.
21. Klink CD, Binnebosel M, Alizai PH, Lambertz A, von Trotha KT, Junker E, et al. Tension of knotted surgical sutures shows tissue specific rapid loss in a rodent model. BMC Surg. 2011;11:36–45.
22. Cheesborough JE, Dumanian GA. Simultaneous prosthetic mesh abdominal wall reconstruction with abdominoplasty for ventral hernia and severe rectus diastasis repairs. Plast Reconstr Surg. 2015; 135:268–76.

23. Jensen KK, Henriksen NA, Jorgensen LN. Endoscopic component separation for ventral hernia causes fewer wound complications compared to open components separation: a systematic review and meta-analysis. Surg Endosc. 2014;228: 3046–52.

24. Luijendijk RW, Hop WC, van den Tol MP, et al. A comparison of suture repair with mesh repair for incisional hernia. N Engl J Med. 2000;343:392–8.

25. Slater NJ, van Goor H, Bleichrodt RP. Large and complex ventral hernia repair using "components separation technique" without mesh results in a high recurrence rate. Am J Surg. 2015;209:170–9.

26. Souza JM, Dumanian GA. Routine use of bioprosthetic mesh is not necessary: a retrospective review of 100 consecutive cases of intraabdominal midweight polypropylene mesh for ventral hernia repair. Surgery. 2013;153:393–9.

27. Iqbal CW, Pham TH, Joseph A, Mai J, Thompson GB, Sarr MG. Long-term outcome of 254 complex incisional hernia repairs using the modified Rives-Stoppa technique. World J Surg. 2007;31:2398–404.

Matthew Z Wilson, Joshua S Winder,
and Eric M Pauli

17.1 Introduction

Parastomal hernia formation, the presence of visceral contents protruding through an abdominal wall defect adjacent to an ostomy, represents a complex problem for the hernia surgeon. When compared to other types of ventral hernias, they occur at a higher rate, they are technically more difficult to repair, and they are associated with higher rates of surgical site occurrences and hernia recurrences. Recent reviews suggest that hernia formation complicates up to 50% of stoma formation [1–6]. The presence of a parastomal hernia also increases the likelihood of a concomitant incisional hernia formation, which further complicates the repair of both hernias [7, 8]. Parastomal hernias have additional morbidity not

Electronic supplementary material: The online version of this chapter (doi:10.1007/978-3-319-27470-6_17) contains supplementary material, which is available to authorized users.

M.Z. Wilson, M.D.
Penn State Milton S. Hershey Medical Center, Hershey, PA, USA

J.S. Winder, M.D.
Department of General Surgery, Division of Minimally Invasive Surgery, Penn State Milton S. Hershey Medical Center, Hershey, PA, USA

E.M. Pauli, M.D. (✉)
Department of Surgery, Division of Minimally Invasive and Bariatric Surgery, Penn State Hershey Medical Center, Hershey, PA, USA
e-mail: epauli@hmc.psu.edu

associated with other hernias, including poorly fitting stoma appliances, parastomal skin breakdown, stoma level obstruction and pain, which results in an overall negative impact on quality of life [9]. This chapter will provide an overview of the various types of open repair of parastomal hernias.

17.2 Risk Factors and Prevention

Multiple factors predispose patients to parastomal hernia formation. Initial stoma placement is perhaps the most critical. Maturation of the stoma through the rectus muscle and above the arcuate line is of primary importance [3, 10, 11]. Stomas that are inadvertently created near or through the linea semilunaris are predisposed to hernia formation due to the thinness of the abdominal wall at this location (Fig. 17.1). Patient factors, such as waist circumference, may play an important role as well. Reports suggest that a waist circumference exceeding 100 cm confers a 75% probability of hernia formation [12]. Pre-operative stoma marking has also been shown to significantly reduce hernia occurrence [13]. The type of stoma being formed also influences the rate of hernia formation, with lower rates of hernias for ileostomy and higher rates for colostomy [14].

Recent literature suggests that staple or mesh reinforcement of the stoma site at the time of creation reduces the risk of hernia formation [15–23]. This topic is further covered in Chapter 23.

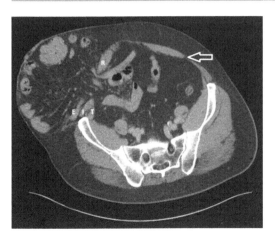

Fig. 17.1 Computed Tomography of a parastomal hernia with loss of domain. The patient's main risk factor for hernia formation was the formation of his end ileostomy through the linea semilunaris. The ostomy disconnected the rectus abdominis (R) from the external oblique (E), internal oblique (I), and the transversus abdominis (T) muscles. The thin contralateral linea semilunaris can also be appreciated (arrowhead)

17.3 Current Repair Strategies

17.3.1 Surgical Technique: Open vs. Laparoscopic

Please see Chapter 23 for an overview of the advantages and disadvantages of each of these techniques in the repair of parastomal hernias.

17.3.2 Surgical Method: Primary Repair vs. Mesh Repair

Primary fascial approximation with sutures alone has a low morbidity and mortality and can be conducted through a peristomal incision alone without the need for a midline laparotomy or laparoscopic access to the abdominal cavity. While technically simple, suture repair of parastomal hernias is discouraged as it has been shown to have a 46–100% recurrence rate, ninefold higher than mesh techniques [24–26]. Given the low overall risk of mesh-related complications, prosthetic reinforcement during parastomal hernia repair is recommended. Suture repair, however, still remains a viable option for repairs

being conducted in circumstances where the surgeon wishes to avoid the morbidity associated with mesh implantation.

17.3.3 Mesh Configuration: Sugarbaker, Keyhole, and Cruciate

Three primary mesh configurations for parastomal hernia repair have been described. The Sugarbaker repair utilizes a large piece of uncut prosthetic mesh placed over the stoma defect and proximal bowel intraperitoneally (underlay) and sutured into position [27, 28]. This approach was initially described using open weave mesh but is modified using polytetrafluoroethylene (PTFE) in order to minimize clinically significant interaction with the bowel (adhesions or erosions) during both open and laparoscopic repairs [29]. This modified Sugarbaker technique is technically simpler and has fewer recurrences compared to the keyhole approach when performed laparoscopically [1, 24, 30]. The major advantage is an uncut piece of mesh which widely overlaps the original stoma and fascial defect (Fig. 17.2a).

Keyhole repairs utilize mesh wrapped circumferentially around the stoma in order to reduce the fascial aperture [31]. The mesh is cut from a free edge toward a central defect giving it the appearance of a keyhole (Fig. 17.2b). This technique is advantageous because it does not require the stoma to be relocated, but does require division of the mesh which predisposes it to retraction and hernia recurrence. Mesh can be placed in an underlay, sublay, or onlay position with this configuration.

Cruciate repairs involve relocation of the stoma within the abdominal wall. The cut end of the bowel is delivered through intersecting linear cuts within the mesh, generally forming an X-shape (Fig. 17.2c) [32]. While this method requires stoma relocation, it permits a very small defect to be made in the mesh to reduce the likelihood of mesh retraction during mesh incorporation. Mesh can also be placed in an underlay, sublay, or onlay position with this configuration.

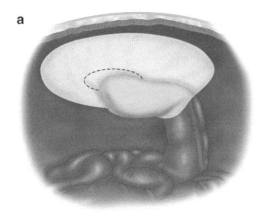

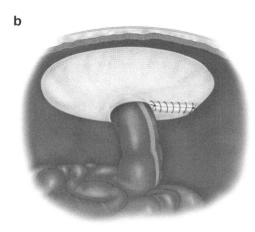

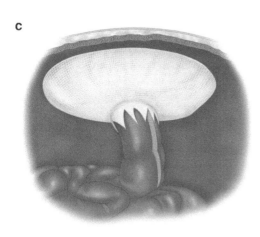

Fig. 17.2 Mesh configurations for open parastomal hernia repair (**a**) Sugarbaker configuration with a large uncut sheet of mesh widely overlapping the hernia defect (*transparent circle*) (**b**) Keyhole configuration mesh is cut, placed around the bowel, and then sewn back together once positioned (**c**) Cruciate mesh configuration permits the bowel to be drawn through a small aperture in the mesh

17.3.4 Mesh Selection: Synthetic vs. Biologic Mesh

Biologic mesh has been widely used in clinical practice in locations susceptible to contamination and is considered in repairs when contamination is present. Evidence does not support the use of biologic mesh over carefully chosen synthetic mesh, even in contaminated fields [33–37]. Data suggests that placement of large pore synthetic mesh (generally light or mid weight polypropylene) in parastomal hernia repairs is safe, effective, and inexpensive [36, 38–41].

17.3.5 Stoma Options: Closure, Relocation, or In Situ Position

Some patients are candidates for ostomy takedown but have not been offered definitive closure because of the complexity of their parastomal hernia (Fig. 17.3). Consideration should be given to closing the ostomy at the time of hernia repair. If a two-staged procedure is indicated (primary stoma takedown with creation of a protecting proximal ileostomy), a bridged hernia repair may be considered at the initial operation followed by definitive abdominal wall reconstruction with ostomy takedown at the second operation.

Many advocate leaving the stoma in situ during parastomal hernia repair [42]. This approach is advantageous because it avoids: the need to transect the bowel, the need to free adhesions to transpose the ostomy to another location, and the additional wound to manage. Disadvantages include: difficulty with primary fascial re-approximation, seroma formation around the ostomy, and the need to use a keyhole mesh configuration which has a higher risk of hernia recurrence than other configurations [1, 30, 33].

Stoma relocation is best performed with the assistance of an enterostomal therapist performing pre-operative marking. As with primary ostomy site localization, a transrectus position is the preferred location. Examination of the patient in standing, sitting, and recumbent positions further facilitates localization by avoiding skin folds or a large pannus. Often, in the case of a large

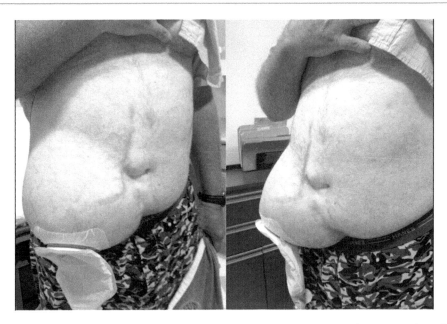

Fig. 17.3 54-year-old male with Crohn's disease who received an emergency end ileostomy and developed a large symptomatic parastomal hernia. The patient was never offered stoma reversal due to his loss of domain, obesity, inflammatory bowel disease, and concomitant midline hernias

parastomal hernia or herniorraphy involving a simultaneous ventral hernia, the pre-operative stoma marking is inadvertently placed away from the rectus abdominis muscle due to lateralization of the rectus muscles from the hernia. In these cases we respect the original cranio-caudal marking, but move the stoma site medial or lateral as necessary to achieve a mid-rectus position following hernia repair with midline re-approximation. Relocation has the advantage of permitting the stoma to be created through a small fascial opening, with a cruciate (not keyhole) mesh configuration in an ideal location for the patient. However, this creates two additional abdominal wounds (old and new stoma sites) and requires transection of the bowel with mobilization of the intestine to reach the new location. Often, especially with a urostomy, there is insufficient bowel length to permit relocation.

17.3.6 Operative Approach: One Team vs. Two Teams

Our group utilizes a two-team approach to parastomal hernia repair. The abdominal wall reconstruction is undertaken by the primary team while a secondary team, typically from the colorectal sur-

gery division, is responsible for intestinal mobilization and reconstruction (as necessary). The patient is seen pre-operatively and the appropriate studies are undertaken to determine the feasibility of stoma takedown. If the patient is a candidate for stoma closure, then the secondary team will perform the reduction of the stoma, anastomosis, and any necessary resections after the lysis of intra-abdominal adhesions by the secondary team. If the patient is not a candidate for stoma closure, the primary team will reduce the stoma after the lysis of adhesions, determine the appropriate placement for a new stoma, and then return to mature the new stoma after the abdominal wall reconstruction is finished. Coordination of two teams can be somewhat difficult. Performing stoma takedown or re-siting can certainly be performed by one team; however, the fatigue factors associated with lengthy reconstructive procedures should not be underestimated.

17.4 Patient Selection

Absolute indications for surgery include obstruction caused by the herniation and incarceration with strangulation. Relative indications for surgery include incarceration, prolapse, stenosis, difficulty with appliance management, intractable dermatitis, large size, pain, and cosmesis [43]. Contraindications to surgical repair include future reversal of the stoma, short life expectancy such as in the case of widely metastatic disease, and other life-threatening diseases such as cardiopulmonary distress that would preclude patients from surgery. A BMI great than 45 is a relative contraindication to elective surgical repair.

When determining the approach to repair (laparoscopic or open) we consider multiple factors. Older patients, those with smaller defects (<6 cm), those with parastomal hernias who are anticipated to have sufficient bowel length to permit a Sugarbaker repair are offered a laparoscopic parastomal repair. Younger patients, those with need for a functional abdominal wall (e.g., patients who perform manual labor), those with defects above 6 cm, those with parastomal defects through or including the linea semilunaris, those with loss of domain hernias, those with simultaneous midline (or other location) hernia, those with a need for additional GI tract procedure, urostomy patients, those who failed prior laparoscopic repair, and those patients in whom laparoscopic repair cannot be performed are offered an open retromuscular repair.

As with other hernia repairs, medical comorbidities must be optimized prior to surgery: management of blood glucose levels, obesity, and pulmonary function should all be addressed in the pre-operative period. Smoking cessation is an absolute.

Because many parastomal hernias occur in the setting of a simultaneous ventral hernia, our preferred method of herniorraphy is open posterior component separation with transversus abdominis release (TAR) [40, 41].

17.5 Surgical Techniques of Open Parastomal Hernia Repair

All patients are marked for new stomas by an enterostomal therapy nurse prior to the procedure. The patient is positioned supine with arms out. A Foley catheter as well as an orogastric tube is placed. All previous scars are marked and gastrointestinal stomas are oversewn and excluded via an iodophor adhesive drape.

Urostomies are sterilely intubated with a Foley catheter for drainage and as an adjunct to identify the conduit intra-operatively.

17.5.1 Sugarbaker Technique

The procedure begins with an exploratory laparotomy and full lysis of adhesions. The stoma is identified and any incarcerated loops of bowel are reduced. The hernia sac is dissected free from the defect and removed. Mesh (typically PTFE-based) is brought to the field and sized such that a minimum of 4 cm of defect overlap is achieved in all directions. The bowel proximal to the stoma is lateralized on the abdominal wall, which may require additional mobilization to prevent kinking of the bowel at the lateral aspect where it arches over the mesh. Transfascial sutures or tacks are placed around the periphery of the mesh at 1 cm intervals to secure it in place (Fig. 17.4).

17.5.2 Anterior Component Separation (External Oblique Release)

A full midline laparotomy is made incorporating the old scar, all visceral adhesions are lysed, and all previous mesh or other foreign bodies are removed. The stoma is then reduced in prepara-

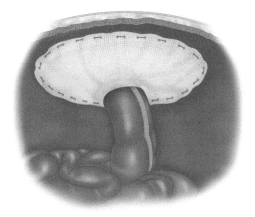

Fig. 17.4 Mesh placement following the Sugarbaker technique with tacks placed at 1 cm intervals around the periphery of the mesh to secure it in place on the abdominal wall

tion for re-siting or anastomosed for restoring continuity and the fascial defect closed with monofilament absorbable suture. At this point, any mobilization of bowel loops in preparation for the new stoma is performed.

The linea alba is identified and lipocutaneous flaps are raised by dissecting the subcutaneous tissue free from the anterior rectus fascia on the side of the parastomal hernia. The flaps are carried laterally to at least 2 cm beyond the linea semilunaris, inferiorly to the inguinal ligament, and superiorly to the coastal margin. Peri-umbilical perforator sparing (PUPS) and endoscopic methods of anterior component separation have been described and are reviewed in Chapters 15–16.

The external oblique aponeurosis is divided 1–2 cm lateral to the linea semilunaris from the costal margin to a point just superior to the inguinal ligament. Care must be taken to not injure the linea semilunaris itself as this can result in the development of a hernia lateral to the rectus muscle. Assessment of the ability to re-approximate the linea alba is made; if the sides can be approximated with no tension, the mesh placement and closure can begin. If tension remains, then the contralateral external oblique aponeurosis can be divided.

The stoma is created through the rectus muscle in a new position and the fascia is closed with a running absorbable monofilament suture. Mesh is placed using an onlay technique, where a closely sized cruciate aperture is made where the stoma will penetrate the mesh. The mesh is secured to the lateral cut edges of the external oblique fascia using monofilament absorbable suture. Several interrupted sutures are placed evenly into the anterior rectus fascia to eliminate dead space. The stoma is now matured and the cutaneous flaps closed in layers over closed suction drains.

17.5.3 Posterior Component Separation (Transversus Abdominis Release)

The initial procedure for a posterior component separation begins identically to that of the ante-

rior component separation. The old scar is removed and an exploratory laparotomy is performed with full lysis of adhesions. The stoma is then reduced in preparation for re-siting or anastomosed for restoring intestinal continuity.

Posterior component separation with TAR is described in detail in Chapter 13. Briefly, using electrocautery, the posterior rectus sheath is incised approximately 5 mm from the medial border and opened superiorly and inferiorly along the entire length of the rectus. Using a combination of blunt dissection and electrocautery, the plane is developed laterally to the linea semilunaris taking care not to injure the neurovascular bundles that penetrate the lateral aspect of the rectus or the epigastric vessels which should remain on the back of the muscle belly. The plane is then developed superiorly into the retrosternal space and interiorly into the space of Retzius. Here blunt dissection can expose the symphysis pubis and Cooper's ligaments bilaterally. There will be a defect in the posterior layer in the location of the previous stoma (Fig. 17.5).

Retrorectus dissection alone is generally insufficient to permit wide mesh overlap lateral to the stoma defect as the rectus sheath ends at the lateral boarder of the rectus muscle. To provide wider lateral overlap, transversus abdominis release is performed. Using cautery, the anterior

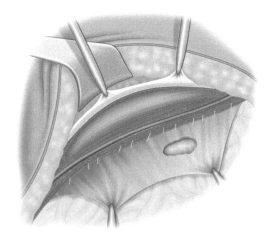

Fig. 17.5 Posterior rectus sheath taken down from the rectus muscles lateral to the linea semilunaris as identified by the traversing neurovascular bundles. There is a defect in the posterior sheath at the location of the old ostomy

aspect of the posterior sheath is incised at a point approximately 5 mm medial to the linea semilunaris, preferably in a more cephalad location where the muscle is better defined and more medial (Fig. 17.6). Using a right angle clamp for assistance, cautery is used to transect the anterior layer of transversalis fascia and the transversus muscle belly, taking care to avoid injury to the peritoneum/posterior transversalis fascia deep to the muscle. Release of the transversus continues inferiorly through the level of the arcuate line. Once the muscle has been divided, blunt dissection can be undertaken laterally to the psoas muscle, superiorly under the costal margin and inferiorly to the myopectineal orifice providing a large sublay space for mesh to be positioned.

Retrorectus dissection on the contralateral side is then undertaken. This is necessary to permit the posterior layers from both sides to be closed together to recreate the visceral sac. The retromuscular space created will permit the mesh to cover the old stoma site and reinforce the midline incision and the new stoma site on the contralateral rectus muscle. If the midline fascia cannot be easily approximated, contralateral release of the transversus abdominis can be accomplished at this juncture. This may be nec-

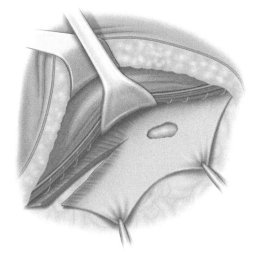

Fig. 17.6 Identification of the transversus abdominis muscle within the posterior rectus sheath is best performed in the upper abdomen, below the costal margin

essary in the case of large parastomal hernias with loss of domain or with simultaneous parastomal and midline ventral hernia repairs.

The posterior layer is then approximated in the midline using running 2-0 absorbable suture. All defects in this layer must be closed to prevent bowel from contacting the mesh or herniating into the space between the posterior layer and the mesh (intra-parietal hernia). Larger holes not amenable to primary suture repair may be patched with vicryl mesh and secured with a running absorbable suture. This may be necessary in the location of the old stoma as the defect here can be quite substantial. Primary closure of the parastomal hernia fascial defect is then performed using 0 monofilament absorbable sutures. Occasionally, the stoma cannot be repositioned to a new location. In these cases, the posterior component separation and transversus abdominis release are still completed with the stoma in situ. The mesh is key-holed around the stoma and then sewn back together laterally in a running fashion.

The aperture for the new stoma is created one layer at a time through closely sized cruciate incisions orienting the stoma properly to avoid kinking. A defect is created in the closed posterior layer and the bowel is delivered into the retromuscular plane taking care to properly orient the mesentery (Fig. 17.7).

The mesh is placed in a diamond configuration and anchored transfascially with absorbable 0 monofilament sutures (Figs. 17.8 and 17.9). We preferentially use medium-weight polypropylene mesh when performing posterior component separation parastomal hernia repairs. This mesh is tightened to a physiologic tension by using a Kocher clamp to pull the linea alba medially toward the midline as the transfascial sutures are placed. This will later allow close approximation of the linea alba without tension. After securing the mesh, a cruciate incision is made at the location of the new stoma and the bowel is delivered through the mesh (Fig. 17.9). A defect is then created in the skin, subcutaneous tissues, anterior rectus sheath and rectus muscle and the bowel delivered through. Drains are placed in the retro muscular space and the dead space of the hernia sac(s) as desired. The linea alba is recreated in

Fig. 17.7 Transversus
abdominis release is
accomplished by dividing the
anterior portion of the
transversalis fascia and the
transversus muscle belly but
leaving the posterior layer of
transversalis fascia and the
peritoneum intact deep to the
muscle

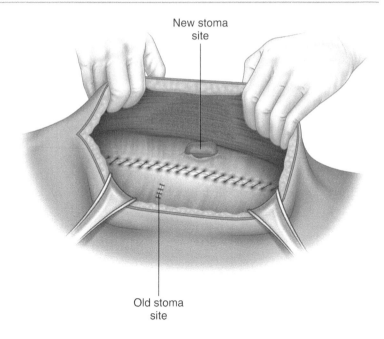

Fig. 17.8 Mesh is placed in a
diamond configuration and
positioned in the retromuscular
space. This covers the old
stoma site and the entire
midline (and any midline
defects) and reinforces the new
stoma location

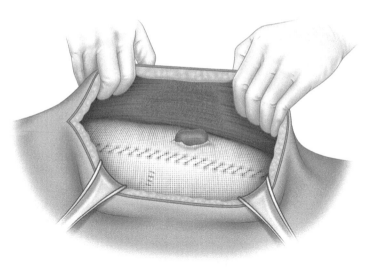

the midline using 0 monofilament absorbable
sutures taking only bites of fascia. The subcutaneous tissues are closed in layers with absorbable
suture and the skin stapled.

17.5.4 Pauli Parastomal Hernia Repair (PPHR)

This novel method of open parastomal hernia repair
avoids ostomy relocation, obviates the need to alter

the mesh with either a cruciate or keyhole incision,
and permits simultaneous coverage of parastomal
and midline defects. This is achieved by combining
posterior component separation and TAR with a
modified Sugarbaker mesh configuration (essentially a retro-muscular Sugarbaker herniorraphy).

The initial steps of the PPHR are completed as
outlined above in the "Posterior Component
Separation" section. Here, however, the TAR is
carefully completed while maintaining the stoma
in situ (Fig. 17.10). With the retromuscular dissec-

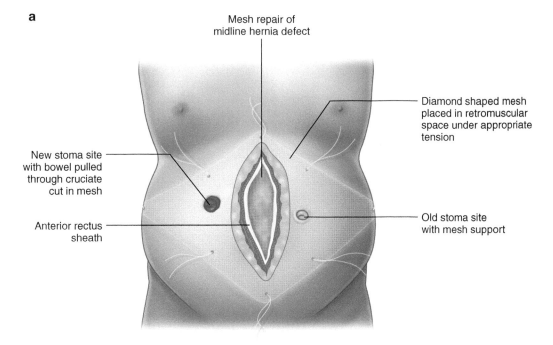

a

Mesh repair of
midline hernia defect

Diamond shaped mesh
placed in retromuscular
space under appropriate
tension

New stoma site
with bowel pulled
through cruciate
cut in mesh

Anterior rectus
sheath

Old stoma site
with mesh support

Eight mesh fixation points

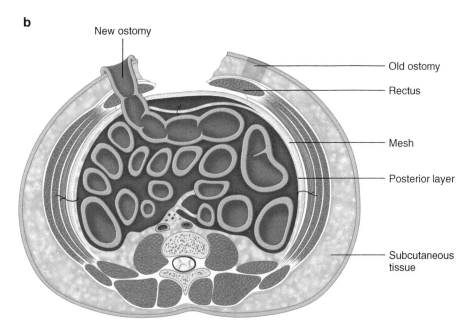

b

New ostomy

Old ostomy

Rectus

Mesh

Posterior layer

Subcutaneous
tissue

Fig. 17.9 The posterior layer of transversalis fascia/peritoneum is closed to recreate the visceral sac. A defect is created at the new ostomy location to deliver the bowel through

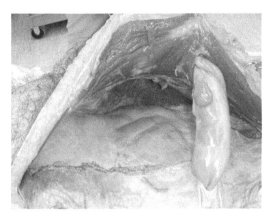

Fig. 17.10 Posterior component separation with TAR completed during PPHR with stoma left in-situ

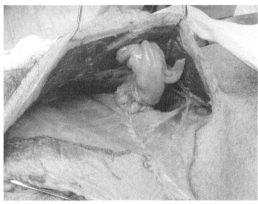

Fig. 17.12 Proximal bowel is delivered through defect into retromuscular plane. The defect is then closed from medial to lateral

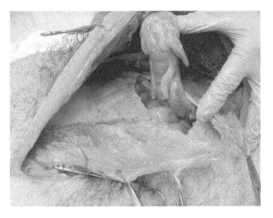

Fig. 17.11 Defect in posterior layer extended laterally

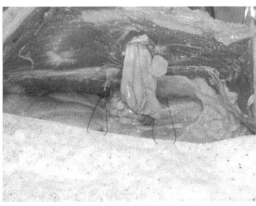

Fig. 17.13 Transfacial sutures are placed on either side of the lateralized bowel to fixate the mesh and create a sling for the stoma

tion extended well beyond the boundaries of the parastomal hernia in all directions, the defect in the posterior layer (through which the stoma exits the abdominal cavity) is intentionally extended laterally (Fig. 17.11). On the contralateral site, retrorectus dissection (or TAR, if needed) is completed. The bowel proximal to the stoma is then delivered into the retromuscular space. The posterior layer is subsequently closed with running absorbable suture simultaneously recreating the visceral sac and lateralizing the location where the proximal bowel enters the retromuscular space (Fig. 17.12).

Mesh is placed in a sublay position within the retromuscular plane with a lateral configuration resembling a Sugarbaker repair. Transfacial sutures are placed in all cardinal directions and on either side of the stoma to create a sling of mesh around the bowel proximal to the stoma (Fig. 17.13). Placing mesh in this fashion provides wide overlap of any additional midline defects while creating a modified Sugarbaker configuration around the stoma that was left in situ (Fig. 17.14). Parastomal and midline defects are primarily closed as described above.

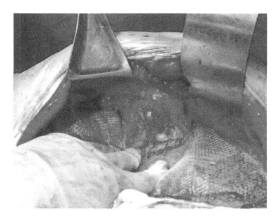

Fig. 17.14 Retromuscular placement of mesh provides wide mesh overlap of any abdominal wall defects and creates a modified Sugarbaker configuration of mesh around the stoma

17.6   Post-operative Care

Parastomal hernia repair patients follow routine post-operative pathways similar to other abdominal wall reconstructive procedures. Antibiotics are routinely stopped at 24 hours and diet is advanced when bowel function has returned. The stoma is observed for any complication and the patient is monitored for signs of infection. Routine venous thromboembolic prophylaxis is mandatory. Abdominal binders are routinely used in the immediate post-operative period. Drains are monitored and typically removed prior to discharge, unless biologic mesh was used, in which case they are maintained for 2 weeks post-op.

17.6.1 Incisional Negative Pressure Wound Therapy

It has been our practice to place negative pressure dressing on the closed midline wound in the operating room when performing open parastomal hernia repair. While this has not been shown to be of benefit for high risk abdominal wall reconstruction incisions, there is support for this practice when performing open colorectal procedures [44, 45]. A narrow strip of petroleum jelly-

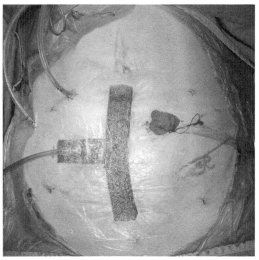

Fig. 17.15 Negative pressure wound dressing applied to the closed midline wound and the loosely closed old stoma site in a T-shaped configuration. Suction is applied over the old stoma site and is set to −75 mmHg

impregnated gauze is applied to the midline wound and loosely closed old stoma site in a T-shaped configuration (Fig. 17.15). This is followed by a similar sized strip of open cell foam. A plastic dressing is applied over top. The suction adaptor is placed over the old stoma site such that the suction will draw to the old ostomy (theoretically the most contaminated wound) and not away from it to the midline wound. Pressure is placed to −75 mmHg suction. This dressing remains in place for 7 days or until discharge. While the exact mechanism of action is not known, one likely benefit is the exclusion of the midline wound from any stoma effluent that may leak around the ostomy appliance and saturate dressings or flow onto the incision.

17.6.2 Mechanical Ventilation

In patients with loss of domain hernias, care must be paid to respiratory mechanics following reconstruction. If plateau airway pressure increases more than 6 mmHg above the baseline level, then intubation is maintained for 24 hours [46]. Neuromuscular blockade is added if plateau airway pressure increases more than 10–11 mmHg after re-approximation of the linea alba [46]. Maintaining urinary and gastric decompression is beneficial in these circumstances to reduce the elevated intra-abdominal pressures that occur following primary fascial re-approximation.

17.7 Results of Open Parastomal Hernia Repair

Results of various types of open parastomal hernia repair are summarized in Table 17.1.

17.8 Complications of Open Parastomal Hernia Repair

General complications of open hernia repair are covered in Chapter 20. Open parastomal hernia repair has some inherent complications not applicable to general open repairs and these will be reviewed here.

17.8.1 Wound Infection

Wound infections following gastrointestinal stoma takedown or relocation remain one of the most common post-operative complications, with rates as high as 41 % [47–50]. This is of particular concern in complex parastomal hernia repair, as wound infections can lead to mesh infection and hernia recurrence (Fig. 17.16). There are a variety of options available for managing the old stoma site, including primary closure (with or without a subcutaneous drain), delayed primary closure, closure by secondary intention and negative pressure wound therapy. The method of closure is partially dependent on the details of the herniorraphy: how large is the subcutaneous dead space, where is the mesh located within the abdominal wall, was the fascia fully closed over the mesh, what type of mesh was used, does the patient have any additional risks for developing a wound infection (immunosuppression, diabetes, malnutrition). Our preference is to close all wounds primarily and place a negative pressure dressing on the closed midline wound and the old stoma site. If there is a large subcutaneous dead space under either of these wounds, a separate closed suction drain may be placed subcutaneously.

17.8.2 Stoma Complications

Complications related directly to the ostomy are unique to parastomal repairs. Rates of these complications are fortunately low, but they can have significant morbidity when they do occur. Stoma ischemia, necrosis, or retractions are often technical complications from tension on the ostomy, twisting of to the mesentery during stoma delivery through the abdominal wall or a tight stoma aperture in the rectus muscle or the mesh (Fig. 17.16). Patient-related factors such as obesity, atherosclerosis, and post-op hypotension can contribute to these complications.

Table 17.1 Results of multiple types of open parastomal hernia repair techniques

Type of repair	Number of patients	Infection% (95% CI)	Mesh infection% (95% CI)	Other complication% (95% CI)	Mortality% (95% CI)	Recurrence% (95% CI)	Mean follow-up (months)
Primary fascial repair[2]	141	9.4 (4.9–15.8)	na	14.1 (8.6–21.3)	2.8 (0.8–7.1)	57.6 (48.4–66.4)	30
Mesh onlay[2]	216	1.9 (0.5–4.7)	1.9 (0.5–4.7)	11.1 (7.3–16.1)	0 (0–1.7)	14.8 (10.2–20.4)	40
Mesh sublay[2]	76	3.9 (0.8–11.1)	0 (0–4.7)	14.5 (7.5–24.4)	0 (0–4.7)	7.9 (3–16.4)	24
Mesh underlay[2]	65	3.1 (0.4–10.7)	1.5 (0–8.3)	15.4 (7.6–24.4)	0 (0–5.5)	9.2 (3.5–19)	38
Mesh sublay[34]	48	31.3	0	25	0	11	13

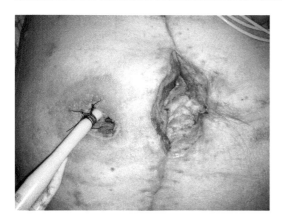

Fig. 17.16 Midline wound infection with exposed synthetic mesh and muco-cutaneous disruption and stoma retraction following a component separation parastomal hernia repair. The stoma output is being managed with a Foley catheter

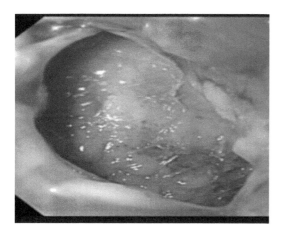

Fig. 17.17 Endoscopic view of polypropylene mesh eroded into the colon following an open parastomal hernia repair

Kinking of the ostomy can result in delayed stoma function or obstruction. This complication can happen with any type of parastomal repair, but is commonly associated with the bowel bending over the lateral edge of the mesh when performing a Sugarbaker repair. It can also occur during posterior component separation with transversus abdominis release if care is not taken to properly align the three individually made holes in the abdominal wall (peritoneum/transversalis layer, mesh layer, rectus muscle/anterior rectus sheath/subcutaneous tissue layer).

Mesh erosion is a rare complication of parastomal hernia repair, but may require stoma takedown and mesh excision. As noted above, placement of synthetic mesh in the vicinity of the stoma is considered safe during both stoma creation and parastomal hernia repair. However, mesh may erode into the bowel if there is significant kinking of the bowel over the edge of the mesh or tension of the bowel over the cut edge of the mesh (Fig. 17.17).

References

1. Hotouras A, et al. The persistent challenge of parastomal herniation: a review of the literature and future developments. Colorectal Dis. 2013;15(5):e202–14.
2. Al Shakarchi J, Williams JG. Systematic review of open techniques for parastomal hernia repair. Tech Coloproctol. 2014;18(5):427–32.
3. Nastro P, et al. Complications of intestinal stomas. Br J Surg. 2010;97(12):1885–9.
4. Rieger N, et al. Parastomal hernia repair. Colorectal Dis. 2004;6(3):203–5.
5. Carne PW, Robertson GM, Frizelle FA. Parastomal hernia. Br J Surg. 2003;90(7):784–93.
6. Israelsson LA. Parastomal hernias. Surg Clin North Am. 2008;88(1):113–25. ix.
7. Timmermans L, et al. Parastomal hernia is an independent risk factor for incisional hernia in patients with end colostomy. Surgery. 2014;155(1):178–83.
8. Powell-Chandler A, Stephenson BM. Avoiding simultaneous incisional and parastomal herniation. Colorectal Dis. 2014;16(12):1020–1.
9. Kald A, et al. Quality of life is impaired in patients with peristomal bulging of a sigmoid colostomy. Scand J Gastroenterol. 2008;43(5):627–33.
10. Sjodahl R, Anderberg B, Bolin T. Parastomal hernia in relation to site of the abdominal stoma. Br J Surg. 1988;75(4):339–41.
11. Al-Momani H, Miller C, Stephenson BM. Stoma siting and the 'arcuate line' of Douglas: might it be of relevance to later herniation? Colorectal Dis. 2014;16(2):141–3.
12. De Raet J, et al. Waist circumference is an independent risk factor for the development of parastomal hernia after permanent colostomy. Dis Colon Rectum. 2008;51(12):1806–9.
13. Baykara ZG, et al. A multicenter, retrospective study to evaluate the effect of preoperative stoma site marking on stomal and peristomal complications. Ostomy Wound Manage. 2014;60(5):16–26.
14. Shah NR, Craft RO, Harold KL. Parastomal hernia repair. Surg Clin North Am. 2013;93(5):1185–98.
15. Serra-Aracil X, et al. Randomized, controlled, prospective trial of the use of a mesh to prevent parastomal hernia. Ann Surg. 2009;249(4):583–7.

16. Wijeyekoon SP, et al. Prevention of parastomal herniation with biologic/composite prosthetic mesh: a systematic review and meta-analysis of randomized controlled trials. J Am Coll Surg. 2010;211(5): 637–45.

17. Figel NA, Rostas JW, Ellis CN. Outcomes using a bioprosthetic mesh at the time of permanent stoma creation in preventing a parastomal hernia: a value analysis. Am J Surg. 2012;203(3):323–6. discussion 326.

18. Hauters P, et al. Prevention of parastomal hernia by intraperitoneal onlay mesh reinforcement at the time of stoma formation. Hernia. 2012;16(6):655–60.

19. Lee L, et al. Cost effectiveness of mesh prophylaxis to prevent parastomal hernia in patients undergoing permanent colostomy for rectal cancer. J Am Coll Surg. 2014;218(1):82–91.

20. Janes A, Cengiz Y, Israelsson LA. Randomized clinical trial of the use of a prosthetic mesh to prevent parastomal hernia. Br J Surg. 2004;91(3):280–2.

21. Janes A, Cengiz Y, Israelsson LA. Preventing parastomal hernia with a prosthetic mesh: a 5-year follow-up of a randomized study. World J Surg. 2009;33(1): 118–21. discussion 122-3.

22. Williams NS, Nair R, Bhan C. Stapled mesh stoma reinforcement technique (SMART)—a procedure to prevent parastomal herniation. Ann R Coll Surg Engl. 2011;93(2):169.

23. Koltun L, Benyamin N, Sayfan J. Abdominal stoma fashioned by a used circular stapler. Dig Surg. 2000; 17(2):118–9.

24. Hansson BM, et al. Surgical techniques for parastomal hernia repair: a systematic review of the literature. Ann Surg. 2012;255(4):685–95.

25. Horgan K, Hughes LE. Para-ileostomy hernia: failure of a local repair technique. Br J Surg. 1986;73(6):439–40.

26. Rubin MS, Schoetz Jr DJ, Matthews JB. Parastomal hernia. Is stoma relocation superior to fascial repair? Arch Surg. 1994;129(4):413–8. discussion 418-9.

27. Sugarbaker PH. Peritoneal approach to prosthetic mesh repair of paraostomy hernias. Ann Surg. 1985;201(3):344–6.

28. Sugarbaker PH. Prosthetic mesh repair of large hernias at the site of colonic stomas. Surg Gynecol Obstet. 1980;150(4):576–8.

29. Mancini GJ, et al. Laparoscopic parastomal hernia repair using a nonslit mesh technique. Surg Endosc. 2007;21(9):1487–91.

30. Tran H, et al. Single-port laparoscopic parastomal hernia repair with modified sugarbaker technique. JSLS. 2014;18(1):34–40.

31. Zacharakis E, et al. Laparoscopic parastomal hernia repair: a description of the technique and initial results. Surg Innov. 2008;15(2):85–9.

32. Raigani S, et al. Single-center experience with parastomal hernia repair using retromuscular mesh placement. J Gastrointest Surg. 2014;18(9):1673–7.

33. Slater NJ, et al. Repair of parastomal hernias with biologic grafts: a systematic review. J Gastrointest Surg. 2011;15(7):1252–8.

34. Lee L, et al. A systematic review of synthetic and biologic materials for abdominal wall reinforcement in contaminated fields. Surg Endosc. 2014;28(9):2531–46.

35. Fleshman JW, et al. A prospective, multicenter, randomized, controlled study of non-cross-linked porcine acellular dermal matrix fascial sublay for parastomal reinforcement in patients undergoing surgery for permanent abdominal wall ostomies. Dis Colon Rectum. 2014;57(5):623–31.

36. Krpata DM, et al. Evaluation of high-risk, comorbid patients undergoing open ventral hernia repair with synthetic mesh. Surgery. 2013;153(1):120–5.

37. Rosen MJ, et al. A 5-year clinical experience with single-staged repairs of infected and contaminated abdominal wall defects utilizing biologic mesh. Ann Surg. 2013;257(6):991–6.

38. Novitsky YW, et al. Transversus abdominis muscle release: a novel approach to posterior component separation during complex abdominal wall reconstruction. Am J Surg. 2012;204(5):709–16.

39. Pauli EM, Rosen MJ. Open ventral hernia repair with component separation. Surg Clin North Am. 2013; 93(5):1111–33.

40. Carbonell AM, et al. Outcomes of synthetic mesh in contaminated ventral hernia repairs. J Am Coll Surg. 2013;217(6):991–8.

41. Carbonell AM, Cobb WS. Safety of prosthetic mesh hernia repair in contaminated fields. Surg Clin North Am. 2013;93(5):1227–39.

42. Hofstetter WL, et al. New technique for mesh repair of paracolostomy hernias. Dis Colon Rectum. 1998;41(8):1054–5.

43. Leslie D. The parastomal hernia. Surg Clin North Am. 1984;64(2):407–15.

44. Pauli EM, et al. Negative pressure therapy for high-risk abdominal wall reconstruction incisions. Surg Infect (Larchmt). 2013;14(3):270–4.

45. Bonds AM, et al. Incisional negative pressure wound therapy significantly reduces surgical site infection in open colorectal surgery. Dis Colon Rectum. 2013; 56(12):1403–8.

46. Blatnik JA, et al. Predicting severe postoperative respiratory complications following abdominal wall reconstruction. Plast Reconstr Surg. 2012;130(4): 836–41.

47. Lahat G, et al. Wound infection after ileostomy closure: a prospective randomized study comparing primary vs. delayed primary closure techniques. Tech Coloproctol. 2005;9(3):206–8.

48. Hackam DJ, Rotstein OD. Stoma closure and wound infection: an evaluation of risk factors. Can J Surg. 1995;38(2):144–8.

49. Vermulst N, et al. Primary closure of the skin after stoma closure. Management of wound infections is easy without (long-term) complications. Dig Surg. 2006;23(4):255–8.

50. van de Pavoordt HD, et al. The outcome of loop ileostomy closure in 293 cases. Int J Colorectal Dis. 1987; 2(4):214–7.

Melissa Phillips LaPinska and Austin Lewis

Overview

Flank hernias represent an interesting challenge to the general surgeon. These are relatively rare, but they are rising in frequency as traumatic avulsions and post-surgical flank complications become more common. Because the location of the costal margin and pelvic brim limits the fixation options available in the repair of flank hernias, surgeons have been forced to evaluate other techniques of mesh overlap in the treatment of these difficult hernias. An understanding of the basic anatomy and tenants of operative repair of these hernias is important for the general surgeon in today's practice. Smaller defects can be addressed laparoscopically, but for larger flank defects or those associated with denervation injuries, the open approach to flank hernia repair offers the surgeon the ability to obtain a mesh fixation with the appropriate overlap to confidently repair these unique hernia defects.

Current Trends in Flank Hernia Repair

Current trends in flank hernia repairs have paralleled the midline incisional hernia repairs for many years. The original repairs involved primary fascial re-approximation closed by suture without reinforcement. With this repair lacking reinforcement, recurrence rates have been particularly high, leading to the trend away from this technique. With the introduction of tension-free mesh repairs, which were introduced as being superior in the inguinal region, open repair of flank hernias was attempted with placement of mesh over the hernia defect, sewing the mesh circumferentially to the fascial edges. This result on the flank as compared to the midline has shown increased diastasis and bulging which has led to this also becoming an unfavorable technique for repair. Additionally, laparoscopic repairs have been attempted, which work well in patients with small fascial defects and no loss of intra-abdominal domain, but are not applicable to a large majority of patients with a flank hernia. Because of this, the "perfect" technique for flank hernia repair remains unclear. Tenants of this ideal open flank hernia repair would include:

Electronic supplementary material: The online version of this chapter (doi:10.1007/978-3-319-27470-6_18) contains supplementary material, which is available to authorized users.

M.P. LaPinska, M.D., F.A.C.S. (✉) • A. Lewis, M.D.
Department of Surgery, University of Tennessee
Health Science Center, Knoxville, TN, USA
e-mail: MSphillips1@utmck.edu

- Durable repair of the fascial defect that would prevent strangulation
- Minimization of patient morbidity and wound complications
- Preservation of native blood supply of the area
- Reconstruction of a functional, innervated abdominal wall

Anatomy Surrounding the Flank Hernia

Flank hernias are broadly divided into those that are congenital and those that are acquired. Congenital hernias are then subclassified into defects involving the superior lumbar triangle (Grynfeltt) versus those involving the inferior lumbar triangle (Petit). More common than the congenital defects are the acquired flank hernias, occurring after many types of surgical interventions including aortic surgery, nephrectomies, retroperitoneal spine exposure cases, orthopedic bone harvest sites, and trauma. Because of the specific details of the original surgery or trauma, the variability in these acquired hernias has made it a difficult task for the general surgeon to find a single technique that applies well to all defects. Because of the location of the fascial defects between the bony prominences of the costal margin and the iliac crest, flank hernias present a challenge in repair because of the lack of options for mesh fixation as well as limited areas available for mesh overlap in this region. Additionally, neurovascular structures contained in the retroperitoneum and pelvic brim provide an increased risk for nerve injury, chronic pain, or numbness related to surgery. The combinations of these anatomic limitations and variety of previous surgical interventions have made it difficult for the general surgeon to find a single "perfect" repair for the flank hernia.

Preoperative Planning

Distinguish Pseudoherniation

The first goal of preoperative patient evaluation is to distinguish a true flank hernia from a pseudohernia of the abdominal wall. Pseudoherniation, also known as diastasis or abdominal wall eventration, comes from a neuromuscular injury to the flank that results in stretching and bulging of the flank without a true fascial defect, as seen in Fig. 18.1. This can be seen in patients with spinal cord injury, previous subcostal incisions cutting through the nerves of the abdominal wall, and after traumatic injury to the ribs/lower thorax. Because this condition is a physiologic bulging rather than a surgically correctable cause, it is important to distinguish this from a true defect because surgical intervention is not needed. CT scan is an effective way of imaging the abdominal wall to make this distinction. Physical therapy can improve but is unlikely to resolve completely pseudoherniation symptoms. Additionally, it is important to make the diagnosis of pseudoherniation in combination with a true fascial defect for preoperative counseling of outcomes. Patients with this combination will often continue to report a bulge of the flank despite adequate repair of the fascial defect following repair and, making it important to address this expectation preoperatively.

Role for Preoperative Imaging

Because of the anatomic limitations detailed above, all patients with a true flank hernia should undergo imaging of the abdominal wall prior to undergoing surgical repair. Detailing the defect size and location is important to planning and appropriate repair. Smaller fascial defects without loss of domain can be addressed laparoscopically [1]. This chapter specifically addresses the open repair of flank hernia which applies well to the following subsets of patients:

- Small fascial defects with large amounts of hernia contents (loss of domain)
- Large fascial defects
- Patients with desire for return of abdominal wall function by muscular re-approximation

Figure 18.2 shows an example of a patient who underwent previous renal transplantation resulting in a lateral fascial defect. As the patient had multiple confounding factors to early hernia repair,

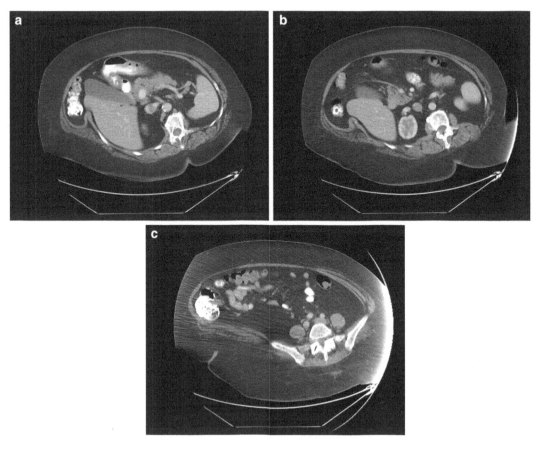

Fig. 18.1 CT scan showing pseudohernia with lateral abdominal wall laxity

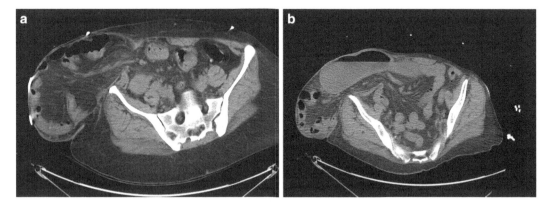

Fig. 18.2 CT scan showing small lateral fascial defect with loss of intra-abdominal domain

including postoperative complications and immu-nosuppression, this fascial defect has remained small but the volume of herniated contents has dra-matically increased. An open repair of the flank hernia (with component separation on the contra-lateral side) is essential in this patient scenario to allow for reduction of the extra-abdominal contents while addressing the fascial defect on the flank.

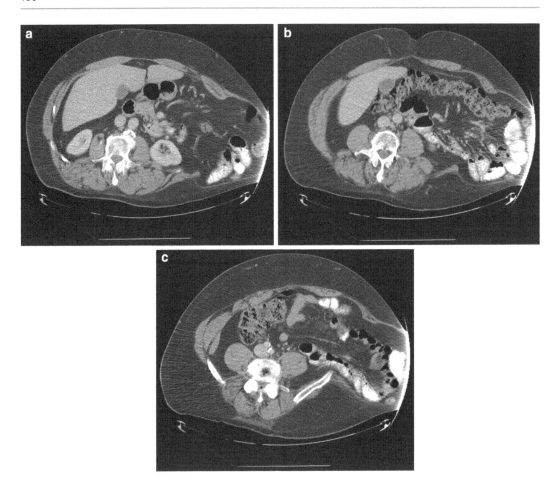

Fig. 18.3 CT scan showing large flank fascial defect after previous orthopedic surgery

Figure 18.3 is an example of a patient with a large fascial defect through a previous surgical incision. Laparoscopic approach to this repair would lead to a large area of mesh without abdominal wall function and, because of that eventration, would lead to a poor cosmetic result for the patient. In assessing patients with this degree of flank hernia, many report problems with balance and walking because of the significant asymmetry of the abdominal contents. Fortunately, this is often corrected with surgical repair.

Patient Optimization

Contradictory to the pressures placed on the surgeon for a quick and expedited repair, the benefit of preoperative optimization of patients will improve both surgical outcomes and patient satisfaction with surgery. With the increasing use of online calculators for surgical risk, a patient's individualized risk profile can be assessed. Time should be spent discussing with patients their risks of undergoing surgery, with specific attention spent on the modifiable risk factors. These modifiable risk factors are not different for flank hernias versus other abdominal hernias and include body mass index, smoking status, diabetic control, immunosuppression, nutritional optimization, infection control, and preoperative exercise status. As has been evidenced in the literature, smoking cession, weight loss, and strict diabetic control can reduce complication rates significantly as well as increase patient participation in his/her medical care.

Specifically with regard to the discussion of infectious risk, depending on the characteristics of the hernia, bony fixation may be required for securement of mesh despite good overlap. Because of the use of bone anchors, patients in this category must be counseled preoperatively about the risks of infection, including osteomyelitis.

Operative Technique

Patient Positioning

Patients with an isolated moderate or large flank defects are best approached from a lateral flank incision [2]. Patients with smaller defects, such as those similar to Fig. 18.2, can be approached through a midline incision with a transversus abdominis release (TAR), as detailed in Chapter 13. Additionally, patients who have a midline defect in combination with a flank defect are often best approached through a midline incision using the TAR procedure so that both areas of fascial defect can be addressed simultaneously.

Patient positioning, as seen in Fig. 18.4, is an important aspect to the open flank repair. Patients must be in the full lateral position and centered on an OR bed that is capable of flexing the patient to optimize the space between the iliac crest and the lower edge of the costal margin. Because of the length of the operation and the movement needed for exposure during the surgery, patients should be well padded, often utilizing a bean bag for support, to prevent injury and secured in multiple locations to reduce the risk of positioning injury. Landmarks that should be included in the operative field include the umbilicus and linea alba anteriorly, spine posteriorly, the costal margin with xiphoid process superiorly, and the pelvic brim with pubic bone inferiorly. These areas will be the edges of mesh placement for larger flank hernias and, thus, the sites of the transfascial fixation sutures.

A transverse incision is made parallel and preferably 3 cm above the superior edge of the iliac crest. If the patient has undergone previous incisions at that location, it is recommended that the old scar be excised to allow for healthier skin edges for postoperative healing. Electrocautery is used to dissect down to the level of the hernia sac, separating the hernia sac as it protrudes through the native fascia. It is important to identify the separate muscular layers of the abdominal wall as these will be closed in layers ventral to the mesh at the completion of the hernia repair. If the patient does not have any reasons for intra-abdominal exploration, such as a history of small bowel obstruction from presumed adhesions, entry into the hernia sac is not needed. If there is a need for intra-abdominal exploration, the hernia sac can be opened and a complete adhesiolysis performed. It is often easier to dissect the hernia

Fig. 18.4 Patient positioning for open flank hernia repair

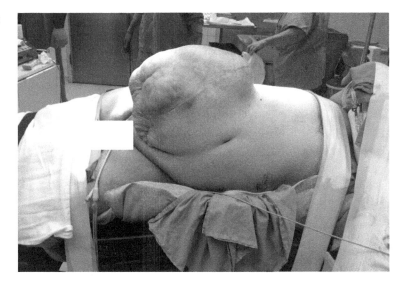

sac down from the fascial edges and use this plane of dissection to enter into the preperitoneal plane after division of the transversus abdominis without entering into the abdomen. In patients with chronic or dense scarring around the hernia sac, it may be impossible to do this without creating a defect through the sac/peritoneum. If a defect is made, the dissection should be continued and the defect will be closed with a #2-0 absorbable, braided suture prior to mesh placement.

Dissection of the Preperitoneal Space

Dissection toward the spine as seen in Fig. 18.5, into the retroperitoneal space, is usually the easiest direction to establish the correct plane. This is a familiar space to many surgeons as it is the same one used for spine exposure or aortic exposure. The intra-abdominal viscera as well as the kidney and adrenal gland are rotated anterior-medially and the psoas muscle is identified. The lateral edge of the psoas muscle should be used as a safety landmark. Along the medial aspect of the psoas muscle are iliac vessels, gonadal vessels, and the ureter. Also present in this area are the genitofemoral, ilioinguinal, iliohypogastric, and lateral femoral cutaneous nerves which must be identified and preserved. Proper identification of these structures during the dissection will also help to avoid injury during transfascial suture placement.

Continuing in the same plane, the dissection is extended toward the pelvis, down into the space of Retzius, mobilizing the bladder and identifying the pubic tubercle. Again, this space is commonly familiar to surgeons from laparoscopic inguinal hernia repair operations. Care should be taken to preserve the inferior epigastric vessels associated with the anterior abdominal wall as well as the vas deferens and gonadal vessels in males. The round ligament in females should be divided to facilitate dissection and subsequent mesh placement. The dissection of the viscera off of the pelvic brim while leaving the neurovascular structures intact on the bony prominence is one of the most important steps in the open repair of a flank hernia. As discussed in the "Anatomic Limitations" section of this chapter, the mesh

overlap beyond the bony structures is really the mainstay of mesh placement as the fascial fixation options are limited. Surgeons should take the time to make sure that this dissection is performed fully; otherwise, the overlap of mesh will not be adequate and the risk of recurrence will be increased.

At this time, rather than proceeding with the more challenging anterior/medial dissection, working on the superior aspect of the dissection next has the advantage of defining the planes. The dissection is carried up to the retroperitoneum with a transition into the preperitoneal plane at the level of the costal margin. The peritoneum can then be removed from the inner aspect of the costal margin and subsequently off the diaphragm. The extent of this dissection up under the costal margin is extremely important in ensuring adequate overlap as shown in Fig. 18.6. All fixation of the upper margin of mesh will be performed below the bony portion of the costal margin and, thus, the attachment of the mesh at this location will be largely dependent on the overlap under the ribs [3]. This dissection in the preperitoneal plane can easily extend 7–10 cm cephalad to the lower edge of the costal margin.

Once these planes have been established, the dissection proceeds medially toward the anterior abdomen. The medial dissection is often the most difficult secondary to the attachment of the peritoneum to the linea alba. If a tear occurs, it is important to recognize this and close the peritoneal defect. Dissection can be carried in this plane to the level of the linea alba. Some authors describe a transition from the preperitoneal space into the retro rectus space after medially crossing the linea semilunaris, performing a reverse transversus abdominis release and entering into the retrorectus position at midline rather than just the preperitoneal space. The "reverse TAR" is difficult technically and should only be used by those trained in advanced abdominal wall surgery. Division of the transversus abdominis too laterally carries with it the risk for injury to the nerves of the abdominal wall, which would result in a diastasis/denervation injury. Additionally, if the landmarks are misidentified and the linea semilunaris is cut during the dissection rather than the transversus abdominis, a full thickness fascial defect is created.

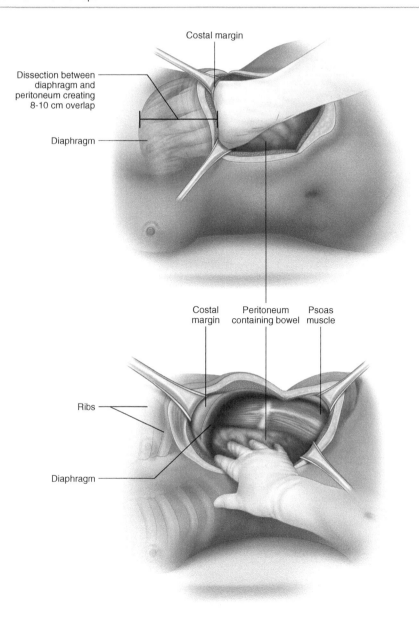

Fig. 18.5   Posterior dissection of the preperitoneal space

Mesh Selection and Insertion

Once the dissection has been completed, any potential rents in the peritoneum or hernia sac should be closed with a #2-0 braided, absorbable suture. This dissected peritoneal layer is not a strength layer but is more intended to prevent contact of the viscera with the mesh and thus must be closed completely. Measurement of the extent of dissection is performed, taking care to appreci-

ate that the mesh will be placed into the area in the shape of a "taco," with folding both anteriorly and posteriorly to the viscera and extending from above the costal margin into the pelvic brim to the pubic tubercle as you can see in the cross section of Fig. 18.7. Similar to the trends in most open hernia repairs, including component separations, mesh used for this repair must be strong enough to hold the strength of the abdominal wall while minimizing the foreign body response. The

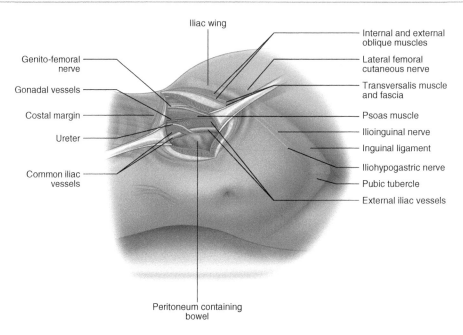

Fig. 18.6 Superior dissection of the preperitoneal space

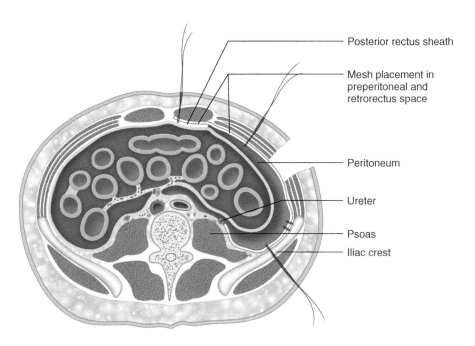

Fig. 18.7 Cross-sectional placement of mesh insertion

authors prefer to use a large (often 30 cm × 30 cm) midweight, macroporous, monofilament mesh. There is no need for an anti-adhesive barrier as is used for intraperitoneal mesh since the peritoneum provides a natural covering to protect the viscera from the mesh. Caution should be given to the use of the lightweight mesh due to risks of excessive bulging and central mesh failures. Some hernia experts even support the use of heavy weight mesh in this situation for this reason. A total of eight transfascial fixation sutures using a #1 absorbable monofilament stitch are placed circumferentially around the mesh as shown in Fig. 18.8. These sutures can be offset up to 10 cm from the edges of the mesh to avoid placement of these sutures around the neurovascular structures near the costal margin and pelvic brim while allowing for additional overlap within these bony structures. Each stitch is passed through a stab incision using a no. 11 blade using a suture passer, securing a 1 cm bite of fascia between each arm of the transfascial suture.

Consideration must be given to the hernia characteristics in determining where to begin with the fixation of the mesh. For a lower flank hernia, it is recommended to begin fixation at the pubic tubercle as this area has the most limitation due to bony structures, and lack of overlap at the inferior side would be the highest risk for recurrence. Additionally, for low flank hernias, one must evaluate the quality of the fascia at the superior edge of the iliac crest when considering the use of bone anchors as illustrated in Fig. 18.9. These devices have been borrowed from the orthopedic surgeons to provide a sturdy fixation point into the anterior superior iliac spine in patients who do not have adequate fascia for mesh securement at this location [4, 5]. A surgi-

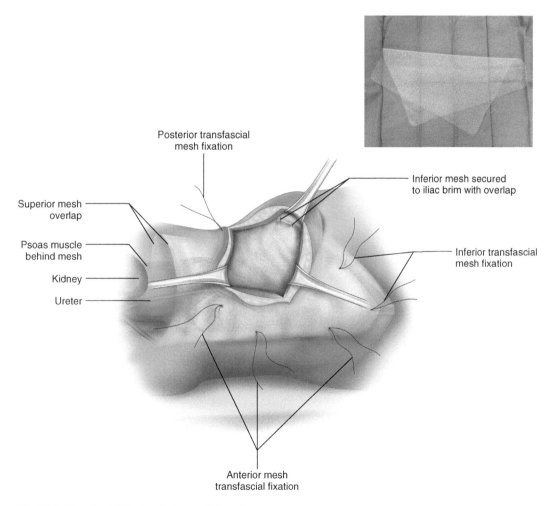

Fig. 18.8 Transfascial fixation during mesh insertion

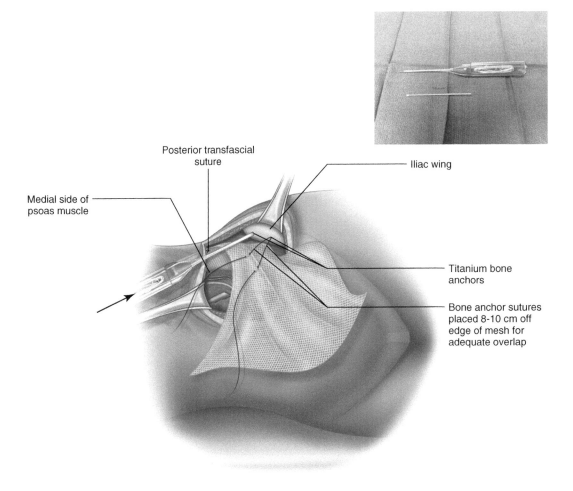

Fig. 18.9 Placement of bone anchors to aid in complex flank hernia mesh placement

cal drill is used to preplace a designated hole at the anterior aspect of the iliac crest. The bone anchor, such as Arthrex Corkscrew® (Arthrex, Naples, FL), which contains a titanium anchor with two attached non-absorbable sutures, is then placed into the predrilled tract. The sutures are then passed through the mesh to secure it to this location at the iliac crest while the mesh drapes down into the pelvis, allowing good overlap with the bony structures. For higher flank hernias, mesh placement should begin at the upper aspect of the defect, securing the mesh to the fascia just below the costal margin while allowing the mesh above the suture to "drape" under the costal margin between the diaphragm and the peritoneum for good overlap in that area.

During the passage of the sutures, it is important to hold tension on each suture directly next to the suture of interest to ensure the location of the stab incision provides correct tension and re-approximation of the mesh to the abdominal wall. After all eight transfascial sutures have been passed, the sutures are tied and cut, allowing the stitch to retract back under the skin.

Closure of the Abdominal Wall

A 15-French drain is placed above the level of the mesh but underneath the primary fascial closure. Fascial closure for recurrent hernias is still a topic of ongoing research, especially with regard to the ratio of suture to incision length. The approach of the authors is to close the flank in a two-layered closure with the transversus and internal oblique in the deep layer and the external oblique through the anterior rectus fascia in the more superficial layer with a #1 absorbable, monofilament suture. In most cases, the fascia can be re-approximated primarily using this technique. It is important to stress the resection of any devitalized tissue, be it subcutaneous fat or excess skin from the previous hernia. A layered closure of the abdominal wall is performed. Although unsupported by literature in the complex hernia population [6], we routinely use a negative pressure dressing (e.g., wound vac) over the closed incision as it has been shown to decrease surgical site infections in other populations following surgery.

Postoperative Care

Surgical drains are left in place until the output is less than 25 ml per day for two consecutive days at which point they are removed in the office. Abdominal distention should be avoided to reduce unnecessary stress on the fascial repair. Abdominal binders are a routine part of recovery following this procedure and are often used for up to 6 weeks. Patients are given lifting restrictions with a maximum of 25 lb for 6 weeks following the surgery, but are encouraged to walk and perform other cardiovascular activities during this time.

Unplanned Challenges

Multiple Fenestrations in the Peritoneal Layer

Rather than a true complication, multiple holes in the peritoneum caused during dissection are a common occurrence in patients with multiple previous operations or with dense adhesions. It is important to recognize and address the presence of the peritoneal defect because the risk of visceral herniation through the peritoneum can lead to direct contact between the bowel and the unpro-

tected mesh, predisposing to intestinal obstructions. Any patient with an early small bowel obstruction, particularly in the setting of a transition point, should be considered for this rare complication. As is true for many situations, prevention is the key. All peritoneal defects should be closed with either a running or an interrupted absorbable suture prior to mesh placement.

Inability to Primarily Close the Fascia

Most large fascial defects using this surgical approach can be closed primarily. Two main factors influence the ability to obtain fascial closure: extent of dissection and tension distribution over the mesh to offload the fascial tension. As detailed above in "Dissection of the Preperitoneal Space," the dissection can extend from 10 cm above the costal margin down to the level of the pubic tubercle and from the spine posteriorly to the linea alba anteriorly. Larger defects will require increased amounts of dissection to distribute the tension of closure over a larger area while smaller defects may not require the entire area to be dissected to allow for adequate closure. After dissection, but before transfascial mesh fixation, Kocher forceps can be placed on the primary fascia and the tension of closure assessed. With regard to the mesh aiding in primary fascial closure, the mesh can help distribute the physiologic tension of the abdominal wall. By using Kocher forceps on the fascia to show re-approximation, an appropriate location for the transfascial stitch can be selected that allows for the correct tension distribution.

Enterotomy with Planned Bony Fixation

This specific situation presents a balancing act between hernia recurrence and the risk for postoperative infection-related complications. In the setting where there has been gross spillage from an enterotomy, the fascia around the iliac crest should be closely evaluated. In some settings, the small fascial rim can be mobilized off the bony prominence. If there is at least 1 cm of intact fascia, we recommend using transfascial fixation sutures through this area rather than placing the bone anchors because of the risk of osteomyelitis of the pelvis.

Pseudohernia with True Fascial Defect

The most important step with this complication is the identification preoperatively on CT imaging. Previous flank incisions are often associated with a neurovascular injury that has resulted in a denervation injury to that portion of the abdominal wall as well as an incisional hernia. Patients who have this combination will often be dissatisfied with the persistent diastasis that is present, even after a technically perfect repair. Patients in this group should be counseled ahead of time to ensure that they appreciate the complexities of this repair and understand that some abdominal wall asymmetry may persist following surgery.

Summary

Flank hernias present an interesting challenge to the general surgeon when compared to the standard midline incisional hernia. The approxima-

tion to bony landmarks makes overlap, rather than fixation, the keys to this open surgical repair. Preperitoneal dissection allows for a wide plane of overlap and protects the intra-abdominal contents from mesh contact. Mesh placement with transfascial fixation reinforces the hernia defect and distributes tension over the abdominal wall, allowing for primary fascial closure. This technique gives a durable repair for the treatment of this challenging type of hernia.

References

1. Heniford BT, Iannitti DA, Gagner M. Laparoscopic inferior and superior lumbar hernia repair. Arch Surg. 1997;132:1141–4.
2. Stumpf M, Conze J, Prescher A, Junge K, Krones C, Klinge U, Schumpelick V. The lateral incisional hernia: anatomic considerations for a standardized retromuscular sublay repair. Hernia. 2009;13(3):293–7.
3. Phillips M, Krpata D, Blatnik J, Rosen M. Retromuscular preperitoneal repair of flank hernias. J Gastrointest Surg. 2012;16(8):1548–53.
4. Carbonell A, Kercher K, Sigmon L, Matthews B, Sing R, Kneisl J, Heniford B. A novel technique of lumbar hernia repair using bone anchor fixation. Hernia. 2005;9(1):22–5.
5. Yee J, Harold K, Cobb W, Carbonell A. Bone anchor mesh fixation for complex laparoscopic ventral hernia repair. Surg Innov. 2008;15(4):292–6.
6. Pauli E, Krpata D, Novitsky Y, Rosen M. Negative pressure therapy for high-risk abdominal wall reconstruction incisions. Surg Infect (Larchmt). 2013;14(3):270–4.

Kent W. Kercher

Introduction

Umbilical hernias are among the more common abdominal wall hernias, accounting for 10% of primary hernias in the adult patient population, with over 270,000 repairs per year in the United States. In children, most are congenital, while umbilical hernias are typically acquired fascial defects in adults and can occur either spontaneously or at the site of prior surgical access, such as those which may develop following laparoscopic port placement at the umbilicus. For the purposes of discussion in this chapter, these two types of umbilical hernias will be classified as either primary or recurrent, with recurrent hernias including small incisional hernias localized to the umbilicus.

While most surgeons generally think of an umbilical hernia as a simple, single primary fascial defect, the repair of which represents one of the more straightforward technical exercises in surgery, there is a wide spectrum of disease and hence a number of surgical options for repair. As a result, a careful analysis of the potential clinical presentations and current options for management reveals a much more challenging clinical dilemma than might be initially recognized.

K.W. Kercher, M.D., F.A.C.S. (✉)
Division of Gastrointestinal and Minimally Invasive
Surgery, Carolinas Medical Center, Charlotte, NC, USA
e-mail: kent.kercher@carolinashealthcare.org

Variables that may play a role in management include defect size, etiology (primary vs. recurrent), body habitus (BMI), fascial integrity (tissue strength and thickness), and patient factors such as steroid use, chronic cough, smoking, ascites, previous surgical site infection, and even vocation. Each of these factors will be addressed in the various management algorithms described in this chapter.

Current Trends

At this point, it is clear that tension-free repair of incisional and inguinal hernias reduces recurrence rates. The impact of mesh for umbilical hernia repair remains a subject of debate. To date, four prospective randomized controlled trials have addressed this question. Three of these studies found lower recurrence rates after mesh (0–2.7%) vs. primary suture repair (11–19%), with the greatest differences identified in cirrhotic patients and those undergoing emergent repair for incarcerated hernias. A number of other observational series have provided similar results (Table 19.1) [1–7]. Pooled data from these studies including one meta-analysis indicate that recurrence rates are lower after mesh, with no significant increased risk for wound or infectious complications.

That being said, most authors agree that the repair of umbilical hernias should be tailored to the individual patient and there remains some

© Springer International Publishing Switzerland 2016
Y.W. Novitsky (ed.), *Hernia Surgery*, DOI 10.1007/978-3-319-27470-6_19

Table 19.1 Summary of selected umbilical hernia repair studies

Author	Study	n			Recurrence (%)			Surgical site infection (%)		
		Total	Suture	Mesh	Suture	Mesh	p	Suture	Mesh	p
Aorroyo	PRCT	200	100	100	11	1	0.0015	3	2	ns
Abdel-Baki	PRCT	42	21	21	19	0	<0.05	14.3	9.5	ns
Ammar	PRCT	72	35	37	14.2	2.7	<0.05	8.5	16.2	ns
Polat	PRCT	50	18	32	11	0	ns	5.6	6.3	ns
Asolati	RCS	229	97	132	7.7	3	ns	NR	NR	–
Sanjay	RCS	100	61	39	11.5	0	0.0007	11.5	0	0.007
Berger	RCS	392	266	126	7.5	5.6	ns	7.9	19.8	<0.01

skepticism that every umbilical hernia requires mesh. To date, no study has firmly identified a method to stratify patients effectively, though some trends do exist [8–10]. Identified risk factors for recurrence include obesity, cirrhosis, defects >3 cm, and recurrent hernias. In lower risk patients, the potential disadvantages of mesh (infection, foreign body sensation, and adhesions) should be carefully weighed against the potential benefits. Since there is no one perfect repair for umbilical hernias, a number of options are presented below and should be included in the surgeon's armamentarium for managing this diverse group of patients.

Options for Surgical Repair of Umbilical Hernias

Primary Repair

Primary repair (using sutures alone) has been the standard method for treating umbilical hernias for many decades. Initially described in 1901, the Mayo repair involved a "vest over pants" fascial closure using two rows of horizontal mattress sutures placed in a transverse orientation (Fig. 19.1) [11]. While popular for many years, recurrence rates of up to 54% have been reported during long-term follow-up. Today, suture repair typically involves closure of the defect with simple interrupted or figure-of-eight permanent sutures used to approximate the fascia in a horizontal fashion.

My personal technique for primary repair is as follows: After induction of general anesthesia, the abdomen is widely prepped and draped in the usual sterile fashion (Fig. 19.2). Intravenous antibiotics are administered [first generation cephalosporin or Vancomycin (if penicillin allergic)]. A small, curvilinear incision is made along the infra-umbilical fold. The hernia sack is circumferentially dissected using Metzenbaum scissors. Dissection from both sides of the umbilicus is critical to achieving complete isolation of the hernia sack such that both sides of the dissection can be connected and the scissors can be easily passed across the midline. Use of a forceps or hemostat can assist in guiding the tips of the scissors around the hernia sack and out of the skin incision on the opposite side. The hernia sack is then divided with either a scalpel or cautery, taking care to avoid a "button hole" in the umbilical skin. Sounding out the depth of the umbilicus with a hemostat prior to hernia sack division can help to prevent this complication. Incarcerated fat within the hernia defect can be reduced or excised as necessary (Fig. 19.3).

The fascial defect should now be easily visualized. The superior and inferior fascial edges are elevated with either Kocher clamps or a hemostat. With judicious use of electrocautery, the anterior fascia is circumferentially cleared of subcutaneous tissue over a distance of 1–2 cm. If the fascia is of good integrity and can easily be approximated without significant tension, three to four figure-of-eight #1 woven nonabsorbable sutures are placed, taking bites of fascia at least 1-cm from edge of the defect (Fig. 19.4). After all sutures are placed, Kocher clamps are removed and sutures are tied down (Fig. 19.5). The wound is irrigated and the

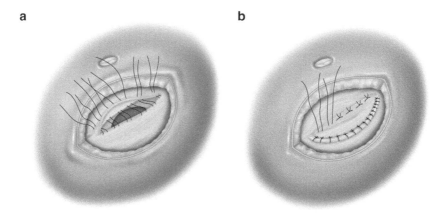

Fig. 19.1 Mayo repair

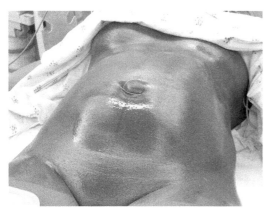

Fig. 19.2 Sterile prep for primary umbilical hernia repair

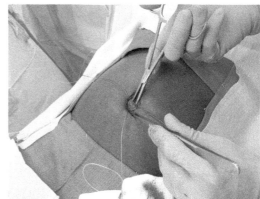

Fig. 19.4 Primary repair with permanent suture

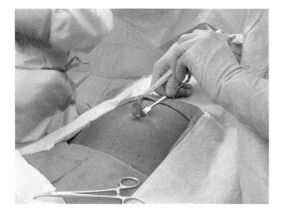

Fig. 19.3 Chronically incarcerated pre-peritoneal fat within umbilical hernia defect

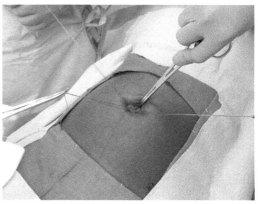

Fig. 19.5 Defect closure

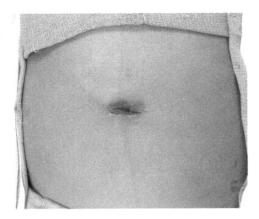

Fig. 19.6 Subcuticular skin closure

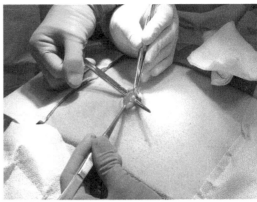

Fig. 19.8 Circumferential dissection and isolation of hernia sack

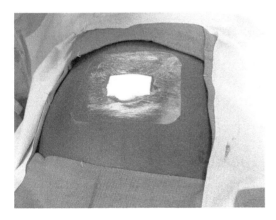

Fig. 19.7 Occlusive pressure dressing

umbilicus tacked down using 3-0 absorbable suture and the skin closed with 4-0 absorbable subcuticular sutures. Skin adhesive is applied and a sterile occlusive pressure dressing is placed (Figs. 19.6 and 19.7). The patient is discharged to home from the recovery room.

Mesh Repair

Open mesh repair generally utilizes a flat sheet of mesh or possibly a mesh plug, though newer mesh patch devices have been designed specifically for treatment of umbilical hernias utilizing a common design that allows for mesh deployment deep to the fascia. As with other mesh-based repairs of abdominal wall defects, there

are a number of options for mesh placement location. These include mesh onlay (over a primary fascial closure), mesh inlay (mesh plug fixated to the fascial ring), and mesh underlay (either in the intra-peritoneal, pre-peritoneal, or retro-muscular space). Two final options for mesh repair are the purely laparoscopic and the laparoscopic-assisted approaches, both of which involve placement of an intra-peritoneal tissue-separating mesh with variable degrees of mesh fixation and varying numbers of laparoscopic ports, with or without primary closure of the hernia defect over the mesh.

Open Techniques

For open mesh repair of umbilical hernias, I prefer a mesh underlay which utilizes one of the three available umbilical hernia patches currently on the market. These include the Proceed Ventral Patch (Ethicon, Inc), the CQur V-Patch (Atrium, Inc.), and the Ventralex-ST Patch (Bard, Inc.). While each of these meshes is equipped with an absorbable tissue-separating layer designed to allow for intra-peritoneal mesh placement, my personal preference is for pre-peritoneal mesh deployment. Preparation of the patient and location of skin incision are identical to that described for the open primary repair. If possible, opening of the hernia sack is avoided during the initial phases of dissection and tissue division (Fig. 19.8). Once the hernia sack is delineated, it is carefully dissected away from the edges of the fascial defect. Fascial edges are again elevated with Kocher clamps, and meticulous dissection is used to enter the pre-peritoneal space using electrocautery. The easiest location to enter the pre-peritoneal space is inferiorly at the interface between the hernia sack and the caudal edge of the fascial defect. Once entered, the pre-peritoneal space is circumferentially developed with a combination of blunt dissection and judicious use of cautery. Care must be taken to elevate the fascia and to divide only the tissue between the fascia and the peritoneum in order to avoid potential injury to the underlying viscera.

After a wide pre-peritoneal pocket has been developed, hemostasis is confirmed. Oozing along the medial umbilical ligaments (at the 5 and 7 o'clock positions) is the most common area of minor but nuisance bleeding. Any holes in the hernia sack are closed with absorbable suture to exclude the viscera from the pre-peritoneal space. Depending upon the size of the hernia defect and width of the pre-peritoneal space achieved, an appropriate mesh size is selected. When possible, my preference is to develop a wide pre-peritoneal pocket that will accommodate an 8-cm hernia patch (Figs. 19.9 and 19.10). The mesh is then deployed into the pre-peritoneal space deep to the muscular layers of the abdominal wall and the anchoring straps are brought out through the hernia defect. The fascia is closed with #1 woven non-absorbable suture using two figure-of-eight sutures on each side and one or two horizontal mattress sutures in the center, incorporating the tails of the mesh with the closure. Fascial sutures are tied down and the tails of the mesh cut just above the fascia. Adjacent scar and fascia are closed over the cut tails of the mesh, the umbilicus is tacked down, and the skin closed with subcuticular suture (Figs. 19.11, 19.12 and 19.13).

If the pre-peritoneal space cannot be developed, then the mesh patch can be deployed deep to the fascial defect into the intra-peritoneal space (Figs. 19.14, 19.15 and 19.16). The anchoring straps on the mesh are again brought out through the hernia defect, allowing the mesh to be pulled up into apposition with the peritoneum (Figs. 19.17, 19.18, 19.19, 19.20 and 19.21). Non-absorbable sutures are utilized

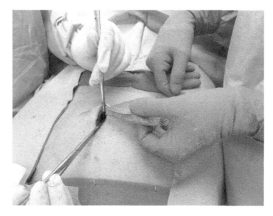

Fig. 19.10 Umbilical hernia patch folded to allow for mesh insertion into pre-peritoneal pocket

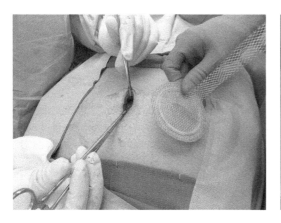

Fig. 19.9 Elevation of fascial edges assists in development of pre-peritoneal space for mesh deployment

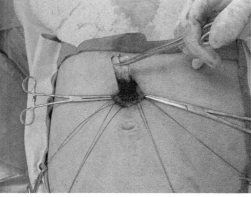

Fig. 19.11 Fascial sutures incorporate mesh tails during defect closure

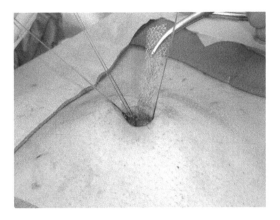

Fig. 19.12 Hernia defect closed over mesh patch

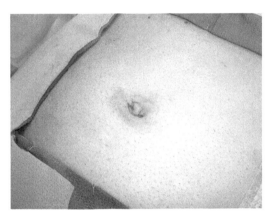

Fig. 19.13 Umbilical skin tacked down and closed

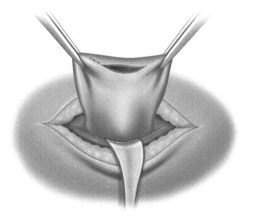

Fig. 19.14 Umbilical hernia sack is circumferentially dissected from the fascia, opened, and resected

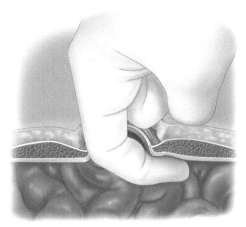

Fig. 19.15 The intra-peritoneal space is cleared of adhesions

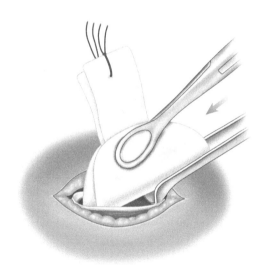

Fig. 19.16 Mesh is deployed into the intra-peritoneal space, just deep to the fascia

to secure the anchoring straps to the fascia. Whether or not to close the defect is at the surgeon's discretion. Some surgeons prefer to separate and fixate the tails of the mesh to the edges of the fascial defect (Fig. 19.22), allowing for a tension-free repair. My personal preference is to close the fascial defect, while incorporating both mesh tails into the fascial closure (as demonstrated in Figs. 19.11 and 19.12). In all cases, the redundant tails of the

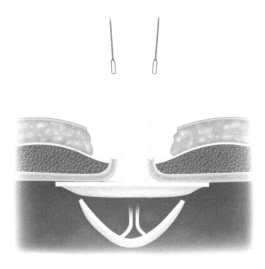

Fig. 19.17 Anchoring straps (mesh tails) are pulled up to bring the mesh patch into direct contact with the abdominal wall

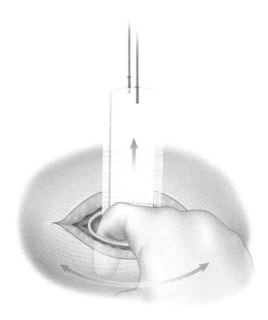

Fig. 19.19 Complete circumferential deployment of the mesh is confirmed

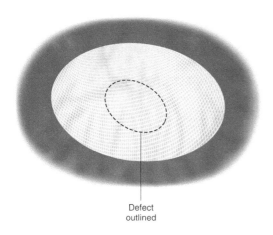

Defect
outlined

Fig. 19.18 Mesh patch provides wide overlap of the hernia defect

mesh are trimmed down to the level of the fascia and the wound is closed in layers. Care is taken to close the scar and the subcutaneous tissue over the cut tails of the mesh in order to exclude the mesh tails from the skin closure (Fig. 19.23).

Although the currently available umbilical hernia patches are designed with a tissue-separating layer to allow for safe insertion into the abdominal cavity, there is the potential for bowel adhesions to the mesh, particularly if the mesh is not well seated against the peritoneal

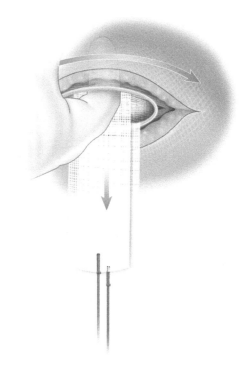

Fig. 19.20 Using the surgeon's finger to circumferentially sweep around the edges of the mesh, the prosthetic is confirmed to lie flat against the parietal side of the abdominal wall

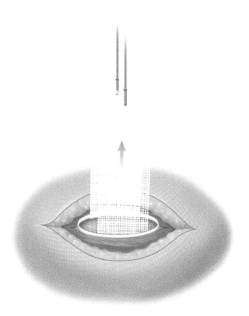

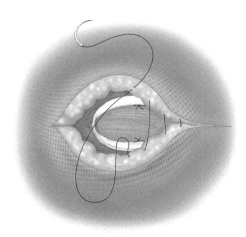

Fig. 19.23 The wound is closed in layers

Fig. 19.21 Mesh tails are gently elevated to bring the mesh into apposition with the abdominal wall. Pulling up too aggressively on the anchoring straps is discouraged, as excessive traction can deform the mesh

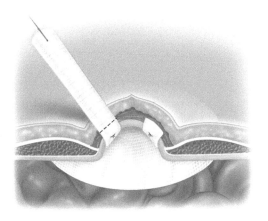

Fig. 19.22 The tails of the mesh are secured to the edges of the defect with permanent suture

surface deep to the abdominal wall muscula-ture. For this reason, many surgeons will take additional steps to fixate the mesh to the perito-neum, either with sutures placed through the hernia defect or by tacking the periphery of the mesh using a laparoscopic-assisted approach. With this technique, the mesh is deployed into

the peritoneal cavity through the umbilical her-nia defect in a standard "open" fashion, but two additional 5-mm laparoscopic ports and a laparoscopic tacker are utilized to fixate the edges of the mesh under pneumoperitoneum using laparoscopic guidance (Fig. 19.24).

Laparoscopic Techniques

While laparoscopic repair of midline incisional/ventral hernias is a standard practice, the laparoscopic approach to umbilical hernias is generally limited to larger defects (>3–5 cm), recurrent umbilical hernias, or fascial defects occurring at the site of prior umbilical surgery, such as the site of a prior laparoscopic access, and would technically be considered small inci-sional hernias. For these larger, more challenging umbilical hernias, two primary approaches can be considered: laparoscopic-assisted repair with mesh and primary defect closure (as described above) or a standard (purely) laparoscopic repair with mesh.

While strategies vary based upon personal preference, my approach for laparoscopic umbilical hernia repair typically involves a 4-port technique that allows for adhesiolysis and intra-peritoneal mesh deployment with wide overlap of at least 5 cm beyond the edges of the hernia defect. A tissue-separating perma-nent synthetic mesh is used and is deployed intra-peritoneal as an underlay. Defect closure

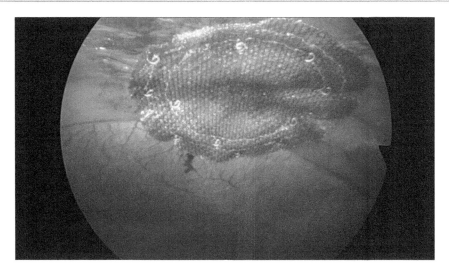

Fig. 19.24   Intra-peritoneal view of umbilical hernia patch and laparoscopic fixation sites

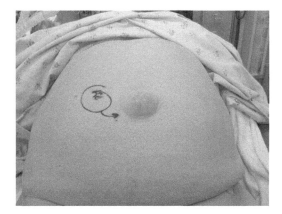

Fig. 19.25   Large chronically incarcerated umbilical hernia prior to repair

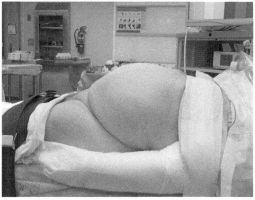

Fig. 19.27   Patient positing for laparoscopic repair with arms padded and tucked

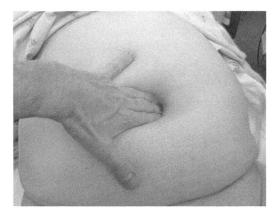

Fig. 19.26   Demonstration of 3–5 cm fascial defect

is optional. Four trans-fascial sutures are used to suspend and secure the mesh in the laparoscopic environment and are reinforced by a double crown of tacks for mesh fixation (Figs. 19.25, 19.26, 19.27, 19.28, 19.29, 19.30 and 19.31).

Algorithms for the Management of Umbilical Hernias

As with any surgical intervention, the specific technique utilized in any given patient must be individualized. Ultimately, decisions are based upon

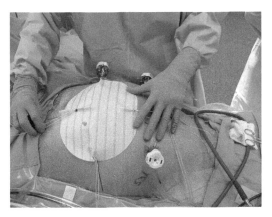

Fig. 19.28 Mesh preparation with four cardinal sutures

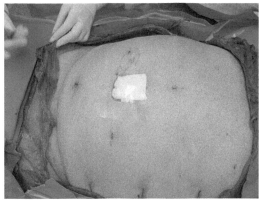

Fig. 19.31 Laparoscopic port and suture fixation sites at conclusion of case

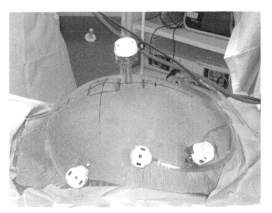

Fig. 19.29 Four-port trocar strategy for laparoscopic umbilical hernia repair

the clinical scenario and the surgeon's own skill set and experience. There are a number of factors to consider in individualizing the treatment of umbilical hernias. These include the etiology of the hernia (primary vs. recurrent/incisional), defect size, body habitus, fascial quality, tension, patient age, vocation, and co-morbidities as well as the risk for wound and or mesh complications.

My general approach to umbilical hernias is as follows: For thin, healthy patients presenting with a small primary umbilical hernia that can be easily approximated without tension, a primary

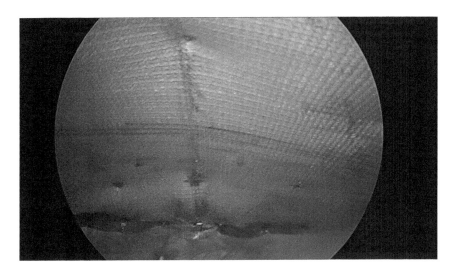

Fig. 19.30 Laparoscopic view of wide intra-peritoneal mesh reinforcement

repair with non-absorbable suture is used. In heavier patients with larger defects and particularly in those who regularly perform strenuous physical labor, I generally recommend mesh reinforcement, utilizing an umbilical hernia patch placed in the pre-peritoneal space. In the morbidly obese patient or in those with large, recurrent hernia defects, a laparoscopic approach often provides for greater mesh overlap and the potential advantage of fewer wound complications. While I believe that it is appropriate to consent every patient for a potential change in operative strategy during the procedure, the algorithms below can guide pre-operative decision-making.

Indications for Primary Repair
– Primary hernia
– "Finger-tip" defect (<1 cm)
– Thin female
– Good fascia
– Minimal tension

Indications for Open Mesh Repair
– Medium-sized defect (2–3 cm)
– Recurrent hernia
– Incisional hernia
– Overweight—mildly obese
– Male
– Laborer
– Thin fascia
– Tension
– Chronic cough

Indications for Laparoscopic Repair with Mesh
– Morbid obesity
– Large defect (>3 cm)
– High risk for wound complications (steroids, diabetes, ascites, smoking)
– Recurrent hernia

Summary

A wide variety of options are available for the repair of umbilical hernias. These surgical techniques range from primary suture repair to rein-

forcement with mesh and can be performed through open and laparoscopic approaches. At present, there is no accepted gold standard for umbilical hernia repair. Recent studies have shown lower rates of recurrence after mesh repair when compared with sutures alone, although conflicting data exist. The potential disadvantages of synthetic mesh placement (including infection, seroma, foreign body sensation, and adhesions to underlying viscera) must be recognized and considered; however, pooled data demonstrate no significant differences in complication rates when comparing mesh to suture repair. Based upon current evidence, primary repair remains reasonable and appropriate for small primary umbilical hernias. Mesh reinforcement should be considered in patients deemed high risk for recurrence. As always, the specific technique for repair should be tailored to the individual patient.

References

1. Arroyo A, Garcia P, Perez F, Anrdreu J, Candela F, Calpena R. Randomized clinical trial comparing suture and mesh repair of umbilical hernia in adults. Br J Surg. 2001;88:1321–3.
2. Abdel-Baki NA, Bessa SS, Abdel-Razek AH. Comparison of prosthetic mesh repair and tissue repair in the emergency management of incarcerated para-umbilical hernia: a prospective randomized study. Hernia. 2007;11:163–7.
3. Ammar SA. Management of complicated umbilical hernias in cirrhotic patients using permanent mesh: randomized clinical trial. Hernia. 2010;14: 35–8.
4. Polat C, Dervisoglu A, Senyurek G, et al. Umbilical hernia repair with the prolene hernia system. Am J Surg. 2005;190:61–4.
5. Asolati M, Huerta S, Sarosi G, et al. Predictors of recurrence in veteran patients with umbilical hernia: single center experience. Am J Surg. 2006;192: 627–30.
6. Sanjay P, Reid TD, Davies EL, Arumugam PJ, Woodward A. Retrospective comparison of mesh and sutured repair for adult umbilical hernias. Hernia. 2005;9:248–51.
7. Berger RL, Li LT, Hicks SC, Liang MK. Suture versus preperitoneal polypropylene mesh for elective umbilical hernia repairs. J Surg Res. 2014;192(2):426–31.
8. Aslani N, Brown CJ. Does mesh offer an advantage over tissue in the open repair of umbilical hernias? A systematic review and meta-analysis. Hernia. 2010;14:455–62.

9. Halm JA, Heisterkamp J, Veen HF, Weidema WF. Long-term follow-up after umbilical hernia repair: are there risk factors for recurrence after simple and mesh repair. Hernia. 2005;9:334–7.

10. Erilymaz R, Sahin M, Tekelioglu MH. Which repair in umbilical hernia of adults: primary or mesh? Int Surg. 2006;91(5):258–61.

11. Mayo WJ. An operation for the radical cure of umbilical hernia. Ann Surg. 1901;34:276–80.

Managing Complications of Open Hernia Repair

Eric M. Pauli and Ryan M. Juza

Introduction

Abdominal wall hernias are becoming increasingly prevalent as the population ages, surgical management of intra-abdominal pathology increases, and medical comorbidities such as obesity, diabetes, and smoking continue to occur with relatively high frequency in surgical populations [1–5]. Ventral hernia repairs occur at a rate of 350,000 cases per year in the United States and are increasing at a rate of 1–2% annually [6, 7]. As such, open ventral hernia repair is one of the most common elective general surgical procedures performed in the United States every year [8].

Despite numerous technical advances and increased awareness of complications of herniorraphy, morbidity following open ventral hernia repair remains common. Managing these complications is an essential skill of the abdominal wall surgeon. For component separation herniorraphy in particular, where 25–50% of patients can be expected to have at least one post-operative occurrence, complication diagnosis and management is a routine part of post-operative care. High complication rates have led to vast research on the topic, including the description of novel management strategies, and the establishment of working groups and risk stratification scores to guide patient selection and better predict complication rates [9–11]. With reimbursement being increasingly tied to outcomes, optimizing patient care in the pre- and post-operative intervals is now as important as the operative care the patient receives.

As a group, complications following open ventral hernia repair are a more common occurrence compared to laparoscopic herniorraphy. This chapter will review the spectrum of common complications following open ventral hernia repair with an emphasis on prevention, diagnosis, and management options.

Risk Factors of Complication

Multiple studies have investigated patient comorbidities and their risk for developing post-operative complication following open hernia repair. The majority of these studies have focused on the development of surgical site infection, as it is well established that wound infection significantly increases the risk of hernia recurrence [12]. Comorbidities shown to increase post-operative

E.M. Pauli, M.D. (✉)
Division of Minimally Invasive and Bariatric Surgery, Department of Surgery, Penn State Hershey Medical Center, Hershey, PA, USA
e-mail: epauli@hmc.psu.edu

R.M. Juza, M.D.
Department of Surgery, Penn State Milton S. Hershey Medical Center, Hershey, PA, USA

© Springer International Publishing Switzerland 2016
Y.W. Novitsky (ed.), *Hernia Surgery*, DOI 10.1007/978-3-319-27470-6_20

complication rates in ventral hernia repair include smoking, diabetes, chronic pulmonary disease, poor nutritional status (low serum albumin), immunosuppression (including steroid use), morbid obesity, coronary artery disease, and advanced age [3, 13, 14].

Our "prehabilitation" strategy for elective open ventral hernia repairs focuses on aggressively managing these comorbidities. Smoking, tobacco and nicotine cessation (including patches and electronic cigarettes) is mandatory, and we routinely check blood and urine for nicotine metabolites prior to scheduling and performing complex open hernia repairs. Long-term control of diabetes is assessed with glycosylated hemoglobin levels (HbA1C), and referrals are made to primary care physicians or endocrinologists as needed to achieve an HbA1C ≤ 7.0. Chronic pulmonary disease (in particular home oxygen use or significant dyspnea on exertion) may preclude herniorraphy. Pulmonary function testing and referral to pulmonary medicine are appropriate for risk modification. Nutritional supplementation and multivitamin administration may be necessary to increase albumen and correct micronutrient deficiencies. The degree to which obesity contributes to hernia recurrence and post-operative wound and pulmonary complications has not been well established and no strict guidelines for a body mass index (BMI) cutoff exist. Our preference is to perform elective repairs on patients with a $BMI \leq 40$ kg/m^2. Referral for medically supervised or surgical weight loss procedure (typically laparoscopic sleeve gastrectomy) may be necessary. Coronary artery disease should be investigated and managed as before any major surgical procedure; cardiology referral, stress testing, and angiography may be necessary.

Complications and Their Management

Surgical Site Occurrences

Wound-related complications such as erythema, infection, seroma, hematoma, dehiscence, and fistula formation occurring within 30 days of the principle operation are included in the definition of surgical site occurrences (SSO) as outlined by the Ventral Hernia Working Group [11]. The term surgical site occurrence was established because of a recognized need for standardization in the reporting of wound complications following hernia repair. Reports before 2010 had non-standardized methodology of reporting these complications and as such, interpretation of the true rates of SSO is often unreliable. Ideally, standardized definitions and reporting will improve the reliability of data as future studies present outcomes in a common language. Unfortunately, there is still a spectrum of complication severity within each of these categories; a minor wound separation and a complete wound separation would both be categorized as a wound dehiscence within this nomenclature, making it difficult to determine major and minor SSO rates. Surgical site occurrences complicate 14% of low risk open hernia repairs, 27% of repairs in patients with comorbid conditions, and 46% of contaminated hernia repairs [10]. The higher rates of SSO in contaminated repairs are largely attributable to infections.

Surgical Site Infection

Surgical site infection (SSI) is one of the most common surgical site occurrences complicating open ventral hernia repair and is the most significant predictor of hernia recurrence (Fig. 20.1) [3]. It is also the most common reason for hospital readmission following open ventral hernia surgery [9, 12, 15]. Open repairs have a significantly higher rate of surgical site infections than laparoscopic repairs [16–18]. SSIs complicate 19% of open ventral hernia repairs, but the incidence varies widely depending on the preoperative hernia grade and method of repair (Table 20.1) [9–11, 16–22].

Surgical site infections are divided into superficial and deep incisional and organ space infections as defined by the Centers for Disease Control [23]. Superficial incisional infections affect the skin and subcutaneous tissue and are diagnosed by local erythema, swelling, pain, or purulent drainage. Deep incisional infections reach the fascial or muscle layers and may be associated with abscess formation, or wound separation exposing the deeper tissue layers. Organ space infections involve non-incisional parts of the operative field; in the case of open ventral hernia repair, this is generally the peritoneal or retroperitoneal spaces.

Management of SSIs follows standard surgical principles. Minor superficial infections can be managed with empiric antibiotics alone, with special consideration given to patients known to carry resistant organisms (e.g. methicillin-resistant *Staphylococcus aureus* (MRSA)). More serious infections may require incision, drainage, packing, and targeted antibiotic therapy based on wound cultures. Deep incisional infections generally require drainage (which may be surgical or

percutaneous) and targeted antibiotic therapy. Non-viable muscle, fascia, and subcutaneous tissue may need to be aggressively debrided to eliminate ongoing sources of infection. Organ space infections are generally treated with percutaneous drainage; however, non-focal infections may require laparotomy to clear the infection and permit peritoneal lavage. Special consideration should be given to a missed enterotomy or leak from intestinal reconstructive work (anastomosis, enterotomy repair) done during the course of herniorrhaphy as the source of an organ space infection.

Development of an SSI is dictated by a multitude of patient-related and surgical variables similar to other general surgical procedures. For open mesh repairs, a prior wound infection is notably not predictive of an SSI [24, 25]. Maneuvers to improve microvascular blood flow and optimize native immunity (e.g. smoking cessation) allow better mesh incorporation. When considering where to place mesh, it therefore makes sense to place it adjacent to well vascularized tissue to provide a robust interface to allow immune recognition and reaction to the foreign body. For incisional infections (both superficial and deep), mesh location within the abdominal wall must be considered in the management strategy. Underlay and sublay mesh may not be involved with the infectious process of incisional infections, whereas onlay mesh is more likely to be (Fig. 20.2). Surgical management of these infections may require mesh removal (see Mesh Infection below).

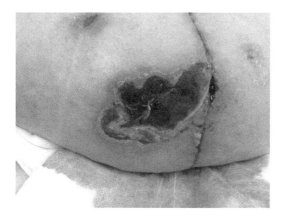

Fig. 20.1 Wound ischemia and deep surgical site infection following anterior component separation with external oblique release (Photo courtesy of Dr. Luis J. Garcia, University of Iowa)

Table 20.1 Surgical site occurrence, rates following open ventral hernia repair

	Anterior component separation	Rectrorectus	Posterior component separation	Bridged
Total wound complications	43% Jensen [17]		26% Krpata [78]	51% Basta [21]
	49% Krpata [78]		24% Novitsky [20]	19% Albino [19]
	16% Albino [19]		6% Albino [19]	
Seroma	13% Jensen [17]	9% Paajanen [22]	5% Albino [19]	8% Basta [21]
	3% Albino [19]	3% Albino [19]		12% Albino [19]
Surgical site infection	13% Jensen [17]	6% Paajanen [22]	7% Novitsky [20]	22% Basta [21]
	15% Albino [19]	7% Albino [19]	7% Albino [19]	12% Albino [19]
Skin dehiscence	0% Jensen [17]			35% Basta [21]
Chronic pain		4% Paajanen [22]		
Skin necrosis	6% Jensen [17]			

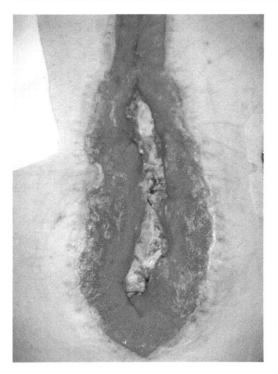

Fig. 20.2 Deep surgical site infection following operative debridement and several days of negative pressure wound therapy. Note the exposed onlay biologic mesh at the base of the wound

Seroma

Seroma formation, the accumulation of sterile serous fluid within the spaces created during herniorraphy, frequently complicates open ventral hernia repair (Fig. 20.3). Seromas occur as a consequence of the extent of tissue mobilization and local inflammatory reactions to mesh and suture material [26, 27]. Surgical dissection creates dead space between anatomic planes which function as a space for transudative fluid to collect. Fluid may collect at a greater rate if the peritonealized hernia sack is left in situ within subcutaneous tissues.

Seroma formation rates vary between 0 and 36% depending on the surgical technique and type of the mesh employed for repair [22, 28–35]. For open ventral hernia repair, the incidence of seroma formation is directly dependent on the surgical technique employed. Placing mesh in the sublay position is superior to onlay mesh placement based on numerous published studies

(Table 20.2). It has been postulated that the superior vascularity in the retrorectus plane reduces the incidence of seroma formation over the poorly vascularized lipocutaneous flaps created in open ventral hernia repairs when the mesh is placed in the onlay position. This theory is supported by studies evaluating the outcomes of endoscopic component separation which avoids creating large devascularized flaps by endoscopically releasing the external oblique. This significantly decreases the wound complications associated with onlay mesh placement [17, 29, 31].

Seroma prevention is based on two main principles: reducing dead space volume and minimizing devascularized tissue. Preoperative patient factors including obesity, smoking, and diabetes have all been shown to increase the rate of seroma formation [25, 33]. Postoperatively, the use of closed suction drains to prevent fluid accumulation is widely practiced during open ventral hernia repair to reduce dead space volume, but management of drains is by no means standardized. Our preference is to leave the drains in place until daily output is less than 30 cc per day for two consecutive days. A recent review of the literature was unable to demonstrate a direct benefit of drains versus no drains; however, this more likely highlights the paucity of high-quality studies directly related to seroma management [36].

Abdominal binders are also a modality widely used to decrease seroma formation by decreasing dead space volume and therefore decreasing fluid accumulation. Effective duration of therapy necessary to prevent seroma formation is not well described and is often limited by patient tolerance. Additionally, less widely practiced methods such as the use of quilting stitches and the application of fibrin sealant to dissected planes theoretically assist physiologic closure of the dead space; however, the literature is mixed regarding the efficacy of these methods and there is no clear evidence to support the use of either regularly [37, 38].

Despite the frequency of seroma formation, this low acuity complication has limited high-level research. Management is largely directed by small studies, case reports, and empiricism. Diagnosis occurs clinically or radiographically.

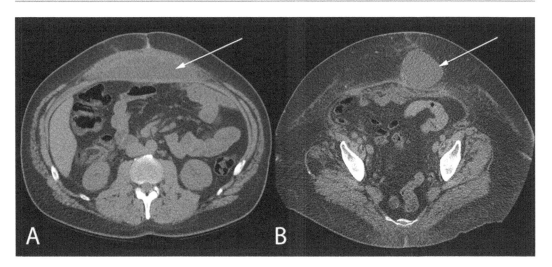

Fig. 20.3 Benign, asymptomatic seromas (*arrows*) (**a**) Seroma surrounding biologic mesh in the retrorectus space. (**b**) Seroma within the subcutaneous dead space created following hernia reduction

Table 20.2 Seroma rates following open ventral hernia repair

	$n=$	Method of repair	Mesh location	Seroma (%)
Harth et al. [29]	22	Anterior component separation	Onlay	5
Albright et al. [30]	14	Anterior component separation	Onlay	36
Giurgius et al. [31]	15	Anterior component separation	Onlay	33
Fox et al. [32]	26	Anterior component separation	Onlay	0
Satterwhite et al. [33]	106	Anterior component separation	Onlay	18
Paajanen et al. [22]	84	Retrorectus	Sublay	9
Rosen et al. [34]	49	Retrorectus	Sublay	0
McLanahan [35]	104	Retrorectus	Sublay	1
Peterson et al. [28]	175	Retrorectus	Sublay	6
Iqbal [12]	254	Retrorectus	Sublay	4

When sterile and asymptomatic, the majority can be observed for spontaneous, albeit potentially protracted resolution over the course of weeks to months. Intervention is indicated when the seroma becomes infected or symptomatic (Fig. 20.4). Although some advocate needle aspirating these collections, this risks inoculating an otherwise sterile collection [39]. Evidence of an infected seroma includes localized and/or systemic reactions. When treatment is required, percutaneous closed suction drainage is the preferred method of management. Open drainage and neg-

ative pressure therapy are additional management strategies for infected seromas not amendable to or failing percutaneous drainage and targeted antibiotic therapy.

Hematoma

Hematomas following open ventral hernia repair are uncommonly reported, but can occur from several sources. Bleeding from named vessels (typically the epigastric vessels) generally occurs as a direct injury not recognized during retrorectus dissection or during transfascial suture place-

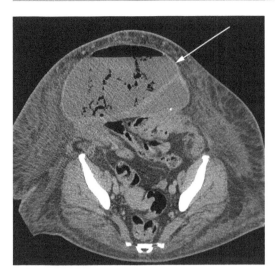

Fig. 20.4 Infected subcutaneous seroma (*arrow*) with loculation, septation, and an air fluid level

ment. Component separation hernia repairs involve transection of myofascial barriers, and bleeding from cut edges of muscles can occur (Fig. 20.5a). Subcutaneous bleeding can also occur into the space created by raising large lipocutaneous flaps during anterior component separation (Fig. 20.5b). Patients with bleeding diathesis, thrombocytopenia, or the need for early post-operative anticoagulation (e.g. mechanical valve patients) are at a higher risk for post-herniorraphy hematoma.

Hematomas are managed conservatively unless bleeding is ongoing or there is hemodynamic instability. Correction of coagulopathy, withholding prophylactic anticoagulation, and pressure dressings may all have benefit. Transfusion may be required for large hematomas. Like seromas, the majority of hematomas can be observed for spontaneous resolution and should only be drained for clinically relevant symptoms or infection.

Wound Dehiscence

Wound dehiscence involves separation of the skin edges in the absence of surgical site infection. Contributing factors include poor blood supply to the skin edges, poor suturing technique or damage to suture material, and radial tension on the wound edges due to tissue loss or body habitus. As with many other post-operative complications, wound dehiscence is poorly reported in the literature (Table 20.1). There is a clear spectrum of complication that can be classified as wound dehiscence ranging from minor separation requiring no dedicated therapy to complete wound disruption and mesh exposure (Fig. 20.6). Wound dehiscence is generally managed with local wound therapy including dressing changes. Mesh exposure from wound dehiscence may warrant mesh removal.

Enterocutaneous Fistulae Formation

Enterocutaneous fistula (ECF) formation has been reported in cases of intraperitoneally placed prosthesis as a consequence of mesh eroding into bowel (Fig. 20.7) [40, 41]. By moving the mesh into the more protected onlay or sublay positions, enterocutaneous fistula formation is a rare complication. Other causative factors in ECF formation include delayed leak from an enteroenterostomy performed during the course of the herniorraphy and underlying patient disease (e.g. Crohn's Disease). Many cases of fistula formation reported in the literature have occurred in contaminated fields where fistula or perforation was already present prior to repair [33, 41–43]. When an ECF develops, management is similar to other ECF in other post-operative settings; sepsis must be controlled, nutrition augmented parenterally (depending on fistula output), and skin cared for aggressively. Extirpation of the mesh is essential to gain control of and excise the involved segment of bowel [41–43].

Other SSOs: Erythema, Ischemia, Granulation Tissue

There are a variety of other minor wound-related issues that fall under the SSO umbrella including wound erythema, wound ischemia, and granulation tissue formation. Erythema may signal an early SSI or may be related to reactions to tape, suture material, or tension from an abdominal binder. No treatment strategies exist, but those potentially related to infection are generally treated with empiric antibiotics. Wound ischemia is not widely reported in the literature, and can take a variety of forms including wound edge ischemia leading to dehiscence (Table 20.1, Fig. 20.6a) or severe full thickness ischemia of a

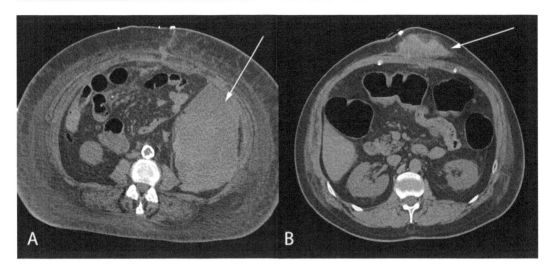

Fig. 20.5 Acute post-operative hematomas (*arrows*) (**a**) retroperitoneal hematoma following posterior component separation with transversus abdominis release. (**b**) Subcutaneous hematoma following retrorectus hernia repair

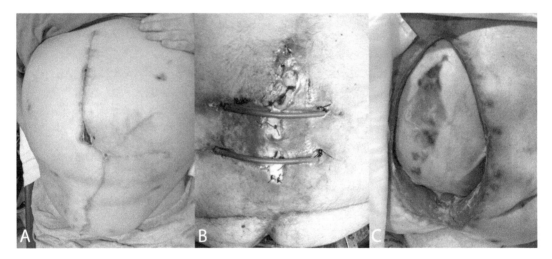

Fig. 20.6 Various degrees of wound dehiscence (**a**) Multiple areas of minor wound dehiscence following component separation hernia repair in a patient with complex intersecting incisions. (**b**) Large area of wound dehis-cence following primary (suture) hernia repair performed under tension. (**c**) Complete wound dehiscence and bio-logic mesh exposure following a bridged repair in a patient with significant wound tension due to morbid obesity

lipocutaneous flap (Fig. 20.1). Management depends on the degree of ischemia and any concerns for an underlying SSI, but wound debridement and dressing changes are typical management strategies. Granulation tissue can take a variety of forms from minor wound edge areas of non-healing, to suture sinus tracts (Fig. 20.8), to large open wounds with chronic mesh infections (Fig. 20.9). Granulation at wound edges can be managed with chemical cautery ablation. Granulation associated with suture sinuses is best treated with local exploration and suture removal. Large areas of granulation tissue associated with mesh exposure are best managed by mesh excision.

Pulmonary Complication

Pulmonary complications following abdominal wall reconstruction are a common and morbid

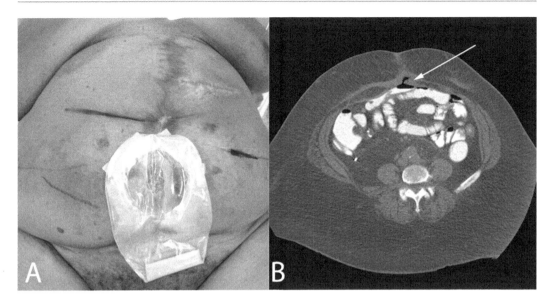

Fig. 20.7 (**a**) Enterocutaneous fistula that developed 5 years following a multiply recurrent incisional hernia repair. At exploration, the fistula was associated with underlay mesh erosion into the jejunum that was noted on pre-operative CT scan (**b**)

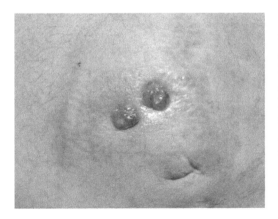

Fig. 20.8 Granulation tissue associated with permanent suture sinuses

complication. Pneumonia, respiratory distress requiring upgrade in care, or intubation and prolonged ventilator dependence are considered serious complications of hernia repair. Such complications are reported in as many as 15–20% of patients undergoing component separation hernia repairs [44–47]. Contributing factors to pulmonary complications include chronic obstructive pulmonary disease, baseline dyspnea, prolonged operative time, and elevated intra-operative airway pressures [44–47].

Patients experiencing postoperative respiratory failure have longer hospital admissions $(21.0 \pm 18.5$ vs. 5.9 ± 5.5 days, $p < 0.001)$, a higher mortality rate $(14.7\%$ vs. $0.1\%, p < 0.001)$, and an added cost of \$60,933 per patient [45, 47]. Pulmonary complications are managed with aggressive pulmonary toilet, non-invasive ventilation, and endotracheal ventilator assistance as necessary. Rarely, tracheostomy is necessary after open hernia repair for prolonged ventilator-dependent respiratory failure.

Predictive models and preventative strategies for pulmonary complications have been described [44, 45]. The greater the change in plateau airway pressure, the greater the risk of developing a respiratory complication with an odds ratio of 8.67 for a change in plateau pressure ≥ 6 cm H_2O and an odds ratio of 11.5 for a change in plateau pressure ≥ 9 cm H_2O [44]. As such, the finding of an elevation in plateau pressure of >6 mmHg following open ventral hernia repair should prompt overnight ventilator support to permit normalization of plateau pressure.

Ileus

Delay in the resumption of intestinal function, or ileus, is a normal physiologic response to open abdominal surgery. For hernia surgery, where

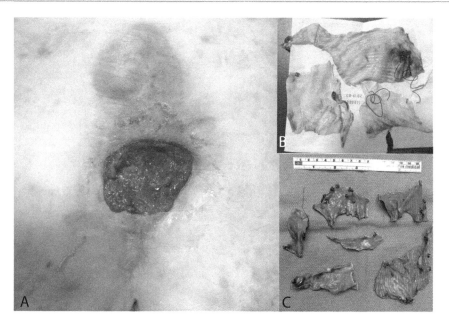

Fig. 20.9 (**a**) Chronic non-healing midline wound resulting from exposure and infection of PTFE mesh that was removed in clinic (**b**) and in the operating room (**c**)

there may be significant bowel manipulation as well as a need for higher dose post-operative narcotics, paralytic ileus is an anticipated part of the normal post-operative recovery that resolves spontaneously. Prolonged ileus may be clinically significant, leading to abdominal pain, vomiting, a need for imaging studies (to differentiate from mechanical bowel obstruction or other post-operative complication such as a missed bowel injury), and results in patient dissatisfaction and a prolonged hospital stay. Ileus is more likely following open ventral hernia surgery than laparoscopic hernia repair and may relate to more significant shifts in fluids and electrolytes, greater degrees of bowel manipulation, and higher post-operative narcotic use.

Ileus is managed conservatively with electrolyte replacement, nasogastric decompression, and patience. Imaging studies help differentiate ileus from small bowel obstruction (Fig. 20.10). Prolonged ileus may necessitate the institution of parenteral nutrition until full bowel recovery is made.

Acute Kidney Injury

Acute kidney injury (AKI), diagnosed as an increase in serum creatinine of ≥ 0.3 within 48 hours or increase in serum creatinine to ≥ 1.5 times baseline within 7 days, is an uncommon, but likely under-reported, complication of abdominal wall reconstruction [48]. Contributing factors to AKI include baseline chronic kidney disease, myoglobinuria (from prolonged operative times and muscle trauma during hernia repair), dehydration and volume shifts associated with open surgery, nephrotoxic drugs administered in the peri-operative period. Despite this, complex abdominal wall reconstruction can be safely conducted even in patients at high risk for AKI [49]. AKI should be managed with supportive therapy including volume resuscitation, withdrawal of nephrotoxic drugs, and renal replacement therapy if indicated.

Intra-Abdominal Hypertension

Heightened awareness of intra-abdominal hypertension (intra-abdominal pressure ≥ 12 mmHg) and abdominal compartment syndrome (intra-abdominal pressure ≥ 20 mmHg) has led to growing attention to the severity of this clinical entity in the context of an acute abdomen from abdominal trauma, pancreatitis, or perforated viscus [50–53]. This entity is increasingly recognized as a common but transient occurrence following

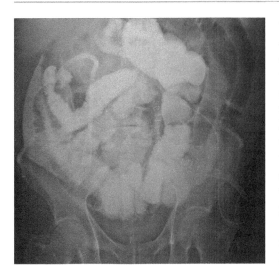

Fig. 20.10 Ileus following parastomal hernia repair with posterior component separation and transversus abdominis release. Contrast administered via the catheter in the stoma (RUQ) traverses the length of the GI tract, filling multiple, dilated loops with no clear transition zone. This resolved spontaneously

complex open ventral hernia repair and its contribution to the post-operative renal and pulmonary complications noted above has been questioned [54]. Intra-abdominal hypertension should likely be viewed as a "permissive" consequence of the procedure that resolves with conservative measures.

Mesh Complications

Mesh Infection

Mesh infection complicates as many as 8% of open ventral hernia repairs, a rate almost ten times higher than laparoscopic repairs [55–57]. There are clear differences between the rates of mesh infections between different methods of herniorraphy and between different locations for mesh placement (underlay vs. sublay vs. onlay). Albino et al. evaluated cases requiring mesh explantation when surgical site infection complicated hernia repair and found significant differences between onlay mesh position (5%) and sublay (retrorectus) position (0.5%) [19]. This is attributable to the large lipocutaneous flaps created for onlay repairs which complicate bacterial clearance when mesh contacts the poorly

vascularized anterior fat layer (Fig. 20.2). Strengthening this argument, Petersen et al. evaluated the effect of placing mesh in a well vascularized space by comparing complete versus incomplete rectus sheath closure when the mesh was placed in the retrorectus plane. Incomplete closure resulted in direct mesh contact with the lipocutaneous layer directly beneath the midline wound. They found a ninefold decrease (2% vs. 18%) in mesh infection when the anterior fascia could be closed over mesh placed in the retrorectus plane [28].

Mesh type also contributes to the rate of infection with multifilament, microporous, and heavy-weight meshes having higher associated rates of infection [58, 59]. Light-weight, macroporous, monofilament meshes elicit a decreased foreign body reaction, permit improved bacterial clearance and better integrate into tissue [60–67].

Mesh infections present in a variety of ways: they can be acute or delayed following the repair; they may present with typical signs of systemic infection or with more subtle signs such as chronic pain or skin changes; they may be associated with a superficial or deep SSI; or they can occur independent of these (Fig. 20.11) [68]. When a mesh-related infection occurs, a synergistic medical and surgical approach of targeted antibiotic therapy and removal of the mesh is the traditional management strategy [39]. This strategy has been modified in recent years, as monofilament, macroporous mesh (polyester, polypropylene) may respond to antibiotics and drainage alone, whereas PTFE infection generally requires complete mesh removal (Figs. 20.9 and 20.12).

Mesh Erosion

Mesh erosion into the GI tract is a well-documented and likely underreported late complication of mesh placement (Fig. 20.7). Intra-peritoneal mesh (especially uncoated mesh) has been associated with erosion and the development of late entero- or colo-cutaneous fistulae (Fig. 20.13) [35, 40, 69–71]. Such fistulae generally do not resolve with conservative measures as the mesh acts as a foreign body responsible for keeping the fistulae open. Partial mesh resection is necessary when managing these fistulae, but

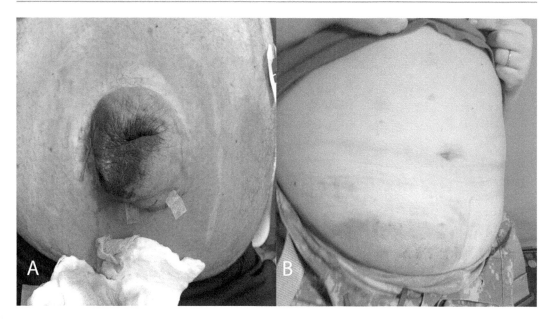

Fig. 20.11 Skin changes resulting from underlying mesh infections. (**a**) Cellulitis, skin ischemia from an acute deep surgical site, and polypropylene mesh infection. (**b**) Erythematous petechial, pruritic rash associated with smoldering PTFE infection

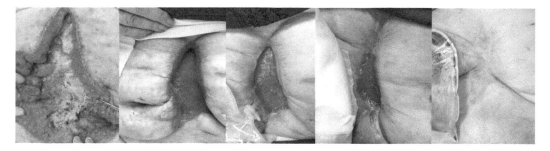

Fig. 20.12 Three-month healing process (*left* to *right*) of exposed, infected light-weight polyprolyene mesh following parastomal hernia repair with component separation. Following initial washout, the mesh was permitted to granulate without the need for systemic antibiotics or mesh removal

complete excision of well incorporated mesh is not mandatory.

Mesh Fracture

The recognition that light-weight, macroporous, monofilament meshes generate improved tissue integration, improved bacterial clearance, decreased foreign body reaction, and cause less chronic pain has resulted in a migration away from the use of their heavy-weight counterparts. This migration, however, has led to an increasing recognition of central mesh failure (CMF) as a mechanism of hernia recurrence (Fig. 20.14).

Initial reports of CMF occurred in cases of light-weight polypropylene use with incomplete closure of the anterior fascial layers [72]. Subsequently, Petro et al. reported a 19% recurrence rate due to CMF when mid-weight monofilament polyester mesh was placed in a sublay position with complete anterior fascial closure [73]. They emphasized cautious use of light-weight meshes, particularly when there is inadequate fascial closure to support the mesh.

Mesh fracture has also been well documented with other devices, most notably the Kugel ventral hernia mesh device which contained a periph-

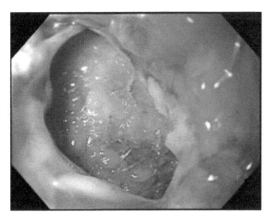

Fig. 20.13 Endoscopic view of polypropylene mesh eroded into the colon following an open parastomal hernia repair

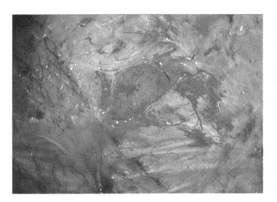

Fig. 20.14 Laparoscopic view of a recurrent incisional hernia as a consequence of central mesh failure (Photo courtesy of Dr. Yuri W. Novitsky, Case Western Reserve University)

eral memory ring composed of polyester held between layers of polypropylene. This device was recalled by the Food and Drug Administration in 2005, due to reports of ring fracture leading to bowel perforation and obstruction. The exact mechanism of polyester ring fracture has not been elucidated.

Mesh fracture typically presents as a hernia recurrence or a complication thereof (such as bowel obstruction) and should be managed as such.

Thromboembolic Complications

There are few studies directly addressing the risk of venous thromboembolism (VTE) following open ventral hernia repair. The risk of VTE following an abdominal wall procedure is quoted at

0.1–0.6%, but this data reflects minor abdominal wall procedures [74]. Complex open abdominal wall reconstructions likely have a higher VTE rate of 0.8–1.7% associated with major general surgery [75]. With higher BMI being a major risk factor for hernia development and recurrence, one must also consider the higher risk classification for VTE that is associated with obesity [76]. VTE prevention, diagnosis, and treatment follow standard protocols and little special consideration needs to be given to the nature of the herniorraphy itself.

Iatrogenic Hernia Formation

As component separation herniorraphy has become increasingly utilized to address complex ventral hernias, there has been greater recognition of the risk of creating iatrogenic hernias with these types of repairs. While uncommon, such iatrogenic hernias can be difficult to address and require mastery of a variety of hernia repair techniques.

Injury to the Linea Semilunaris

Full thickness injury to the semilunar line can occur during anterior component separation with

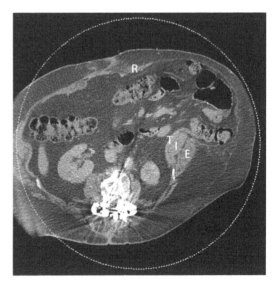

Fig. 20.15 Lateral hernia resulting from a full thickness injury to the linea semilunaris during an anterior component separation with external oblique release. The lateral musculature (Transversus Abdominis (T), Internal Oblique (I) and External Oblique (E)) have been disconnected from the rectus abdominis muscle (R)

Fig. 20.16 Iatrogenic lateral hernias (*arrowheads*) resulting from full thickness injury to the linea semilunaris during robotic posterior component separation. The lateral musculature (L) has been disconnected from the rectus muscles (R) bilaterally (Photo courtesy of Dr. Yuri W. Novitsky, Case Western Reserve University)

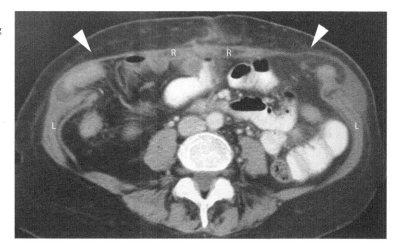

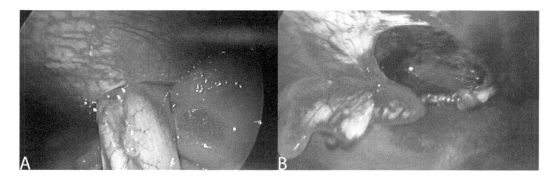

Fig. 20.17 Laparoscopic view of acutely incarcerated small bowel (**a**) within an intra-parietal hernia defect (**b**) following posterior component separation with transversus abdominis release. Note the location of the hernia is between the posterior rectus sheath and the sublay-positioned polypropylene mesh (Photo courtesy of Dr. Yuri W. Novitsky, Case Western Reserve University)

external oblique release (Fig. 20.15) or during posterior component separation (Fig. 20.16) if care is not taken to respect correct myofascial boundaries. Such defects can span the entire length of the rectus muscle, from costal margin to inguinal ligament. Recent reports suggest that posterior component separation utilizing transversus abdominis release can successfully address this type of iatrogenic hernia [77].

Posterior Layer Defects

Failure to adequately recreate a closed visceral sac during any of the posterior component separation herniorraphies can result in defects that permit bowel to herniate between this layer and the mesh layer (Fig. 20.17). Such intra-parietal hernias can present acutely as an early small

bowel obstruction requiring surgical re-intervention. A high index of suspicion must be maintained to correctly diagnose this complication. Fortunately, laparoscopy can often be used to reduce the bowel and to reinforce the posterior layer defect with mesh. This avoids midline wound re-exploration, anterior fascial opening, and mesh transection or removal.

References

1. Henriksen NA, et al. Risk factors for incisional hernia repair after aortic reconstructive surgery in a nation-wide study. J Vasc Surg. 2013;57(6):1524–30. 1530 e1–3.
2. Hoer J, et al. Factors influencing the development of incisional hernia. A retrospective study of 2,983 lapa-

rotomy patients over a period of 10 years. Chirurg. 2002;73(5):474–80.

3. Martindale RG, Deveney CW. Preoperative risk reduction: strategies to optimize outcomes. Surg Clin North Am. 2013;93(5):1041–55.

4. Sorensen LT, et al. Smoking is a risk factor for incisional hernia. Arch Surg. 2005;140(2):119–23.

5. Yahchouchy-Chouillard E, et al. Incisional hernias. I. Related risk factors. Dig Surg. 2003;20(1):3–9.

6. Ross SW, et al. Components separation in complex ventral hernia repair: surgical technique and postoperative outcomes. Surg Technol Int. 2014; 24:167–77.

7. S., F. Abdominal wall defects: the magnitude of the problem. In: Abdominal wall reconstruction 2011 consortium. 2011. Washington, DC.

8. Jin J, Rosen MJ. Laparoscopic versus open ventral hernia repair. Surg Clin North Am. 2008;88(5):1083–100. viii.

9. Berger RL, et al. Development and validation of a risk-stratification score for surgical site occurrence and surgical site infection after open ventral hernia repair. J Am Coll Surg. 2013;217(6):974–82.

10. Kanters AE, et al. Modified hernia grading scale to stratify surgical site occurrence after open ventral hernia repairs. J Am Coll Surg. 2012;215(6):787–93.

11. Ventral Hernia Working Group, Breuing K, Butler CE, Ferzoco S, Franz M, Hultman CS, Kilbridge JF, Rosen M, Silverman RP, Vargo D. Incisional ventral hernias: review of the literature and recommendations regarding the grading and technique of repair. Surgery. 2010;148(3):544–58.

12. Iqbal CW, et al. Long-term outcome of 254 complex incisional hernia repairs using the modified Rives-Stoppa technique. World J Surg. 2007;31(12): 2398–404.

13. Dunne JR, et al. Abdominal wall hernias: risk factors for infection and resource utilization. J Surg Res. 2003;111(1):78–84.

14. Mangram AJ, et al. Guideline for prevention of surgical site infection, 1999. Hospital Infection Control Practices Advisory Committee. Infect Control Hosp Epidemiol. 1999;20(4):250–78. quiz 279–80.

15. Nguyen MT, et al. Readmission following open ventral hernia repair: incidence, indications, and predictors. Am J Surg. 2013;206(6):942–8. discussion 948–9.

16. Liang MK, et al. Outcomes of laparoscopic vs open repair of primary ventral hernias. JAMA Surg. 2013;148(11):1043–8.

17. Jensen KK, Henriksen NA, Jorgensen LN. Endoscopic component separation for ventral hernia causes fewer wound complications compared to open components separation: a systematic review and meta-analysis. Surg Endosc. 2014;28(11):3046–52.

18. Arita NA, et al. Laparoscopic repair reduces incidence of surgical site infections for all ventral hernias. Surg Endosc. 2014;29(7):1769–80.

19. Albino FP, et al. Does mesh location matter in abdominal wall reconstruction? A systematic review of the literature and a summary of recommendations. Plast Reconstr Surg. 2013;132(5):1295–304.

20. Novitsky YW, et al. Transversus abdominis muscle release: a novel approach to posterior component separation during complex abdominal wall reconstruction. Am J Surg. 2012;204(5):709–16.

21. Basta MN, Fischer JP, Kovach SJ. Assessing complications and cost-utilization in ventral hernia repair utilizing biologic mesh in a bridged underlay technique. Am J Surg. 2014;209(4):695–702.

22. Paajanen H, Hermunen H. Long-term pain and recurrence after repair of ventral incisional hernias by open mesh: clinical and MRI study. Langenbecks Arch Surg. 2004;389(5):366–70.

23. Horan TC, et al. CDC definitions of nosocomial surgical site infections, 1992: a modification of CDC definitions of surgical wound infections. Infect Control Hosp Epidemiol. 1992;13(10):606–8.

24. Hicks CW, et al. History of methicillin-resistant *Staphylococcus aureus* (MRSA) surgical site infection may not be a contraindication to ventral hernia repair with synthetic mesh: a preliminary report. Hernia. 2014;18(1):65–70.

25. Blatnik JA, et al. Does a history of wound infection predict postoperative surgical site infection after ventral hernia repair? Am J Surg. 2012;203(3):370–4. discussion 374.

26. Watt-Boolsen S, et al. Postmastectomy seroma. A study of the nature and origin of seroma after mastectomy. Dan Med Bull. 1989;36(5):487–9.

27. Agrawal A, Ayantunde AA, Cheung KL. Concepts of seroma formation and prevention in breast cancer surgery. ANZ J Surg. 2006;76(12):1088–95.

28. Petersen S, et al. Ventral rectus fascia closure on top of mesh hernia repair in the sublay technique. Plast Reconstr Surg. 2004;114(7):1754–60.

29. Harth KC, Rosen MJ. Endoscopic versus open component separation in complex abdominal wall reconstruction. Am J Surg. 2010;199(3):342–6. discussion 346–7.

30. Albright E, et al. The component separation technique for hernia repair: a comparison of open and endoscopic techniques. Am Surg. 2011;77(7):839–43.

31. Giurgius M, et al. The endoscopic component separation technique for hernia repair results in reduced morbidity compared to the open component separation technique. Hernia. 2012;16(1):47–51.

32. Fox M, et al. Laparoscopic component separation reduces postoperative wound complications but does not alter recurrence rates in complex hernia repairs. Am J Surg. 2013;206(6):869–74. discussion 874–5.

33. Satterwhite TS, et al. Outcomes of complex abdominal herniorrhaphy: experience with 106 cases. Ann Plast Surg. 2012;68(4):382–8.

34. Rosen MJ, et al. Evaluation of surgical outcomes of retro-rectus versus intraperitoneal reinforcement with bio-prosthetic mesh in the repair of contaminated ventral hernias. Hernia. 2013;17(1):31–5.

35. McLanahan D, et al. Retrorectus prosthetic mesh repair of midline abdominal hernia. Am J Surg. 1997;173(5):445–9.
36. Gurusamy KS, Allen VB. Wound drains after incisional hernia repair. Cochrane Database Syst Rev. 2013;12:CD005570.
37. Bercial ME, et al. Suction drains, quilting sutures, and fibrin sealant in the prevention of seroma formation in abdominoplasty: which is the best strategy? Aesthetic Plast Surg. 2012;36(2):370–3.
38. Kohler G, et al. Prevention of subcutaneous seroma formation in open ventral hernia repair using a new low-thrombin fibrin sealant. World J Surg. 2014;38(11):2797–803.
39. Falagas ME, Kasiakou SK. Mesh-related infections after hernia repair surgery. Clin Microbiol Infect. 2005;11(1):3–8.
40. Kaufman Z, Engelberg M, Zager M. Fecal fistula: a late complication of Marlex mesh repair. Dis Colon Rectum. 1981;24(7):543–4.
41. Kunishige T, et al. A defect of the abdominal wall with intestinal fistulas after the repair of incisional hernia using Composix Kugel Patch. Int J Surg Case Rep. 2013;4(9):793–7.
42. Krpata DM, et al. Outcomes of simultaneous large complex abdominal wall reconstruction and enterocutaneous fistula takedown. Am J Surg. 2013; 205(3):354–8. discussion 358-9.
43. Carbonell AM, et al. Outcomes of synthetic mesh in contaminated ventral hernia repairs. J Am Coll Surg. 2013;217(6):991–8.
44. Blatnik JA, et al. Predicting severe postoperative respiratory complications following abdominal wall reconstruction. Plast Reconstr Surg. 2012; 130(4):836–41.
45. Fischer JP, et al. Validated model for predicting postoperative respiratory failure: analysis of 1706 abdominal wall reconstructions. Plast Reconstr Surg. 2013;132(5):826e–35.
46. Ma Q, Xue FS, Li RP. Analysis of risk factors, morbidity, and cost associated with respiratory complications following abdominal wall reconstruction. Plast Reconstr Surg. 2015;135(2):459e–60.
47. Fischer JP, et al. Analysis of risk factors, morbidity, and cost associated with respiratory complications following abdominal wall reconstruction. Plast Reconstr Surg. 2014;133(1):147–56.
48. Levey AS, et al. Definition and classification of chronic kidney disease: a position statement from Kidney Disease: Improving Global Outcomes (KDIGO). Kidney Int. 2005;67(6):2089–100.
49. Yussim A, Yampolski I, Greif F, Mor E. Acute kidney injury after complex incisional hernia in transplant recipients. Transplant Proc. 2012;94(10S):1024.
50. Kirkpatrick AW, et al. Intra-abdominal hypertension and the abdominal compartment syndrome: updated consensus definitions and clinical practice guidelines from the World Society of the Abdominal Compartment Syndrome. Intensive Care Med. 2013;39(7):1190–206.
51. Cheatham ML, et al. Results from the International Conference of experts on intra-abdominal hypertension and abdominal compartment syndrome. II. Recommendations. Intensive Care Med. 2007; 33(6):951–62.
52. Malbrain ML, et al. Results from the International Conference of experts on intra-abdominal hypertension and abdominal compartment syndrome. I. Definitions. Intensive Care Med. 2006;32(11): 1722–32.
53. Malbrain ML, et al. Incidence and prognosis of intraabdominal hypertension in a mixed population of critically ill patients: a multiple-center epidemiological study. Crit Care Med. 2005;33(2):315–22.
54. Petro C, Raigani S, Orenstein S, Klick J, Rowbottom J, Novitsky Y, Rosen M. Permissive abdominal hypertension following open incisional hernia repair: a novel concept. Hernia. 2014;18 Suppl 1:S78.
55. Cobb WS, et al. Incisional herniorrhaphy with intraperitoneal composite mesh: a report of 95 cases. Am J Surg. 2003;69(9):784–7.
56. Petersen S, et al. Deep prosthesis infection in incisional hernia repair: predictive factors and clinical outcome. Eur J Surg. 2001;167(6):453–7.
57. Heniford BT, et al. Laparoscopic repair of ventral hernias: nine years' experience with 850 consecutive hernias. Ann Surg. 2003;238(3):391–9. discussion 399–400.
58. Bellon JM, et al. Macrophage response to experimental implantation of polypropylene prostheses. Eur Surg Res. 1994;26(1):46–53.
59. Amid PK. Classification of biomaterials and their related complications in abdominal wall hernia surgery. Hernia. 1997;1:15–21.
60. Cobb WS, Kercher KW, Heniford BT. The argument for lightweight polypropylene mesh in hernia repair. Surg Innov. 2005;12(1):63–9.
61. Cobb WS, et al. Textile analysis of heavy weight, mid-weight, and light weight polypropylene mesh in a porcine ventral hernia model. J Surg Res. 2006;136(1):1–7.
62. Schmidbauer S, et al. Heavy-weight versus low-weight polypropylene meshes for open sublay mesh repair of incisional hernia. Eur J Med Res. 2005;10(6):247–53.
63. Orenstein SB, et al. Comparative analysis of histopathologic effects of synthetic meshes based on material, weight, and pore size in mice. J Surg Res. 2012;176(2):423–9.
64. Blatnik JA, et al. In vivo analysis of the morphologic characteristics of synthetic mesh to resist MRSA adherence. J Gastrointest Surg. 2012;16(11): 2139–44.
65. Sanders D, et al. An in vitro study assessing the effect of mesh morphology and suture fixation on bacterial adherence. Hernia. 2013;17(6):779–89.

66. Asarias JR, et al. Influence of mesh materials on the expression of mediators involved in wound healing. J Invest Surg. 2011;24(2):87–98.

67. Nguyen PT, Asarias JR, Pierce LM. Influence of a new monofilament polyester mesh on inflammation and matrix remodeling. J Invest Surg. 2012;25(5): 330–9.

68. Mavros MN, et al. Risk factors for mesh-related infections after hernia repair surgery: a meta-analysis of cohort studies. World J Surg. 2011;35(11): 2389–98.

69. Balen EM, et al. Repair of ventral hernias with expanded polytetrafluoroethylene patch. Br J Surg. 1998;85(10):1415–8.

70. Leber GE, et al. Long-term complications associated with prosthetic repair of incisional hernias. Arch Surg. 1998;133(4):378–82.

71. Vrijland WW, et al. Intraperitoneal polypropylene mesh repair of incisional hernia is not associated with enterocutaneous fistula. Br J Surg. 2000;87(3):348–52.

72. Zuvela M, et al. Central rupture and bulging of low-weight polypropylene mesh following recurrent incisional sublay hernioplasty. Hernia. 2014;18(1): 135–40.

73. Petro CC, Nahabet EH, Criss CN, Orenstein SB, von Recum HA, Novitsky YW, Rosen MJ. Central failures of lightweight monofilament polyester mesh causing hernia recurrence: a cautionary note. Hernia. 2015;19(1):155–9.

74. Samama CM, et al. Venous thromboembolism prevention in surgery and obstetrics: clinical practice guidelines. Eur J Anaesthesiol. 2006; 23(2):95–116.

75. Huber O, et al. Postoperative pulmonary embolism after hospital discharge. An underestimated risk. Arch Surg. 1992;127(3):310–3.

76. Westling A, et al. Incidence of deep venous thrombosis in patients undergoing obesity surgery. World J Surg. 2002;26(4):470–3.

77. Pauli EM, Wang J, Petro CC, Juza RM, Novitsky YW, Rosen MJ. Posterior component separation with transversus abdominis release successfully addresses recurrent ventral hernias following anterior component separation. Hernia. 2015; 19(2):285–91.

78. Krpata DM, et al. Posterior and open anterior components separations: a comparative analysis. Am J Surg. 2012;203(3):318–22. discussion 322.

David M. Krpata and Yuri W. Novitsky

Introduction

Ventral herniorrhaphies are among the most commonly performed operations by general surgeons throughout the world. Incisional hernias, with a reported incidence of up to 20%, have become an increasing problem due to the increasing number of laparotomies performed. In the United States, approximately 175,000 ventral abdominal hernias are repaired each year. Surgical approaches to ventral herniorrhaphy have been a subject of research and technical modifications for many years. Although the routine use of prosthetic reinforcement for the repair of herniations in adults has been contested, existing evidence strongly supports tension-free hernia repairs in most patients [1, 2]. With the development and popularization of tension-free repairs using prosthetic meshes, the recurrence rates are typically less than 20% [1, 2].

Large abdominal incisions and wide tissue dissection with the creation of large flaps are needed for open placement of adequately sized mesh [3]; however, this dissection may result in high incidence of postoperative morbidity and wound complications. Not surprisingly, with the advent of minimally invasive surgery, the use of laparoscopy for ventral hernia repairs has become standard [4–7]. The mesh is placed as an intra-peritoneal underlay with wide coverage of the hernia defect. Avoidance of large incisions has substantially reduced wound complications [4, 6]. Overall, the clinical benefits of laparoscopic ventral hernia repair (LVHR) include a faster convalescence, fewer complications and, importantly, a low recurrence rate [4–7]. Additionally, the laparoscopic approach can be employed for the management of more complex hernia locations, such as suprapubic ventral hernias. In this chapter, we will discuss the technical aspects of the traditional laparoscopic repairs and address potential pitfalls and contraindications.

Preoperative preparation and patient selection

The workup of a ventral hernia patient includes a thorough history and physical examinations. It is important to obtain all old operative reports. All pertinent comorbidities, including smoking, diabetes, and obesity, must be optimized. Bowel preparation is not given. Abdominal imaging (with Ultrasound or CT scan) is essentially uniform

D.M. Krpata, M.D. (✉)
General Surgery, Cleveland Clinic Comprehensive Hernia Center, Cleveland, OH, USA
e-mail: krpatad@ccf.org

Y.W. Novitsky, M.D., F.A.C.S.
Department of Surgery, Case Comprehensive Hernia Center, University Hospitals Case Medical Center, Cleveland, OH, USA

© Springer International Publishing Switzerland 2016
Y.W. Novitsky (ed.), *Hernia Surgery*, DOI 10.1007/978-3-319-27470-6_21

except for small defects. Information gleaned from abdominal imaging may not only allow to delineate the defect(s), but may also affect a given patient's suitability for a laparoscopic repair. In our practice, relative contraindications to a laparoscopic approach include hernias wider than 8–10 cm, significant overlying skin changes, previous intra-peritoneal mesh, as well as repairs in clean-contaminated or contaminated settings.

Techniques of Laparoscopic VHR

After general anesthesia is induced, the patient is positioned supine with the arms adducted and "tucked" at the sides (Fig. 21.1). This allows for adequate space for both primary surgeon and an assistant on the same side of the patient. We use two monitors placed on each side of the patient. In most cases, the bladder and stomach are decompressed with catheters. An antibiotic, usually a first-generation cephalosporin, is given prophylactically before the incision was made and repeated if the operation lasts longer than 4 hours. We routinely use an Ioban™ drape (3M Company, St. Paul, MN) to minimize mesh contact with the patient skin. Laparoscopic hernia repair is performed by using a 30° angled laparo-

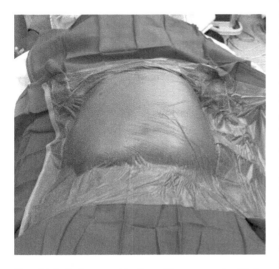

Fig. 21.1 Patient positioning. The arms should be "tucked" to allow for operating surgeon and assistant to stand on the same side and minimize potential interference of the outstretched arms with instrument handles

scope, 5-mm bowel graspers, scissors, and clip appliers.

Safe access to the peritoneal cavity is a key first step in LVHR. The access is gained using either a cut-down technique, an optical trocar, or a Veress needle. Regardless of the method chosen, access to the abdominal cavity must be performed away from any previous incisions. A window of access is usually present, even in the multiply operated abdomen, at the costal margin between the mid-clavicular or anterior axillary lines. We prefer an optical trocar technique in the left upper quadrant just off the rib. Once access is established, it is imperative to confirm that no inadvertent injuries to the abdominal organs or vessels occurred. Any uncertainties must be followed by a laparoscopic exploration. One should have a very low threshold to convert to open if the safety of the initial access cannot be confirmed.

After pneumoperitoneum is established, we typically place an additional 5-mm trocar under direct vision laterally along the anterior-to-mid-axillary line. If adhesions are extensive, a third 5-mm trocar is placed to allow for two working ports and a camera on the same side. Furthermore, two additional 5-mm trocars are placed on the contralateral side to facilitate intra-abdominal mesh introduction and fixation. This strategy involves utilization of five 5-mm trocars (Fig. 21.2). For smaller defects, the number of the access ports could be reduced. However, fewer working ports result in poor triangulation, reduced efficiency, and difficulties with mesh positioning and tacking. Given a very low morbidity and scarring associated with a 5-mm port, additional access sites are well worth it. We strongly advise to have at least two trocars on each side of the abdomen for most, if not all, cases.

Following trocar placement, adhesiolysis is performed sharply with limited use of electrosurgery or ultrasonic coagulators. This is another critical step for a safe LVHR. Inadvertent and unrecognized bowel injuries can cause significant morbidity and even mortality. Missed enterotomy during LVHR remains the most common reason for malpractice litigation. Reduction of the hernia contents is performed using blunt graspers and sharp dissection from the inside and

Fig. 21.2 Typical trocar strategy for our standard laparoscopic ventral hernia repair

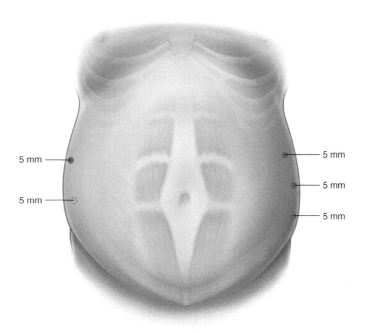

5 mm

5 mm

5 mm

5 mm

5 mm

5 mm

is facilitated by manual compression from the outside. The hernia sac is usually left in situ.

Once the adhesiolysis is completed, the hernia defect is measured to determine an appropriate size of a prosthetic mesh. The borders of the defect are delineated with a combination of laparoscopic vision and external palpation. The edges of the defect are marked externally. We utilize trans-abdominal spinal needles to obtain precise dimensions of the hernia defect (Fig. 21.3). This maneuver is especially important in obese patients with large defects as the externally measured defect size can be dramatically overestimated. A ruler is placed through a 5-mm port, and the dimensions of the hernia defect are measured directly. Additionally, defect closure could be performed and is addressed in detail in Chapter 22.

The mesh is then tailored to overlap all margins of the hernia by at least 5 cm. Our general rule of thumb is to obtain overlap of 25–30% of the defects size on each side. Once the mesh is cut to the desirable size, four size-0 permanent monofilament or ePTFE sutures are placed at the mid-point of each side of the mesh. Points of reference on the mesh and corresponding points

on the abdominal wall are marked to aid in orienting the mesh after its introduction into the abdomen. The mesh is rolled up and pushed or pulled into the abdomen through an additional 12 or 15-mm trocar. This port is placed near the hernia defect so that the mesh covers the site, negating the need for fascial closure and minimizing the risks of trocar-site hernia (Fig. 21.4). Alternatively, (and less desirable in our opinion), any of the lateral trocars could be up-sized to allow for mesh introduction.

The mesh is rolled from both edges to facilitate the unfolding step. If the defect size requires a very large prosthetic, it is usually introduced in the abdominal cavity by pulling with the grasper passed through the contralateral trocar (Fig. 21.5). It is important to maintain the appropriate mesh orientation during the insertion and unfolding of the mesh. Modern positioning devices have significantly facilitated this step, allowing for rapid and accurate mesh placement. After the mesh is oriented intra-corporeally, the sutures are pulled through the abdominal wall with a suture passer (Fig. 21.6). Adequate mesh/defect overlap is once again confirmed using spinal needles, similarly to that described above.

Fig. 21.3 Intra-corporeal (direct) measurement of a hernia defect. Spinal needles allow for more precise identification of the edges of the defect. Additional spinal needles may be used for defects larger than the length of a ruler

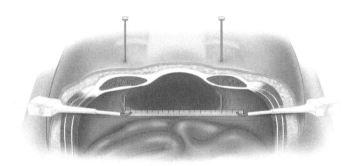

Fig. 21.4 Instead of enlarging a 5-mm lateral port, the additional 12-mm port, used for mesh introduction, is placed close to the edge of the hernia to allow for subsequent mesh coverage of the trocar site

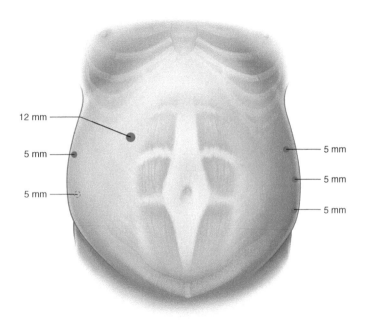

The top or bottom suture is pulled first. We recommend beginning with the point closest to the bony margin (xiphoid, pubis, iliac crest, costal margin, etc.). We subsequently pull the suture that is opposite to the first one. Once sufficient overlap is confirmed, we tie both sutures with the knots buried in the subcutaneous tissues. The other two lateral sutures are then pulled transabdominally and tied ensuring that the overlap is sufficient. We recommend starting with the lateral stitch ipsilateral to the camera (#3 in Fig. 21.6). To facilitate this step, we move the camera to the superior-most trocar. We routinely reduce pneumoperitoneum to 7–8 mmHg to ensure the mesh is taut and doesn't wrinkle after desuflation. Once again, having at least two trocars on each side of the abdomen allows for easy and precise mesh positioning. After correct positioning is confirmed, the fourth stitch is pulled through and all stitches are tied.

The perimeter of the mesh is then attached to the peritoneum with tacks, at approximately 1 cm intervals to prevent intestinal herniation. Placing the tacks is facilitated by the external manual

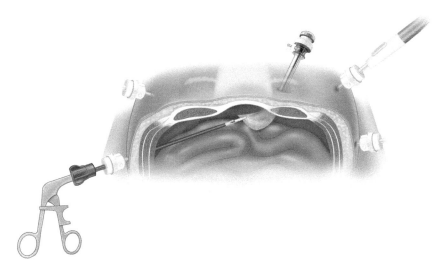

Fig. 21.5 The mesh could be introduced by "pulling" it in to the abdomen through a trocar

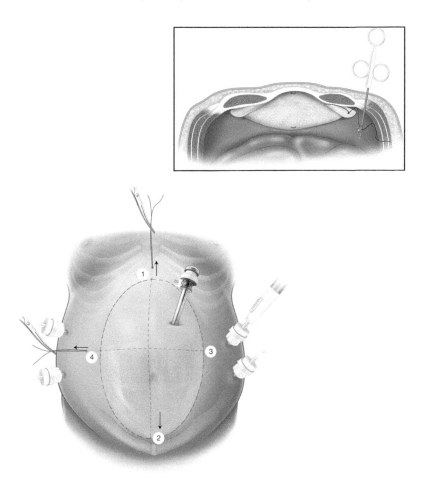

Fig. 21.6 Mesh fixation. Inferior and superior sutures are pulled first, followed by the lateral sutures

palpation of the tacker's tip (Fig. 21.7). Tactile feedback is particularly important for tacking the mesh in the lower abdomen to ensure that the tacks are placed superiorly to the inguinal ligament. Similarly, for upper abdominal hernias, manual counter palpation is paramount to ensure that the tacks are placed below the costal margin. Failure to do so may lead to pulmonary and pericardial injuries. If the mesh extends cephalad to the costal margin and xiphoid process, that portion of the mesh should not be tacked and should be affixed to the peritoneum with sutures or glue.

Although some investigators have advocated a "double-crown" technique of mesh fixation, we strongly believe additional suture fixation is critical to ensure the long-term durability of the repair. Additional full-thickness stitches are placed circumferentially every 5–8 cm by using the suture passer (Fig. 21.8). This transabdominal fixation is crucial to ensure that the mesh will not be displaced over time. The knots are tied in the subcutaneous tissues. The skin is released to avoid dimpling.

Postoperative Care

While some patients may be suited for LVHR on an outpatient basis, most patients with moderate defects require at least a 1–2 day hospitalization.

This is done to ensure adequate pain control and resolution of ileus. Factors influencing longer recovery include extensive adhesiolysis, large incarcerated defects, and multiple transabdominal sutures. We advocate a clear or soft diet for the first 3–5 days following the repair to provide for adequate return of normal bowel function. The abdominal binders are encouraged, especially in the first 2 weeks. Activities are not restricted and are guided by patients' discomfort.

Complications and Outcomes

While LVHR has its benefits with relation to wound morbidity compared to open techniques, it is not without potential complications. In general, these complications can be categorized into intra-operative, postoperative, and long-term. Some complications are associated with laparoscopy and some with ventral hernia repair; the following discussion focuses on complications that are somewhat unique to LVHR.

Wound and mesh infections are known complications of any hernia repair. Many investigators have shown that laparoscopy is associated with an extremely low rate of wound infections and very rare mesh infections [5–7]. Modern meshes without an ePTFE component have reduced infectious complications of LVHR even further. However,

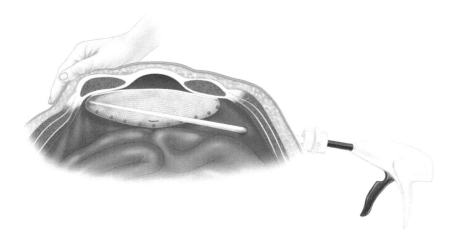

Fig. 21.7 Placement of tack is done circumferentially along the whole length of the mesh to avoid bowel incarceration. External palpation of the abdominal wall facili- tates placement of the tacks and helps to avoid tacking the mesh below the inguinal ligament and above costal margins

Fig. 21.8 Trans-abdominal suture fixation of the mesh

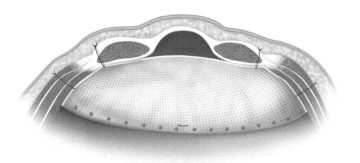

any persistent cellulitis and/or persistent fluid collection around the intra-peritoneal mesh should be a point of concern for acute or chronic prosthetic infection, especially if ePTFE-based mesh was used. Open exploration, mesh removal, primary hernia repair, and delayed formal reconstruction are the best and safest ways to approach infected mesh after LVHR.

Intra-operative complications such as bleeding or injury to surrounding intra-abdominal structures are rare. Nonetheless, an enterotomy or missed enterotomy will significantly impact the outcome of surgery. An enterotomy identified during surgery with spillage of enteric content within the abdomen should cause the surgeon to re-evaluate the operative plan. The enterotomy can be repaired laparoscopically if it is well visualized and ports are optimally placed. If there is any question about the integrity of laparoscopic repair of the enterotomy, conversion to a laparotomy is mandatory. With gross spillage of enteric content, a formal hernia repair should be delayed. Missed enterotomy or a delayed bowel injury from electrocautery resulting in intra-abdominal sepsis and mesh infection would require laparotomy, repair of the bowel injury, and complete excision of the mesh. Failure to completely remove the mesh would almost certainly lead to persistent intra-abdominal infection.

Seroma formation is one of the most common complications after LVHR [6]. Failure to obliterate the potential space within the hernia sac frequently leads to fluid accumulation in the hernia sac. The seroma may present as a bulge which patients may commonly perceive as a hernia recurrence. Careful physical exam should easily differentiate between the two. If the diagnosis is in question, ultrasound or CT scan evaluation can be used to differentiate between diagnoses. Management of a seroma should follow a conservative pathway as it will typically resolve without intervention. For persistent seromas, sterile aspiration can be performed in the office. However, fluid may re-accumulate in the potential space after aspiration necessitating additional aspirations. It is important to realize that any aspiration and subsequent aspirations put a patient at risk for converting a sterile seroma into an abscess. Closing the defect during LVHR with the "shoelace" technique (Chapter 22) can significantly reduce or even eliminate the risk of seroma formation.

In the early postoperative period, patients may complain of pain at the trans-abdominal suture sites. Conservative management with NSAIDs may resolve the patient's pain; however, persistent pain may require injection with local anesthetics. The use of slowly absorbable sutures for mesh fixation could be associated with reduced postoperative pain, but that has not been proven in prospective trials. While the use of absorbable tacks has been proposed to reduce chronic pain, their utilization has been shown to have no effect on postoperative pain.

Arguably, the most important complication from an LVHR is a hernia recurrence, as this is the primary outcome measure of long-term success of the surgery. Recurrence rates in the literature vary from 2 to 20% with the largest series demonstrating recurrence rates around 5% [6, 7]. Long-term, the best chance for a successful

LVHR without recurrence, in our opinion, is to maximize coverage of the hernia defect and securely fixate the mesh to the abdominal wall with both tacks and trans-abdominal sutures.

Conclusion

LVHR is associated with decreased perioperative pain, reduced hospital stay, and faster recovery. Minimal wound morbidity, however, appears to be its biggest advantage over most open repairs. Overall, numerous studies demonstrate that laparoscopic ventral hernia repair is an effective and safe approach to the abdominal wall hernia. It can be performed in complex surgical patients with a low rate of conversion to open surgery, a short hospital stay, and a low risk of recurrence. Modern modifications with mesh-positioning devices and laparoscopic defect closure have further advanced the results of LVHR. Appropriate patient selection, safe abdominal access, adhesiolysis, precise mesh positioning, and fixation are key factors that ensure a safe and effective laparoscopic repair of most ventral defects.

References

1. Burger JW, Luijendijk RW, Hop WC, Halm JA, Verdaasdonk EG, Jeekel J. Long-term follow-up of a randomized controlled trial of suture versus mesh repair of incisional hernia. Ann Surg. 2004;240 (4):578–83.
2. Luijendijk RW, Hop WC, van den Tol MP, et al. A comparison of suture repair with mesh repair for incisional hernia. N Engl J Med. 2000;343(6):392–8.
3. Stoppa RE. The treatment of complicated groin and incisional hernias. World J Surg. 1989;13(5):545–54.
4. DeMaria EJ, Moss JM, Sugerman HJ. Laparoscopic intraperitoneal polytetrafluoroethylene (PTFE) prosthetic patch repair of ventral hernia. Prospective comparison to open prefascial polypropylene mesh repair. Surg Endosc. 2000;14(4):326–9.
5. Carbajo MA, Martin del Olmo JC, Blanco JI, et al. Laparoscopic treatment vs open surgery in the solution of major incisional and abdominal wall hernias with mesh. Surg Endosc. 1999; 13(3):250–2.
6. Heniford BT, Park A, Ramshaw BJ, Voeller G. Laparoscopic repair of ventral hernias: nine years' experience with 850 consecutive hernias. Ann Surg. 2003;238(3):391–9.
7. Novitsky YW, Cobb WS, Kercher KW, Matthews BD, Sing RF, Heniford BT. Laparoscopic ventral hernia repair in obese patients: a new standard of care. Arch Surg. 2006;141(1):57–61.

Sean B. Orenstein and Yuri W. Novitsky

Introduction

Both open and laparoscopic techniques are efficacious for repairing a variety of ventral defects; however, laparoscopic ventral hernia repair (LVHR) offers the advantages of reduced wound morbidity including infection, quicker return of bowel function, reduced length of stay, and improved cosmesis [1–6]. While restoration of the abdominal wall by reapproximating the midline is thought to be a mainstay of open VHR, this philosophy has not become standard practice for laparoscopic repairs. Instead, LVHR commonly results in mesh placed as an underlay, essentially bridging one or multiple defects. In an effort to provide a more durable repair, laparoscopic defect closure was introduced to create a more functional repair by combining primary fascial closure with mesh reinforcement (as with open repairs), while still preserving the benefits of minimally invasive surgery.

Electronic supplementary material: The online version of this chapter (doi:10.1007/978-3-319-27470-6_22) contains supplementary material, which is available to authorized users.

S.B. Orenstein, M.D. (✉)
Oregon Health & Science University,
3181 SW Sam Jackson Park Rd, L223A,
Portland, OR 97239, USA
e-mail: orenstei@ohsu.edu

Y.W. Novitsky, M.D., F.A.C.S.
Department of Surgery, UH Case Medical Center,
11100 Euclid Avenue, Cleveland, OH 44106, USA
e-mail: Yuri.Novitsky@UHhospitals.org

Abdominal Wall Mechanics

While bridging may be successful for some repairs, it is not uncommon to see postoperative CT images demonstrating a mesh-lined hernia sac. One way to reduce mesh "eventration" from occurring is to ensure adequate mesh fixation with multiple trans-abdominal sutures. Still, even with wide mesh overlap and suture fixation, the Law of LaPlace ($T = P \times R/W$) dictates that there will be increased tension on the mesh directly underneath unclosed defect(s) [7–10] (Fig. 22.1). While the Law of LaPlace and Pascal's Principle (pressure equalization within a closed vessel) are advantageous for hernia repairs utilizing underlay and sublay mesh placement by keeping the mesh pressed up against the abdominal wall or preperitoneal inguinal sites, this negatively affects sites directly under hernia defects. The only way to equalize the tension on the abdominal wall is to close the areas with greater radius, that is, the hernia defects. This concept may be more important now given the severe rise in obesity, with ultimate ramifications for LVHR. Increased abdominal girth and intra-abdominal mass may lead to increased intra-abdominal pressure. Abdominal wall thickness affects tension, with a thinner-walled region above the hernia defect resulting in increased tension at that site. Additionally, differing abdominal wall thickness adjacent to hernia defects may lead to shear stress transmitted to the mesh as a result of abrupt tension changes within the vicin-

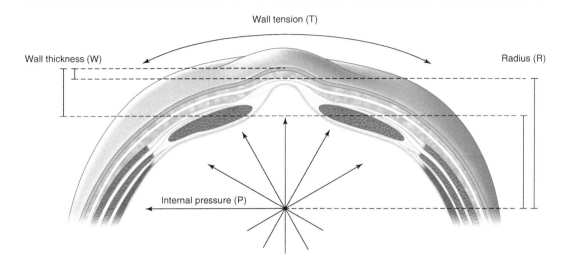

Fig. 22.1 Law of LaPlace. A simplified equation for LaPlace's Law is $T = P \times R/W$, whereby T is the tension exerted on the abdominal wall; P is the intra-abdominal pressure, which, according to Pascal's principle, is equal throughout the abdominal cylinder or sphere; R is the radius; W is the wall thickness

ity of defects. Thus, the increased width (radius), wall thickness, and pressure will bode unfavorably at sites of abdominal wall defects, possibly leading to worse outcomes following traditional LVHR with bridging as our population continues to increase in size.

Concept of Defect Closure

Functional, Dynamic Repair

Restoring a patient's displaced musculature and fasciae to near-native anatomy to improve functionality are important goals for most abdominal wall reconstructions (AWR). One of the key facets of AWR is medialization of the rectus abdominis muscles by restoring the linea alba, the major insertion point of abdominal wall musculature [11, 12]. By restoring to near-native anatomy, a more functional and dynamic abdominal wall is likely to be created. While this is routinely discussed for open repairs, there is limited conversation for laparoscopic repairs. If it makes sense to restore the abdominal wall to a more native and functional level in open repairs, then why not use the same philosophy for laparoscopic repairs? Instead, traditional LVHR solely relies on the support of a bridged defect with mesh prosthetic, which may be detrimental to the patient. Mesh bridging may result in regions of friction and shear force at the edges of the defect with excessive pressure centrally, leading to mesh instability, stretching of the sutures causing increased postoperative pain, as well as bulging [13]. Additionally, without direct contact between the anterior abdominal wall and the mesh, there can be no ingrowth at sites of hernia defects. Closing the defect not only leads to equalization of pressure and tension along the mesh and abdominal wall but also allows complete incorporation of the mesh prosthetic for a more durable repair.

Laparoscopic defect closure combines the tenants of primary fascial closure along with prosthetic mesh reinforcement. Primary closure alone for open hernia repairs carries a very high recurrence rate, with recurrences seen in 18–63% of repairs in the long term. The use of mesh has markedly reduced recurrence rates down to 2–32% [14–18], thus making mesh reinforcement a necessary component of successful repairs. However, even with mesh placement and routine trans-abdominal fixation, significant tension may still exist along the primary fascial closure site. As discussed in our initial experience with defect "shoelacing," because of the increased tension on the fascial closure, additional trans-abdominal sutures are placed to off-load some of that tension [19]. By placing interrupted buttress-ing sutures on either side of the shoelace closure, tension is transferred from the shoelace repair to the mesh itself. Of note, while some surgeons argue for double-crown tacking as the sole source of fixation during LVHR, this certainly would not apply to laparoscopic defect closure, as trans-abdominal fixation remains an essential compo-nent for defect closure repairs.

Patient Selection

Among other factors such as comorbidities, her-nia grade and wound class, the size, quality, and location of the defect greatly determine whether laparoscopic repair with or without shoelace clo-sure is feasible. In general, if the defect is too large or complex for shoelace repair, then other means of repair, including traditional (non-shoelace) LVHR or open repair, should be strongly considered. While there is no strict cut-off for width of defect able to be closed, we rou-tinely close defects up to 6 cm in width and selectively for defects 6–8 cm. Large or multiple "Swiss-cheese" type of defects or those with poor skin/tissue integrity should be considered for open repair or traditional LVHR without defect closure.

Hernia location is another determination for defect closure. Flank hernias may be amenable to defect closure; however, care must be taken to secure the mesh appropriately with adequate overlap which may require bone anchors for secure fixation. Parastomal hernias can be repaired utilizing a Sugarbaker technique, using defect closure as an adjunct with LVHR. In this setting, the defect size is reduced enough to allow adequate room for bowel prior to placement of mesh. On the other hand, subxiphoid defects are often not amenable to defect closure due to their proximity to the costal margin, resulting in an inability to adequately reapproximate the fascial edges as well as risk of injury to subcostal neuro-vascular structures.

Advantages and Drawbacks

Smaller Mesh

A frequent question of hernia defect closure is "Do you implant a mesh sized for the original defect or the newly closed defect?" While the vertical dimensions of the mesh will be same, shoelace closure does allow for somewhat smaller width meshes to be placed. A generous overlap of at least a 5 cm is still recommended; therefore defect closure still requires at least a 10 cm wide mesh. For example, a 5 cm wide defect may be repaired using a 10–12 cm wide mesh following defect closure instead of 15 cm or larger mesh. Less foreign body theoretically reduces fibrotic reactions and ensuing scar plate formation on the lateral abdominal wall, thus improving patients' symptoms and mobility. While it is unclear what the true clinical signifi-cance in the long term is as there is limited rigor-ous data thus far, we strive to use only what is necessary when it comes to implanted foreign bodies.

Recurrence

The benefit of reduced recurrence rate has not been completely elucidated due to the lack of any randomized trials and only a small number of comparative studies; however, recent data is encouraging. In their review paper of the 11 stud-ies involving LVHR with defect closure, Nguyen et al. describe recurrence rates of 0–7.7% [20]. Three of those studies retrospectively compared closure vs nonclosure and discovered significant reductions in recurrence rates, with recurrence rates of 0–5.7% for defect closure, compared to a range of 4.8–16.7% for traditional bridged LVHR [21–23].

Dead Space Elimination

Additional benefits of laparoscopic defect clo-sure are based on obliteration of the dead space that is typically present in traditional bridged LVHRs. Reduction of the dead space results in decreased seromas and the potential infectious complications of seromas. We previously described our cohort of 47 patients that underwent laparoscopic shoelace closure, none of whom returned with seroma or hernia recurrence [19]. Likewise, all other studies, with the exception of one, demonstrate low seroma rates, ranging from 0 to 11.4% [20]. However, one study demonstrated increased seroma formation following defect closure when compared to nonclosure of the defect (11 vs. 4%) [23]. While it is unclear what the cause of this outlier value is, this study utilized braided suture for defect closure, as opposed to monofilament. Comparatively, LVHR without defect closure results in seroma rates of up to 32% though many are not clinically significant [20, 24].

Additionally, if wound infections should arise requiring wound opening or if the skin dehisces, defect closure provides an additional barrier of tissue above the mesh, thus limiting mesh exposure and possible contamination or infection. Finally, shoelace defect closure may offer a cosmetic advantage in the long term. While initial postoperative wounds tend to demonstrate bunched up tissue under the skin, the lax tissues anterior to the defect tend to tighten up as myofibroblast contraction takes place, resulting in a reduction in subjective bulging and a more cosmetically appealing repair.

Laparoscopic Shoelace Closure Technique

- *Setup*: Laparoscopic defect closure employs a combination of primary fascial closure of the hernia sites along with mesh prosthetic placement for reinforcement. The case is initiated using standard LVHR technique, as discussed in Chapter 21. Positioning the patient supine with arms tucked aids in adhesiolysis and tacking from various angles around the patient. Nasogastric tubes are typically reserved only for incarcerated bowel or procedures requiring extensive lysis of adhesions.

For suprapubic or low midline defects, we typically place a 3-way Foley catheter preoperatively for instillation of saline to assist in bladder identification.

- *Access*: Access is typically achieved using optical trocar entry via left upper subcostal entry. 5-mm accessory trocars are placed under direct visualization, with eventual bilateral trocar placement after sufficient adhesiolysis. Eventually, a 12- or 15-mm trocar will need to be placed for mesh insertion. We typically place this trocar as close to midline as possible without going directly through the hernia sac. This allows for subsequent mesh coverage of the port site, thus reducing the chance of a trocar site hernia.
- *Shoelacing Supplies:*
  - #11-blade scalpel
  - Spinal needles
  - Marking pen and ruler
  - Suture passer (e.g., Carter-Thomason, Cooper Surgical, Inc., Trumbull, CT, USA)–Disposable device recommended as reusable devices tend to have dull tips over time, and multiple passes are necessary.
  - Suture: Multiple #1 permanent monofilament sutures (e.g., Prolene) with needles cut off.
  - Hemostats
  - Laparoscopic grasper (e.g., Maryland dissector)
- *Shoelacing Technique*: (Fig. 22.2)
- An external vertical line is drawn on the skin through the central portion of the defect(s). Using spinal needles, the superior and inferior edges are identified and marked. Sites for figure-of-eight sutures are marked approximately every 3 cm on the vertical line.
- Prepare each #1 Prolene suture by cutting the needle off, placing a hemostat on one end to prevent pull-through, and grasping the other end with the suture passer.
- Starting at one end, a stab incision is made with the #11 blade. Under direct visualization, using the suture passer, the first #1 Prolene suture is passed through the stab incision centrally, then advanced through one fascial edge approximately 1 cm from the edge.

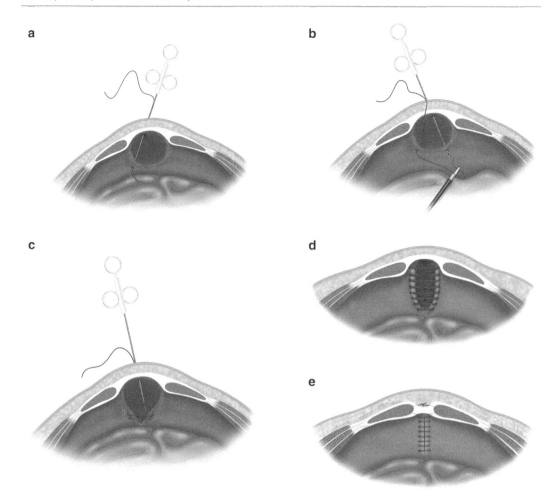

Fig. 22.2 Shoelace closure technique (Please see text for details regarding steps)

A Maryland dissector is used to grasp the suture from the suture passer.

- Using the same stab incision, advance the suture passer through the contralateral fascial edge, passing the suture from the Maryland dissector to the suture passer. Withdraw it externally leaving the suture within the suture passer so that it is ready for the next pass.
- Again, using the same stab incision, advance the suture passer with suture into the ipsilateral fascial edge, advancing approximately 1 cm along the midline. After passing the suture to the Maryland dissector, replace the suture passer in the contralateral fascia, grasping the suture and withdrawing it externally. Grasp both ends of the suture with the pre-

placed hemostat, thus completing placement of one figure-of-eight suture. Sutures will be tied after all have been placed.

Tip: Instead of advancing the suture passer/ suture through the skin and fascia in one motion, advance it in two steps. Initially, pass the suture passer/suture through the skin centrally vertically through the hernia sac, down in the abdominal cavity without incorporating any fascia. Then, back the suture passer tip up into the hernia cavity before entering the fascial edge. This helps limit oblique passing of the suture through the sack and puckering the skin.

- Continue placing additional figure-of-eight sutures along the length of the pre-marked line every 3 cm in an identical manner. Take care to avoid locking subsequent sutures on previously placed figure-of-eights. Gentle outward traction of previously placed sutures may help by reducing excess suture within the hernia cavity.

– Hernia defect closure proceeds after placement of all figure-of-eight sutures. In order to facilitate defect closure, ensure the patient has received adequate paralysis prior to tying sutures down. To reduce tension on the central aspect, knots are tied sequentially, starting at the superior and inferior ends and advancing centrally. Knots are buried in the subcutaneous tissue; after cutting the suture tails, the skin/dermis is released with the tip of a hemostat or with tooth graspers to prevent dermal and skin puckering (see Fig. 22.3).

Tip: Pneumoperitoneum should be released to reduce tension on the abdominal wall and facilitate closure. However, bowel or omentum can entrap itself within your closure, causing visceral injury. One method of preventing this is to maintain a very low pneumoperitoneum (e.g., 3–5 mmHg), and tie each knot down under direct laparoscopic visualization.

• *Mesh Placement*: Defect closure allows placement of smaller meshes, though at least a 5 cm overlap is still recommended. For mesh insertion, the 12- or 15-mm trocar should be placed close to midline without disrupting the closed defect. The central location allows adequate mesh overlap of the large trocar site, thus preventing trocar site herniation. Using the suture passer, the site is closed in a simple or figure-of-eight fashion with #1 resorbable monofilament suture (PDS or Maxon). This can be tied down at this time. Initially, the mesh is fixated to the abdominal wall using standard LVHR technique with tacks and trans-abdominal sutures as discussed in Chapter 21.

• *Buttressing Sutures*: To relieve tension on the newly reapproximated midline, additional buttressing sutures are placed alongside the shoelace closure. Using permanent monofilament sutures (#1 Prolene), full-thickness trans-abdominal (including mesh) simple U-stitches are placed every 4–5 cm bilaterally, approximately 1–2 cm lateral to the midline (Fig. 22.4) Use caution when tying these sutures down–they should be snug but not so tight as to buckle the mesh. Figure 22.5 demonstrates the completed closure and placement of all sutures with mesh in situ.

– *Tip*: Passing both the suture passer with the suture in its grasping tip can create a wider hole in the mesh than if the suture passer was

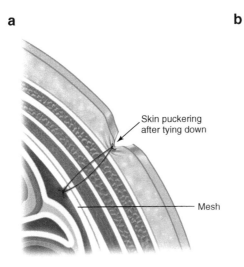
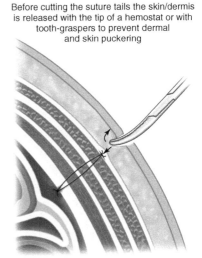

Skin puckering after tying down

Mesh

Before cutting the suture tails the skin/dermis is released with the tip of a hemostat or with tooth-graspers to prevent dermal and skin puckering

Fig. 22.3 Skin puckering and release of a dimple

Fig. 22.4 Buttressing sutures (Please see text for details regarding steps)

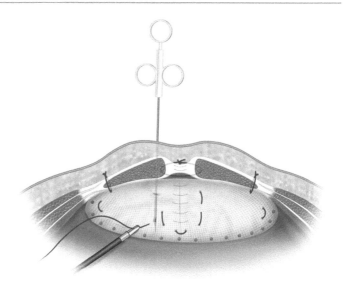

not grasping suture. Therefore, the suture is initially placed intracorporeally through an accessory trocar with a laparoscopic grasper, then passed to the empty suture passer below the mesh and pulled from the inside out. The empty suture passer is then passed through same skin incision and through the mesh 1–2 cm away from the previous pass, grasping the second end of the stitch to pull out.

- *Case Completion and Analgesia*:
  - No drains are used.
  - All stab incision sites are closed with a topical adhesive.
  - Trocar sites are closed with absorbable subcuticular or deep dermal suture.
  - We infuse local anesthetic at all trans-abdominal suture sites, including the shoelace closure. If available, 72-hour long-acting liposomal bupivacaine (EXPAREL, Pacira Pharmaceuticals, Parsippany, NJ, USA) is a useful adjunct for pain control. One vial of this long-active local analgesic can be diluted, allowing wide infusion at all trans-abdominal suture sites.

- *Other Techniques for Defect Closure*: Common themes of current literature describing defect closure favor the use of permanent suture for closure of the hernia defects as well as placement of multiple interrupted sutures.

Additionally, most studies demonstrate extra-corporeal suture placement using percutaneous suture-passer devices. However, other techniques have been described with similar rates of success. Instead of percutaneous interrupted closure, Palanivelu et al. describe closure by running a monofilament nylon suture intracorporeally [25]. Zeichen et al. closed defects in three ways using braided polyester: percutaneously with a suture passer, intracorporeally using standard laparoscopic needle drivers as well as intracorporeally using an EndoStitch device (Covidien, Dublin, Ireland) [23]. In two papers, Agarwal et al. described their unique "double-breasted" defect closure using two spinal needles as suture passers to force the medial edges of fascia and rectus muscles to overlap, with no recurrences reported at a mean of 34 and 58 months [13, 26].

Drawbacks

Any technique that is novel or without randomized trials has its potential shortcomings, and not every patient is a candidate for laparoscopic defect closure. First, defect closure can result in significant fascial tension. While trans-abdominal

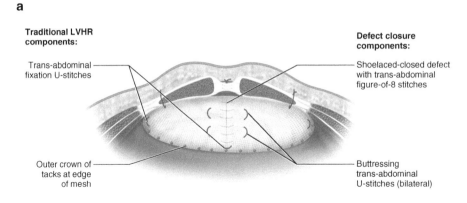

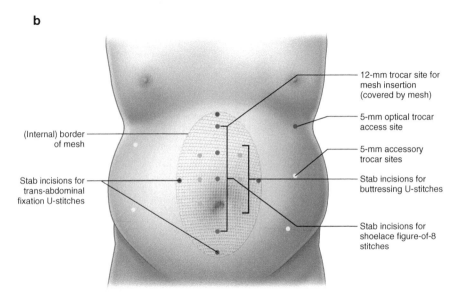

Fig. 22.5 Defect closure completion. (a) *Intracorporeal*—Internal view following completion, demonstrating traditional LVHR and shoelace compo-nents of repair. (b) *Extracorporeal*—External view of tro-car sites and multiple stab incisions for suture and mesh placement.

buttressing sutures are placed to offload tension onto the mesh, closure of large defects or abdomi-nal walls without significant laxity may result in excessive tension. This fascial strain may result in fascial dehiscence and possible hernia recurrence if insufficient mesh overlap exists. Also, because of the increased need for permanent trans-abdom-inal sutures, there lies a greater risk for suture granuloma formation and possible suture abscess. It is, therefore, important to ensure all sutures are tied down appropriately and buried deeply within the subcutaneous tissue to reduce abscesses.

Cosmetically, initial postoperative wounds may display signs of bunched up tissue over the repair. As discussed above, while this typically flattens out over time, it should be noted cosmetic benefits might not be apparent for weeks to months fol-lowing repair. Intraoperatively, there is an increased risk of bowel injury as viscera can become entrapped within the hernia sac and sutures. Astute attention is required to reduce vis-ceral entrapment. One of the possible strategies is to tie the knots down under direct visualization using low insufflation pressures. Finally, defect closure can result in significant postoperative pain as a result of fascial tightening as well as additional trans-abdominal sutures. Therefore, adequate multimodal analgesia is an essential part of postoperative management. Except for small defects, we routinely admit patients for at least 1 night to ensure adequate pulmonary function and adequate pain control prior to discharge.

Summary

Laparoscopic ventral hernia repair with shoelace defect closure offers a more functional and dynamic repair, akin to open ventral hernia repairs, while preserving the benefits of minimally invasive surgery. Compared to traditional "bridged" laparoscopic repairs, defect closure allows the use of somewhat smaller mesh prosthetics; it obliterates the dead space resulting in fewer seromas with less bulging, and early data demonstrate reduced recurrences. However, not every ventral hernia is destined for laparoscopic repair with defect closure. Hernias in the immediate subxiphoid location may be difficult to close during LVHR. Furthermore, complex defects that are large, made of multiple Swiss cheese-like defects with poor tissue integrity should be considered for open repair. While prospective randomized trials are necessary to truly demonstrate long-term durability and clinical advantages, defect closure may be the next logical step in producing beneficial outcomes for our patients undergoing laparoscopic ventral hernia repair.

References

1. Poulose BK, Shelton J, Phillips S, Moore D, Nealon W, Penson D, Beck W, Holzman MD. Epidemiology and cost of ventral hernia repair: making the case for hernia research. Hernia. 2012;16:179–83.
2. Heniford BT, Park A, Ramshaw BJ, Voeller G. Laparoscopic repair of ventral hernias: nine years' experience with 850 consecutive hernias. Ann Surg. 2003;238:391–9. discussion 399–400.
3. Itani KM, Hur K, Kim LT, Anthony T, Berger DH, Reda D, Neumayer L. Comparison of laparoscopic and open repair with mesh for the treatment of ventral incisional hernia: a randomized trial. Arch Surg. 2010;145:322–8. discussion 328.
4. Sauerland S, Walgenbach M, Habermalz B, Seiler CM, Miserez M (2011) Laparoscopic versus open surgical techniques for ventral or incisional hernia repair. Cochrane Database Syst Rev:CD007781
5. Salvilla SA, Thusu S, Panesar SS. Analysing the benefits of laparoscopic hernia repair compared to open repair: a meta-analysis of observational studies. J Minim Access Surg. 2012;8:111–7.
6. Zhang Y, Zhou H, Chai Y, Cao C, Jin K, Hu Z. Laparoscopic versus open incisional and ventral hernia repair: a systematic review and meta-analysis. World J Surg. 2014;38:2233–40.
7. Giancoli DC. Physics : principles with applications. 4th ed. Englewood Cliffs, N.J.: Prentice Hall; 1995.
8. Sabiston DC, Townsend CM. Sabiston textbook of surgery : the biological basis of modern surgical practice. 18th ed. Philadelphia: Saunders/Elsevier; 2008.
9. Brown CN, Finch JG. Which mesh for hernia repair? Ann R Coll Surg Engl. 2010;92:272–8.
10. Srivastava A, Sood A, Joy PS, Mandal S, Panwar R, Ravichandran S, Sarangi S, Woodcock J. Principles of physics in surgery: the laws of mechanics and vectors physics for surgeons-part 2. Indian J Surg. 2010;72:355–61.
11. Breuing K, Butler CE, Ferzoco S, Franz M, Hultman CS, Kilbridge JF, Rosen M, Silverman RP, Vargo D. Incisional ventral hernias: review of the literature and recommendations regarding the grading and technique of repair. Surgery. 2010;148:544–58.
12. Novitsky YW, Elliott HL, Orenstein SB, Rosen MJ. Transversus abdominis muscle release: a novel approach to posterior component separation during complex abdominal wall reconstruction. Am J Surg. 2012;204:709–16.
13. Agarwal BB, Agarwal S, Gupta MK, Mishra A, Mahajan KC. Laparoscopic ventral hernia meshplasty with "double-breasted" fascial closure of hernial defect: a new technique. J Laparoendosc Adv Surg Tech A. 2008;18:222–9.
14. Luijendijk RW, Hop WC, van den Tol MP, de Lange DC, Braaksma MM, JN IJ, Boelhouwer RU, de Vries BC, Salu MK, Wereldsma JC, Bruijninckx CM, Jeekel J. A comparison of suture repair with mesh repair for incisional hernia. N Engl J Med. 2000;343:392–8.
15. Burger JW, Luijendijk RW, Hop WC, Halm JA, Verdaasdonk EG, Jeekel J. Long-term follow-up of a randomized controlled trial of suture versus mesh repair of incisional hernia. Ann Surg. 2004;240:578–83. discussion 583–575.
16. Sauerland S, Schmedt CG, Lein S, Leibl BJ, Bittner R. Primary incisional hernia repair with or without polypropylene mesh: a report on 384 patients with 5-year follow-up. Langenbecks Arch Surg. 2005;390:408–12.
17. Lomanto D, Iyer SG, Shabbir A, Cheah WK. Laparoscopic versus open ventral hernia mesh repair: a prospective study. Surg Endosc. 2006;20:1030–5.
18. Rosen MJ, Jin J, McGee MF, Williams C, Marks J, Ponsky JL. Laparoscopic component separation in the

single-stage treatment of infected abdominal wall prosthetic removal. Hernia. 2007;11:435–40.

19. Orenstein SB, Dumeer JL, Monteagudo J, Poi MJ, Novitsky YW. Outcomes of laparoscopic ventral hernia repair with routine defect closure using "shoelacing" technique. Surg Endosc. 2011;25:1452–7.

20. Nguyen DH, Nguyen MT, Askenasy EP, Kao LS, Liang MK. Primary fascial closure with laparoscopic ventral hernia repair: systematic review. World J Surg. 2014;38:3097–104.

21. Banerjee A, Beck C, Narula VK, Linn J, Noria S, Zagol B, Mikami DJ. Laparoscopic ventral hernia repair: does primary repair in addition to placement of mesh decrease recurrence? Surg Endosc. 2012;26:1264–8.

22. Clapp ML, Hicks SC, Awad SS, Liang MK. Transcutaneous Closure of Central Defects (TCCD) in laparoscopic ventral hernia repairs (LVHR). World J Surg. 2013;37:42–51.

23. Zeichen MS, Lujan HJ, Mata WN, Maciel VH, Lee D, Jorge I, Plasencia G, Gomez E, Hernandez AM. Closure versus non-closure of hernia defect during laparoscopic ventral hernia repair with mesh. Hernia. 2013;17:589–96.

24. Turner PL, Park AE. Laparoscopic repair of ventral incisional hernias: pros and cons. Surg Clin North Am. 2008;88:85–100. viii.

25. Palanivelu C, Jani KV, Senthilnathan P, Parthasarathi R, Madhankumar MV, Malladi VK. Laparoscopic sutured closure with mesh reinforcement of incisional hernias. Hernia. 2007;11:223–8.

26. Agarwal BB, Agarwal S, Mahajan KC. Laparoscopic ventral hernia repair: innovative anatomical closure, mesh insertion without 10-mm transmyofascial port, and atraumatic mesh fixation: a preliminary experience of a new technique. Surg Endosc. 2009;23:900–5.

Laparoscopic Parastomal Hernia Repair

23

Erin M. Garvey and Kristi L. Harold

Overview

Stoma creation is necessary for a number of elective and emergent gastrointestinal and urological procedures. Unfortunately, parastomal hernia (PH) can be a ubiquitous complication which poses a great challenge for general, colorectal, and urological surgeons.

Definition and Classification

PH is often defined as a protrusion in proximity to a stoma or the abnormal protrusion of abdominal cavity contents through the abdominal wall defect resulting from colostomy, ileostomy, or ileal conduit creation [1, 2]. There are a number of PH classification systems based on clinical, radiographic, or intraoperative criteria; however, no classification system is universally agreed upon [3–6].

Electronic supplementary material: The online version of this chapter (doi:10.1007/978-3-319-27470-6_23) contains supplementary material, which is available to authorized users.

E.M. Garvey, M.D. • K.L. Harold, M.D. (✉)
Division of General Surgery, Mayo Clinic Arizona,
5779 E Mayo Boulevard, MCSB SP 3-522 Gen Surg,
Phoenix, AZ 85054, USA
e-mail: Garvey.erin@mayo.edu;
Harold.kristi@mayo.edu

Risk Factors

A number of risk factors for PH development relating to patient, disease, and surgical factors have been proposed. Female gender is associated with a greater risk of PH [7, 8]. Increasing patient age, defined in some studies as age >60 years, is also a risk factor [7–12]. Body mass index (BMI) is a controversial risk factor as studies have shown a higher rate of PH in patients with a waist circumference >100 cm and a doubling in the rate of PH when comparing patients with a BMI ≥30 versus <30, while another study showed no significant risk when comparing PH development with waist circumference or BMI [8, 13, 14]. Other comorbidities including chronic obstructive pulmonary disease, hypertension, and ascites have been shown to be independent risk factors for PH development [7, 15]. Risk factors for surgical site infection or wound dehiscence in general, specifically smoking, diabetes mellitus, cardiovascular or pulmonary comorbidities, amount of blood loss, and type of surgery performed, should also be kept in mind [16]. Patients with inflammatory bowel disease commonly undergo stoma creation procedures, and those patients with Crohn's disease have a higher rate of PH formation compared to those patients with ulcerative colitis [17]. The type of stoma created also has an impact on the rate of PH development with the highest rates occurring after colostomy creation and the lowest rates occurring after loop ileostomy creation [18, 19].

Incidence

The incidence of PH can vary greatly (0–80%) based on the definition used, diagnostic technique, and surgical approach at the time of stoma creation [20–22]. The incidence of PH for end and loop colostomies is as high as 48% and 38%, respectively, while the rates of PH are notably lower for end and loop ileostomies at 1.8–28.3% and 0–6.2%, respectively [18].

Diagnosis

PH diagnosis is often made by a history and physical exam with various imaging modalities serving as an adjunct to clinical diagnosis. The median time between formation of the stoma and detection of PH was 44 months in one study while others believe that most PHs develop within the first 2 years of stoma creation [5, 23]. A review of the French federation of ostomy patients determined 76% of patients with PH were symptomatic citing pain, difficulty with appliance fit, and leakage [12]. In another series, 85% of patients with a clinically detectable PH were also symptomatic [5]. Physical examination may uncover a fascial defect or reveal parastomal bulging with a Valsalva maneuver [24]. Imaging can increase the rate of PH detection, however, some PH may not be detectable by CT scan [5, 8, 24, 25]. Intrastomal ultrasonography may also be utilized to evaluate for PH while magnetic resonance imaging is rarely used for this purpose [26, 27].

Complications

PH complications can range from mild abdominal discomfort to intestinal perforation requiring emergent laparotomy [24]. Repeat surgical intervention is required in approximately 30% of patients with PH often due to bleeding, poor appliance fit, obstruction, and/or strangulation [28, 29]. Less severe symptoms may be managed nonoperatively. Expert consultation with a stoma nurse, if available, can often be helpful. It is

recommended that the aperture size should be tailored to leave no more than a 2–3 mm rim around the stoma [30]. Flexible appliances can mold to uneven contours of the skin, and protective skin sealants may optimize appliance adherence [30–32]. Stoma belts may also improve appliance security and abdominal binders may help to relieve abdominal discomfort [32].

Operative Management

Laparoscopic Approach

One of the main benefits of laparoscopy is limiting the potential sites for new hernia formation. Similar to the open intraperitoneal repairs, the modified Sugarbaker and keyhole techniques are utilized in addition to the sandwich technique which is a combination of the two approaches. For the sandwich technique, one piece of mesh is placed in a keyhole configuration while a second piece of mesh covers the first piece and the remaining abdominal wall [33]. A 2012 review of laparoscopic PH repairs demonstrated a 2.7% mesh infection rate, 3.6% rate of conversion to open, 4.1% iatrogenic bowel injury, and an overall morbidity of 17.2% [34]. The recurrence rate was significantly lower in the Sugarbaker technique at 11.6% versus 34.6% for the keyhole technique (Odds Ratio 2.3, 5% CI 1.2–4.6, $p=0.016$) [34]. The recurrence rate for the sandwich technique was 2.1% but this was based solely on one series of 47 patients [34]. Table 23.1 details the outcomes of laparoscopic parastomal hernia repairs for studies with greater than 15 patients.

Our Approach

Operative Technique

It is our preference to perform the laparoscopic modified Sugarbaker technique for PH and recurrent PH repairs. A first generation cephalosporin is given within 1 hour of the incision. Laparoscopic monitors and surgeon position

Table 23.1 Outcomes of laparoscopic parastomal hernia repairs from studies with greater than 15 patients

Study	Technique and mesh	No. of repairs	Conversion (%)	Recurrence (%)	Complications excluding recurrence (%)	Infection (%)	Median follow-Up (range)
Berger and Bientzle (2007) [33]	Sugarbaker/Sandwich ePTFE and Polyvinylidene fluoride	66	1.5	12	10.6	4.5	24 (3–72)
Mancini et al. (2007) [52]	Sugarbaker ePTFE	25	0	4	12	8	19 (2–38)
McLemore et al. (2007) [53]	Sugarbaker/Keyhole ePTFE	19	–	10.5	63	11	20[a]
Craft et al. (2008) [54]	Sugarbaker/Keyhole ePTFE	21 (incl. 9 IC)	0	4.8	48	14	14 (1–36)
Berger and Bientzle (2009) [55]	Sandwich Polyvinylidene fluoride	47 (+297 IH)	0	2	–	1.2% (for entire 344 pt cohort)	20
Hansson et al. (2007, 2009) [56, 57]	Keyhole ePTFE	54	14.5	37	14.4	3.6	36 (12–72)
Liu et al. (2011) [58]	CK parastomal patch	24	25	4.2	33	0	27[a] (6–39)
Wara and Andersen (2011) [59]	Keyhole Polypropylene and PTFE	72	4	3	22	4.2	36 (6–132)
Mizrahi et al. (2012) [60]	Keyhole Bard CK parastomal hernia patch Polypropylene and ePTFE	29 (incl. 1 IC)	6.9	46.4	17.2	3.4	30 (12–53)

[a]Studies reporting mean follow-up

ePTFE expanded polytetrafluoroethylene, *incl.* including, *IC* ileal conduit, *IH* incisional hernia, *pts* patients are shown in Fig. 23.1. After induction of general anesthesia, the patient is placed in the supine position with both arms tucked. A Foley catheter is placed into the bladder, if the operation is expected to take longer than 1 hour. An additional Foley catheter (16 French) is placed directly into the ostomy and 10 mL of sterile water is placed in the Foley balloon (Fig. 23.2a). This allows for easy identification of the loop of intestine terminating in the stoma which can be helpful in the case of dense adhesions. The abdomen, stoma, and additional Foley catheter are prepped and then covered by an Ioban drape (3M Company, St. Paul, MN) (Fig. 23.2b). The peritoneal cavity is accessed with a Veress needle placed subcostally in the left upper quadrant in the midclavicu-

lar line. Once adequate pneumoperitoneum is obtained (15 mmHg of carbon dioxide), a 5 mm Optiview port is used to enter the peritoneal cavity laterally, on the side opposite to the stoma. Two additional 5 mm trocars are placed in the lateral position near the Optiview port (Fig. 23.3). External manipulation of the Foley catheter in the ostomy can help to identify the correct loop of bowel ending in the ostomy and can guide lysis of adhesions accordingly (Fig. 23.4). Once adhesiolysis is complete, the hernia contents, with the exception of the stoma, are reduced. The entire abdominal wall and the hernia defect, including any coexisting ventral or incisional hernia defects, can then be visualized and measured. Four spinal needles are used to mark the extent of

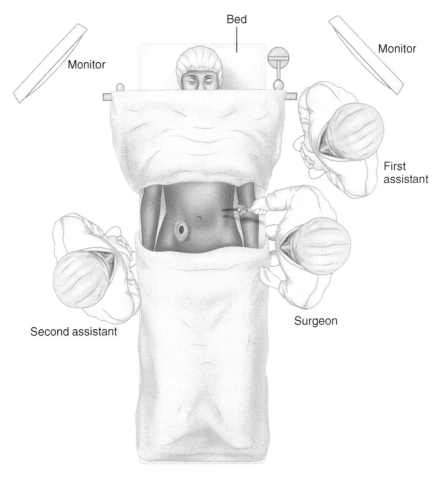

Fig. 23.1 Laparoscopic monitors are positioned on either side of the patient. The surgeon (S) and the first assistant (FA) stand on the side opposite the stoma and the second assistant (SA) stands on the side of the stoma. The camera is placed in the most cephalad lateral port and is driven by the FA

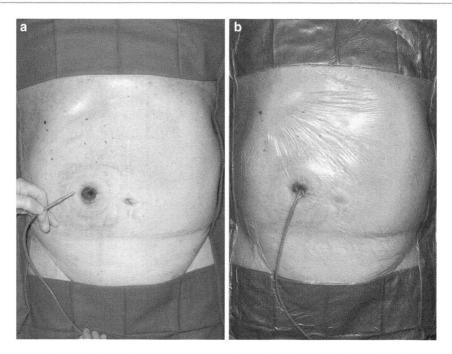

Fig. 23.2 A 16 French foley is placed into the stoma so as to help with lysis of adhesions (**a**). The abdomen is prepped with an Ioban drape (**b**)

Fig. 23.3 Trocar placement consists of three 5 mm trocars placed laterally on the side opposite of the stoma. Later, a fourth 5 mm port will be placed on the ipsilateral side of the stoma

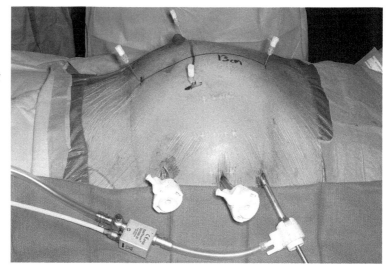

the defect at the superior, inferior, and lateral-most aspects. A laparoscopic ruler is then inserted to measure the extent of the defect from the superior to inferior spinal needles for length and between lateral spinal needles for width (Fig. 23.5a). The defect is also measured and marked on the patient's abdominal skin to assist with cen-tering the prosthesis later in the procedure (Fig. 23.5b). The size of mesh is selected based on the defect measurements and allowing for a 5 cm overlap beyond all fascial edges. The mesh is then trimmed to the appropriate size. It is our preference to utilize ePTFE (Gore DUAL-MESH; W.L. Gore, Flagstaff, AZ). The textured

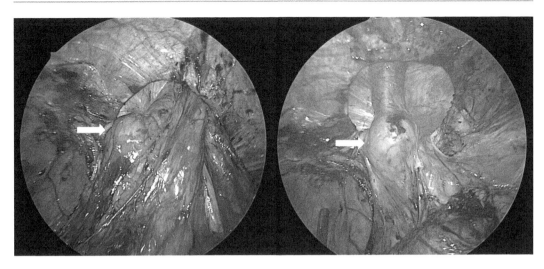

Fig. 23.4 External manipulation of the intrastomal foley catheter helps to identify the loop of bowel terminating in the stoma and facilitates lysis of adhesions (*white arrow* marks the intrastomal foley balloon)

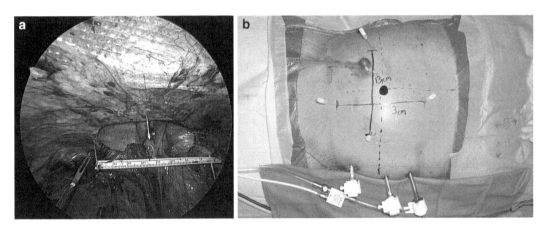

Fig. 23.5 Spinal needles are used to demarcate the superior, inferior, and lateral borders of the hernia defect. A laparoscopic ruler is used to measure the defect (**a**). Mesh size is selected based on the internal measurement allowing for an overlap of 5 cm in all directions. The defect is also measured externally with the center of the defect marked (*black circle*) so as to allow for centering of the mesh by placing sutures on the *dashed lines* for the superior, inferior, and contralateral side to the stoma (**b**)

surface of the mesh is marked to identify the superior and inferior portions of the mesh. A single Gore-Tex transfascial suture (CV-0) is placed at the edge of the mesh on three of the four sides that are not associated with the stoma. Two Gore-Tex transfascial sutures are placed on the fourth side on either side of where the stoma will lay creating a mesh flap valve. Two knots are tied at the time of each suture placement to secure each suture to the mesh. A 5 mm trocar is then placed in the lateral abdomen on the ipsilateral side of

the stoma. A 12 mm trocar is placed through the hernia defect where it will later be covered by the mesh repair to minimize the risk of trocar site hernia. The Gore-Tex suture tails are arranged in the middle of the mesh, and the two marked edges of the mesh (superior and inferior) are rolled tightly toward one another. A grasper is placed through the ipsilateral trocar and is brought out through the 12 mm trocar to grasp the rolled mesh helping to guide it into the abdomen (Fig. 23.6a). The 12 mm trocar may need to

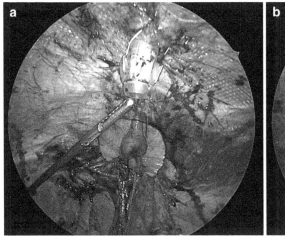
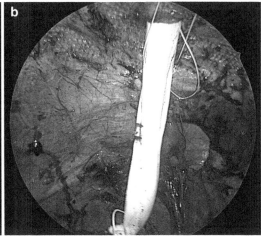

Fig. 23.6 A locking grasper is inserted through a 12 mm port placed through the fascial defect to grasp the rolled mesh and guide it into the abdomen (**a**). The 12 mm port may need to be removed to allow for mesh entry pending size of the mesh (**b**)

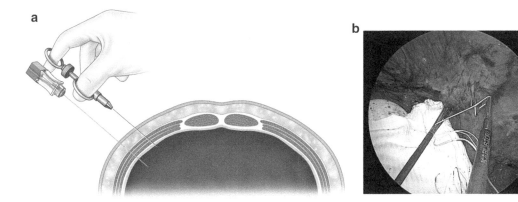

Fig. 23.7 A transfascial suture device is inserted into the abdomen (through the *dotted line* shown in Fig. 23.5b) following the angle of the spinal needle to retrieve the tails of the Gore-Tex suture (**a**). A grasper is used to identify and hand the correct tail to the suture passer, one at a time (**b**)

be removed if the mesh size prohibits its passage through the trocar (Fig. 23.6b). The mesh is unrolled utilizing two graspers and oriented according to the earlier markings. The open jaws of an atraumatic bowel grasper are used to measure a 5 cm overlap from the edge of each of the fascial defects and these areas are marked with new spinal needles. Following the direction of the spinal needle, a suture passer is used to pass the transfascial sutures through the sites marked by the spinal needles while being careful to avoid the stoma as it traverses the edge of the mesh

(Fig. 23.7). The mesh flap valve is crafted such that the stoma crosses the lateral or inferior edge. The transfascial sutures are secured with hemostats rather than tied until the most ideal mesh coverage and placement has been achieved. A laparoscopic tacker is used to secure the mesh in place circumferentially with the exception of the area around the stoma (Fig. 23.8a). Additional Gore-Tex transfascial sutures are placed with a suture passer every 4 to 5 cm around the mesh (Fig. 23.8b). The transfascial sutures are tied with ten knots in the subcutaneous tissues and the

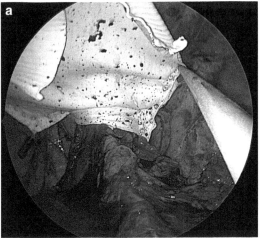

Fig. 23.8 Once all sutures are tied after achieving ideal mesh placement, a laparoscopic tacker is used to circumferentially secure the mesh, with the exception of around the stoma (**a**). The secured mesh creates a flap valve allowing the stoma to pass through the lateral edge (**b**)

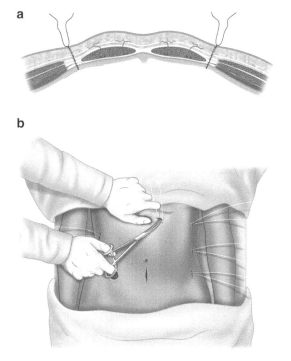

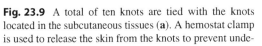

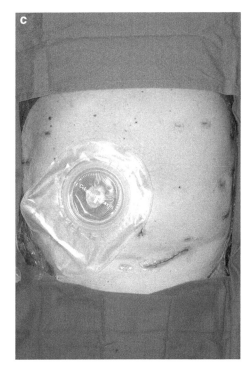

Fig. 23.9 A total of ten knots are tied with the knots located in the subcutaneous tissues (**a**). A hemostat clamp is used to release the skin from the knots to prevent unde-sirable skin puckering at the incision sites (**b**). The skin is closed with suture and adhesive bandage. This patient also had an open left inguinal hernia repair (**c**)

skin is freed from the knot with a hemostat so as to prevent dimpling (Fig. 23.9a). The trocar sites are closed with 4-0 monocryl suture and the stab incisions from the suture passer are closed with skin adhesive (Fig. 23.9b).

Recurrent Parastomal Hernia

Data on recurrent PH is limited, and repair of recurrent PH presents the same challenges as initial PH repair. Failure of primary fascial repair is reported as high as 100% [3]. Stoma relocations fair only slightly better with a failure rate of 71% [3]. Prosthetic mesh repair failure has a lower recurrence rate of 33%, however, in Sugarbaker's original description, six of his seven patients had recurrent PHs and he reported 100% success rate [3, 35]. It is our preference to approach recurrent PH the same as for initial PH with a laparoscopic modified Sugarbaker technique as described above.

Current Trends

Parastomal Hernia Prevention

Although not a new concept, the prevention of PH with prophylactic mesh has been the focus of recent and ongoing research. The idea was first introduced by Bayer et al. in 1986 who reported no PH over a four-year follow-up period in 43 patients who had Marlex mesh (Phillips Petroleum Company, Bartlesville, OK) placed at the time of colostomy creation [36]. Following Bayer's initial success, there have since been many observational studies evaluating the efficacy and safety of prophylactic mesh placement. Figel et al. demonstrated no mesh complications or PH recurrences in 16 patients who underwent placement of a bioprosthetic mesh with a median 38-month follow-up [37]. Gogenur et al. demonstrated no infectious complications, an 8% rate of minor complications, and an 8% rate of PH recurrence in 25 patients who had an onlay of polypropylene mesh with a median follow-up of 12 months [38]. A small series of intraperitoneal onlay of polyvinylidene mesh during laparoscopic abdomino-perineal resection (APR) showed no mesh-related complications, infections, or PH recurrence at a mean follow-up of 6 months [39]. A study by Nagy et al. evaluated the polypropylene hernia system large device in 14 cases after APR with sigmoid colostomy and noted no PH recurrence in the first postoperative year [40]. Marimuthu et al. studied a polypropylene monofilament mesh with a circle cut in it for the stoma placed in the preperitoneal space without stitches in 18 patients and found no PH at a

mean follow-up of 16 months. One patient did require revision for stoma necrosis on postoperative day 1 and subsequently developed a wound infection, but no other complications were noted [41]. A prospective study of preperitoneal polypropylene mesh placed in 42 patients with a mean follow-up of 31 months demonstrated an incidence of 10% for PH [42]. Cost-effectiveness of mesh prophylaxis has also been studied by Lee et al. They looked at mesh prophylaxis in 60 year olds who underwent APR with end colostomy for rectal cancer and found mesh prophylaxis to be less costly and more effective compared to no mesh for those patients with stage I-III rectal cancers [43]. Another RCT found significantly decreased presence of radiological PH in patients who had a lightweight intraperitoneal/onlay mesh placed for laparoscopic APR compared to those without mesh (50% versus 94%, $p = 0.008$) [44].

The three RCTs by Hammond, Janes, and Serra-Aracil are the most cited papers on the topic of PH prevention. In 2008, Hammond et al. published a RCT of 20 patients undergoing defunctioning stomas with a porcine-derived collagen implant placed in the sublay position in 10 patients. With a median follow up of 6.5 months, there were no complications and there were no PHs in the mesh group compared to 30% in the non-mesh group [45]. Janes et al. evaluated 54 patients undergoing permanent colostomy creation (27 patients with a conventional stoma and 27 with placement of a sublay large-pore lightweight polypropylene and polyglactin mesh). They found a lower rate of PH in the mesh group compared to the non-mesh group at 12-month follow-up (4.8% vs 50%). There were no infectious complications [46]. A five-year follow-up study again revealed a lower rate of PH in the mesh group 13.3% versus 81%): ($p < 0.001$) [22]. The RCT by Serra-Aracil evaluated 54 patients undergoing end colostomy for distal rectal cancer and utilized a sublay lightweight mesh in 27 patients. At a median 29-month follow-up, there were fewer PHs in the mesh group 14.8% (4/27) compared to 40.7% (11/27) in the non-mesh group ($p = 0.03$). Importantly, the morbidity between the two groups was similar [47]. In

2012, Sajid et al. and Shabbir et al. performed systematic reviews of the RCT literature. Sajid et al. analyzed the three RCTs by Janes, Hammond, and Serra-Aracil encompassing 128 patients who underwent colorectal resections with stoma creation (64 patients in the mesh group versus 64 patients in the non-mesh group), and found significantly decreased odds for developing a PH with the use of mesh without added morbidity [48]. Shabbir et al. reviewed 27 RCTs and excluded all but the same three RCTs as the Sajid paper. This review demonstrated an incidence of PH in 13% in the mesh group compared to 53% in the control group ($p<0.0001$). There were no differences in mesh-related complications between the two groups [49]. A similar systematic review that included the same three RCTs, but also three prospective observational studies and one retrospective study, found a lower rate of PH in the mesh group [50]. All three systematic reviews concluded the use of prophylactic mesh at the time of stoma creation can reduce the incidence of PH. In contrast, a recently published prospective multicenter randomized controlled trial examined the utility of porcine-derived acellular dermal matrix reinforcement at the time of end-stoma creation in 55 patients compared to 58 control patients without mesh reinforcement. They found a similar incidence of PH for both groups at 12.2% for the mesh group and 13.2% for the control group [51]. The ideal technique including mesh selection and operative approach for PH prevention remains to be determined.

Conclusion

Parastomal hernias commonly develop after stoma creation, and the sequelae can range from mild to severe necessitating repeat operative intervention. Open and laparoscopic repairs with mesh are preferable to non-mesh repairs. For the open approach, a sublay or intraperitoneal placement of mesh is favored, and for the laparoscopic approach, the Sugarbaker technique has been shown to have a lower recurrence rate. It is our preference to perform a laparoscopic modified Sugarbaker technique. The use of prophylactic prosthetic mesh decreases the rate of PH development and is not associated with increased infectious complications.

References

1. Janes A, Cengiz Y, Israelsson LA. Randomized clinical trial of the use of a prosthetic mesh to prevent parastomal hernia. Br J Surg. 2004;91(3):280–2.
2. Smietanski M, Szczepkowski M, Alexandre JA, Berger D, Bury K, Conze J, et al. European Hernia Society classification of parastomal hernias. Hernia. 2013;18(1):1–6.
3. Rubin MS, Schoetz Jr DJ, Matthews JB. Parastomal hernia. Is stoma relocation superior to fascial repair? Arch Surg. 1994;129(4):413–8. discussion 8–9.
4. Devlin HB, Kingsnorth AN. Management of abdominal hernias. London: Hodder Arnold; 1998.
5. Moreno-Matias J, Serra-Aracil X, Darnell-Martin A, Bombardo-Junca J, Mora-Lopez L, Alcantara-Moral M, et al. The prevalence of parastomal hernia after formation of an end colostomy. A new clinico-radiological classification. Colorectal Dis. 2009;11(2):173–7.
6. Gil G, Owski MS. A new classification of parastomal hernias—from the experience at Bielanski Hospital in Warsaw. Pol Przegl Chir. 2011;83(8):430–7.
7. Sohn YJ, Moon SM, Shin US, Jee SH. Incidence and risk factors of parastomal hernia. J Kor Soc Coloproctol. 2012;28(5):241–6.
8. Hong SY, Oh SY, Lee JH, Kim do Y, Suh KW. Risk factors for parastomal hernia: based on radiological definition. J Korean Surg Soc. 2013;84(1):43–7.
9. Leong AP, Londono-Schimmer EE, Phillips RK. Life-table analysis of stomal complications following ileostomy. Br J Surg. 1994;81(5):727–9.
10. Londono-Schimmer EE, Leong AP, Phillips RK. Life table analysis of stomal complications following colostomy. Dis Colon Rectum. 1994;37(9):916–20.
11. Pilgrim CH, McIntyre R, Bailey M. Prospective audit of parastomal hernia: prevalence and associated comorbidities. Dis Colon Rectum. 2010;53(1):71–6.
12. Ripoche J, Basurko C, Fabbro-Perray P, Prudhomme M. Parastomal hernia. A study of the French federation of ostomy patients. J Visc Surg. 2011;148(6):e435–41.
13. Schreinemacher MH, Vijgen GH, Dagnelie PC, Bloemen JG, Huizinga BF, Bouvy ND. Incisional hernias in temporary stoma wounds: a cohort study. Arch Surg. 2011;146(1):94–9.
14. De Raet J, Delvaux G, Haentjens P, Van Nieuwenhove Y. Waist circumference is an independent risk factor for the development of parastomal hernia after permanent colostomy. Dis Colon Rectum. 2008;51(12):1806–9.
15. Carne PW, Frye JN, Robertson GM, Frizelle FA. Parastomal hernia following minimally invasive stoma formation. ANZ J Surg. 2003;73(10):843–5.

16. Sorensen LT, Hemmingsen U, Kallehave F, Wille-Jorgensen P, Kjaergaard J, Moller LN, et al. Risk factors for tissue and wound complications in gastrointestinal surgery. Ann Surg. 2005;241(4): 654–8.

17. Carlstedt A, Fasth S, Hulten L, Nordgren S, Palselius I. Long-term ileostomy complications in patients with ulcerative colitis and Crohn's disease. Int J Colorectal Dis. 1987;2(1):22–5.

18. Carne PW, Robertson GM, Frizelle FA. Parastomal hernia. Br J Surg. 2003;90(7):784–93.

19. Rullier E, Le Toux N, Laurent C, Garrelon JL, Parneix M, Saric J. Loop ileostomy versus loop colostomy for defunctioning low anastomoses during rectal cancer surgery. World J Surg. 2001;25(3):274–7. discussion 7–8.

20. Helgstrand F, Rosenberg J, Kehlet H, Jorgensen LN, Wara P, Bisgaard T. Risk of morbidity, mortality, and recurrence after parastomal hernia repair: a nationwide study. Dis Colon Rectum. 2013;56(11): 1265–72.

21. Israelsson LA. Preventing and treating parastomal hernia. World J Surg. 2005;29(8):1086–9.

22. Janes A, Cengiz Y, Israelsson LA. Preventing parastomal hernia with a prosthetic mesh: a 5-year follow-up of a randomized study. World J Surg. 2009;33(1):118–21. discussion 22–3.

23. Rieger N, Moore J, Hewett P, Lee S, Stephens J. Parastomal hernia repair. Colorectal Dis. 2004;6(3):203–5.

24. Cingi A, Cakir T, Sever A, Aktan AO. Enterostomy site hernias: a clinical and computerized tomographic evaluation. Dis Colon Rectum. 2006;49(10): 1559–63.

25. Gurmu A, Matthiessen P, Nilsson S, Pahlman L, Rutegard J, Gunnarsson U. The inter-observer reliability is very low at clinical examination of parastomal hernia. Int J Colorectal Dis. 2011;26(1):89–95.

26. Gurmu A, Gunnarsson U, Strigard K. Imaging of parastomal hernia using three-dimensional intrastomal ultrasonography. Br J Surg. 2011;98(7):1026–9.

27. Smietanski M, Bury K, Matyja A, Dziki A, Wallner G, Studniarek M, et al. Polish guidelines for treatment of patients with parastomal hernia. Pol Przegl Chir. 2013;85(3):152–80.

28. Burgess P, Matthew V, Devlin H. A review of terminal colostomy complications following abdominoperineal resection for carcinoma. Br J Surg. 1984;71:1004.

29. Burns F. Complications of colostomy. Dis Colon Rectum. 1970;13:448–50.

30. Rolstad BS, Boarini J. Principles and techniques in the use of convexity. Ostomy Wound Manage. 1996;42(1):24–6. 8–32; quiz 3–4.

31. Armstrong E. Practical aspects of stoma care. Nurs Times. 2001;97(12):40–2.

32. Kane M, McErlean D, McGrogan M, Thompson MJ, Haughey S. Clinical protocols for stoma care: 6. Management of parastomal hernia. Nurs Stand. 2004;18(19):43–4.

33. Berger D, Bientzle M. Laparoscopic repair of parastomal hernias: a single surgeon's experience in 66 patients. Dis Colon Rectum. 2007;50(10):1668–73.

34. Hansson BM, Slater NJ, van der Velden AS, Groenewoud HM, Buyne OR, de Hingh IH, et al. Surgical techniques for parastomal hernia repair: a systematic review of the literature. Ann Surg. 2012;255(4):685–95.

35. Sugarbaker PH. Peritoneal approach to prosthetic mesh repair of paraostomy hernias. Ann Surg. 1985;201(3):344–6.

36. Bayer I, Kyzer S, Chaimoff C. A new approach to primary strengthening of colostomy with Marlex mesh to prevent paracolostomy hernia. Surg Gynecol Obstet. 1986;163(6):579–80.

37. Figel NA, Rostas JW, Ellis CN. Outcomes using a bioprosthetic mesh at the time of permanent stoma creation in preventing a parastomal hernia: a value analysis. Am J Surg. 2012;203(3):323–6. discussion 6.

38. Gogenur I, Mortensen J, Harvald T, Rosenberg J, Fischer A. Prevention of parastomal hernia by placement of a polypropylene mesh at the primary operation. Dis Colon Rectum. 2006;49(8):1131–5.

39. Martinek L, Dostalik J, Gunkova P, Gunka I, Mazur M. Prevention of parastomal hernia using laparoscopic introduction of a prosthetic mesh--initial experience. Rozhl Chir. 2012;91(4):216–8.

40. Nagy A, Kovacs T, Bognar J, Mohos E, Loderer Z. Parastomal hernia repair and prevention with PHSL type mesh after abdomino-perineal rectum extirpation. Zentralbl Chir. 2004;129(2):149–52.

41. Marimuthu K, Vijayasekar C, Ghosh D, Mathew G. Prevention of parastomal hernia using preperitoneal mesh: a prospective observational study. Colorectal Dis. 2006;8(8):672–5.

42. Vijayasekar C, Marimuthu K, Jadhav V, Mathew G. Parastomal hernia: Is prevention better than cure? Use of preperitoneal polypropylene mesh at the time of stoma formation. Tech Coloproctol. 2008;12(4):309–13.

43. Lee L, Saleem A, Landry T, Latimer E, Chaudhury P, Feldman LS. Cost effectiveness of mesh prophylaxis to prevent parastomal hernia in patients undergoing permanent colostomy for rectal cancer. J Am Coll Surg. 2013;29.

44. Lopez-Cano M, Lozoya-Trujillo R, Quiroga S, Sanchez JL, Vallribera F, Marti M, et al. Use of a prosthetic mesh to prevent parastomal hernia during laparoscopic abdominoperineal resection: a randomized controlled trial. Hernia. 2012;16(6):661–7.

45. Hammond TM, Huang A, Prosser K, Frye JN, Williams NS. Parastomal hernia prevention using a novel collagen implant: a randomised controlled phase 1 study. Hernia. 2008;12(5):475–81.

46. Janes A, Cengiz Y, Israelsson LA. Preventing parastomal hernia with a prosthetic mesh. Arch Surg. 2004;139(12):1356–8.

47. Serra-Aracil X, Bombardo-Junca J, Moreno-Matias J, Darnell A, Mora-Lopez L, Alcantara-Moral M, et al.

Randomized, controlled, prospective trial of the use of a mesh to prevent parastomal hernia. Ann Surg. 2009;249(4):583–7.

48. Sajid MS, Kalra L, Hutson K, Sains P. Parastomal hernia as a consequence of colorectal cancer resections can prophylactically be controlled by mesh insertion at the time of primary surgery: a literature based systematic review of published trials. Minerva Chir. 2012;67(4):289–96.

49. Shabbir J, Chaudhary BN, Dawson R. A systematic review on the use of prophylactic mesh during primary stoma formation to prevent parastomal hernia formation. Colorectal Dis. 2012;14(8):931–6.

50. Tam KW, Wei PL, Kuo LJ, Wu CH. Systematic review of the use of a mesh to prevent parastomal hernia. World J Surg. 2010;34(11):2723–9.

51. Fleshman JW, Beck DE, Hyman N, Wexner SD, Bauer J, George V, PRISM Study Group. A prospective, multicenter, randomized, controlled study of non-cross-linked porcine acellular dermal matrix fascial sublay for parastomal reinforcement in patients undergoing surgery for permanent abdominal wall ostomies. Dis Colon Rectum. 2014;57(5):623–31.

52. Mancini GJ, McClusky 3rd DA, Khaitan L, Goldenberg EA, Heniford BT, Novitsky YW, et al. Laparoscopic parastomal hernia repair using a nonslit mesh technique. Surg Endosc. 2007;21(9):1487–91.

53. McLemore EC, Harold KL, Efron JE, Laxa BU, Young-Fadok TM, Heppell JP. Parastomal hernia: short-term outcome after laparoscopic and conventional repairs. Surg Innov. 2007;14(3):199–204.

54. Craft RO, Huguet KL, McLemore EC, Harold KL. Laparoscopic parastomal hernia repair. Hernia. 2008;12(2):137–40.

55. Berger D, Bientzle M. Polyvinylidene fluoride: a suitable mesh material for laparoscopic incisional and parastomal hernia repair! A prospective, observational study with 344 patients. Hernia. 2009;13(2):167–72.

56. Hansson BM, de Hingh IH, Bleichrodt RP. Laparoscopic parastomal hernia repair is feasible and safe: early results of a prospective clinical study including 55 consecutive patients. Surg Endosc. 2007;21(6):989–93.

57. Hansson BM, Bleichrodt RP, de Hingh IH. Laparoscopic parastomal hernia repair using a keyhole technique results in a high recurrence rate. Surg Endosc. 2009;23(7):1456–9.

58. Liu F, Li J, Wang S, Yao S, Zhu Y. Effectiveness analysis of laparoscopic repair of parastomal hernia using CK Parastomal patch. Zhongguo Xiu Fu Chong Jian Wai Ke Za Zhi. 2011;25(6):681–4.

59. Wara P, Andersen LM. Long-term follow-up of laparoscopic repair of parastomal hernia using a bilayer mesh with a slit. Surg Endosc. 2011;25(2):526–30.

60. Mizrahi H, Bhattacharya P, Parker MC. Laparoscopic slit mesh repair of parastomal hernia using a designated mesh: long-term results. Surg Endosc. 2012;26(1):267–70.

Laparoscopic Subxiphoid and Suprapubic Hernia Repair

William S. Cobb

Background

Subxiphoid defects can be congenital or incisional, usually following coronary bypass procedures or subcostal incisions for liver or foregut procedures (Fig. 24.1). Congenital epigastric defects can approach the xiphoid as well. Frequently, epigastric defects can be multiple and well suited for laparoscopy to avoid missed defects. Solitary defects can be addressed in an open fashion either with suture alone or mesh reinforcement. The incidence of subxiphoid hernias is unknown, as most authors do not routinely separate these types of defects in their reports.

Suprapubic hernias are almost always incisional in nature. Fascial defects that are within 5 cm of the symphysis pubis are considered suprapubic (Fig. 24.2). These types of hernias are more common in females due to gynecologic procedures via a lower midline or Pfannenstiel approach. Additionally, colorectal procedures and urologic procedures through a lower midline incision can result in suprapubic-type defects. The true incidence of suprapubic hernias is not

Electronic supplementary material: The online version of this chapter (doi:10.1007/978-3-319-27470-6_24) contains supplementary material, which is available to authorized users.

W.S. Cobb, M.D. (✉)
Department of Surgery, Greenville Health System, Greenville, SC, USA
e-mail: wcobb@ghs.org

well reported, as the definition varies by author. In our database of 860 laparoscopic ventral repairs, 15% required bladder mobilization and were classified as suprapubic [2].

Many times the subxiphoid or suprapubic areas are approached during a routine incisional defect that involves the midline. For incisions that course from "stem to stern," incisional hernias may result that are both subxiphoid and suprapubic. These are especially challenging when it comes to placing sutures for mesh fixation. In this chapter, I will discuss the nuances of the laparoscopic approach to subxiphoid and suprapubic hernias.

Preoperative Considerations

By definition, a subxiphoid or suprapubic hernia is one in which the extent of the fascial defect is within 5 cm of the bony prominence. Preoperative imaging of the abdomen and pelvis using computed tomography (CT) is critical to plan one's approach. On CT imaging, it is important to measure the number of "cuts" from the xiphoid down to the superior aspect, or from the symphysis up to the inferior-most point of the fascial defect. This determination is more important for suprapubic defects because preoperative knowledge will prompt the surgeon to plan for potential saline infusion of the bladder prior to draping. This technique will be described in further detail in the "Technical Considerations" section.

Apart from imaging, all other preoperative concerns mimic those of any incisional hernia

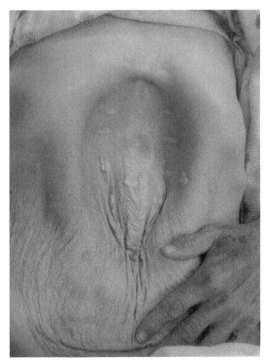

Fig. 24.1 Upper midline hernia involving a subxiphoid region

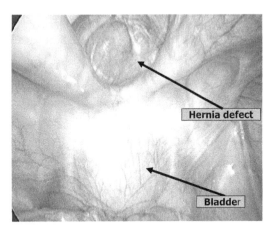

Fig. 24.2 Intra-operative view of the suprapubic hernia

patient that is being considered for a laparoscopic approach. The patient must be able to tolerate general anesthesia. Preoperative optimization should include tobacco cessation, management of blood glucose, and reasonable weight control.

Following laparoscopic repair of subxiphoid and suprapubic hernias, pain management is definitely an issue. The subxiphoid repair is especially uncomfortable due to placement of sutures and fixation constructs along the sensitive costal margin. Proper preoperative consent should address this concern with patients. Non-narcotic measures for pre-emptive pain control should be considered and addressed preoperatively, not after the fact. The use of preoperative "pain cocktails" to include intravenous non-steroidal analgesics, epidural catheters to assist with postoperative analgesia, and low-dose ketamine infusions can be utilized to improve patient satisfaction and pain control postoperatively. A collaborative approach with anesthesiology can help to establish enhanced recovery pathways for a better patient experience.

Technical Considerations

Subxiphoid

For epigastric and subxiphoid hernias, it is not critical to tuck the patient's arms. The surgeon will be positioned typically at the patient's lower quadrant and working cephalad. We recommend always tucking the arms, however, to avoid any potential unexpected surprises like adhesions extending down to the inferior aspect of the midline, or an unanticipated umbilical defect.

For adhesiolysis during a subxiphoid hernia, the transverse colon should always be identified. Once its location is established and shown to be well away from the defect, takedown of adhesions can proceed rather quickly. The liver and stomach can be involved in subxiphoid defects; however, they typically reduce easily and are much easier to deal with if injuries occur to them. Once the upper abdomen is cleared of adhesions, the falciform should be taken down. This maneuver requires energy for hemostasis, which is why confirmation of the location of the transverse colon is critical. Monopolar or ultrasonic energy can be used to mobilize the falciform ligament at its juncture with the abdominal wall. This dissection should extend to at least 5 cm superior to the edge of the defect to allow for flush mesh placement. Not infrequently, the falciform ligament may be involved in the hernia defect. It should be grasped and brought into the abdominal cavity to visualize its insertion point into the underside of the fascia.

Mesh Orientation and Fixation

For atypical location hernias, placement of the mesh can be the most difficult step of the operation. Due to the bony structures and the vicinity of important structures like diaphragm, pericardium, iliac vessels, etc., placement of sutures and orientation of the mesh can be tricky. Some additional time should be given to these steps to avoid improper overlap and potential recurrences long term.

Following safe adhesiolysis, the defect is prepared for mesh placement. Spinal needles can be used to mark the edges of the defect in a lateral and cephalad-to-caudad orientation. Many techniques to measure the size of the defect can be employed. We use an internal metric ruler to determine the distance between the edges of the defect. Umbilical tape or suture can be stretched between the two marks as well. Some measure while the abdomen is desufflated. The midpoints of the defect should be determined and marked externally on the patient. These marks will be important to position the mesh precisely.

Particular note should be made of the distance from the superior aspect of the defect and the tip of the xiphoid process. The determination of mesh size and location of the superior suture (if used) will be based on this measurement. If the superior aspect of the hernia defect is at the xiphoid, in order to achieve a 5-cm mesh overlap, the superior suture should be placed 5 cm off the mesh edge. For example, if the defect is 10 cm long, a mesh that is 20 cm in length will be selected. However, if the superior aspect of the defect is 3 cm from the xiphoid process, the overlap will be calculated to allow for 5 cm of overlap onto the ribs in addition to the distance from the xiphoid. So, for the same 10 cm long defect, a mesh that is 23 cm in length would be chosen. It

is also important to note the distance from the lateral edges of the defect and the costal margin. For patients with steeply sloped ribs, sutures at the lateral edge may have to be placed away from the mesh edge to avoid passing them through the chest wall.

Once the mesh is introduced into the abdominal cavity through a trocar, the mesh is unfurled. The first suture to be retrieved is the superior suture at the level of the xiphoid. One of the lateral sutures is then placed along the grid that was created earlier. The assistant pulls up on these two sutures and the mesh is stretched inferiorly to gauge the location of the inferior suture. The same technique is used to place the final lateral suture. Once the sutures are secured, tacks are placed. The decision to use permanent versus absorbable tacks is surgeon dependent. However, the use of absorbable tacks does not change the fact that no fixation constructs should be placed above the costal margin! A double-crown approach may be utilized as long as all tacks are caudal to the costal margin. The superior aspect of the mesh is left to be held in place by the liver, by holding the mesh in place during desufflation of the abdominal cavity. Frequently, suturing the edge of the mesh or utilization of the glue is needed to ensure that no bowel is trapped between the mesh and the diaphragm. No tacks should be used cephalad to the costal margin and xiphoid process in order to avoid devastating cardiopulmonary injuries (Fig. 24.3).

Suprapubic

Positioning of the patient is more critical in suprapubic hernia repairs. The arms must be carefully padded and tucked at the side of the patient. Given that the fascial defect is inferior and the surgeon will be standing at the patient's head, both arms should be tucked to prevent harm to the patient's arm while leaning against the arm board. Tucking the arms will also prevent undue stress on the surgeon's back that results from twisting and other gyrations used to avoid the outstretched arm. The patient should be secured to the bed with the waist strap and additional tape

Fig. 24.3 Mesh placement for subxiphoid hernias. Note, no tacks are placed cephalad to the costal margin and xiphoid process

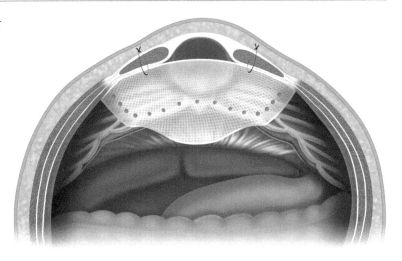

around the thighs if necessary. During dissection, steep Trendelenburg positioning helps to assist with retraction of the intestinal contents. Pads that minimize sliding of the patient can be considered as well.

Intra-operative bladder infusion is critical to facilitate its safe dissection. A three-way urinary catheter should be placed and the bladder infusion should be set up prior to draping. Standard intravenous infusion tubing is attached to the infusion port using the luer-lock tip. When it is time for bladder infusion, the nurse should place a clamp on the tubing that drains the urinary catheter close to the catheter. This clamp should not be placed on the urinary catheter itself or the tubing. Experience has taught us to instruct the nurse prior to prepping and draping where to place the clamp to avoid any confusion during the case. We infuse 250–500 cm^3 of Normal saline into the bladder to identify its superior extent so that the peritoneal flap can be safely developed superior to this margin. Signs of injury to the bladder include visualization of the urinary catheter balloon, excessive bleeding, or a rush of fluid. Once the peritoneal flap is raised, the remaining portion of the dissection to develop the space of Retzius is largely blunt. There may be small venous tributaries to the bladder, but these are easily controlled with light touches of the cautery. Even in multiply operated patients, keeping the dissection close to the abdominal

wall when lowering the bladder flap will help to avoid injury. The bladder is much thicker than the peritoneum. If the dissection does not progress bluntly, or if the tissue that is being dissected is very thick or bleeds a lot, the surgeon should reassess the plane. Once the pubic symphysis is visualized, dissection should continue for 1–2 cm inferior to symphysis to allow for subsequent mesh overlap. Cooper's ligaments should be identified bilaterally (Fig. 24.4). At the lateral edge of Cooper's ligament, the entrance to the femoral canal and iliac vessels has to be identified. Careful dissection of the medial aspect of the myopectineal orifice is essential for sufficient mesh overlap, but extreme caution in that area is necessary to avoid devastating injuries to major vascular structures.

Bladder injuries can occur. Usually, cystotomy results from impatience and not instilling the bladder with saline. Injuries should be repaired based on the comfort level of the surgeon. A two-layer repair with absorbable suture is ideal. Since the injury occurs at the dome of the bladder, large bites can be taken without concern for compromising the bladder lumen or injuring the ureters. The decision to proceed with the hernia repair is again the choice of the surgeon. Urine is technically sterile, and multiple reports describe repair of the bladder laparoscopically and completion of the hernia repair without any infectious complications. This approach is our

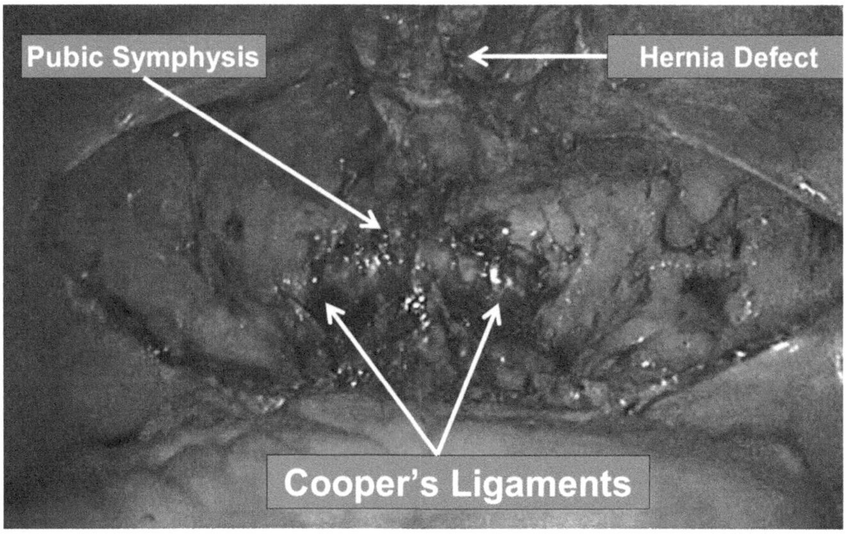

Fig. 24.4 Laparoscopic suprapubic hernia repair. The urinary bladder needs to be mobilized to expose both Cooper's ligaments and pubic symphysis to allow for subsequent adequate mesh overlap

preference, but it is also acceptable to abandon the repair and bring the patient back to the operating room in 3–5 days to complete the repair and place the mesh. This time frame is chosen because adhesions will not have formed and there will be enough time to clear any bacterial contamination.

Once bladder mobilization is complete, the defect size is assessed as described earlier. The distance from the symphysis to the inferior aspect of the fascial defect should be determined. In contrast to the subxiphoid hernia, the inferior suture in the suprapubic defect will need to be positioned at a distance from the mesh edge to allow for appropriate overlap onto the pubis. By leaving 5 cm of overlap beyond the symphysis, the mesh can be secured to Cooper's ligaments bilaterally. The potential weak point of the repair of suprapubic defects is inferior. Recurrences are more likely inferior due to improper mesh overlap and/or fixation. In our experience, those recurrences are due to failure to take down the bladder flap. The surgeon is then unable to provide adequate mesh overlap or fixation due to fear of injury to the bladder. By identifying the bladder upfront, injuries from sutures and fixation constructs can be avoided.

Mesh Orientation and Fixation

After introducing the mesh, the preplaced inferior suture is retrieved first just off the pubic symphysis (Fig. 24.5). The superior suture should be the next one to be pulled up. The site for suture placement is determined by stretching the mesh taut. An alternative method of mesh fixation is to utilize a mesh-positioning system. For suprapubic defects, placement of additional inferior sutures is critical. Once the sutures are secured, circumferential tacks are placed. Permanent, metallic tacks are preferred here as they more reliably penetrate the ligaments along the superior ramus. Absorbable tacks may be also used if placed just superior to the ramus and not into the bone directly. Tacks may be placed in a double crown configuration with the inner row around the hernia orifice. One additional suture is then placed on either side of the inferior, cardinal suture for more secure fixation inferiorly. It is important not to put any tacks below Cooper's ligaments (Fig. 24.6). Also, the inferior-lateral aspect of the mesh could be in the "Triangles of Doom and Pain". No tack fixation should be done in that area. This is accomplished by identifying

Fig. 24.5 Mesh coverage and fixation of the suprapubic hernia. The inferior-most stitch should be placed first, just off the pubic symphysis. Please note that the stitch should be preplaced 2–5 cm off the lower edge of the mesh

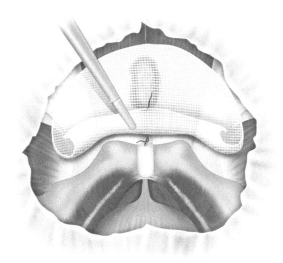

Fig. 24.6 Tacking the mesh. No tacks should be placed below the Cooper's ligaments in the area of the neurovascular structures within myopectineal orifices

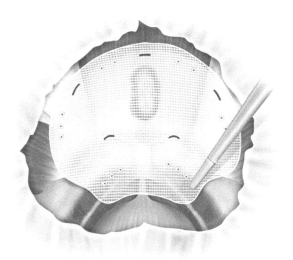

the iliopubic tract and providing external palpation for EVERY tack in that area. Fibrin glue is a very helpful adjunct for fixation of the inferior aspect of the mesh. Following mesh fixation, the bladder is desufflated and the flap left in situ. There is no need to attempt to re-approximate the flap, since a barrier-coated mesh was used. Incomplete closure of the flap may actually create potential openings that may result in internal hernias involving the small bowel.

For large defects or recurrent defects in the suprapubic position, more secure fixation can be provided by bone anchors [3]. A small, stab incision is made over the pubic symphysis. The bone guide is placed through the skin incision and rested against the symphysis. A pilot hole is

Fig. 24.7 Bone anchors

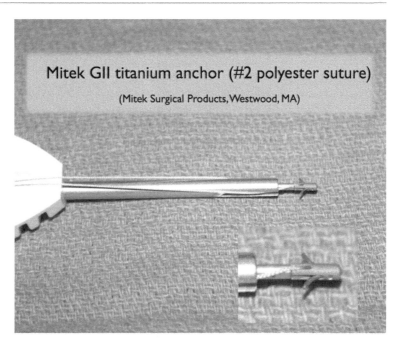

Mitek GII titanium anchor (#2 polyester suture)

(Mitek Surgical Products, Westwood, MA)

created with the drill, and the bone anchor is inserted into the symphysis. The bone anchors contain a double-armed braided suture (Fig. 24.7). The needles are cut off and the tails of the suture are passed through the stab incision and into the mesh. Additional anchors may be placed along the superior ramus as well.

series of stab incisions and figure-of-eight sutures in a "shoelace" fashion (Chapter 22). Intracorporeal suturing of the defect has also been described, including recent modification with the use of the robot. Fascial closure of the subxiphoid defects can be attempted as well, however, the benefit is not as great and the trade-off is increased pain.

Postoperative Concerns

For the most part, the postoperative management of the patient undergoing laparoscopic subxiphoid or suprapubic hernia repair is similar to standard laparoscopic ventral hernia repair. All patients are admitted predominantly for pain control. The concerns for ileus versus small bowel obstruction, seroma, and infection are the same as with all ventral hernia repairs. Early ambulation and generous use of analgesics is encouraged. Urinary catheters are removed on the morning of postoperative day one unless there was a bladder injury that required repair.

Seromas frequently complicate suprapubic repairs. Attempts to close the defect laparoscopically at the time of repair may help mitigate some of this concern. The defect may be closed with a

Conclusion

Laparoscopic approach to repair of subxiphoid and suprapubic defects represents an additional challenge. Familiarity and proficiency with laparoscopic repairs of routine to midline ventral defects is mandatory prior to embarking on the repair of the atypical defects. Understanding of anatomic nuances of both the upper and lower abdomen is paramount to avoid visceral and vascular injuries as well as providing durable and lasting repairs. Understanding and implementation of strategies for safe urinary bladder identification and mobilization is critical for suprapubic repairs. Mesh placement in both locations should be aimed to extend beyond the bony margins with fixation performed off the edge of the mesh. Importantly, maintaining the xiphoid process and costal margin as cranial safety margins for safe tacker/suture placement is absolutely necessary to avoid pulmonary/cardiac injuries. Defect closure may be of particular use for suprapubic defects to minimize postoperative seromas and bulging. Overall, suprapubic and subxiphoid defects can be effectively repaired laparoscopically, provided the important principles of safe dissection and mesh positioning described in this chapter are always maintained.

References

1. Cobb WS, Kercher KW, Heniford BT. Laparoscopic repair of incisional hernias. Surg Clin North Am. 2005;85(1):91–103.
2. Carbonell AM, Kercher KW, Matthews BD, Sing RF, Cobb WS, Heniford BT. The laparoscopic repair of suprapubic ventral hernias. Surg Endosc. 2005;19(2):174–7.
3. Yee JA, Harold KL, Cobb WS, Carbonell AM. Bone anchor fixation for complex laparoscopic ventral hernia repair. Surg Innov. 2008;15(4):292–6.

Ciara R. Huntington and Vedra A. Augenstein

Introduction and Background

Flank Hernia Definition and Anatomy

Flank hernias, including lumbar and parailiac hernias, are hernias of the lateral abdominal wall which occur between the 12th rib and iliac crest. The lateral abdominal wall is constructed of several large muscle groups from the back and abdomen including the latissimus dorsi, serratus posterior, external and internal oblique muscles, and transversus abdominis. Flank hernias occur within anatomic areas termed the "superior" and "inferior lumbar triangles." The majority of spontaneous and incisional hernias occur in the superior triangle, while congenital hernias are usually found in the inferior triangle [1].

The superior lumbar triangle (Fig. 25.1) is formed with a base as the 12th rib, posterior border formed by the erector spinae muscles and anterior border of the external oblique muscle. The triangle's floor is formed by the transversus abdominis, and its apex touches the iliac crest. This triangle is found in 82% of humans; in a recent cadaver study, 18% did not exhibit this triangle, and instead, the natural space of the triangle, which usually contains only the aponeurosis of the transversus abdominis, was covered by the external abdominal oblique and erector spinae muscles [2].

The inferior lumbar triangle (Fig. 25.2) is formed with the iliac crest as its base, the medial border of the external oblique, posterior/lateral border of the latissimus dorsi, and a floor formed by the internal oblique.

Hernias occurring within the superior and inferior triangles account for 95% of flank hernias; "diffuse" hernias, which occur on the flank without a specific relation to these anatomic triangles, account for the remaining 5% [3, 4].

C.R. Huntington, M.D.
Department of Surgery, Carolinas Medical Center,
1025 Morehead Medical Drive, Suite 300, Charlotte,
NC 28204, USA
e-mail: Ciara.huntington@carolinas.org

V.A. Augenstein, M.D., F.A.C.S. (✉)
Division of Gastrointestinal and Minimally Invasive
Surgery, Carolinas Medical Center,
1025 Morehead Medical Drive, Suite 300, Charlotte,
NC 28204, USA
e-mail: Vedra.augenstein@carolinas.org

Related Anatomy of the Posterolateral Abdominal Wall

Despite advances in laparoscopy and endovascular surgery, open access to the lateral abdominal wall for nephrectomies, adrenalectomies, back surgery, iliac graft harvests, retroperitoneal aortic surgery, advanced abdominal wall reconstruction and component separation techniques, and repair

© Springer International Publishing Switzerland 2016
Y.W. Novitsky (ed.), *Hernia Surgery*, DOI 10.1007/978-3-319-27470-6_25

Fig. 25.1 Superior lumbar triangle: The superior lumbar triangle (Grynfeltt's triangle) is formed by the erector spinae muscles, internal oblique muscles, and 12th rib. Its floor is the transversus abdominis

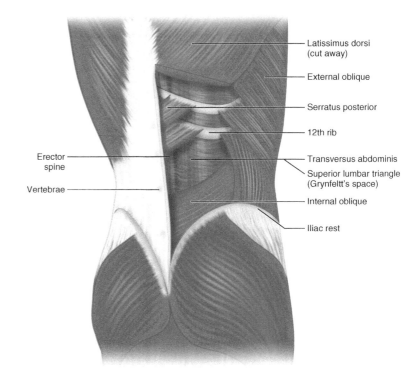

Latissimus dorsi (cut away)

External oblique

Serratus posterior

12th rib

Transversus abdominis

Superior lumbar triangle (Grynfeltt's space)

Internal oblique

Iliac rest

Erector spine

Vertebrae

Fig. 25.2 Inferior lumbar triangle: The inferior lumbar triangle (Petit's triangle) is formed by the latissimus dorsi muscle, external oblique muscle, and iliac crest. Its floor is the internal oblique muscle

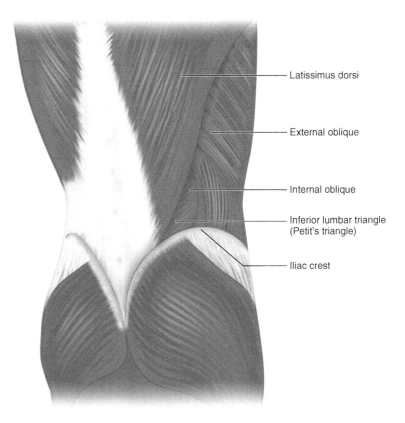

Latissimus dorsi

External oblique

Internal oblique

Inferior lumbar triangle (Petit's triangle)

Iliac crest

of retroperitoneal traumatic injuries is still common. Prevention and repair of flank hernias rely on good understanding of the anatomy. Avoiding injury to surrounding structures and careful fixation of the mesh are key to good quality of life outcomes.

The flank is the intersection of the back and abdominal musculature, several of which fuse to form aponeuroses. The deep fascia of the back, also known as lumbodorsal or thoracolumbar fascia, is formed by the fused aponeuroses of the latissimus dorsi, internal oblique, and transversus abdominis muscles [5]. The internal oblique muscles and transversus abdominis muscle join together at the lateral edge of the erector spinae muscles, and this aponeurosis extends to cover portions of the bony spine [5]. A surgeon can judge the depth of an incision here by the fact that the internal oblique muscle fibers begin at the edge of the erector spinae muscles while the transversus abdominis muscle fibers continue to be aponeurotic laterally [5].

The quadratus lumborum muscle lies anterior to the deep fascia, and the subcostal, iliohypogastric, and ilioinguinal nerves pass laterally and anterior to this muscle before entering the plane between the transversus abdominis and internal oblique muscles to course towards the anterior midline [5]. Superficial to the quadratus lumborum, contained within Gerota's fascia, lays the kidney and adrenal glands with their attendant vascular structures. The ureter also starts proximally with the renal vessels before moving in a curvilinear path in the retroperitoneum to the ureteropelvic junction at approximately the level of L2, then moves anteriorly along the psoas muscle [6]. It crosses under the gonadal vein and crosses over the iliac vessels at the bifurcation of the common iliac into the external and internal iliac vessels [7]. The ureter is found medial to the sacroiliac joint before moving laterally into the pelvis [6].

When performing a hernia repair, constant awareness of one's dissection and proximity to pelvic nerves, vasculature, and the ureter is necessary; moreover, lateral positioning can further distort anatomy leading to injury.

Brief History of Flank Hernias

The flank hernia was first described in the literature in 1672 by the Dutch anatomist and surgeon Paul Barbette [8]. Physicians Dolée in 1703 and Budgeon in 1728 are also credited with early descriptions, and Garangeot (1731) described the first report of a strangulated flank hernia, which was reduced after the patient's death [9]. In 1750, the first surgical reduction and repair was reported by Ravanton [9]. The anatomical boundaries of the inferior lumbar triangle were again described by the French physician Petit in 1783, and the hernia of that space now bears his eponym [10]. Hernias of the superior lumbar triangle are named by the surgeon Grynfeltt, who described the space in 1866 [11]. He was a contemporary with the German physician Lesshaft who defined the triangle independently in 1870, and the superior lumbar triangle hernia is sometimes referred to as a Grynfeltt–Lesshaft hernia [9].

Flank hernias are rare with only an estimated 300 cases reported in the literature [12]. Laparoscopic case series are similarly scarce. The first laparoscopic repair of a traumatic flank hernia was reported by Burick et al. in 1996 [13] and the first laparoscopic primary flank hernia repair by Heniford et al. in 1997 [14].

Epidemiology

Flank hernias account for 1.5–2% of abdominal wall defects [4]. The majority (2/3) of flank hernias occur in men [14]. Incarceration risk is estimated to be approximately 25%, with 8% chance of strangulation [3, 4]. Overall, 20–25% of flank hernias are congenital, and 55% are primary. Primary or spontaneous flank hernias are most common in the fifth to seventh decades of life and are associated with states that promote herniation of the abdominal contents through the weakened superior lumbar triangle, such as obesity, chronic illness, advanced age, polio, and local muscle weakness [3, 12]. There are reports of herpes zoster contributing to eventration leading to herniation [15].

Incisional or traumatic hernias have become more prevalent than in decades past and now account for 25–30% of flank hernias [3, 12]. Faro et al. reported that 7 out of 850 patients who received CT scan imaging for acute abdominal trauma were diagnosed with traumatic lumbar hernia [16]. CT scan has a 98% sensitivity for traumatic flank hernias which can be easily missed by physical exam on trauma survey but are commonly associated with intra-abdominal injuries (61%) [17]. Traumatic flank hernias are more often diffuse or located within the inferior lumbar triangle [17]. Seat belt injury via rapid deceleration and shearing of the iliac crest and associated muscles can be associated with traumatic flank herniation [17].

Similar to ventral hernias, incidence of incisional hernias in the flank is about 20–30% [12]. Eventration can occur as a result of iatrogenic injury of the 12th subcostal nerve, which runs anterior to the quadratus lumborum muscle, enters through the transversalis fascia, and runs under the internal oblique muscles before joining the iliohypogastric nerve [18]. When injured, the lateral abdominal wall muscles will weaken and eventrate. In one study of patients undergoing radical nephrectomy, 34 of 70 (49%) reported persistent flank bulging 1 year postoperatively; the authors did not differentiate between eventration and herniation in this study [18].

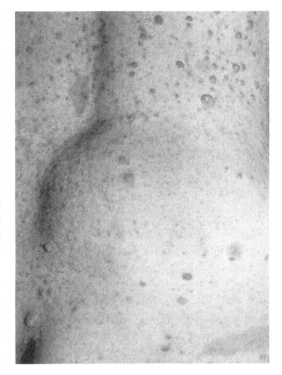

Fig. 25.3 Flank hernia on exam: This patient with neurofibromatosis has a posterior bulge on Valsalva consistent with a primary flank hernia

Surgical Approach

Preoperative Workup

Patients with flank hernias often present with posterolateral bulges (Fig. 25.3) that are exacerbated by Valsalva maneuver and resolved with lying flat. A history is taken with careful attention to precipitating factors such as illness, trauma, or surgery. Symptoms of small bowel obstruction, colon obstruction, and urinary obstruction are pertinent. Physical exam is performed in standing and lateral laying positions, noting the presence of previous surgical scars in the region, the approximate size of the flank hernia defect, reducibility of hernia contents, and

proximity to the iliac crest. Auscultation and palpation may reveal incarcerated colon, bowel, or even the kidney. Though ultrasound may be helpful because of the ability to recognize the presence of the hernia and any contents within the sac, CT scanning is routinely recommended [3, 12, 14]. A CT scan differentiates between muscle laxity and true flank herniation and provides preoperative identification of the contents of the hernia sac, defect location, and which layers of muscle may be atrophied or contracted (Figs. 25.4 and 25.5). The size of the defect and the presence of a previous hernia repair can influence the decision to proceed with an open or laparoscopic approach (Table 25.1). Moreno-Egea et al. published the first prospective trial of laparoscopic versus open repair of 16 incisional lumbar hernias. They reported reduced mean operating time, postoperative complications, mean length of stay, quicker return to activities, and lower associated costs with the laparoscopic repair compared to open, though the laparo-

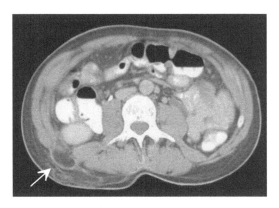

Fig. 25.4 CT scan flank hernia—Axial view: This preoperative CT scan demonstrates a *right* sided flank hernia

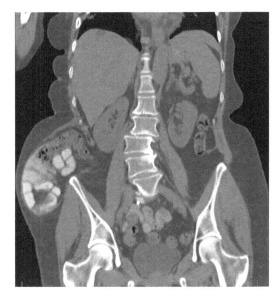

Fig. 25.5 CT scan flank hernia—Coronal view: Another patient with a large, *right*-sided flank hernia containing colon

Table 25.1 Factors influencing operative approach to flank hernia repair

Operative approach to repair of flank hernias
Consider open approach
Very large defects where muscle approximation is desired
Numerous previous repairs ± mesh
Inability to tolerate pneumoperitoneum
Extensive intra-abdominal adhesions
Large unappealing scar with atrophic skin
Consider laparoscopic approach
Smaller defects where muscle approximation is less important
Morbidly obese patients
Diabetic patients
Tobacco users who necessitate repair
Immunocompromised patients
Patients with high risk of wound complications

scopic group had a smaller average defect size [19]. In a follow-up of this study in 2013, Moreno-Egea et al. confirmed these findings and recommended a laparoscopic approach for those with a hernia defect size of less than 15 cm, especially if the hernia was located within one of the lumbar triangles [20]. However, preoperative evaluation and discussion with the patient regarding repair techniques are key in choosing the best approach for repair. Long- and short-term patient goals are important; data from large ventral hernia series indicates that laparoscopic repairs may have more initial pain but fewer wound complications compared to open repairs [21].

Regardless of surgical approach, the patient's risk of wound complications and hernia recurrence can be optimized by smoking cessation 4–6 weeks prior to surgery, weight loss depending on patient BMI, and improving glucose control in patients with diabetes [22–24]. Cardiac and medical clearance may be appropriate for elderly or patients with significant comorbidities [25]. Involving the transplant team in the hernia operation for patients who have a kidney transplant can be very valuable in identification and prevention of transplanted ureter or kidney injury. Consultation with an orthopedic surgeon for placement of bone anchors in cases where there is no fascia on the bone is recommended.

For patients with contracted muscles and large defects, preoperative injection of Botulinum toxin A (Botox) under CT or U/S guidance into the transversus abdominis, internal oblique, and/or external oblique muscles should be considered. The injection is done approximately 1 month prior to surgery. In small non-randomized studies on ventral hernias, preoperative injections of Botox have been shown to paralyze lateral muscles, reduce transverse hernia defects, decrease intra-abdominal pressure and muscle tension, and allow easier surgical closure [26]. This method has been utilized by our group with good results for an open repair in a patient with recurrent flank hernia after partial nephrectomy (unpublished data, Heniford 2014). Muscles will retain laxity for approximately 3 months postoperatively, which may give the appearance of persistent herniation.

Positioning and Trocar Placement

Patient positioning is crucial to a successful operation. Before moving the patient from the supine position, the patient's midline, hernia defect and intended trocar sites should be marked with a marking pen, as the abdomen will be distorted with positioning. The patient is then placed in a semilateral position with 45° elevation of the side ipsilateral to the hernia with flexion at the hip (Fig. 25.6) [27]. This position allows the patient to be rolled flat or in full lateral position to opti-

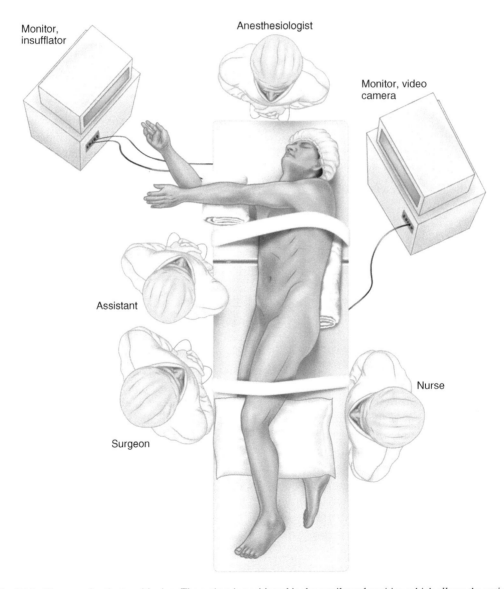

Fig. 25.6 Diagram of patient positioning. The patient is positioned in the semilateral position which allows the patient to be rolled flat or in full lateral position to optimize exposure

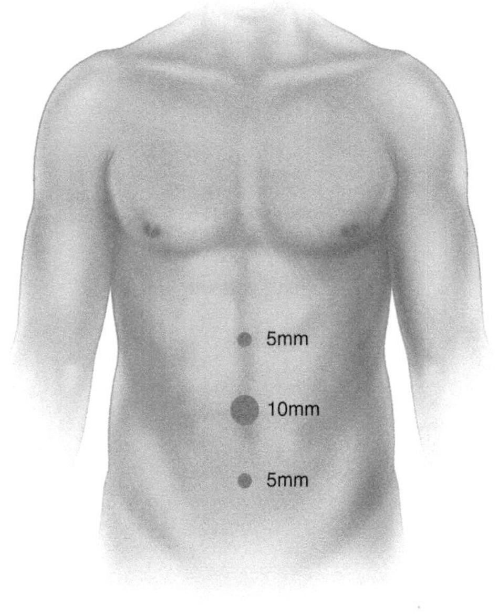

Fig. 25.7 Trocar placement. Three trocars are placed in the midline, depending on the patient's body habitus, location of the hernia defect, and presence of previous surgical incisions

mize exposure. In the semilateral position, the viscera fall away from hernia. Adding a kidney rest will further open the space between the iliac crest and costal margin. The patient should be adequately padded and secured to the operating table so that positioning can be changed during the operation safely and as needed.

Trocar positioning depends on the location and size of the defect, presence of other surgical scars, and patient body habitus [26]. One option is to place a 10 mm trocar at the umbilicus. Two additional 5 mm trocars can be placed anteriorly along the midline infraumbilically and supraumbilically, 5–6 cm from the umbilical port (Fig. 25.7).

Hernia Repair

Defining the Hernia Defect

After insufflation and brief survey of the abdomen, adhesiolysis with sharp and blunt dissection commences. Energy devices are used infrequently

due to the risk of iatrogenic injury. Mobilization of the colon is generally required [14]. This is performed by incision of the peritoneum along the white line of Toldt with cautery or endoscopic scissors [14]. Occasionally, mobilization of the kidney is also needed [14]. Any incarcerated contents are reduced laparoscopically.

With the takedown of adhesions and mobilization of the colon, the retroperitoneum including the psoas and erector spinae muscles becomes accessible [28]. Superiorly, the dissection is carried to allow mesh fixation to the costal margin, but care must be taken to avoid violation of the thoracic cavity, diaphragm, or pericardium [28]. Similarly, inferior dissection to expose Cooper's ligament and the iliopubic tract is necessary for larger defects [28]. As noted previously, meticulous identification of the ureter, iliac vessels, spermatic cord, and pelvic nerves is required [27, 28].

After the hernia defect is visualized, it is measured intracorporeally to plan for appropriate mesh coverage. A disposable ruler can be introduced via the 10 mm port or a laparoscopic instrument of known size (such as the open jaws of an endoscopic grasper) can be used for reference. Alternatively, spinal needles can be introduced through the skin at cardinal directions surrounding the defect. A piece of suture is used to measure the distance between needles (as the defect size is reduced within the abdominal cavity) and provides the dimensions of the hernia defect (Fig. 25.8). An adequate overlap generally requires 4–6 cm overlap at the hernia edge.

Securing the Mesh

Mesh used for laparoscopic intra-abdominal placement should have an adhesion barrier and should be selected according to criteria similar for laparoscopic ventral hernia repairs. Transfascial sutures and tacks attach the mesh to the abdominal wall, and both absorbable and nonabsorbable materials may be used.

Adequate mesh coverage is paramount for successful repair of the flank hernia. The posterior suture attaches the mesh far posteriorly to the

Fig. 25.8 Measuring the defect laparoscopically. The figure demonstrates one method for measuring the hernia defect. Spinal needles are placed through the skin to mark the edges of the defect. Two laparoscopic graspers span the distance from one spinal needle to the other using a piece of suture, then the suture length is measured extracorporeally

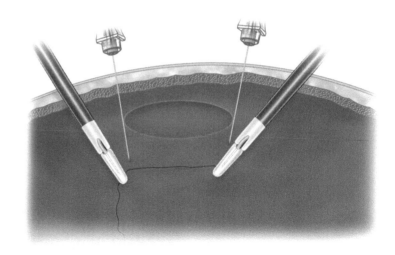

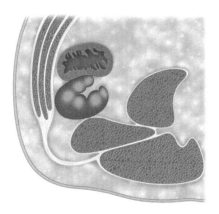 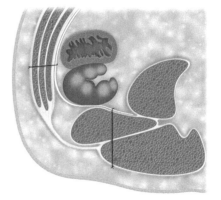

Fig. 25.9 Mesh positioning. The mesh is placed retroperitoneally, posterior to the kidney. Depending on the size of the defect, the mesh may cover from the abdominal *midline* to the psoas muscle, and from the iliac crest to the coastal region, behind the liver

erector spinae fascia and muscles and the anterior suture will depend on the size and area of the defect. Superiorly, the mesh can be secured to the costal margin as needed but can extend beyond this and drape over liver or spleen for increased overlap. Inferiorly, the mesh is secured above the iliac crest or to the Cooper's ligament.

The mesh is secured using tacks and sutures where the number depends on the size of mesh and defect as with ventral hernias. Making sure that the mesh is taut and in good contact with the abdominal wall is important to help with incorporation. Sutures are usually secured to the mesh extracorporeally and with the knots on the side that opposes the abdominal wall. The mesh is then rolled and inserted into the abdomen. It is laid out to overlap the defect adequately and then sutures are exteriorized using a suture passer (Figs. 25.9a, b and 25.10). The mesh is secured superiorly by suture through the rib, avoiding fixation to the diaphragm, and to the iliac crest inferiorly by passing the suture through the periosteum of the bone. Use of bone anchors in the iliac crest to fix the mesh inferiorly [27, 29] or fixation of the mesh to Cooper's ligament and the iliopubic tract with tacks [28] can be performed.

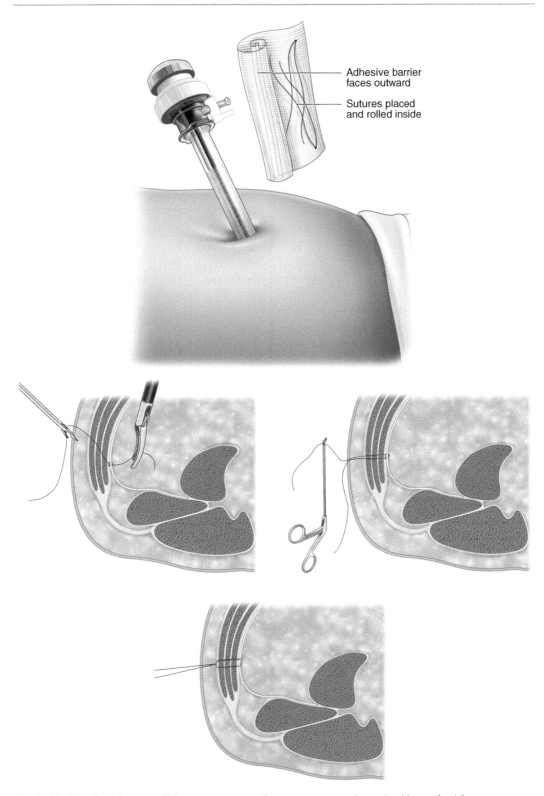

Fig. 25.10 Transfascial sutures. Using a suture passer, the surgeon secures the mesh with transfascial sutures

Regardless of which method is chosen, no tacks or sutures should be placed below the iliopubic tract to avoid injury to neurovascular structures.

If a portion of the peritoneum is taken down, it may be used as long as there is no space left for internal herniation of bowel [20]. To secure the mesh, laparoscopic tacks are utilized approximately every 2 cm. Adequate posterior positioning of the mesh is critical. Edwards et al. suggest examining preoperative CT scans closely to ensure patients have adequate paraspinal muscles to allow for hernia repair [28]. Some authors are cautious about tacks along the psoas due to the nearby presence of the iliohypogastric, ilioinguinal, or genitofemoral nerves and prefer to utilize intracorporeal suturing to attach the mesh to the investing fascia in this region [30]. The lateral edge of the psoas muscle should be considered the border for safety in order to avoid critical nerves. Regardless of the method, generous overlap of the defect with mesh coverage into the retroperitoneum should be the goal. Sutures do not have to be at the edges of the mesh, but can be closer to the center if needed to facilitate secure placement.

After fixation of the mesh, the surgical field is examined and then the trocars are removed under direct visualization. Trocar sites greater than 5 mm are closed at the fascial level. Injecting suture sites with local anesthetic is strongly recommended intraoperatively.

Primary Closure

Though laparoscopic repair does not generally include primary fascial closure, this should be a consideration in repair. The surgeon should discuss options with the patient indicating the pros and cons of closing the defect [20]. Our preference is to close the defect when possible to establish better mesh overlap and restore abdominal wall functionality; researchers have demonstrated that in patients undergoing laparoscopic ventral hernia repair, there is no internal or external oblique muscle hypertrophy unless the midline fascia is closed [31]. If an incision

over the defect is required to accomplish muscle and defect closure, the patient will lose some of the benefits of laparoscopy such as a lower rate of wound complications. However, hernia sac resection and primary myofascial reapproximation may not be feasible via a laparoscopic approach.

Postoperative Care and Quality of Life Considerations

In our practice, preoperative epidurals are routinely performed especially in patients with large defects, and where an epidural is not possible or refused, a patient-controlled analgesia (PCA) pump is used. The patient's diet is advanced as tolerated postoperatively. Early mobilization, within 6–8 hours of surgery, is strongly encouraged. A single dose of preoperative antibiotics is administered, as well as a subcutaneous injection of heparin in the preoperative holding area for venous thromboembolic (VTE) prophylaxis. Chemoprophylaxis and sequential compression devices (SCDs) are utilized from postoperative day 0 to prevent VTE events. Subfascial drains are removed prior to discharge, while prefascial drains are left in place until the output has decreased in quantity to less than 30 cc/day for 2 days.

In Edwards et al.'s series of laparoscopic flank hernia repairs ($n=27$), patients stayed in the hospital for an average of 3.1 days (range 0–6 days) and had no wound complications or recurrence at mean 3.6 month follow-up (range 1–10 months) [28]. However, three patients did report persistent pain at their hernia site at follow-up.

Moreno-Egea et al. published long-term results on 55 patients who either underwent laparoscopic ($n=35$) or open ($n=20$) flank hernia repair [20]. The patients in the laparoscopic group were more obese (mean BMI 31.2 vs. 28.2) but had smaller hernias (average defect 11.7 cm² vs. 14.5 cm²) than the open group. Overall, 2.9% of the laparoscopic repairs ($n=1$) and 13% of open repairs ($n=3$) developed recurrence (NS, $p=0.13$). Compared to open repairs, the laparoscopic group had more hematomas (11.4% vs. 0%), but fewer seromas (20% vs. 40%). The laparoscopic group returned to normal activities much faster (average 14 vs. 27 days). At 1 and 6 months, via a visual analog scale, pain was lower in the laparoscopic group ($p < 0.001$). By 1 year, the groups were the same with 88.2% of the laparoscopic and 90% of the open repair groups reporting no pain [20].

Quality of life after flank hernia repair has been examined using the prospective International Hernia Mesh Registry. Of 62 patients who underwent flank hernia repair—12 laparoscopic and 50 open—the majority of patients reported pain, movement, and mesh sensation postoperatively (Unpublished data, Heniford 2014, see Table 25.2). Using the Carolinas Comfort Scale (CCS), a hernia-specific quality of life assessment tool, there was no significant difference between operative approaches, but a trend towards more pain in laparoscopy (Unpublished data, Heniford 2014). Between 11.2 and 33.3% of patients continue to report pain 1 year after laparoscopic flank hernia repair (Unpublished data, Heniford 2014). This is an important element of preoperative counseling, especially for patients who present because of pain.

Table 25.2 Quality of life outcomes for laparoscopic vs. open flank hernia repair

	Lap	Open	p value
Pain			
1 Month	60.0	37.5	0.17
6 Months	50.0	40.0	0.58
12 Months	33.3	29.4	0.81
Movement limitation			
1 Month	53.3	37.5	0.33
6 Months	33.3	25.0	0.7
12 Months	35.7	23.5	0.46
Mesh sensation			
1 Month	43.8	23.1	0.25
6 Months	25.0	25.0	1
12 Months	35.7	36.8	0.95

Represented as percentage of patients with symptoms. QOL determined via Carolinas Comfort Scale (CCS)
Data from the International Hernia Mesh Registry on 62 patients undergoing flank hernia repair (12 laparoscopic, 50 open repairs). *CCS* Carolinas Comfort Scale, a hernia-specific quality of life assessment tool

Summary

Flank hernia is a rare entity but can be successfully treated laparoscopically. Careful preoperative preparation and patient counseling are important. Intraoperatively, mesh should be placed with wide coverage of the hernia defect, often stretching from the costal margin to the iliac crest, and from the anterior abdomen to the erector spinae muscles and psoas muscles. A thorough anatomical awareness of the flank region is important to avoid damage to the surrounding structures, such as the ureter, pelvic nerves, spermatic cord, and vascular structures.

References

1. Orcutt TW. Hernia of the superior lumbar triangle. Ann Surg. 1971;173(2):294–7. Epub 1971/02/01.
2. Loukas M, El-Zammar D, Shoja MM, Tubbs RS, Zhan L, Protyniak B, et al. The clinical anatomy of the triangle of Grynfeltt. Hernia. 2008;12(3):227–31. Epub 2008/02/20.
3. Suarez S, Hernandez JD. Laparoscopic repair of a lumbar hernia: report of a case and extensive review of the literature. Surg Endosc. 2013;27(9):3421–9. Epub 2013/05/03.
4. Alcoforado C, Lira N, Kreimer F, Martins-Filho ED, Ferraz AA. Grynfelt hernia. Arq Bras Cir Dig. 2013;26(3):241–3. Epub 2013/11/06.
5. Scott-Conner CE, Dawson DL. Operative Anatomy. 3rd ed. Philadelphia: Lippincott Williams & Wilkins; 2009.
6. Anderson JK, Kabalin JN, Cadeddu JA. Surgical anatomy of retroperitoneum, adrenals, kidneys, and ureters. In: Wein AJ, editor. Campbell-Walsh Urology. 9th ed. Philadelphia: Saunders Elsevier; 2007. p. 37.
7. Wu YM. Cadaveric donor nephrectomy and renal transplantation. In: Carol EH, Scott-Conner DLD, editors. Operative anatomy. 3rd ed. Philadelphia: Lippincott Williams & Wilkins; 2009.
8. Barbette P. Opera chirurgico-anatomica. Ad circularem sanguinis motum, aliaque recentiorum inventa, accommodata. Accedit de peste tractatus observationibus illustratus. Leiden: Gelder; 1672.
9. Goodman EH, Speese J. Lumbar hernia. Ann Surg. 1916;63(5):548–60.
10. Petit J. Traite des maladies chirurgicales, et des operations qui leur convenient. TF Dido. 1774;2:256–9.
11. Grynfeltt J. Quelques mots sur la hernie lombaire. Montp Med. 1866;16:323.
12. Moreno-Egea A, Baena EG, Calle MC, Martinez JA, Albasini JL. Controversies in the current management of lumbar hernias. Arch Surg. 2007;142(1):82–8. Epub 2007/01/17.

13. Burick AJPS. Laparoscopic repair of a traumatic lumbar hernia: a case report. J Laparoendosc Surg. 1996;6:259–62.

14. Heniford BT, Iannitti DA, Gagner M. Laparoscopic inferior and superior lumbar hernia repair. Arch Surg. 1997;132(10):1141–4. Epub 1997/10/23.

15. Hindmarsh A, Mehta S, Mariathas DA. An unusual presentation of a lumbar hernia. Emerg Med J. 2002;19(5):460. Epub 2002/09/03.

16. Faro SH, Racette CD, Lally JF, Wills JS, Mansoory A. Traumatic lumbar hernia: CT diagnosis. AJR Am J Roentgenol. 1990;154(4):757–9. Epub 1990/04/01.

17. Burt BM, Afifi HY, Wantz GE, Barie PS. Traumatic lumbar hernia: report of cases and comprehensive review of the literature. J Trauma. 2004;57(6):1361–70. Epub 2004/12/31.

18. Chatterjee S, Nam R, Fleshner N, Klotz L. Permanent flank bulge is a consequence of flank incision for radical nephrectomy in one half of patients. Urol Oncol. 2004;22(1):36–9. Epub 2004/02/19.

19. Moreno-Egea A, Torralba-Martinez JA, Morales G, Fernandez T, Girela E, Aguayo-Albasini JL. Open vs laparoscopic repair of secondary lumbar hernias: a prospective nonrandomized study. Surg Endosc. 2005;19(2):184–7. Epub 2004/12/02.

20. Moreno-Egea A, Alcaraz AC, Cuervo MC. Surgical options in lumbar hernia: laparoscopic versus open repair. A long-term prospective study. Surg Innov. 2013;20(4):331–44. Epub 2012/09/08.

21. Colavita PD, Tsirline VB, Belyansky I, Walters AL, Lincourt AE, Sing RF, et al. Prospective, long-term comparison of quality of life in laparoscopic versus open ventral hernia repair. Ann Surg. 2012;256(5):714–22; discussion 22–3. Epub 2012/10/26.

22. Colavita PD, Zemlyak AY, Burton PV, Dacey KT, Walters AL, Lincourt AE, Tsirline VE, Kercher KW, Heniford BT. The expansive cost of wound complications after ventral hernia repair. Washington DC: American College of Surgeons; 2013.

23. Finan KR, Vick CC, Kiefe CI, Neumayer L, Hawn MT. Predictors of wound infection in ventral hernia repair. Am J Surg. 2005;190(5):676–81. Epub 2005/10/18.

24. Medina M, Sillero M, Martinez-Gallego G, Delgado-Rodriguez M. Risk factors of surgical wound infection in patients undergoing herniorrhaphy. Eur J Surg. 1997;163(3):191–8. Epub 1997/03/01.

25. Feely MA, Collins CS, Daniels PR, Kebede EB, Jatoi A, Mauck KF. Preoperative testing before noncardiac surgery: guidelines and recommendations. Am Fam Physician. 2013;87(6):414–8. Epub 2013/04/04.

26. Ibarra-Hurtado TR, Nuno-Guzman CM, Echeagaray-Herrera JE, Robles-Velez E, de Jesus Gonzalez-Jaime J. Use of botulinum toxin type a before abdominal wall hernia reconstruction. World J Surg. 2009;33(12):2553–6. Epub 2009/09/23.

27. Arca MJ, Heniford BT, Pokorny R, Wilson MA, Mayes J, Gagner M. Laparoscopic repair of lumbar hernias. J Am Coll Surg. 1998;187(2):147–52. Epub 1998/08/15.

28. Edwards C, Geiger T, Bartow K, Ramaswamy A, Fearing N, Thaler K, et al. Laparoscopic transperitoneal repair of flank hernias: a retrospective review of 27 patients. Surg Endosc. 2009;23(12):2692–6. Epub 2009/05/23.

29. Woodward AM, Flint LM, Ferrara JJ. Laparoscopic retroperitoneal repair of recurrent postoperative lumbar hernia. J Laparoendosc Adv Surg Tech A. 1999;9(2):181–6. Epub 1999/05/11.

30. Salameh JR, Salloum EJ. Lumbar incisional hernias: diagnostic and management dilemma. JSLS. 2004;8(4):391–4. Epub 2004/11/24.

31. Silva GD. Comparative radiographic analysis of changes in the abdominal wall musculature morphology after open posterior component separation or bridging laparoscopic ventral hernia repair. J Am Coll Surg. 2014;218(3):353–7.

Robotic Ventral Hernia Repair

26

Conrad Ballecer and Eduardo Parra-Davila

General Overview

In 2004, the American Hernia Society concluded in their consensus statement that the Rives-Stoppa repair of ventral hernias was the standard by which all open hernia repairs should be judged [1, 2]. While shown to be a durable repair, wound complications often times result in unacceptable patient morbidity. To defend against wound morbidity, laparoscopic ventral hernia repair (LVHR) emerged. In fact, laparoscopic repair of incisional hernias, first introduced in 1992 [3, 4], leads to markedly improved wound morbidity, shorter hospital stay, and lower overall complication rates. Published recurrence rates have been reduced, ranging from 0 to 9% [5–8]. These recurrences have been attributed primarily to improper positioning of the mesh (with <3 cm overlap of mesh and fascia) and to the use of tacking or stapling devices as sole fixation without permanent suture fixation [8, 9].

Electronic supplementary material: The online version of this chapter (doi:10.1007/978-3-319-27470-6_26) contains supplementary material, which is available to authorized users.

C. Ballecer, M.D., FACS (✉)
Arrowhead Medical Center, Banner Thunderbird Medical Center, Peoria, AZ, USA
e-mail: cballecer1@icloud.com

E. Parra-Davila, M.D., F.A.C.S., F.A.S.C.R.S.
General Surgery/Colorectal, Celebration, FL, USA
e-mail: eduardo.parradavila@flhosp.org

Although laparoscopic repair has been associated with improved outcomes compared to the open technique, there continues to be a significant incidence of postoperative pain. Several authors [7, 10–13] have reported a 2% incidence of significant postoperative pain lasting more than 2–8 weeks after repair. The pain is described by patients as a point of constant burning in a dermatomal pattern at the points of transabdominal sutures or tackers and has been attributed to tissue and nerve entrapment.

The da Vinci robot (Intuitive Surgical, Sunnyvale, CA, USA) offers numerous advantages when compared to laparoscopy, including several degrees of motion, three-dimensional (3D) imaging, and superior ergonomics that enable easy and precise intracorporeal suturing. Other reports have demonstrated the ease of intracorporeal suturing of the mesh to the abdominal wall [10]. Thus, this device is an ideal tool for intracorporeal suturing of mesh to the posterior fascia of the anterior abdominal wall for ventral hernia repair. Whereas previous reports have confirmed the need to suture the mesh at 2 to 5-cm intervals [7–9] as a means of reducing the recurrence rates associated with laparoscopic hernia repairs, we believe that continuous circumferential suturing applies those principles while evenly distributing the tension throughout the mesh.

Limitations of the robot-assisted technique are obvious. Large ventral hernias, as they approach the working ports and camera, make this technique technically challenging for the robotic arms to be placed and to be able to work with the angulations needed or when the amount of redundant skin is large and removal of soft tissue is indicated.

Traditionally, the steps of LVHR involve three primary steps: gaining safe access to the abdomen, adhesiolysis, and placement and fixation of a tissue separating mesh. Adhesiolysis is the Achilles heel of this procedure due to its technical difficulty, especially in recurrent hernia and in patients with previous intraperitoneal mesh placement. This difficulty is accentuated by poor ergonomics and the demands of applying non-articulating instruments high on the anterior abdominal wall. Secondly, bridging defects may predispose to migration or eventration of the mesh into the defect and seroma formation. Thirdly, the requirement for circumferential tacks and multiple full thickness transfascial sutures to adequately secure the intraperitoneal onlay mesh (IPOM), predispose to both acute and chronic pain [13, 14]. Lastly, in a certain group of patients, leaving mesh in the intraperitoneal area may complicate future surgical intervention [15].

Robotic ventral hernia repair (RVHR) may overcome these shortcomings by allowing the operator to offer traditional open repair techniques through minimally invasive incisions. The robotic repair of ventral hernias was first described in 2002 by Ballantyne [16]. Boasting the benefits of improved visualization, tremorless precision, and superior ergonomics has stimulated the emergence of robotic techniques in the hernia field. In this chapter, we will detail perioperative considerations and technical pearls of RVHRs.

Preoperative Considerations

Obtaining a thorough history and physical is mandatory to coordinate an operative plan. Specifically, comorbidities such as diabetes, obesity, smoking, and collagen vascular disease may critically affect the operative plan. A CT scan of the abdomen and pelvis is critical to preoperative planning and remains the gold standard imaging test. This imaging modality can delineate the size and location of the hernia defect, the content of the hernia sac, and possibly the position of previously placed mesh. A complete medical history along with imaging offers the opportunity for surgeons to construct a risk/benefit ratio. This scale may then be presented to the patients so they can make an informed decision regarding the repair that would be best to address their specific hernia.

Techniques

Hernia repair techniques amenable to the robotic approach include:

- IPOM bridge
- IPOM after primary closure of the defect
- Preperitoneal placement of mesh
- Placement of retromuscular mesh with or without posterior components separation

These individual techniques are chosen based on location of the hernia defect, size of defect, and perhaps most importantly, surgeon experience. This chapter will provide a detailed instruction on each individual technique along with author insight, where applicable.

Intraperitoneal Onlay Mesh After Primary Closure of the Defect

Patient Positioning, Trocar Placement, and Docking

For the majority of patients with defects in the midline, supine positioning with the arms tucked is preferred, unless trocar access to the lateral abdomen is obscured by this position. In this situation, the arm is placed on a board set at 90° from the trunk. For mid-abdominal hernias, the trocars should be placed at the most extreme lateral, cranial, and caudal positions possible. The most lateral position of the camera and two instrument arms will allow for a full range of motion, which

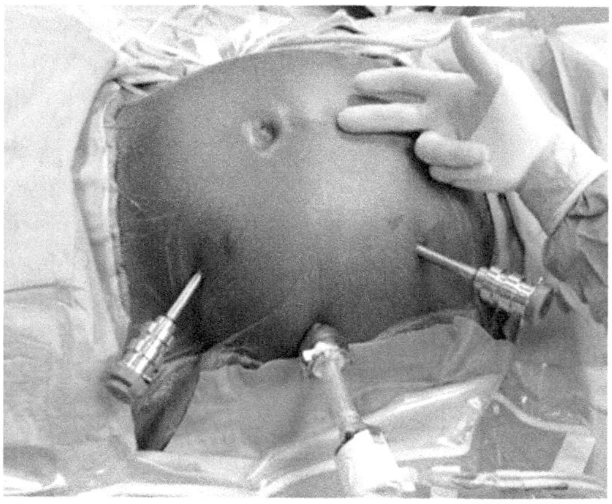

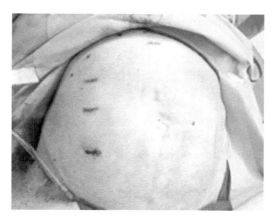

Fig. 26.1 Trocar position for midline abdominal wall hernias

Fig. 26.2 Subxiphoid accessory port

facilitates dissection and suturing on the anterior abdominal wall.

Gaining safe intra-abdominal access remains the first important step in minimally invasive surgery. This can be difficult in the multiply operated abdomen. Sites of previous operative intervention will certainly influence the strategy to gain initial access. Optical entry with a 5 mm trocar with or without initial Veress needle insufflation in the left upper quadrant is generally safe. A 12 or 8 mm trocar for the camera is placed as far lateral to the ipsilateral edge of the defect as possible. This, in most cases, obviates the need to place trocars on the contralateral abdomen when securing the mesh to the ipsilateral abdominal wall. An 8 mm dV trocar is placed in the lower lateral abdomen and the initial 5 mm optical trocar is then replaced with an 8 mm dV trocar or by the camera trocar (Fig. 26.1).

Another consideration is the accessory port. The accessory port is used to aid with the mesh introduction and orientation, suture introduction and removal, and suture cutting. We found that using the accessory trocar for the larger mesh introduction under direct visualization was safer and more efficient than introducing the mesh and sutures through the 12 mm camera port. The accessory port is less useful for the repair of smaller ventral hernias, where the orientation of the mesh and the retraction of the mesh for exposure during suture placement are less cumbersome.

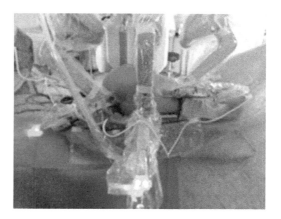

Fig. 26.3 Robot docking

The accessory port location must also be determined in relationship to the three da Vinci arms. The optimal positions are located opposite the defect between one instrument arm and the camera arm trocar and also at the subxiphoid or suprapubic area; that way it may serve for both sides if needed (Fig. 26.2). It is crucial to place the accessory port as far from the defect as possible to allow for increased range of motion and effectiveness (Fig. 26.3).

Generally, for mid-abdominal hernias, a neutral supine position is sufficient. Any patient position manipulation, however, must be performed prior to docking of the robot. The robotic cart is driven directly over the abdomen and in-line with the trocar sites.

Instrumentation

For right-handed surgeons, a dV prograsp (or fenestrated bipolar) is placed in arm #2, 8 mm or 12 mm 30° up camera in the camera port, and the dV monopolar scissors is placed in arm #1.

The dV SutureCut needle driver is used to primarily close the hernia defect as well as fixating the mesh to the abdominal wall. A fenestrated bipolar grasper instead of the prograsp might be used (Fig. 26.4).

Essential Steps

Adhesiolysis

The essential steps of robotic hernia repair are analogous to that of conventional laparoscopic repair. Adhesiolysis of the abdominal wall to isolate the hernia defect must be performed meticulously to avoid iatrogenic injury to the abdominal viscera. The dV platform facilitates adhesiolysis through its 3-D visualization, extended range of motion, tremor-less precision, and superior ergonomics.

One important distinction between conventional laparoscopy and the robotic platform is that in the latter, the surgeon is stationed at a remote location from the patient. Therefore, it is mandatory for the surgeon to always have the instruments in view. Injudicious movements of instruments outside the visual field may lead to serious iatrogenic injury.

For direct bowel handling, the dV fenestrated bipolar grasper is less traumatic to bowel serosa. It is important to emphasize the loss of haptic feedback when performing robotic surgery. This shortcoming is overcome by the improved ability to visualize individual stretch fibers. Special attention is therefore required to prevent iatrogenic bowel injury and excessive bleeding by way of atraumatic handling and judicious use of energy devices. Complete adhesiolysis is mandatory to ensure adequate evaluation of the abdominal wall. If necessary, the falciform ligament is taken down to allow for the flush placement of mesh against the abdominal wall. In the setting of dense adhesions, the robotic harmonic scalpel or dV vessel sealer may facilitate hemostasis.

Primary Closure of the Defect

Successful primary closure of the defect is facilitated by the use of the barbed V-loc suture (Covidien) or Stratafix (Ethicon Inc). Preoperative studies including physical examination, evaluation of abdominal wall compliance, and CT evaluation generally suffice in determining the feasibility of primary closure. The ability to primarily close defects without component separation is based on the principles of Ramirez regarding width and location of the hernia defect [17]. However, this is clearly based on open technique and not while working against the forces of pneumoperitoneum. As a general rule, however, a defect less than 10 cm in the mid-abdomen is amenable to primary closure. It is important to

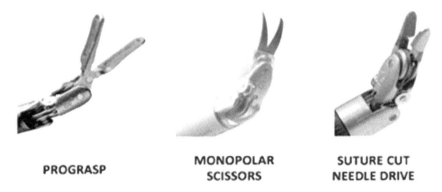

PROGRASP   MONOPOLAR   SUTURE CUT
                            SCISSORS   NEEDLE DRIVE

Fig. 26.4 Instrumentation

note that subxiphoidal and suprapubic defects are more difficult to close. Desufflating the abdominal cavity to 6–8 mmHg pneumoperitoneum may be necessary. The suture is introduced into the intra-abdominal cavity through the 8 mm dV trocar or the accessory port. It is recommended to straighten the needle to facilitate both introduction and subsequent removal through an 8 mm trocar.

Mesh Placement and Fixation

A tissue separating mesh is utilized when placed in the intraperitoneal underlay position. The sizing of the mesh is similar to the principles of traditional laparoscopy, maintaining at least 5 cm overlap in all directions. For larger defects, where primarily closure may be under moderate tension, a wider mesh is employed. Depending on the size of the prosthetic, it can be introduced through the 8 mm dV trocar, camera port, or accessory 10–15 mm port.

There are a myriad of options to secure the mesh to the abdominal wall including reproducing standard LVHR technique with a combination of tacks and full thickness transfascial sutures versus intracorporeal partial thickness suture fixation, or securing the mesh to the abdominal wall with circumferential suture fixation. With the mesh positioned on the abdominal wall by using a scroll technique or using mesh equipped with a positioning device (Ventralight ECHO, CR Bard, Cranston, RI), a full length nonabsorbable 00 or 0 monofilament suture is introduced into the intra-abdominal cavity through the same trocar as the needle holder. The external end of the suture situated outside the trocar is secured with a hemostat. This technique avoids excessive suture in the intra-abdominal cavity, thereby facilitating fixation. In a running fashion, the suture is then placed around the circumference of the mesh. It may be necessary to use more than one suture for larger prosthetics. Upon completion of mesh fixation, the robot is undocked. Only the 10–12 mm trocar fascial sites are closed with a suture passer under direct laparoscopic vision.

Robotic TAPP Ventral Hernia Repair

Exploiting the layers of the abdominal wall is made possible by the precision the dV robot affords. While feasible using conventional laparoscopy, working high on the anterior abdominal wall remains technically demanding and ergonomically challenging. Placing mesh in the preperitoneal space obviates the need for a more costly tissue separating mesh, allows the mesh to incorporate directly on fascia, and theoretically decreases the need for sutures or tack fixation. This, in turn, should reduce postoperative pain, and likely minimize complications inherent with leaving mesh in the intraperitoneal position, e.g., bowel erosion, fistula or severe adhesions.

The robotic transabdominal preperitoneal (TAPP) VHR was developed based on the TAPP inguinal hernia repair and involves dissection of the preperitoneal plane, reduction of the hernia sac, primary closure of the defect, placement of mesh, and reperitonealization of the mesh (Fig. 26.5).

Essential Steps

Patient positioning, trocar placement, docking, and instrumentation are analogous to that described above.

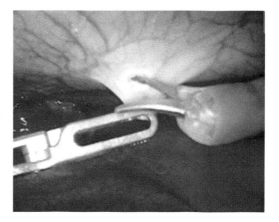

Fig. 26.5 Peritoneal incision

Developing a Preperitoneal Plane

The peritoneum is incised at least 5 cm from the hernia defect on the side of the abdomen ipsilateral to the trocar sites (Fig. 26.5). Peritoneal incision is best made in proximity of the preperitoneal fat underlying the rectus fascia. A preperitoneal plane is then developed widely with a combination of blunt and sharp technique. Care is taken to avoid disrupting the posterior fascia. In the event the posterior fascia is breached and the rectus muscle is visible, it is subsequently closed with suture. The hernia sac is reduced and dissection continues distal to the defect, thereby allowing for placement of an adequately sized mesh. Wide distal dissection allows for the creation of a large mobile flap to completely reperitonealize the mesh. If the preperitoneal space is inaccessible, the approach is modified to placement of an intraperitoneal mesh subsequent to primary closure of the defect.

Primary Closure of the Defect

The hernia defect is closed with 0 or 1 V-loc running barbed permanent or long-term absorbable suture. Desufflation of the abdominal cavity may need to be employed to facilitate closure of the hernia defect (Fig. 26.6).

Mesh Placement, Fixation, and Reperitonealization

The mesh is introduced into the intra-abdominal cavity and placed flat on the abdominal wall. Large overlap of the closed defect (5 cm mini-

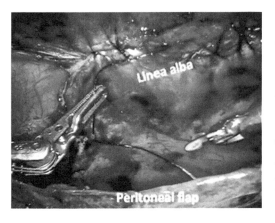

Fig. 26.6 Defect closure

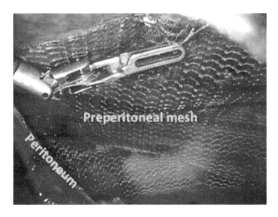

Fig. 26.7 Mesh placement

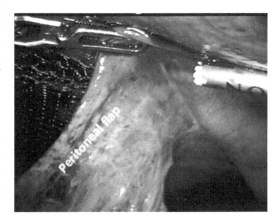

Fig. 26.8 Reperitonealization of mesh

mum in all directions) is insured. The mesh is secured to the abdominal wall with four absorbable tacks placed at the cardinal points of the mesh or with sutures as per surgeon's preference. Once adequate fixation and hemostasis is achieved, the peritoneal flap is re-approximated to cover the mesh with a continuous 00 absorbable running suture or tacks (Fig. 26.8).

Subxiphoid Hernias

Traditionally, subxiphoidal hernias have been difficult to repair laparoscopically because of the difficulty in reliably securing the mesh to the lower thoracic outlet. The preperitoneal technique obviates the need for full thickness transfascial sutures because the mesh is effectively sandwiched between the abdominal wall and peritoneum which allows the mesh to incorporate on both faces. The technique itself is analogous to that of the TAPP ventral hernia for mid-abdominal defects which involves dissecting a large preperitoneal plane, reducing the hernia sac, primary closure of the defect, mesh placement, and reperitonealization. Takedown of the falciform ligament and associated peritoneum assists in mobilizing a large flap for subsequent reperitonealization of the mesh. If the preperitoneal space is inaccessible an IPOM can be easily achieved. The mesh is secured by suturing it to the abdominal wall and diaphragm, carefully avoiding the cardiac bare area.

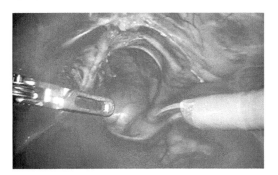

Fig. 26.9 Suprapubic hernia

Patient Positioning, Trocar Placement, and Docking

The patient is placed in a supine position with the arm tucked. The strategy again is to place the camera trocar at least 15–20 cm from the caudal aspect of the defect. Depending on body habitus and torso length, an infraumbilical incision for initial access generally works well. Two or three dV 8 mm trocars are placed in line with the 12 mm trocar with at least 6–10 cm of space between trocars. Patient positioning must be completed prior to docking of the robot. The robot is then docked over the right or left shoulder.

Suprapubic Hernias

The challenges of laparoscopic suprapubic hernia repair include the requisite mobilization of the bladder, creating a pelvic dissection within the space of Retzius, and fixating the mesh along the pelvic rim. Robotic preperitoneal repair facilitates bladder mobilization, visualization of the pelvic rim, and creation of a large preperitoneal space to accommodate overlapping mesh that is especially difficult in the setting of recurrent hernias or in patients with previous open prostatectomy (Fig. 26.9).

Patient Positioning, Trocar Placement, and Docking

The patient is placed in a supine lithotomy position. A three-way Foley catheter is placed which is used to distend the bladder for proper identification. The patient is positioned in a slight Trendelenburg position. A 12 mm camera trocar is placed in a supraumbilical location for initial access. The camera port must be at least 15–20 cm from the superior aspect of the hernia defect. Two or three dV 8 mm trocars are placed in line with the camera trocar and the robot is docked in between the legs.

Essential Steps

A preperitoneal plane is incised a minimum of 5 cm cephalad to the superior aspect of the hernia defect. A wide plane of dissection is necessary to accommodate a large sheet of overlapping mesh. The hernia defect is reduced. The superior dome of the bladder may occupy the hernia sac and therefore, great care and meticulous dissection is performed to avoid bladder injury. This is facilitated by instilling 300 cc of sterile saline into the bladder for easy identification. The retroinguinal space (space of Bogros) is developed bilaterally to expose Cooper's ligament. Dorsal mobilization of the bladder reveals the space of Retzius (Fig. 26.10). This space can be dissected inferiorly to ensure adequate overlap of mesh inferior to the caudal aspect of the hernia defect.

The hernia defect is primarily closed with 0 or #1 V-loc barbed suture as described above. Partial desufflation of the abdominal cavity may be required to adequately close the defect. The dome of the defect may also be incorporated into the closure in order to obliterate the dead space, thereby reducing the risk of seroma formation. An adequately sized light or medium weight polypropylene mesh is introduced into the abdominal cavity (Fig. 26.11). Absorbable tacks or sutures are placed to secure the mesh to the abdominal wall. Then, 00 or 0 prolene suture is used to secure the mesh to Cooper's ligament bilaterally as well as to the symphysis pubis. Upon completion of mesh fixation, the mesh is reperitonealized with 00 running absorbable suture or tacks.

Parastomal Hernia

The trocar strategy relies on the same principles as described above. The trocars are placed as far lateral as possible opposite the ostomy to ensure sufficient distance for medial mesh overlap during Sugarbaker repair (Figs. 26.12 and 26.13). After adhesiolysis, exposing the defect, and identifying the bowel limb of the ostomy, the defect is closed with 0 or 1 barbed permanent or long-term absorbable V-loc suture. We then lateralize the segment of bowel to the wall with 00 absorbable monofilament suture. The mesh is introduced through the 12–15 mm trocar depending on the size the mesh. Using mesh with a positioning device (ECHO, CR Bard) significantly facilitates

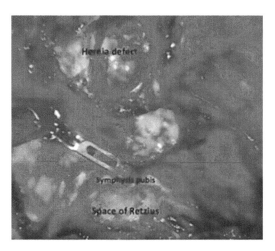

Fig. 26.10 Dissection of suprapubic space (Emailed figure 26.10)

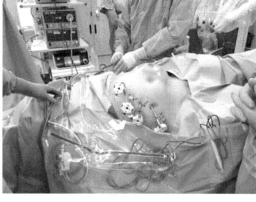

Fig. 26.12 Trocar placements in parastomal hernia repair

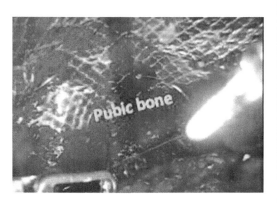

Fig. 26.11 Suture fixation to the pelvic rim

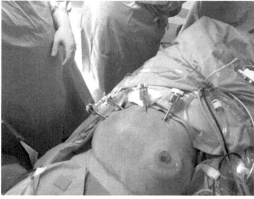

Fig. 26.13 Trocar placements in parastomal hernia repair

this step. The details of laparoscopic Sugarbaker technique are described in Chapter 23.

Robotic Rives-Stoppa Repair with Bilateral Transversus Abdominis Muscle Release

The retromuscular hernia repair as described by Rives is considered by many to be the standard by which all hernia repairs are judged [1, 2, 18]. The posterior component separation (PCS) technique allows for the closure of large hernia defects with wide prosthetic mesh overlap. These two techniques performed in tandem have traditionally been exclusive to open hernia repair.

The retromuscular repair, as described by Rives, uses the natural myofascial planes of the abdominal wall while preserving the integrity of the subcutaneous tissue [18]. In this technique, mesh is secured in the retrorectus position, sandwiched by closure of the anterior fascia above and by the posterior fascia below. With recurrence rates reported to be in the range of 0–4%, many consider this technique of open ventral hernia repair as the gold standard for all hernia repairs [1, 2]. The limitation of the Rives-Stoppa repair is that the maximal transverse diameter of the mesh is confined to the lateral edge (linea semilunaris) of the rectus muscles.

The transversus abdominis muscle release (TAR), as described by Novitsky, involves posterior sheath mobilization off the rectus, incision of the lateral posterior sheath, identification and division of the transversus abdominis, and dissection of the preperitoneal space [2]. This technique is described in detail in Chapter 13. TAR allows for wide release and advancement of the posterior rectus sheath and peritoneum below the arcuate line, preservation of the neurovascular bundle serving the rectus abdominis, and wide lateral dissection to the level of the lateral border of the psoas muscle. In the setting of large incisional hernias, this technique allows for reconstruction of the linea alba, re-approximation of the rectus to the midline, and placement of a large overlapping mesh beyond the confines of the linea semilunaris.

While considered an effective and durable technique associated with low recurrence rates, trauma to the abdominal wall via open hernia repair is associated with a high incidence of wound complications including mesh infection which may lead to unacceptable patient morbidity [13, 14]. Utilization of the daVinci robot has enabled minimally invasive replication of this technique traditionally reserved for open repair.

General Considerations

Abdominal wall reconstruction by way of PCS mandates dissection of individual layers of the abdominal wall intended to primarily close large hernia defects, create a large space for the placement of a reinforcing prosthetic mesh, and ultimately restore the anatomy and physiology of the abdominal wall. Therefore, a thorough knowledge of the anatomy of the abdominal wall is critical to optimizing patient outcome. Hernia repair by way of abdominal wall reconstruction and component separation should be highly regarded as the ultimate definitive repair for large hernias. Therefore, it is mandatory that surgeons performing robotic TAR are not only experienced in the open counterpart, but also deemed experts with the robotic platform.

It is also important to consider that robotic TAR is a technique that continues to evolve. Although larger defects have been closed in our early experience, general recommendations for hernia width remain between 10 and 16 cm. Candidates most amenable to robotic abdominal wall reconstruction are patients with large mid-abdominal wall defects. Factors which preclude robotic abdominal wall reconstruction include hernias with loss of domain, defects which extend from flank to flank or subxiphoid to pubis, and significant overlying skin issues—those patients would generally benefit from traditional open repair. Inability to gain adequate laparoscopic access is another contraindication to the robotic repair.

Patient Positioning, Trocar Placement, and Docking

For the majority of patients with large defects in the midline, supine positioning with the arms tucked is preferred, unless trocar access to the lateral abdomen is obscured. In this setting, the arms are situated at a 90° angle relative to the trunk. Trocars are placed in the lateral abdomen similar to conventional laparoscopic repair. Optical trocar technique, preferably in a location remote to previous surgical intervention is used to gain initial access. An 8–12 mm trocar is placed in the lateral abdomen and then two 8 mm trocars follow on each side of this trocar (Fig. 26.14). It is also important to consider, if you are utilizing the da Vinci SI, that this procedure requires a double docking technique. All effort should be made to communicate with the anesthesiologist and surgical staff that the patient will require 180° rotation to access the contralateral abdomen.

Essential Steps

Posterior Sheath Incision
The anterior abdominal wall is cleared of all adhesions to adequately define and size the hernia defect. The retromuscular space is accessed by incision and subsequent mobilization of the posterior sheath. Below the arcuate line, the peritoneum and transversalis fascia are mobilized in a similar fashion. The degree of cranial-caudal dissection is based on the size of the defect, assuring a bare minimum of 5 cm overlap (Fig. 26.15).

Transversus Abdominis Release
The uniform retraction afforded by pneumoperitoneum allows dissection within an avascular plane to the level of the linea semilunaris. The neurovascular bundle serving the rectus is exposed and preserved. An incision is made in the lateral posterior sheath in the upper third of the abdomen where the medial fibers of the transversus abdominis muscle are most prominent. The muscle is exposed and divided along the extent of posterior sheath and peritoneal dissection (Figs. 26.16, 26.17, 26.18 and 26.19). This step allows entry and dissection into the preperitoneal space resulting in wide release of both the posterior and anterior fascial layers.

Once sufficient posterior sheath release has been achieved, the robot is undocked, mirror image trocars are placed on the contralateral abdomen, and the patient is rotated 180° and the robot is re-docked. This step is eliminated by the rotational capability of the daVinci Xi. The contralateral posterior sheath is then dissected and the steps above are repeated.

Closure of the Anterior Sheath, Mesh Placement, and Posterior Sheath Closure
Closure of the anterior sheath is accomplished utilizing a 0 V-loc suture in a running fashion. The subcutaneous tissue and hernia sac are incor-

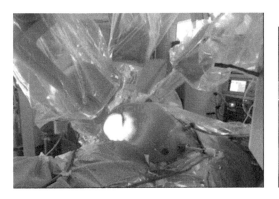

Fig. 26.14 Double docking technique and port position

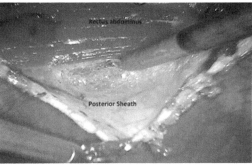

Fig. 26.15 Posterior sheath mobilization

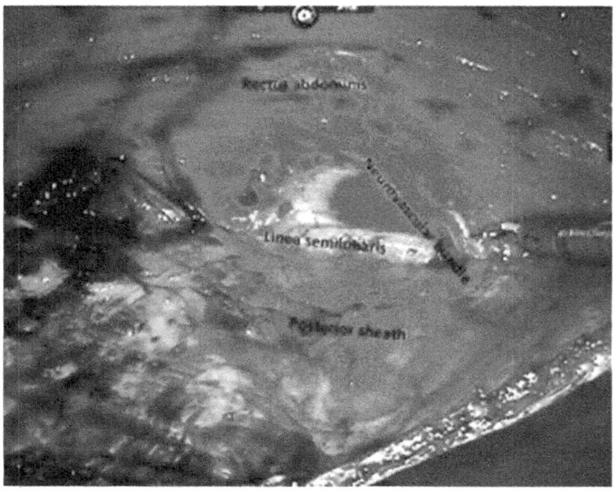

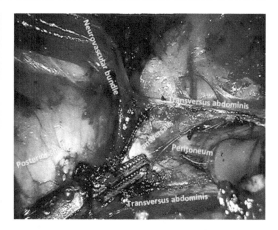

Fig. 26.16 Posterior sheath mobilization

Fig. 26.18 Division of transversus abdominis and preperitoneal plane

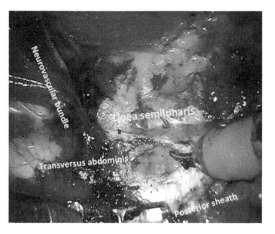

Fig. 26.17 Division of the transversus abdominis muscle and preperitoneal plane

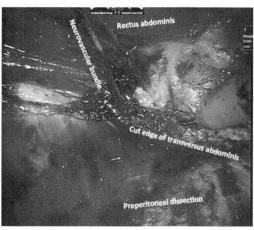

Fig. 26.19 Preperitoneal dissection

porated into the closure to obliterate the anterior dead space. This step restores the linea alba and mobilizes the rectus abdominis muscle in its correct anatomical and physiologic position.

The extent of dissection is then measured in cranial caudal and axial dimensions to choose an appropriately sized mesh. It is important that the associated length and width of the mesh completely covers the area of dissection. A single central transfascial suture is utilized to position the light or mid-weight polypropylene mesh in the retromuscular position (Fig. 26.20). Circumferential fixation is accomplished with an

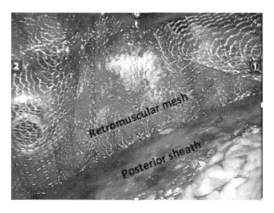

Fig. 26.20 Retromuscular mesh placement

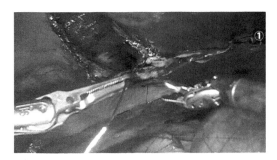

Fig. 26.21 Posterior sheath closure

absorbable tacker or suture. The posterior sheath is then re-approximated using 0 V-loc suture (Fig. 26.21). It is often helpful to incorporate a bite of mesh to elevate the two leaves of the posterior sheath away from the intra-abdominal viscera. The peritoneum is re-approximated below the arcuate line.

Drain Placement

Secondary to pneumoperitoneum, the retromuscular space represents a large potential space for seroma formation. Trocars are withdrawn from the intraperitoneal cavity and positioned into the retrorectus space under laparoscopic guidance. In this position, adequate hemostasis can be confirmed and two 19F drains are placed. Alternatively, a sequence of fascial closure which more closely resembles the open technique may be employed. This involves re-approximation of the posterior sheath after bilateral TAR is accomplished. Mesh is then placed overlying the posterior sheath along the extent of dissection. The anterior fascia is then re-approximated thereby restoring the linea alba.

Summary

The technique of robot-assisted laparoscopic incisional hernia repair with intracorporeal closure of the fascial defect and continuous circumferential suturing for mesh fixation is feasible and may reduce postoperative pain by eliminating transfascial sutures. The component separation techniques performed robotically may decrease the incidence of surgical site infection

in this difficult group of patients. Long-term data is lacking to truly assess the benefit to the patient and, therefore, further evaluations and studies are required.

References

1. Jin J, Rosen MJ. Laparoscopic versus open ventral hernia repair. Surg Clin North Am. 2008;88:1083–100.
2. Novitsky YW, Elliott HL, Orenstein SB, et al. Transversus abdominis muscle release: a novel approach to posterior component separation during complex abdominal wall reconstruction. Am J Surg. 2012;204:709–16.
3. Heniford BT, Park A, Ramshaw BJ, Voeller G. Laparoscopic repair of ventral hernias: nine years' experience with 850 consecutive hernias. Ann Surg. 2003;238:391–9.
4. Perrone JM, Soper NJ, Eagon JC, et al. Perioperative outcomes and complications of laparoscopic ventral hernia repair. Surgery. 2005;138:708–15.
5. Carbajo MA, Martin de Olmo JC, Blanco JI, et al. Laparoscopic treatment vs open surgery in the solution of major incisional and abdominal wall hernias with mesh. Surg Endosc. 1999;13:250–2.
6. Franklin ME, Dorman JP, Glass JL, et al. Laparoscopic ventral and incisional hernia repair. Surg Laparosc Endosc. 1998;8:294–9.
7. Heniford BT, Ramshaw BJ. Laparoscopic ventral hernia repair: a report of 100 consecutive cases. Surg Endosc. 2000;14:419–23.
8. Heniford BT, Park A, Ramshaw BJ, et al. Laparoscopic ventral and incisional hernia repair in 407 patients. J Am Coll Surg. 2000;190:645–50.
9. Sanders LM, Flint LM, Ferrara JJ. Initial experience with laparoscopic repair of incisional hernias. Am J Surg. 1999;177:227–31.
10. Ballantyne GH, Hourmont K, Wasielewski A. Telerobotic laparoscopic repair of incisional ventral hernias using intraperitoneal prosthetic mesh. JSLS. 2003;7:7–14.
11. Earle D, Seymour N, Fellinger E, et al. Laparoscopic versus open incisional hernia repair: a single-institution analysis of hospital resource utilization for 884 consecutive cases. Surg Endosc. 2006;20:71–5.
12. Harrell AG, Novitsky YW, Peindl RD, et al. Prospective evaluation of adhesion formation and shrinkage of intraabdominal prosthetics in a rabbit model. Am Surg. 2006;72:808–13.
13. McKinlay RD, Park A. Laparoscopic ventral incisional hernia repair: a more effective alternative to conventional repair of recurrent incisional hernia. J Gastrointest Surg. 2004;8:670–4.
14. Heniford BT, Carbonell AM, Harold K, et al. Local Injection for the Treatment of Suture Site Pain after Laparoscopic Ventral Hernia Repair. Am Surg. 2003;69:688–91.

15. Lange JF, Halm JA, de Wall LL, et al. Intraperitoneal polypropylene mesh hernia repair complicates subsequent abdominal surgery. World J Surg. 2003;31(2):423–9.
16. Ballantyne GH. Robotic surgery, telerobotic surgery, telepresence, and telementoring: review of early clinical results. Surg Endosc. 2002;16:1389–402.
17. Ramirez OM, Ruas E, Dellon AL. "Components separation" method for closure of abdominal-wall defects: an anatomic and clinical study. Plast Reconstr Surg. 1990;86:519–26.
18. Rives J, Pire JC, Flament JB, et al. Treatment of large eventrations. New therapeutic Indications apropos of 322 cases. Chirurgie. 1985;111:215–25.

Further Reading

Mudge M, Hughes LE. Incisional hernia: a 10-year prospective study of incidence and attitudes. Br J Surg. 1985;72:70–1.

LeBlanc KA, Heniford BT, Voeller GR. Innovations in ventral hernia repair. Contemp Surg 2006:1–8

Van der Linden FT, Van Vroonhoven TJ. Long-term results after surgical correction of incisional hernia. Neth J Surg. 1988;40:127–9.

Stoppa RE. The treatment of complicated groin and incisional hernia. World J Surg. 1989;13:545–54.

Laber GE, Garb JL, Alexander AI, et al. Long-term complications associated with prosthetic repair of ventral hernias. Arch Surg. 1998;133:378–82.

White TJ, Santos MC, Thompson JS. Factors affecting wound complications in repair of ventral hernias. Am Surg. 1998;64:276–80.

Berger D, Bientzle M, Muller A. Postoperative complications after laparoscopic incisional hernia repair. Surg Endosc. 2002;16:1720–3.

Bansal VK, Misra MC, Kumar S, et al. A prospective randomized study comparing suture mesh fixation versus tacker mesh fixation for laparoscopic repair of incisional and ventral hernias. Surg Endosc. 2011;25:1431–8.

Dubay DA, Wang X, Kirk S, et al. Fascial fibroblast kinetic activity is increased during abdominal wall repair compared to dermal fibroblasts. Wound Repair Regen. 2004;12:539–45.

Giulianotti PC, Coratti A, Angelini M, et al. Robotics in general surgery: personal experience in a large community hospital. Arch Surg. 2003;138:777–84.

LeBlanc KA, Booth WV. Laparoscopic repair of incisional abdominal hernias using expanded polytetrafluoroethylene: preliminary findings. Surg Laparosc Endosc. 1993;3:39–41.

Schluender S, Conrad J, Divino CM, et al. Robot-assisted laparoscopic repair of ventral hernia with intracorporeal suturing. Surg Endosc. 2003;17:1391–5.

Tayar C, Karoui M, Cherqui D, et al. Robot-assisted laparoscopic mesh repair of incisional hernias with exclu-

sive intracorporeal suturing: a pilot study. Surg Endosc. 2007;21:1786–9.

LeBlanc KA. The critical technical aspects of laparoscopic repair of ventral and incisional hernias. Am Surg. 2001;67:809–12.

Sorensen LT, Hemmingsen UB, Kirkeby LT, et al. Smoking is a risk factor for incisional hernia. Arch Surg. 2005;140:119–23.

Sauerland S, Walgenbach M, Habermalz B et al. Laparoscopic versus open surgical techniques for ventral or incisional hernia repair. Cochrane Database Syst Rev. 2011; (3):CD007781.

Forbes SS, Eskicioglu C, McLeod RS, et al. Meta-analysis of randomized controlled trials comparing open and laparoscopic ventral and incisional hernia repair with mesh. Br J Surg. 2009;96:851–8.

Sajid MS, Bokhari SA, Mallick AS, et al. Laparoscopic versus open repair of incisional/ventral hernia: a meta-analysis. Am J Surg. 2009;197:64–72.

Beldi G, Wagner M, Bruegger LE, et al. Mesh shrinkage and pain in laparoscopic ventral hernia repair: a randomized clinical trial comparing suture versus tack mesh fixation. Surg Endosc. 2011;25:749–55.

Allison N, Tieu K, Snyder B, Pigazzi A, Wilson E. Technical feasibility of a robotic assisted ventral hernia repair. World J Surg. 2012;36(2):447–52.

Bower CE, Reade CC, Kirby LW, Roth JS. Complications of laparoscopic incisional-ventral hernia repair: the experience of a single institution. Surg Endosc. 2004;18:672–5.

Cadiere GB, Himpens J, Germay O, Izizaw R, Degueldre M, Vandromme J, Capelluto E, Bruyns J. Feasibility of robotic laparoscopic surgery: 146 cases. World J Surg. 2001;25:1467–77.

Corcione F, Esposito C, Cuccurullo D, Settembre A, Miranda N, Amato F, Pirozzi F, Caiazzo P. Advantages and limits of robot-assisted laparoscopic surgery: preliminary experience. Surg Endosc. 2005;19:117–9.

Earle D, Seymour N, Fellinger E, Perez A. Laparoscopic versus open incisional hernia repair: a single-institution analysis of hospital resource utilization for 884 consecutive cases. Surg Endosc. 2006;20:71–5.

Heniford BT, Park A, Ramshaw BJ, Voeller G. Laparoscopic ventral and incisional hernia repair in 407 patients. J Am Coll Surg. 2000;190:645–50.

LeBlanc KA. Current considerations in laparoscopic incisional and ventral herniorrhaphy. JSLS. 2000;4:131–9.

LeBlanc KA. The critical technical aspects of laparoscopic repair of ventral and incisional hernias. Am Surg. 2001;67:809–12.

McKinlay RD, Park A. Laparoscopic ventral incisional hernia repair: a more effective alternative to conventional repair of recurrent incisional hernia. J Gastrointest Surg. 2004;8:670–4.

Park A, Birch DW, Lovrics P. Laparoscopic and open incisional hernia repair: a comparison study. Surgery. 1998;124:816–22.

Perrone JM, Soper NJ, Eagon JC, Klingensmith ME, Aft RL, Frisella MM, et al. Perioperative outcomes and complications of laparoscopic ventral hernia repair. Surgery. 2005;138:708–15.

Robbins SB, Pofahl WE, Gonzalez RP. Laparoscopic ventral hernia repair reduces wound complications. Am Surg. 2001;67:896–900.

Rudmik LR, Schieman C, Dixon E, Debru E. Laparoscopic incisional hernia repair: a review of the literature. Hernia. 2006;10:110–9.

Talamini MA, Chapman S, Horgan S, Melvin WS. A prospective analysis of 211 robotic-assisted surgical procedures. Surg Endosc. 2003;17:1521–4.

Tani KM, Neumayer L, Reda D, Kim L, Anthony T. Repair of ventral incisional hernia: the design of a randomized trial to compare open and laparoscopic surgical techniques. Am J Surg. 2004;188:22S–9.

Van't RM, Vrijland WW, Lange JF, Hop WC, Jeekel J, Bonjer HJ. Mesh repair of incisional hernia: comparison of laparoscopic and open repair. Eur J Surg. 2002;168:684–9.

Bageacu S, Blanc P, Breton C, Gonzales M, Porcheron J, Chamber M, Balique JG. Laparoscopic repair of incisional hernia: a retrospective review of 159 patients. Surg Endosc. 2002;16:345–8.

Bucknall TE, Cox PJ, Ellis H. Burst abdominal and incisional hernia: a prospective study of 1129 major laparotomies. Br Med J. 1982;284:931–3.

Carbajo MA, de Olmo JC M, Blanco JI, de la Cuesta C, Toledano M, Martin F, et al. Laparoscopic treatment vs open surgery in the solution of major incisional and abdominal wall hernias with mesh. Surg Endosc. 1999;13:250–2.

Franklin ME, Dorman JP, Glass JL, Balli JE, Gonzalez JJ. Laparoscopic ventral and incisional hernia repair. Surg Laparosc Endosc. 1998;8:294–9.

Heniford BT, Ramshaw BJ. Laparoscopic ventral hernia repair: a report of 100 consecutive cases. Surg Endosc. 2000;14:419–23.

Hesselink VJ, Luijendijk RW, Heide R, Jeekel J. An evaluation of risk factors in incisional hernia recurrence. Surg Gynecol Obstet. 1993;176:228–34.

Holzman MD, Purut CM, Reintgen K, Eubanks S, Pappas TN. Laparoscopic ventral and incisional hernia repair. Surg Endosc. 1997;11:32–5.

Kyzer S, Alis M, Aloni Y, Charuzi I. Laparoscopic repair of postoperation ventral hernia. Surg Endosc. 1999;13:928–31.

LeBlanc KA, Booth WV, Whitaker JM, Bellanger DE. Laparoscopic incisional and ventral herniorrhaphy: our initial 100 patients. Hernia. 2001;5:41–5.

Luxembourger O, Regairaz C. La cure des hernies et eventrations ombilicales et sous-ombilicales sous celioscopie: a propos de 22 cas. Lyon Chir. 1997;2: 130–1.

Ramshaw BJ, Esartic P, Schwab J, Mason EM, Wilson RA, Duncan TD, Miller J, Lucas GW, Promes J. Comparison of laparoscopic and open ventral herniorrhaphy. Am Surg. 1999;65:827–31.

Renier JF, Bokobza B, Leturgie C, Merveille M, Selamn M, Sfihi A. Cure des eventrations soud laparoscopie par plaque intraperitoneal d'ePTFE: technique et resultants, apropos de 135 cases. J Coeliochir. 1999; 32:63–7.

Sanders LM, Flint LM, Ferrara JJ. Initial experience with laparoscopic repair of incisional hernias. Am J Surg. 1999;177:227–31.

Thoman DS, Phillips EH. Current status of laparoscopic ventral hernia repair. Surg Endosc. 2002;16(932–942): 1395.

Evidence-Based Optimal Fixation During Laparoscopic Hernia Repair: Sutures, Tacks, and Glues

H. Reza Zahiri and Igor Belyansky

Introduction

Mesh fixation during ventral and inguinal hernia repair is a critical step which should aim to secure the mesh in place, and prevent hernia recurrence while promoting rapid ingrowth and reducing associated pain, formation of adhesions, and mesh shrinkage [1]. Additional consideration should be given to the prevention of seroma, infection, and fistula during this important step. Correctly selecting the appropriate mesh and fixation device contributes significantly towards these goals. For example, a macroporous mesh paired with a smaller fixation device will inevitably lead to an inadequate mesh/device interface and weak securing of the mesh.

At present, seventeen various devices may be used for mesh fixation, which may be divided into four categories: Nonabsorbable tacks, absorbable tacks, sutures, and glues [1]. There are also a variety of mesh products available on the market, including two with self-adhering properties. Nevertheless, the focus of this chapter is on fixation options, and a detailed discussion of mesh types is beyond the scope of this chapter.

Fixation Products

Nonabsorbable Tacks

Three products exist under this category and it is the most common technique for securing mesh in place during hernia repair due to strength and facility of use [1]. The ProTack™ (Covidien Corp., Mansfield, MA) is the most popular of the three and utilizes helical titanium tacks with a diameter of 5 mm and length of 3.8 mm. The EndoAnchor™ (Ethicon Endosurgery, Inc., Cincinnati, OH) uses a double-armed nickel titanium tack with a length of 5.9 mm. Finally, the PermaFix™ (Bard Davol, Warwick, RI) uses hollow core tacks made of polymer blend with a 6.8 mm penetration depth.

Current evidence, regarding both nonabsorbable and absorbable tacks, if used as an exclusive means of fixation, supports application in a double row or "double crown" fashion (an outer row 0.5 cm from the mesh edge, and an inner row around the fascial defect) [2]. Tacks should not be spaced more than 1–2 cm apart. Figure 27.1 illustrates the "double crown" technique with two rows of fixation.

Absorbable Tacks

Six products exist under this category [1]. Securestrap™ (Ethicon EndoSurgery, Inc., Cincinnati, OH) is designed to resemble a strap

H.R. Zahiri, D.O. • I. Belyansky, M.D. (✉)
Department of Surgery, Anne Arundel Medical
Center, Annapolis, MD, USA
e-mail: igor.belyansky@gmail.com

© Springer International Publishing Switzerland 2016
Y.W. Novitsky (ed.), *Hernia Surgery*, DOI 10.1007/978-3-319-27470-6_27

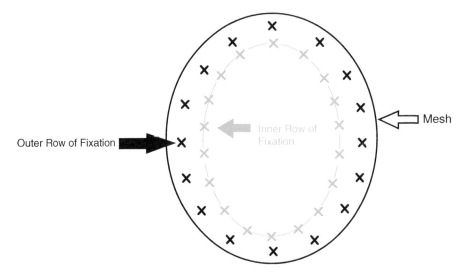

Fig. 27.1 The "double crown" technique of mesh fixation with two rows of tacks, an outer and an inner layer

with two points of fixation that are 6.7 mm long. Its absorption time is 12 months. AbsorbaTack™ (Covidien Corp., Mansfield, MA) is designed like a screw with 4 mm of penetration and an absorption time of 6–12 months. Sorbafix™ (Bard Davol, Warwick, RI) is designed with a hollow core and blunt edge, promising enhanced tissue integration. Its reach after deployment is 6.8 mm and is absorbed after 1 year. I-Clip™ (Covidien Corp, Mansfield, MA) is 7.5 mm in length and also completes absorption in 1 year. PermaSorb™ (Bard Davol, Warwick, RI) utilizes a needle as an introducer to facilitate mesh and tissue entry, reaching 5 mm of depth with an absorption time of 16 months. Finally, the iMesh Tacker™ (Easy-Lap, Wrentham, MA) uses an articulating tip to deliver helical tacks that reach 6.3 mm with an unknown absorption time.

Adhesives

Tissue sealants may be utilized as atraumatic fixators of mesh products [1]. This category can be further divided into synthetic, biologic, and genetically engineered polymer protein glues. Under the synthetic products sub-category, cyanoacrylate, marketed as Histoacryl™ (B. Braun

Melsungen AG, Melsungen, Germany) and Glubran II™ (GEM, Viareggio, Italy), reacts with water to polymerize and join adjacent surfaces within 60 s. In time, the hardened glue will undergo hydrolysis and degradation allowing for tissue ingrowth. Thus, limited targeted use is recommended to prevent delays in tissue integration while adequately fixing mesh. Under the biologic glue sub-category, fibrin sealant is marketed as EVICEL® (Ethicon EndoSurgery, Inc., Cincinnati, OH), Tisseel™, Tissucol™, and Artiss™ (Baxter, Deerfield, IL) comprise a sealer protein solution and a thrombin solution. These are mixed at the time of fixation to duplicate the terminal coagulation reaction and generate polymerized fibrin. Applied to mesh, it can serve as a fixator, with 3 min required for reaction completion. Another product, Bioglue™ (CryoLife Inc., Kennesaw, GA), combines bovine serum albumin and glutaraldehyde to provide stable adhesion lasting 12 months prior to breakdown. Finally, genetically engineered polymer protein glues mainly have applications in the laboratory due to cost, but efforts persist to incorporate their use in the clinical settings in the near future.

Table 27.1 is a summary of various fixation devices and their properties.

Table 27.1 Comparison of fixation products

Fixation device	Image	Company	Type	Material	Depth of penetration (mm)
ProTack™		Covidien (Mansfield, MA)	Nonabsorbable	Titanium	3.8
EndoAnchor™		Ethicon (Cincinnati, OH)	Nonabsorbable	Nickel	5.9
PermaFix™		Bard Davol (Warwick, RI)	Nonabsorbable	Molded polymer blend	6.8
Securestrap™		Ethicon (Cincinnati, OH)	Absorbable	Polydioxanone/L(−)-Lactide/Glycolide	6.7
AbsorbaTack™		Covidien (Mansfield, MA)	Absorbable	Polyester from lactic and glycolic acid copolymers	4
SorbaFix™		Bard Davol (Warwick, RI)	Absorbable	Poly (D,L) lactide material	6.8
I-Clip™	Not Available	Covidien (Mansfield, MA)	Absorbable	Poly (D,L) lactide material	7.5
iMesh™	Not Available	Easy-Lap (Wrentham, MA)	Absorbable	Polyester from lactic and glycolic acid copolymers	6.3

continued

Fixation device	Image	Company	Type	Material	Depth of penetration (mm)
Hisoacryl™		B. Braun Melsungen AG (Melsungen, Germany)	Adhesive	Cyanoacrylate based	N/A
Glubran II™		GEM (Viareggio, Italy)	Adhesive	Cyanoacrylate based	N/A
Evicel™		Ethicon (Cincinnati, OH)	Adhesive	Fibrin sealant; 2-component: sealer protein and thrombin	N/A
Tisseel™/Tissucol™/Artiss™		Baxter (Deerfield, IL)	Adhesive	Fibrin sealant; 2-component: sealer protein and thrombin	N/A
Bioglue™		CryoLife (Kennesaw, GA)	Adhesive	2-Component: bovine serum albumin and glutaraldehyde	N/A

Source: Harslof SS, Wara P and Friis-Andersen H. Fixation Devices in Laparoscopic Ventral Hernia Repair: A Review. Surg Technol Int. 2014. Mar;24:203–13

Sutures

Both absorbable and nonabsorbable sutures may be used to fix mesh to the abdominal wall [1]. Generally, these are applied transfascially after reduction of intraperitoneal pressure (roughly 8 mmHg down from 12 mmHg), incorporating the abdominal wall musculoaponeurotic layers. A suture passer is often utilized to guide sutures through the wall. Suture selection, quantity, and placement are widely variable among surgeons with no favored evidence-supported technique.

Current Evidence

Laparoscopic Ventral/Incisional Hernia Repair

Currently, most surgeons secure the mesh to the abdominal wall using a combination of sutures and tacks [3]. Incidence of hernia recurrence after laparoscopic surgery is cited in the literature as ranging from 0 to 17.6% [4–9]. The incidence of postoperative short-term pain (<4 weeks) may range from 2.5 to 35% [10–13]. Chronic pain (>4 weeks) after surgery affects 0.7–20% of patients depending on method of fixation [10, 12, 14–24].

Several randomized prospective studies have been conducted to determine the ideal mesh fixation in laparoscopic ventral or incisional hernia repair. In 2013, the WoW trial (with or without sutures) analyzed "double crown" tack vs. suture and tack fixation techniques in a randomized prospective clinical trial with 76 patients enrolled [25]. In this trial, hernia recurrence was determined to be 7.9% after 24 months of follow-up with no statistically significant difference between the groups. Additionally, pain post hernia repair was compared as the primary outcome using the validated visual analog scale (VAS) [26, 27] at rest and with coughing at 4 hours, 1 month, and 3 months. Pain was significantly higher when sutures were used at 4 hours and at 3 months compared to tacks alone. In another randomized prospective study, Eriksen and associates followed 34 patients for 12 months after

laparoscopic ventral/umbilical hernia repair with fibrin sealant vs. titanium tack fixation [28]. Although the study was not adequately powered, the authors observed a high overall hernia recurrence rate of 17% with an increased trend in the fibrin sealant group. *Bansal et al.* compared suture to tack fixation in two randomized prospective studies [29, 30]. They found no difference in recurrence rates between the groups with up to 32.2 months of follow-up. Pain was significantly higher with tacks up to 3 months post surgery, but was not different between the groups at 32 months of follow-up. A randomized clinical trial by Beldi et al., in 2011, analyzed nonabsorbable suture vs. tacks in 36 patients with 8 cm hernia defects over a 6-month period [31]. They found no difference in recurrence rates between the two groups. Pain was higher with sutures at 6 weeks but no significant difference at 6 months was detected. Finally, Wassenaar et al. prospectively compared three groups (absorbable sutures with tacks, tacks alone, and nonabsorbable sutures with tacks) in a randomized fashion [32]. They concluded no difference in postoperative pain and complications between the three groups.

Studies analyzing various mesh fixation methods include, most recently, a meta-analysis looking at 25 retrospective and prospective trials comparing fixation with tacks and sutures vs. tacks alone vs. nonabsorbable sutures alone determined an overall hernia recurrence rate of 2.7% (95% CI [1.9–3.4%]) and no statistically significant difference in recurrence rates between the compared groups [33]. Furthermore, while pain in both the early postoperative period (<4 weeks) and long term (>1 month) were increased with any type of invasive mesh fixation, sutures were associated with more pain compared to tacks. In a 2013 retrospective study, nonabsorbable titanium and absorbable tacks were compared for mesh fixation in 38 patients [34]. No difference in recurrence rates or pain at 30 days was found, with one patient having hernia recurrence in each group after mean follow-up of 10.7–14.6 months. In a review of the literature, Turner and Brill determined that the superiority of suture fixation in terms of recurrence or prolonged pain was not supported compared to tacks and staples alone and infection rates rose with the use of sutures through the abdominal wall [35].

While some studies have found increased infections [2, 35] and decreased mesh shrinkage [31] with transfascial sutures, no consistent difference has been found with respect to seroma formation [30, 36], fixation strength [37–49], and adhesion formation [37, 38, 42, 50–54].

Laparoscopic Inguinal Hernia Repair

Both transabdominal (TAPP) or total extraperitoneal (TEP) laparoscopic techniques have been used to address inguinal hernias beginning in the 1990s [55]. While patients have benefited from diminished pain and faster recovery compared to the open approach, 22.5% of patients still develop chronic pain after laparoscopic inguinal hernia repair [56]. Pain may be neurogenic secondary to nerve impingement or nonneurogenic from periosteal injury, both caused by fixation device. Thus, there have been efforts to secure mesh less invasively during inguinal hernia repair.

Several randomized prospective studies have been conducted to analyze fixation methods of mesh for laparoscopic inguinal hernia repair. Melissa et al. compared fibrin sealant to stapling in TEP repairs [57]. They studied postoperative acute and chronic pain, recurrence incidence, seroma formation, analgesic requirements, quality of life, and costs. They found that fibrin sealant was associated with lower post operative day 1 pain and hospitalization costs but was comparable to staples in every other category with 6 months of follow-up. Another study in 2012 looked at fibrin sealant vs. staple mesh fixation in TAPP repair with 1 year of follow-up [58]. This study found no difference in pain, quality of life, or recurrence between the study groups. In a 2007 study, Lovisetto et al. compared fibrin glue to staples in TAPP repairs in 197 patients and found the fibrin sealant group had significantly less pain, faster recovery, and better quality of life at 1 month with no difference in recurrence rates after 12 months of follow-up [59]. In a 2005 study, 93 patients were randomized to either fibrin sealant or stapling for mesh fixation [60]. The primary

endpoints were pain, analgesic requirements, and seroma formation. Secondary endpoints included length of hospital stay, time to recovery, recurrences, and chronic pain. This study found that, in comparison to the staple group, the fibrin sealant group used significantly less analgesics post surgery, but also had significantly higher rates of seroma formation (17.4% vs. 5.3%, $p=0.009$). No other statistically significant differences were found between the groups.

In 2011, Belyansky et al. reported on quality of life outcomes of 2086 patients who underwent inguinal hernia repair. This study demonstrated that use of more than ten tacks, recurrent hernia repairs, and bilateral hernia repairs were significant predictors of postoperative pain. The number of tacks used varied significantly, where in 18.1% of TAPP and 2.3% of TEP cases surgeons used more than ten tacks ($P=0.005$). The incidence of hernia recurrences was equivalent and the number or type of tacks utilized did not impact recurrence rates [61].

In a 2012 meta-analysis study, 662 TEP repairs were analyzed comparing fibrin sealant to staple/tack mesh fixation [55]. This study found significantly higher pain at 3 months post surgery in the staple/tack group compared to fibrin sealant with no difference in operating time, seroma development, length of hospitalization, or time to recovery between the groups.

Authors Practice and Recommendations

After laparoscopic repair of ventral/incisional hernias, patients' postoperative pain is proportional to the amount of invasive fixation material (tacks or sutures) used, which has an impact on their recovery. Currently in our practice, smaller defects (<4 cm in greatest diameter) are addressed with primary closure using a transfascial suture fixation device and then reinforced with mesh via the laparoscopic approach. In such cases, mesh is secured with tackers only.

For large abdominal defects (5–10 cm in greatest diameter), we aim for at least 4–5 cm of defect overlap with a prosthetic device. Of note, an attempt is still made to close the defect primarily with a transfascial suture fixation device when possible. During mesh placement, the authors use at least four axis transfascial sutures at the 12, 3, 6, and 9 o'clock points. After positioning, tackers are used in a double crown fashion to secure the periphery of the mesh to the anterior abdominal wall. Tackers are positioned approximately 1 cm away from each other. It should be noted that the need for axial sutures to position the mesh may soon be unnecessary with the recent advent of various laparoscopic devices to assist with mesh placement.

For cases with defects greater than 10 cm in diameter, the authors use transfascial sutures to prevent potential migration of the mesh. With older heavy weight prosthetic materials, mesh contraction is a real risk and extra suture fixation may play an important role in the long run to prevent mesh migration. With newer lightweight materials, we have observed higher rates of mesh eventration after repair of larger defects. Therefore, in our practice, we attempt laparoscopic vs. open approach for primary closure of all larger defects. In addition, primary closure of the large defects may improve abdominal wall functionality, although no current level one data exists to support this notion. When dealing with incisional/ventral hernia defects, adhesive sealants are not used by the authors to secure the mesh as higher trends of hernia recurrence have been observed in such cases.

When performing laparoscopic inguinal hernia repairs, the authors typically secure the mesh with tacks ensuring that there is at least two points of fixation to prevent mesh rotation or migration in the early postoperative period. Care is taken not to place tacks in the Triangles of Doom and/or Pain to avoid injuring iliac vessels and sensory nerve structures. Use of adhesive sealants is a good alternative to tackers in such cases without inadvertent increase in inguinal hernia recurrence rates.

Conclusions

Overall, the current literature does not consistently support any particular fixation technique over another for laparoscopic hernia repair. Even

for well-conducted randomized prospective studies, there is limited long-term follow-up data. Therefore, any definitive conclusions regarding best fixation technique are not possible. While there is some indication that sutures add additional stability to fixation of mesh, they may also be associated with more acute and chronic pain. Tacks and staples may reduce pain compared to sutures, but may not prevent mesh shrinkage and migration and are more invasive than glue fixation. Glue fixation has not been definitively shown to be inferior to other fixation modalities, although data indicates its trend towards higher recurrence rates.

Acknowledgment We would like to thank Mr. Ivan George and Mr. Paxton Paganelli for all their help and efforts in preparing our graphics and figure illustrations.

References

1. Harslof SS, Wara P, Friis-Andersen H. Fixation devices in laparoscopic ventral hernia repair: a review. Surg Technol Int. 2014;24:203–13.
2. Morales-Conde S, Cadet H, Cano A, et al. Laparoscopic ventral hernia repair without sutures-double crown technique: our experience after 140 cases with a mean follow-up of 40 months. Int Surg. 2005;90:S56–62.
3. Heniford BT, Park A, Ramshaw BJ, et al. Laparoscopic repair of ventral hernias: nine Years' experience with 850 consecutive hernias. Ann Surg. 2003;238:391–400.
4. Garcea G, Ngu W, Neal CP, et al. Results from a consecutive series of laparoscopic incisional and ventral hernia repair. Surg Laparosc Endosc Percutan Tech. 2012;21:173–80.
5. Itani KM, Hur K, Kim LT, et al. Veterans affairs ventral incisional hernia investigators. Comparison of laparoscopic and open repair with mesh for the treatment of ventral incisional hernia: a randomized trial. Arch Surg. 2010;145:322–8.
6. Lahon M, Simoens C, Thill V, et al. A retrospective study of 74 laparoscopic repair of incisional hernias. Acta Chir Belg. 2009;109:595–601.
7. Carbajo MA, del Olmo JCM, Blanco JI, et al. Laparoscopic treatment versus open surgery in the solution of major incisional and abdominal wall hernias with mesh. Surg Endosc. 1999;13:250–2.
8. Barbaros U, Asoglu O, Seven R, et al. The comparison of laparoscopic and open ventral hernia repairs: a prospective randomized study. Hernia. 2007;11:51–6.
9. Bencini L, Sanchez LJ, Boffi B, et al. Incisional hernia repair: retrospective comparison of laparoscopic and open techniques. Surg Endosc. 2003;17:1546–51.

10. Stickel M, Rentsch M, Clevert DA, et al. Laparoscopic mesh repair of incisional hernia: an alternative to the conventional open repair? Hernia. 2007;11:217–22.

11. Gananadha S, Samra JS, Smith GS, et al. Laparoscopic ePTFE mesh repair of incisional and ventral hernias. ANZ J Surg. 2008;78:907–13.

12. Chelala E, Thoma M, Tatete B, et al. The suturing concept for laparoscopic mesh fixation in ventral and incisional hernia repair: mid-term analysis of 400 cases. Surg Endosc. 2007;21:391–5.

13. Palanivelu C, Jani KV, Senthilnathan P, et al. Laparoscopic sutured closure with mesh reinforcement of incisional hernias. Hernia. 2007;11:223–8.

14. Carbajo MA, del Olmo JCM, Blanco JI, et al. Laparoscopic approach to incisional hernia. Surg Endosc. 2003;17:118–22.

15. Reitter DR, Paulsen JK, Debord JR, et al. Five-year experience with the "four-before" laparoscopic ventral hernia repair. Am Surg. 2000;66:465–9.

16. Parker 3rd HH, Nottingham JM, Bynoe RP, et al. Laparoscopic repair of large incisional hernias. Am Surg. 2002;68:530–4.

17. Cobb WS, Kercher KW, Matthews BD, et al. Laparoscopic ventral hernia repair: a single center experience. Hernia. 2006;10:236–42.

18. Saber AA, Elgamal MH, Rao AJ, et al. A simplified laparoscopic ventral hernia repair: the scroll technique. Surg Endosc. 2008;22:2527–31.

19. Olmi S, Brba L, Magnone S, Bertolini A, et al. Prospective clinical study of laparoscopic treatment of incisional and ventral hernia using a composite mesh: indications, complications and results. Hernia. 2006;10:243–7.

20. Baccari P, Nifosi J, Ghirardelli L, et al. Laparoscopic incisional and ventral hernia repair without sutures: a single-center experience with 200 cases. J Laparoendosc Adv Surg Tech A. 2009;19:175–9.

21. Bencini L, Sanchez LJ, Bernini M, et al. Predictors of recurrence after laparoscopic ventral hernia repair. Surg Laparosc Endosc Percutan Tech. 2009;19:128–32.

22. Moreno-Egea A, Bustos JA, Girela E, et al. Long-term results of laparoscopic repair of incisional hernias using an intraperitoneal composite mesh. Surg Endosc. 2010;24:359–65.

23. Theodoropoulou K, Lethaby D, Hill J, et al. Laparoscopic hernia repair: a two-port technique. JSLS. 2010;14:103–5.

24. Alkhoury FHS, Ippolito R. Cost and clinical outcomes of laparoscopic ventral hernia repair using intraperitoneal nonheavyweight polyprolene mesh. Surg Laparosc Endosc Percutan Tech. 2011;21:82–5.

25. Muysoms F, Vander-Mijnsbrugge G, Pletinckx P, et al. Randomized clinical trial of mesh fixation with "double crown" versus "sutures and tackers" in laparoscopic ventral hernia repair. Hernia. 2013; 17:603–12.

26. DeLoach LJ, Higgins MS, Caplan AB, et al. The visual analog scale in the immediate postoperative period: intrasubject variability and correlation with a numeric scale. Anesth Analg. 1998;86:102–6.

27. Gallagher EJ, Bijur PE, Latimer C, et al. Reliability and validity of a visual analog scale for acute abdominal pain in the ED. Am J Emerg Med. 2002;20:287–90.

28. Eriksen JR, Bisgaard T, Assaadzadeh S, et al. Fibrin sealant for mesh fixation in laparoscopic umbilical hernia repair: 1-year results of a randomized controlled double-blinded study. Hernia. 2013; 17(4):511–4.

29. Bansal VK, Misra MC, Babu D, et al. Comparison of long-term outcome and quality of life after laparoscopic repair of incisional and ventral hernias with suture fixation with and without tacks: a prospective, randomized, controlled study. Surg Endosc. 2012;26(12):3476–85.

30. Bansal VK, Misra MC, Kumar S, et al. A prospective randomized study comparing suture mesh fixation versus tacker mesh fixation for laparoscopic repair of incisional and ventral hernias. Surg Endosc. 2011;25(5):1431–8.

31. Beldi G, Wagner M, Bruegger LE, et al. Mesh shrinkage and pain in laparoscopic ventral hernia repair: a randomized clinical trial comparing suture versus tack mesh fixation. Surg Endosc. 2011;25:749–55.

32. Wassenaar E, Schoenmaeckers E, Raymakers J, et al. Mesh-fixation method and pain and quality of life after laparoscopic ventral or incisional hernia repair: a randomized trial of three fixation techniques. Surg Endosc. 2010;24:1296–302.

33. Reynvoet E, Deschepper E, Rogiers X, et al. Laparoscopic ventral hernia repair: is there Ann optimal mesh fixation technique? a systematic review. Langenbecks Arch Surg. 2014;399:55–63.

34. Cavallaro G, Campanile FC, Rizzello M, et al. Lightweight polypropylene mesh fixation in laparoscopic incisional hernia repair. Min Inv Ther. 2013;22:283–7.

35. Brill JB, Tuner PL. Long-term outcomes with transfascial sutures versus tacks in laparoscopic ventral hernia repair: a review. Am Surg. 2011;4:458–65.

36. Olmi S, Cesana G, Sagutti L, et al. Laparoscopic incisional hernia repair with fibrin glue in select patients. JSLS. 2010;14:240–5.

37. Hollinsky C, Kolbe T, Walter I, et al. Tensile strength and adhesion formation of mesh fixation systems used in laparoscopic incisional hernia repair. Surg Endosc. 2010;24:1318–24.

38. LeBlanc KA, Stout RW, Kearney MT, et al. Comparison of adhesions formation associated with pro-tack (US surgical) versus a new mesh fixation device, salute (ONUX medical). Surg Endosc. 2003;17:1409–17.

39. Melman L, Jenkins ED, Deeken CR, et al. Evaluation of acute fixation strength for mechanical tacking devices and fibrin sealant versus polypropylene suture for laparoscopic ventral hernia repair. Surg Innov. 2010;17:285–90.

40. Dilege E, Deveci U, Erbil Y, et al. N-butyl cyanoacrylate versus conventional suturing for fixation of meshes in an incisional hernia model. J Invest Surg. 2010;23:262–6.

41. Hollinsky C, Kolbe T, Walter I, et al. Comaprison of a new self-gripping mesh with other fixation methods for laparoscopic hernia repair in a rat model. J Am Coll. 2009;208:1107–14.

42. Clarke T, Katkhouda N, Mason RJ, et al. Fibrin glue for Intraperitoneal laparoscopic mesh fixation: a comparative study in a swine model. Surg Endosc. 2011;25:737–48.

43. van't Riet M, de vos van Steenwijk PJ, Kleinrensink GJ, et al. Tensile strength of mesh fixation methods in laparoscopic incisional hernia repair. Surg Endosc. 2002;16:1713–6.

44. Petter-Puchner AH, Fortelny R, Mitter-mayr R, et al. Fibrin sealing versus stapling of hernia meshes in an onlay model in the rat. 2005;9:322–9.

45. Jenkins ED, Melman L, Desai S, et al. Evaluation of intraperitoneal placement of absorbable and nonabsorbable barrier coated mesh secured with fibrin sealant in a New Zealand white rabbit model. Surg Endosc. 2011;25:604–12.

46. Gruber-Blum S, Petter-Puchner AH, Mika K, et al. A comparison of a bovine albumin/glutaraldehyde glue versus fibrin sealant for hernia mesh fixation in experimental onlay and IPOM repair in rats. Surg Endosc. 2010;24:3086–94.

47. Fortelny RH, Petter-Puchner AH, Walder N, et al. Cyanoacrylate tissue sealant impairs tissue integration of macroporous mesh in experimental hernia repair. Surg Endosc. 2007;21:1781–5.

48. Ladurner R, Drosse I, Burklein D, et al. Cyanoacrylate glue for intra-abdominal mesh fixation of polypropylene-polyvinylidene fluoride meshes in a rabbit model. J Surg Res. 2011;167:e157–62.

49. Losi P, Burchielli S, Spiller D, et al. Cyanoacrylate surgical glue as an alternative to suture threads for mesh fixation in hernia repair. J Surg Res. 2010;163:e53–8.

50. Reynvoet E, Berrevoet F, De Somer F, et al. Tensile strength testing for resorbable mesh fixation systems in laparoscopic ventral hernia repair. Surg Endosc. 2012;26(9):1–8.

51. Eriksen JR, Bech JI, Linnemann D, et al. Laparoscopic intraperitoneal mesh fixation with fibrin sealant (Tisseel) vs. titanium tacks: a randomised controlled experimental study in pigs. Hernia. 2008;12:483–91.

52. Zinther NB, Wara P, Friis-Andersen H. Intraperitoneal onlay mesh: an experimental study of adhesion formations in a sheep model. Hernia. 2010;14:283–9.

53. Byrd JF, Agee N, Swan RZ, et al. Evaluation of absorbable and permanent mesh fixation devices: adhesion formation and mechanical strength. Hernia. 2011;15:553–8.

54. Petter-Puchner AH, Walder N, Redl H, et al. Fibrin sealant (Tissucol) enhances tissue integration of condensed polytetrafluoroethylene meshes and reduces early adhesion formation in experimental intraabdominal peritoneal onlay mesh repair. J Surg Res. 2008;150:190–5.

55. Kaul A, Hutfless S, Le H, et al. Staple versus fibrin glue fixation in laparoscopic total extraperitoneal repair of inguinal hernia: a systematic review and meta-analysis. Surg Endosc. 2012;26:1269–78.

56. Hindmarsh AC, Cheong E, Lewis MPN, et al. Attendance at a pain clinic with severe chronic pain after open and laparoscopic inguinal hernia repairs. Br J Surg. 2003;90:1152–4.

57. Melissa CS, Yuen Bun TA, Wing CK, et al. Randomized double-blinded prospective trial of fibrin sealant spray versus mechanical stapling in laparoscopic total extraperitoneal hernioplasty. Ann Surg. 2014;259(3):432–7.

58. Fortelny RH, Petter-Puchner AH, May C, et al. The impact of atraumatic fibrin sealant vs. staple mesh fixation in TAPP hernia repair on chronic pain and quality of life: results of a randomized controlled study. Surg Endosc. 2012;26(1):249–54.

59. Lovisetto F, Zonta S, Rota E, et al. Use of human fibrin glue (Tissucol) versus staples for mesh fixation in laparoscopic transabdominal preperitoneal hernioplasty: a prospective randomized study. Ann Surg. 2007;245(2):222–31.

60. Lau H. Fibrin sealant versus mechanical stapling for mesh fixation during endoscopic extraperitoneal inguinal hernioplasty. Ann Surg. 2005;242 (5):670–4.

61. Belyansky I, Tsirline VB, Klima DA, et al. Prospective, comparative study of postoperative quality of life in TEP, TAPP, and modified Lichtenstein repairs. Ann Surg. 2011;254(5):709–15.

Karan Chopra and Devinder Singh

Introduction

The resection of a panniculus was first described in 1890 by Demars and Marx who performed the operation in conjunction with large umbilical hernia repair [3]. It was later described in the USA, in 1892, by Kelly who performed the operation to facilitate not only hernia repair, but also gynecologic operations [4]. There are obvious aesthetic and functional benefits to performing panniculectomy (abdominal dermolipectomy), such as improved ambulation and decreased rashing. Another important benefit relates to the potential increase in perfusion to the abdominal skin. Adipose tissue is known to be relatively ischemic as compared to skin and muscle; therefore the presence of abundant adipose tissue can lead to a microvascular "steal" phenomenon resulting in decreased perfusion to healing

Electronic supplementary material: The online version of this chapter (doi:10.1007/978-3-319-27470-6_28) contains supplementary material, which is available to authorized users.

K. Chopra, M.D. (✉)
Department of Plastic Surgery, School of Medicine, Johns Hopkins University, Baltimore, MD, USA
e-mail: kchopra4@jhmi.edu

D. Singh, M.D.
Chief of Plastic Surgery, Anne Arundel Medical Center, Annapolis, MD, USA
e-mail: dsingh@smail.umaryland.edu

midline incisions. While the addition of a transverse waistline incision may at first appear to increase the burden of healing, it is truly beneficial to overall tissue perfusion, reduction in excess weight and tension, and possible decreases in deadspace and resultant seromas. There is now evidence in the plastic surgery literature that patients undergoing hernia repair with simultaneous panniculectomy suffer from fewer major wound and overall complications [5–8]. When used in conjunction with ventral hernia repair, concomitant panniculectomy is a powerful adjunctive procedure with the ability to reduce postoperative morbidity during abdominal wall reconstruction.

There are conceptual overlaps between the panniculectomy operation and abdominoplasty operation, but there are important distinctions. The panniculectomy operation (abdominal dermolipectomy), in the traditional sense involves simply performing a "wedge excision" of abdominal skin and fat, without umbilicoplasty or fascial plication, followed by primary closure. An abdominoplasty, on the other hand, involves not only removal of pannicular abdominal skin and fat, but also entails significant undermining of the upper abdominal skin, transposition of the umbilicus, and fascial plication prior to closure. When performing concomitant panniculectomy at the time of ventral hernia repair, undermining is still often performed in order to access the fascial defect, particularly with onlay mesh placement. Further confusion may arise with respect to the fascial closure. When performing panniculec-tomy at the time of hernia repair there is closure of the fascial defect, however fascial plication is not performed. The decision to preserve the umbilicus is often based on surgeon preference and intraoperative viability of the umbilicus.

Indications

The decision to perform concurrent panniculec-tomy with ventral hernia repair is based on the surgeon's desire to improve the patient's overall complication profile and reduce the likelihood of postoperative complications resulting from a midline vertical incision placed within exces-sive lipodystrophy at the surgical site. Other indications for performing panniculectomy relate to functional limitations resulting from the presence of a large abdominal pannus (Table 28.1). These include frequent rashes and intertrigo resistant to conservative management with medicated powder or cream. Severe cases may even affect activities of daily living such as bathing, functional mobility, and personal hygiene. However, performing a panniculec-tomy cannot overcome medical and metabolic derangements that also affect wound healing and therefore patients must be appropriately selected and medically optimized prior to the operation.

Table 28.1 Indications/Contraindications

Panniculectomy
Indications
• Excess skin and subcutaneous tissue
• Presence of rashes and ulcers
• Chronic infection and intertrigo
• Functional limitation (immobility, inadequate hygiene, massive localized lymphedema)
Relative contraindications
• Smoking
• Intraperitoneal truncal obesity
• Previous abdominal scars compromising blood flow

Contraindications

The presence of a large upper transverse scar (i.e., open cholecystectomy incision) is a contra-indication to panniculectomy. Other relative con-traindications to performing panniculectomy at the time of surgery include: active nicotine use and excess intraperitoneal truncal obesity.

Prior Incisions

There are several incisions used to perform oper-ations of abdominal organs and viscera. These transverse upper abdominal incisions can inter-rupt critical blood supply to the abdominal wall skin and may be a relative contraindication to performing panniculectomy. The incisions and the vascular zones of the abdominal wall will be discussed below.

Nicotine

Smoking tobacco has a well-documented impact on overall postoperative outcomes. Specifically relating to ventral hernia repair, Finan et al. reviewed 1505 ventral hernia repair cases and found that smoking is a statistically significant pre-dictor for postoperative wound infection [9, 10]. Furthermore, a smoker's cough in the postopera-tive period leads to large increases in intra-abdominal pressure that can weaken surgical repair and lead to recurrence of the hernia and dehiscence of the wound closure. Although smok-ing cessation techniques are beyond the scope of this chapter, the senior author emphasizes the importance of smoking cessation for at least 4 weeks prior to surgery and at least 4 weeks postoperatively.

Excess Abdominal Contents

Excess abdominal content can complicate hernia repair and pose an issue with abdominal wall pli-cation at the time of panniculectomy. The increased intra-abdominal pressure resulting from midline plication may not only increase the likelihood of developing abdominal compart-ment syndrome, but may also elevate the patient's diaphragm leading to worsened pulmonary func-tion, particularly in patients with chronic obstruc-tive pulmonary disease (COPD). Furthermore, the increased intra-abdominal pressure decreases venous return via the common iliac veins and increases the risk of deep vein thrombosis (DVT) and pulmonary embolism. Patients with a history of thromboembolic events should undergo thorough evaluation to determine the safety of undergoing the operation or the need for vena cava filter placement.

Preoperative Evaluation

A thorough patient history and physical exam is important prior to performing the operation. This includes a discussion about previous weight loss, symptoms related to the panniculus, prior panniculectomy or abdominal incisions, and a thorough understanding of the patient's prior hernia repair history. On physical exam, observation of the abdominal wall and questioning the patient about scars on the abdomen assists in identifying the presence of incisions that can impair wound healing or lead to skin-flap necrosis if wide undermining is performed. These incisions include the chevron, or Kocher's incision. The presence of infrapannicular rashes, ulceration, malodor, and intertrigo should be documented in the medical record, and adequately treated since the lower incision for panniculectomy is commonly through the area most commonly affected by intertrigo. Palpation of the abdominal wall will identify areas of abdominal wall laxity or presence of hernia that may require repair at the time of surgery. Lastly, the surgeon should review any available computed tomography (CT) imaging to assess the size of the abdominal wall defect.

Operative Approach

Soft Tissue and Muscular Anatomy

An understanding of the abdominal wall tissue layers is necessary to appreciate the complex anatomy of the region. From superficial to deep these include the skin and subcutaneous tissue, Scarpa's fascia, deep investing fascia, muscles of the abdominal wall, and peritoneum [11]. The muscu-

lar anatomy of the abdominal wall is addressed in introductory chapters of the textbook, but is summarized here as consisting of the paired midline rectus abdominis and the lateral tri-layered muscular complex—*external oblique, internal oblique* and *transversus abdominis* (Fig. 28.1).

Vascular Anatomy

In 1979, Huger defined the vascular zones of the abdominal skin [12]. This theory of superficial cutaneous blood supply was later supported by anatomic studies performed by Taylor [13]. In Huger's classification scheme, zone I is located medially and supplied by small perforating blood vessels from the deep inferior and superior epigastric system. Zone II consists of the lower abdominal skin and is supplied by the common femoral system via the superficial inferior epigastric artery, the superficial external pudendal artery, and the superficial circumflex iliac arteries. Zone III is lateral and supplied by the intercostal and subcostal arteries [12] (Fig. 28.2). The three zones are interconnected through an arcade of anastomoses between the blood vessels and through the presence of choke vessels. The importance of understanding the vascular anatomy of the superficial abdominal skin to optimize would healing cannot be overstated.

Often, after resection of the pannus and to facilitate closure of the wound or improve hernia repair exposure, the upper abdominal skin is undermined, thereby creating an abdominoplasty-type flap. The Zone I blood supply is divided when undermining the superior abdominal skin flap. The femoral blood supply (Zone II) is divided by the low transverse waistline incision. The result of dividing Zone I perforators and Zone II blood supply is that the superior flap is solely supplied by laterally based blood supply (Zone III). Therefore, if the zone III vessels were interrupted with a prior scar such as a subcostal open cholecystectomy incision then abdominal wall skin inferomedial to the scar is at risk for necrosis. Limiting lateral dissection while exposing the hernia defect is critical for protecting the remaining lateral blood supply.

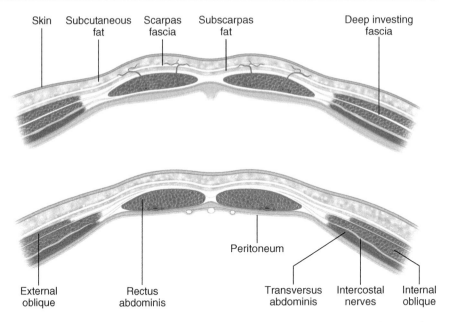

Fig. 28.1 Abdominal wall: paired midline rectus abdominis and the lateral tri-layered muscular complex—external oblique, internal oblique and transversus abdominis

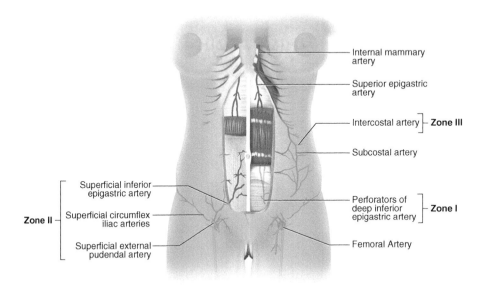

Fig. 28.2 Huger's vascular classification scheme for skin perfusion in the abdomen: Zone I is located medially and supplied by small perforating blood vessels from the deep inferior and superior epigastric system. Zone II consists of the lower abdominal skin and is supplied by the common femoral system via the superficial inferior epigastric artery, the superficial external pudendal artery, and the superficial circumflex iliac arteries. Zone III is lateral and supplied by the intercostal and subcostal arteries

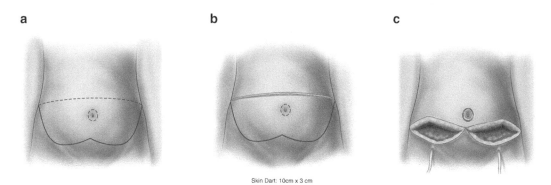

Skin Dart: 10cm x 3 cm

Fig. 28.3 In the panniculectomy patient, an exaggerated triangle of skin is made on the inferior flap to help reduce the unavoidable tension on the wound closure which may otherwise lead to increased ischemia of the skin and result in skin and fat necrosis, or dehiscence

Patient Markings

Markings include a midline symmetry mark from the sternal notch to the pubic symphysis. The inferior incision is marked with excess skin stretched upwards, as a line from one anterior superior iliac crest to the other with an exaggerated skin dart at the midpoint, which is a triangle with a height of 3 cm and a base of 10 cm (Fig. 28.3). With the patient in the diver's pose, excess abdominal soft tissue is assessed and the superior margin is marked, again spanning from ASIS to ASIS and this marking is reassessed intraoperatively with the operating table flexed.

We have previously reported our results in reducing wound healing complications by employing the use of an expanded skin triangle (i.e., "Skin Dart") upon closure of breast reduction sites in massively obese patients [14]. We also believe that similar benefits exist when employing the use of this skin triangle to off-load tension at the time of closure during panniculectomy. In the panniculectomy patient, an exaggerated triangle of skin is made on the inferior flap to help reduce the unavoidable tension on the wound closure which may otherwise lead to increased ischemia of the skin and result in skin and fat necrosis, or dehiscence.

Panniculectomy

The operation begins with intraoperative confirmation of preoperative markings. Next, the operation proceeds with incising the superior mark of the proposed elliptical excision being careful not to undermine the superior skin flap. The inferior mark of the elliptical excision is then incised and dissection proceeds to the rectus fascia. Our preference is to leave the subscarpal inguinal fat down as an attempt to maintain the inguinal lymphatics in that region and potentially reduce seroma formation [15, 16]. The periumbilical dissection proceeds straight down to the level of the rectus fascia ensuring that adequate fat remains attached to the umbilicus to preserve blood supply. Details of umbilical management are discussed in a separate section below.

Although classic descriptions of panniculectomy include excision of adipocutaneous tissue in a "wedge" fashion, with virtually no undermining, when combining panniculectomy with abdominal wall reconstruction undermining has advantages. Therefore, we encourage appropriate skin-flap undermining to provide improved exposure to the hernia defect and aid in mesh placement. For instance, if placing the mesh posteriorly, the use of undermining spares the need for transcutaneous stab incisions to secure the mesh in place. Conversely, with anteriorly placed mesh, undermining is a requirement in order to place the mesh or to perform anterior component separation. If performing upper abdominal skin undermining during panniculectomy, we strongly emphasize limited lateral undermining. Extended skin undermining in the lateral direction increases the risk of dividing the Huger Zone III blood supply which is the sole blood supply to the entire panniculectomy skin flap. This in turn can dramatically increase the risk of flap necrosis and wound breakdown. This simple modification aids in reducing the likelihood of hypoperfusion to the flap. This effect can be seen intraoperatively with perfusion analysis techniques such as indocyanine green (ICG) laser angiography (LA) which allows quantitative assessment of ischemic areas of the abdominal flap.

After the panniculectomy specimen is resected, the fascial defect is closed based on the appropriate technique selected for the size and type of defect. If component separation is selected, the panniculectomy is often advantageous and allows excellent exposure to release the external oblique muscles.

Closure of the superior flap proceeds with placement of progressive tension sutures (PTS) which have two functions (1) obliterate deadspace like quilting sutures and (2) advance the skin flaps on the fascia resulting in a decreased tension at the waistline closure. The PTS are placed between the Scarpa's fascia of the skin flap and the fascia of the abdominal wall (see Fig. 28.4 and Video 28.1). This is a technique

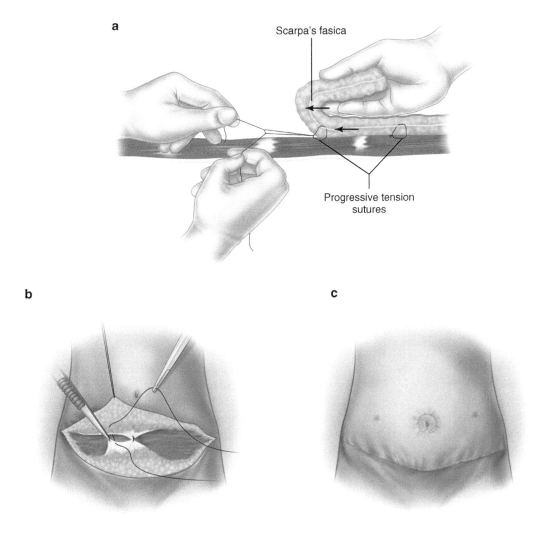

Fig. 28.4 Closure of the superior flap proceeds with placement of progressive tension sutures (PTS) which have two functions (1) obliterate deadspace like quilting sutures and (2) advance the skin flaps on the fascia result- ing in a decreased tension at the waistline closure. The PTS are placed between the Scarpa's fascia of the skin flap and the fascia of the abdominal wall

a   b

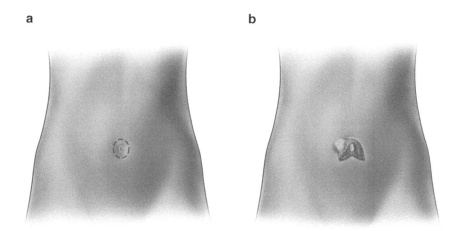

Fig. 28.5 The technique of umbilicoplasty is surgeon dependent, but we find that the "upside down Pac-man" technique is simple to learn, and has an excellent postoperative appearance. The presence of a small skin triangular dart inferiorly aids in reducing cicatricial scar contracture similar to a Z-plasty

that facilitates closure and assists in obliteration of deadspace and reduction in seroma formation [17]. At this point, the umbilicus is clinically assessed for viability based on the presence or absence of dermal bleeding, and with or without the adjunctive use of ICG-laser angiography. In our practice we have a low threshold to resect the umbilicus, but when it is preserved our preferred method for umbilicoplasty is the "upside down Pac-man" (Fig. 28.5).

Our Preferred Method of Umbilicoplasty

The technique of umbilicoplasty is surgeon dependent, but we find that the "upside down Pac-man" technique is simple to learn, and has an excellent postoperative appearance. The presence of a small skin triangular dart inferiorly aids in reducing cicatricial scar contracture similar to a Z-plasty. The marking is demonstrated in the associated video.

Closure of Abdominal Wound

Prior to closure of the wound, closed-suction drains are placed through the lateral aspects of

the incision. Closed-suction drains are routinely placed because of the risk seroma from the dissection in various anatomic planes. Our practice is to maintain drains for at least a week and remove them based on the amount of output (less than 30 cc/day for 3 consecutive days). The abdominal wound closure is a multilayered closure beginning with the Scarpa's layer. This layer provides strength to the closure, reduces tension, reduces the likelihood of an acute postoperative wound dehiscence, and improves scarring.

Techniques for Optimizing Results

Although it may appear counterintuitive that the addition of a large transverse incision will improve would healing, the removal of the hypovascular adipose tissue can paradoxically lead to improved perfusion to the skin flaps and consequently improve healing. Obese patients often suffer from high rates of postoperative complications, such as seroma, surgical site infections, skin and fat necrosis, dehiscence, and hernia recurrence [18]. Management of these complications is challenging even for experienced surgeons and therefore achieving an optimal outcome is technique dependent and can be improved with the appropriate use of adjuncts such as PTS, closed-suction drains, and the DART technique. Below, we will discuss two additional adjuncts that are also effective at optimizing postoperative outcomes.

Indocyanine Green: Laser Angiography

Prior to closure, areas concerning for decreased perfusion are excised to maximize the chances of achieving wound closure with well-vascularized tissue. However the clinical criteria (color, warmth, dermal bleeding, capillary blanching, and refill) can be misleading or underestimate the true extent of hypovascularity. In high-risk patients, the authors elect to employ laser-assisted near-infrared angiography with intravenous indocyanine green (ICG) dye (SPY Intraoperative Imaging Systems; Novadaq Technologies, Inc., Mississauga, Ontario, Canada). ICG angiography provides real-time intraoperative information about soft-tissue perfusion through the detection of plasma protein-bound ICG molecules that fluoresce when illuminated by a low-energy laser [19]. The correlation between tissue perfusion and necrosis has been demonstrated by several animal and clinical studies [20, 21]. Specific to hernia repair, we have previously published on the ability ICG angiography to reduce postoperative wound complications after complex ventral hernia repair using components separation [19].

Incisional Negative Pressure Wound Therapy

Another important adjunctive technique to optimize outcomes is the use of closed incision-negative pressure therapy (ci-NPT). The relatively novel use of negative pressure wound therapy (NPWT) over closed incisions to support primary healing differs from the traditional use of NPWT which commonly aids healing of open wounds by secondary intention. The benefits of closed incision negative pressure therapy for high-risk incisions is well documented across multiple surgical disciplines including cardiac surgery, colorectal

surgery, hernia surgery, orthopedics, and vascular surgery [20]. These benefits include overall decreased likelihood of surgical site infection and wound dehiscence. The proposed mechanism is likely related to increased blood flow [22, 23], reduction of edema [24], and a splinting effect of the wound [25, 26]. This splinting effect is likely the most important since the negative pressure reduces tension across high-risk incisions. Clinical experience with ci-NPT has demonstrated that it can significantly reduce the rate of overall wound complications and skin dehiscence after abdominal wall reconstruction [18]. In our practice we employ ci-NPT on most of our patients presenting with large complex abdominal hernia.

Postoperative Care

Our standard abdominal binder protocol does not involve the use of an abdominal binder until postoperative day (POD) #7 because the undermined skin is at risk from ischemia and tension from closure. When the ci-NPT dressing is removed on POD#7 and the incision is intact, we apply a loose fitting abdominal binder. Over the next 2 weeks, as the closed-suction drains are removed, we suggest progressively tightening the binder especially once the last drain is removed. At this point, the abdominal binder serves to prevent seroma formation by applying external pressure on the skin flaps to the fascia. We understand that traditionally an abdominal binder may assist with pulmonary toilet, but in our experience we have had excellent patient recovery despite the lack of abdominal binder in the early postoperative period.

Early postoperative care involves DVT prophylaxis by sequential compression stockings and early ambulation at the minimum but can also involve the use of chemoprophylaxis. It is our usual practice to administer a dose of prophylactic antibiotics 30–60 min preoperatively and ensure adequate redosing based upon the pharmacologic half-life of the antibiotic used. It is discouraged to routinely continue antibiotics simply as prophylaxis for the duration that the drains remain in place. Instead, we use chlorhexidine-impregnated patches around the drain site and believe this may offer adequate prophylaxis against drain-related infection.

Managing Complications

Although careful and deliberate use of the various techniques above such as protection of lateral (zone III) blood supply, obliteration of deadspace with closed-suction drains, on-table evaluation of skin-flap vascularity with ICG-LA, and application of incisional NPWT to splint the wound, complications can still occur.

Wound Breakdown and Flap Necrosis

The medial aspect of the incision is most prone to ischemia because it is often under the greatest amount of tension at the time of closure and because it is furthest away from the remaining, laterally based zone III blood supply. Although careful redistribution of tension during closure, use of the expanded skin dart technique, PTS, and incisional NPWT can reduce the likelihood of flap necrosis it is still possible and requires adequate management. Skin breakdown may initially be managed with wet-to-dry gauze dressings or NPWT. Early intervention with these moist dressings is especially important if there is exposed biologic matrix at the base of the wound since desiccation should be avoided. Other cases of wound breakdown may require operative debridement of devitalized wound margins, and reclosure. If cellulitis or frank purulent infection has developed, then patients should be admitted to the hospital for management, including possible initiation of appropriate intravenous antibiotics. For full-thickness flap necrosis where biologic mesh is threatened, the authors encourage early operative debridement to healthy wound edges as dictated clinically, or with the use of indocyanine green laser angiography. This also may require mesh removal and placement of open NPWT.

Seroma

Seroma may be managed with sterile and serial aspiration or percutaneous drain placement. If these approaches are unsuccessful then reoperation may be required to excise the pseudobursa that may have formed. In cases where reoperation is performed, one may elect to employ the use of quilting sutures or fibrin sealants.

Conclusion

Concomitant panniculectomy can safely be performed during the hernia operation, can optimize surgical exposure during the hernia repair, and improve postoperative wound healing. Successful repair and good outcomes are highly technique-sensitive and require appropriate patient selection, optimization of medical status and nutrition. Adjunctive techniques presented in this chapter may assist surgeons in optimizing their patient outcomes.

References

1. Flegal KM, Carroll MD, Kit BK, Ogden CL. Prevalence of obesity and trends in the distribution of body mass index among US adults, 1999–2010. JAMA. 2012;307(5):491–7.
2. Petty P, Manson PN, Black R, Romano JJ, Sitzman J, Vogel J. Panniculus morbidus. Ann Plast Surg. 1992;28(5):442–52.
3. Demars M, Marx M. Surgical treatment of obesity. Prog Med. 1890;11:283.
4. Kelly H. Excision of the fat of the abdominal wall lipectomy. Surg Gynecol Obstet. 1910;10(229):18.
5. Shermak MA. Hernia repair and abdominoplasty in gastric bypass patients. Plast Reconstr Surg. 2006;117(4):1145–50; discussion 1151–2.
6. Iljin A, Szymanski D, Kruk-Jeromin J, Strzelczyk J. The repair of incisional hernia following roux-en-Y gastric bypass-with or without concomitant abdominoplasty? Obes Surg. 2008;18(11):1387–91.
7. Koolen PG, Ibrahim AM, Kim K, et al. Patient selection optimization following combined abdominal procedures: analysis of 4925 patients undergoing panniculectomy/abdominoplasty with or without concurrent hernia repair. Plast Reconstr Surg. 2014; 134(4):539e–50e.
8. Saxe A, Schwartz S, Gallardo L, Yassa E, Alghanem A. Simultaneous panniculectomy and ventral hernia

repair following weight reduction after gastric bypass surgery: is it safe? Obes Surg. 2008;18(2):192–5; discussion 196.

9. Finan KR, Vick CC, Kiefe CI, Neumayer L, Hawn MT. Predictors of wound infection in ventral hernia repair. Am J Surg. 2005;190(5):676–81.

10. Krupski WC. The peripheral vascular consequences of smoking. Ann Vasc Surg. 1991;5(3):291–304.

11. Moore KL, Dalley AF, Agur AM. Clinically oriented anatomy. Philadelphia: Lippincott Williams & Wilkins; 2013.

12. Huger Jr WE. The anatomic rationale for abdominal lipectomy. Am Surg. 1979;45(9):612–7.

13. Taylor GI, Palmer JH. The vascular territories (angiosomes) of the body: experimental study and clinical applications. Br J Plast Surg. 1987;40(2):113–41.

14. Chopra K, Tadisina KK, Conde-Green A, Singh DP. The expanded inframammary fold triangle: improved results in large volume breast reductions. Indian J Plast Surg. 2014;47(1):65–9.

15. Le Louarn C, Pascal JF. High superior tension abdominoplasty. Aesthetic Plast Surg. 2000;24(5):375–81.

16. Le Louarn C, Pascal J. High superior tension abdominoplasty—a safer technique. Aesthet Surg J. 2007;27(1):80–9.

17. Pollock H, Pollock T. Progressive tension sutures: a technique to reduce local complications in abdominoplasty. Plast Reconstr Surg. 2000;105(7):2583–6.

18. Conde-Green A, Chung TL, Holton 3rd LH, et al. Incisional negative-pressure wound therapy versus conventional dressings following abdominal wall reconstruction: a comparative study. Ann Plast Surg. 2013;71(4):394–7.

19. Wang H, Singh D. The use of indocyanine green angiography to prevent wound complications in ventral hernia repair with open components separation technique. Hernia. 2013;17(3):397–402.

20. Gurtner GC, Jones GE, Neligan PC, et al. Intraoperative laser angiography using the SPY system: Review of the literature and recommendations for use. Ann Surg Innov Res. 2013;7(1):1.

21. Holm C, Mayr M, Höfter E, Becker A, Pfeiffer U, Mühlbauer W. Intraoperative evaluation of skin-flap viability using laser-induced fluorescence of indocyanine green. Br J Plast Surg. 2002;55(8):635–44.

22. Erba P, Ogawa R, Ackermann M, et al. Angiogenesis in wounds treated by microdeformational wound therapy. Ann Surg. 2011;253(2):402–9.

23. Atkins BZ, Tetterton JK, Petersen RP, Hurley K, Wolfe WG. Laser doppler flowmetry assessment of peristernal perfusion after cardiac surgery: beneficial effect of negative pressure therapy. Int Wound J. 2011;8(1):56–62.

24. Karlakki S, Brem M, Giannini S, Khanduja V, Stannard J, Martin R. Negative pressure wound therapy for management of the surgical incision in orthopaedic surgery: a review of evidence and mechanisms for an emerging indication. Bone Joint Res. 2013;2(12):276–84.

25. Wilkes RP, Kilpad DV, Zhao Y, Kazala R, McNulty A. Closed incision management with negative pressure wound therapy (CIM): biomechanics. Surg Innov. 2012;19(1):67–75.

26. Kairinos N, Solomons M, Hudson DA. Negative-pressure wound therapy I: the paradox of negative-pressure wound therapy. Plast Reconstr Surg. 2009;123(2):589–98; discussion 599–600.

Lauren Chmielewski, Michelle Lee,
and Hooman Soltanian

Background

Abdominal wall defects are some of the most commonly encountered reconstructive challenges. Goals of abdominal wall reconstruction include providing stable soft-tissue coverage, restoring fascial integrity, preventing hernia, protecting abdominal viscera, and restoring function [1]. The fascia and the soft-tissue envelope of the abdominal wall should be considered as two separate units. Each unit should be reconstructed using the "like with like" principle of reconstructive surgery. In general, dead space should be eliminated, skin undermining should be minimized, and the reconstructive choice should reduce potential for bowel adhesions, fistulization, and perforation [1]. It is important to distinguish whether the defect in the abdominal wall is due to skin, subcutaneous tissue, or musculofascial insufficiency. Musculofascial defects are often repaired by reconstruction techniques such as component separation and mesh repair [2]. In cases of abdominal skin/subcutaneous tissue deficiency, primary closure of the skin flaps under tension will result in tissue ischemia, wound dehiscence, and possible exposure/contamination of biomaterials used to reconstruct the musculofascial defects. Deficiency in the skin/subcutaneous tissue can be repaired by a variety of methods: (1) primary closure, if there is minimal tension between the wound edges, (2) rearrangement of existing tissue such as skin grafts, local flaps, regional flaps, and free flaps and (3) expanding the existing tissue with tissue expansion.

One of the earliest reports of the use of abdominal wall tissue expansion was described by Byrd et al. in 1989 for congenital defects of the lower abdominal wall [3]. For skin and subcutaneous tissue deficits, tissue expansion remains a powerful tool to increase the amount of abdominal skin/subcutaneous tissue with subsequent skin flaps closure without tension. It involves insertion of a silicone balloon under the skin and subcutaneous tissue. The balloon is serially inflated by gradual injection of sterile saline via a remote or integrated port to inflate the skin and subcutaneous tissues over the expander. This can provide well-vascularized, autologous skin, subcutaneous tissue, and abdominal fascia for the repair of large defects [1].

L. Chmielewski, M.D.
Plastic Surgery, University Hospitals Case Medical
Center, Cleveland, OH, USA

M. Lee, M.D.
Plastic and Reconstructive Surgery, Beth Israel
Deaconess Medical Center, Harvard Medical School,
Boston, MA, USA

H. Soltanian, M.D., F.A.C.S. (✉)
Department of Plastic Surgery, Case Medical Center,
Cleveland, OH, USA
e-mail: Hooman.Soltanian@UHHospitals.org

© Springer International Publishing Switzerland 2016
Y.W. Novitsky (ed.), *Hernia Surgery*, DOI 10.1007/978-3-319-27470-6_29

Physiology of Expansion

The physiology of tissue expansion is based on the dynamic response of tissues to mechanical stresses placed on them [4]. The intrinsic viscoelastic properties of skin on which the principle of tissue expansion is based are stress relaxation and creep. Stress relaxation is defined as the decrease in the amount of force necessary to maintain a fixed amount of skin stretch over time. Creep is the gain in skin surface area that results when a constant load is applied [5]. The physiologic basis for these properties lies in the fact that as force is applied to a leading skin edge, tissue thickness decreases because of extrusion of fluid and mucopolysaccharides, dermal collagen bundles realign, elastic fibers undergo microfragmentation, and skin stretches mechanically [5].

Tissue expansion can be achieved by the placement of internal or external expanders. Internal expanders are prosthetic devices placed in the subcutaneous plane that enlarge by volume expansion. This technique is generally performed over 3–6 months with inflation performed at weekly intervals [6]. Expansion should be continued until the expanded flap is approximately 20% larger than the size of the defect in order to account for tissue recoil after removal of the expander [5]. External tissue expansion involves placing continuous tension at the wound edge. The skin and the subcutaneous planes are expanded until the wound edges are close enough for primary closure. External expansion should also undergo a period of consolidation to account for tissue recoil.

Expanded tissues demonstrate predictable changes. An increase in epidermal thickness is noted during expansion, which tends to return to initial levels within 4–6 weeks, although some thickness persists for many months. Melanocyte activity is also increased during expansion, but returns to normal within several months after completion of reconstruction. Thinning of the dermis occurs within the first several weeks of expansion and persists throughout the expansion process. This dermal thinning persists for at least

9 months after completion of expansion [4]. Significant muscle atrophy occurs during the expansion process, regardless of whether the expander is placed above or below a specific muscle. Expanded tissue demonstrates increased vascularity with a significant number of new vessels formed adjacent to the expander capsule. It is thought that the observed angiogenesis occurs secondary to the ischemia produced during the expansion process [4] [Table 29.1].

Tissue expansion can contribute to a variety of treatment options: full thickness skin grafts, local flaps adjacent to the lesion, or expansion of a free flap. Advantages of tissue expansion include the ability to create and recruit tissue having similar esthetics of color, texture, thickness, and hair production [6]. Expansion can be associated with the risks of infection, flap ischemia, extrusion, implant failure, patient intolerance/pain, and scar widening. Each of these complications may necessitate prosthesis removal [6]. A representative defect that best suits repair by insertion of a tissue expander is one that is well-defined, healed, and stable. Areas that have undergone irradiation, burns, previous excision and skin grafting, scar contracture, or areas with open or chronically draining wounds are not appropriate for tissue expansion.

Technical points critical for successful expansion include:

1. Adequate preoperative planning to permit ideal incision to facilitate sufficient safe tissue expansion
2. Proper choice of size and shape of the expander
3. Correct positioning of the expander

Incisions are incorporated into tissue that will become one margin of the flap. They should be

Table 29.1 Effects of tissue expansion

	Tissue expansion	
Epidermal thickening	Increased melanocytic activity	Thinning of dermis
Increased vascularity		Muscle atrophy

Fig. 29.1 Various shapes and sizes of the implants are available with both external and internal fill ports. Accuspan® & Integra® Tissue Expanders (PMT Corporation: http://www.pmtcorp.com/tissue_expanders.html, accessed 12/2014)

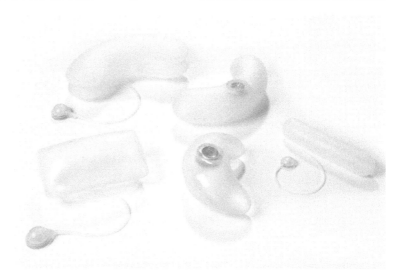

planned to minimize tension on the suture line and thus decrease the risk of extrusion. Tension from inflation will be less when incisions are perpendicular to the suture line, rather than parallel [7]. Expanders are available in a variety of shapes and sizes (rectangular, circular, or elliptical) and can even be custom fabricated to any dimension (Fig. 29.1). They include remote or integrated ports. Integrated ports are composed of self-sealing silicone rubber backed by stainless steel and can be located through the skin by magnetic sensing devices. Ideally, the length of the expander should match the length of the wound and the height of the expander should match the width. Specific fill volume is not vital because expanders are designed to tolerate overfilling. Placement of the expander is usually situated adjacent to the long access of the defect. They are usually placed beneath the skin and subcutaneous tissue above the fascia (Fig. 29.2). However, when the subcutaneous tissue is thin or the risk of extrusion is high, expanders may be placed below the muscle (Fig. 29.3). They should be placed away from sensitive areas, bony prominences, and areas subjected to pressure to minimize patient discomfort. In certain cases, the use of multiple small expanders is better than the use of one large expander. Multiple expanders inflate and expand the tissue more rapidly and complications are fewer [7].

Indications for Using TE for Abdominal Wall Reconstruction

Tissue expansion should be considered in abdominal wall reconstruction when there is a deficiency in abdominal skin and subcutaneous tissue and a clean wound. An inability to primarily close the abdominal wall skin and subcutaneous tissue can be due to a wide range of etiologies, such as large skin resection, serial debridements for infections (such as necrotizing fasciitis), congenital absence of abdominal wall (such as omphalocele), massive distention of the bowels and/or retroperitoneal structures secondary to resuscitation, or may be a result of florid sepsis or active infection [8]. In order to replace the missing abdominal wall skin and subcutaneous tissue, the surgeon needs to either rearrange surrounding skin and subcutaneous tissue with local, regional, and free flaps or increase the area of the remaining abdominal wall skin and subcutaneous tissue with tissue expansion.

Tissue expanders are most commonly placed above the abdominal wall fascia and serially inflated to increase the amount of abdominal skin available for primary closure. Tissue expanders can also be placed between the internal and external oblique and used to expand the abdominal

Fig. 29.2 *Top panel*:
Placement of the tissue
expander in the
subcutaneous layer about
the fascia and muscle layers.
Lower panel: Inflated
subcutaneous expander.
Both the superficial skin and
fat and the deep muscular
layers are affected

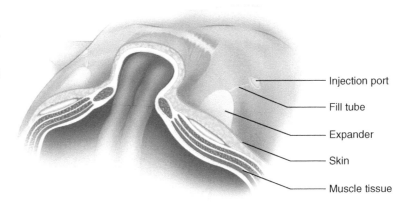

Deflated expander placed subcutaneously

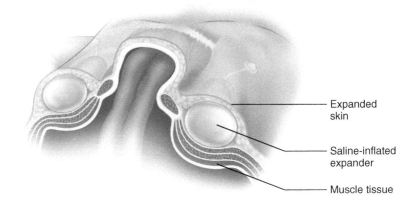

Inflated expander demonstrating expanded skin

Fig. 29.3 Submuscular
placement of the tissue
expander deep to the external
oblique layer and superficial to
the internal oblique layer

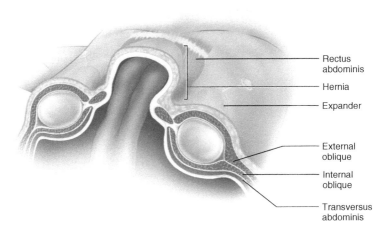

wall fascia. In 1989, Byrd et al. described the first interfascial expansion by placing the expander between the internal oblique and transversus abdominis. However, this technique has been largely abandoned because the expander is not placed on a rigid platform and expansion will occur both outward as well as inward [9]. Bidirectional expansion will be less effective in expanding the desired tissue (abdominal wall fascia/external oblique) and can increase the intraperitoneal pressure unnecessarily. As a result, defects in the abdominal wall fascia are treated with various abdominal hernia repair techniques such as component separation. Those techniques are discussed in other chapters.

In addition to increasing the volume of skin, tissue expanders can incite a fibrous reaction that interposes an additional connective tissue layer on the anterior abdominal wall. This vascularized capsule, combined with any existing anterior rectus sheath can be used to reconstruct abdominal wall defects [3]. The use of prosthetic mesh in conjunction with tissue-expanded skin provides a durable abdominal closure and is technically simpler than flap closure methods [10]. Donor site morbidity is minimized relative to musculofascial techniques. Tissue expansion even allows excision of unsightly scars and skin grafts while providing excellent color and texture match. It also provides well-vascularized skin and soft-tissue coverage over the prosthetic mesh [10].

Techniques of TE for Abdominal Wall Reconstruction

There are wide varieties of expanders differing in shape, texture, and expansion mechanism. Selection of expanders and placement of expander should be tailored to the individual defect. Preoperatively, the surgeon must take into consideration previous scars, postoperative scars, flap movement in relation to the defect, and potential distortion of surrounding structures. Most abdominal wall expanders are used to expand abdominal skin and are placed underneath the skin and subcutaneous tissue, but above the fascia.

Preoperative considerations should include a physical exam assessing the patient's general medical condition, abdominal wall integrity, extent and location of abdominal wall abnormalities, and the presence of scars. Using these principles, Livingston et al. described their technique for providing soft-tissue coverage for traumatic abdominal wall defects. The open abdomen wounds are first temporized with a split thickness skin graft which forms a skin bridge. Once the skin graft demonstrates substantial mobility from the underlying viscera, the patients are deemed to be candidates for tissue expander placement, usually at a minimum of 6 months [8]. The tissue expanders are inserted in the subcutaneous plane above anterior rectus fascia with retention of split thickness skin graft. Expansion is then carried out weekly or biweekly over approximately 6 weeks. After adequate expansion, the tissue expander is removed and the split thickness skin graft is de-epithelialized to form a "connective tissue bridge" (deep layer) over which the expanded subcutaneous tissue and skin is closed [8]. The expanded tissue may need to undergo capsulotomies or capsulectomies of the expander pocket for greater tissue movement [10]. It is important to note that this does not address the hernia itself, but only provides adequate skin and subcutaneous tissue coverage for the defect and/or prosthetic. Potential disadvantages to abdominal wall reconstruction with mesh and tissue expansion includes a possibility of skin breakdown and resultant mesh exposure and infection [10]. However, increased vascularity in the expanded tissue may decrease the potential skin flap ischemia, necrosis, and subsequent wound breakdown and mesh infection [10].

Another drawback of TE is that the typical expansion technique involves staged operations over a period of several weeks or months and multiple postoperative visits. Tissue expanders have the potential to become infected or exposed during expansion. In fact, complications related to using tissue expanders have been reported to be about 15% [10]. Rates of complication vary in relation to the site of implantation. Expansion over bony prominences, burn scars, or previous incision sites tends to have the highest morbidity [10].

Unlike internal expanders, external expanders stretch the skin and subcutaneous tissue by providing constant dermatraction at the wound edges. This can be achieved by placing an elastic vessel loop at the wound edges and adjusting the tension of the vessel loop postoperatively. Commercially available external tissue expanders, such as the Dermaclose™ (Wound Care Technologies Inc. Chanhassen, MN), provide constant and continuous tension at the wound edges. The wound edges should be adequately undermined prior to the application of the external dermatraction device to allow for appropriate movement of the skin flaps.

Conclusion

Tissue expansion can be a valuable tool in the reconstructive armamentarium. Its applications in abdominal wall reconstruction have been thoroughly reviewed in this chapter. Appropriate indications for expansion of the abdominal wall are when there is a deficiency in abdominal skin and subcutaneous tissue and a clean wound. Advantages of tissue expansion include the ability to create and recruit tissue having similar aesthetics of color, texture, thickness, and hair production. However, these advantages must be balanced with the downside that expansion requires staged operations over a period of several weeks or months and multiple postoperative visits. Additionally, expansion can be associated with the risks of infection, flap ischemia, extrusion, implant failure, patient intolerance, pain, and scar widening. Each of these complications may necessitate prosthesis removal. For these reasons, judicious use of tissue expanders is recommended as just one of many tools for abdominal wall reconstruction.

References

1. Althubaiti G, Butler CE. Abdominal wall and chest wall reconstruction. Plast Reconstr Surg. 2014;133: 688e–701.
2. Ramirez OM, Ruas E, Dellon AL. "Components separation" method for closure of abdominal-wall defects: an anatomic and clinical study. Plast Reconstr Surg. 1990;86:519–26.
3. Byrd HS, Hobar PC. Abdominal wall expansion in congenital defects. Plast Reconstr Surg. 1989;84: 347–52.
4. Weinzweig J, Weinzweig N. Plastic surgery techniques (Chapter 5). In: Guyuron B, editor. Plastic surgery indications and practice. Saunders/Elsevier: Edinburgh; 2009. p. 90–108.
5. Leedy JE, Janis JE, Rohrich RJ. Reconstruction of acquired scalp defects: an algorithmic approach. Plast Reconstr Surg. 2005;116:54e–72.
6. Arneja JS, Gosain AK. Giant congenital melanocytic nevi. Plast Reconstr Surg. 2007;120:26e–40.
7. Marks MW, Argenta LC. Principles and applications of tissue expansion (Chapter 27). In: Neligan PC, editor. Plastic surgery. London: Saunders/Elsevier; 2012. p. 621–31.
8. Livingston DH, Sharma PK, Glantz AI. Tissue expanders for abdominal wall reconstruction following severe trauma: technical note and case reports. J Trauma. 1992;32:82–6.
9. Tran NV, Petty PM, Bite U, et al. Tissue expansion assisted closure of massive ventral hernias. J Am Coll Surg. 2003;196:484–8.
10. Paletta CE, Huang DB, Dehghan K, Kelly C. The use of tissue expanders in staged abdominal wall reconstruction. Ann Plast Surg. 1999;42:259–65.

Flap Reconstruction of the Abdominal Wall

30

Donald P. Baumann and Charles E. Butler

Introduction

Soft-tissue flap reconstruction of the abdominal wall implies the inability to recruit local tissue to resurface the abdominal wall defect. Since the majority of abdominal wall defects can be reconstructed with the surrounding redundant tissue from the torso, these defects represent a more complex subset of abdominal wall reconstructions. Indications for flap coverage vary by etiology, defect characteristics, and timeline for closure. Multiple clinical scenarios can lead to a loss of abdominal wall soft-tissue requiring flap reconstruction, including massive ventral hernia with loss of domain, traumatic injury, soft tissue infection, oncologic resection, and the open abdomen.

The surface area of soft-tissue loss and the amount of wound coverage able to be performed with local skin advancement must be factored into the reconstructive plan. Abdominal wall defects requiring soft-tissue flap coverage can be classified as partial thickness defects involving the skin and subcutaneous tissue only or full-thickness composite defects which involve loss of the abdominal wall musculofascia in addition to the overlying skin and subcutaneous tissue.

D.P. Baumann, M.D., F.A.C.S.
C.E. Butler, M.D., F.A.C.S. (✉)
Plastic and Reconstructive Surgery,
University of Texas MD Anderson Cancer Center,
Houston, TX, USA
e-mail: cbutler@mdanderson.org

The indications for soft-tissue flap coverage in abdominal wall reconstruction also depend on the chronicity of the wound defect with some defects benefiting from early flap coverage, others best treated by delayed flap coverage. Certain other defects are more appropriately managed with chronic wound care and healing by secondary intention.

Historically, abdominal wounds were treated with wound care and allowed to heal over time by secondary intention or were reconstructed with a skin graft after the local wound environment was optimized. This resulted in a prolonged course of care and significant morbidity. In time, the concept of delayed-primary closure gained popularity allowing certain patients with favorable wound characteristics to undergo closure after a short period of wound care instead of being committed to weeks or months of open wound care. This enabled patients to achieve definitive wound closure without a skin-grafted surgical site and associated donor site morbidity [1].

Early soft-tissue flap reconstruction offers significant advantages over delayed-primary or secondary healing wound closure. Flap reconstruction is performed as a single stage procedure obviating the need for chronic wound management. Flap reconstruction can often be performed at the same time as the musculofascial reconstruction. Flap reconstruction offers immediate and definitive wound closure, effectively ending the local tissue injury and inflammatory response seen in chronic open wounds. These two factors are critical in reconstructions involving abdominal wall reinforcement with bioprosthetic mesh. When bioprosthetic mesh is interposed between two well-vascularized tissue planes (posterior abdominal wall/peritoneal cavity and a soft tissue flap superficially), bidirectional vascular ingrowth can be achieved accelerating the period of bioprosthetic mesh revascularization and incorporation. In addition, a closed wound environment diminishes the pro-inflammatory state of an open wound, which limits the degree of enzymatic degradation of the bioprosthetic mesh during the incorporation phase [2].

Over the last 20 years, the role of negative-pressure wound therapy (NPWT) has revolutionized the approach to wound care, particularly in the management of abdominal wall defects. NPWT allows preservation of the wound environment by managing fluid and protein losses, decreasing bacterial contamination and accelerating granulation tissue formation. In abdominal wall reconstruction, this translates in preserving the option for delayed-primary closure or delayed flap reconstruction [3].

Composite, full-thickness loss of the abdominal wall musculofascia and overlying soft-tissue represent the most complicated abdominal wall reconstructions, sometimes requiring multiple staged reconstructive procedures. Re-establishment of musculofascial continuity is paramount to setting the stage for a durable abdominal wall reconstruction. Reconstituting the deficient musculofascia with a mesh inlay converts the open abdomen to a more manageable abdominal wall wound. For midline defects, early abdominal closure with primary rectus musculofascial re-approximation over bioprosthetic mesh provides superior outcomes to bridging the fascial defect with bioprosthetic mesh. The risk of developing a hernia increases sevenfold when bridging fascial repairs are performed instead of reinforced mesh repairs [4]. All attempts should be made to achieve fascial coaptation as bridging repairs are far more likely to develop hernias. When early fascial closure is not an option owing to ongoing debridement of the musculofascia or the need to perform a second-look laparotomy, a temporizing abdominal wall closure can be utilized such as the

NPWT system. A static bridging wound dressing protects and insulates the viscera while controlling fluid loss in the wound bed. NPWT also provides abdominal stability in the early postoperative period for patients undergoing mechanical ventilation and later when they ambulate and undergo physical therapy.

When both the soft-tissue and musculofascia require reconstruction, it is preferred to reconstruct these two components independently, rather than using the fascia of the flap for musculofascial reconstruction. Historically, before the introduction of mesh material for use in contaminated cases, flaps such as the tensor fascia lata flap were used to reconstruct full-thickness abdominal wall defects, especially in the setting of wound contamination [5]. Selecting a single flap to restore the musculofascial integrity and resurface the skin defect can compromise durability of the hernia repair as well as lead to a perfusion-related complication (wound dehiscence, flap necrosis) at the skin level. The current approach to these defects includes mesh and often component separation release to re-establish a physiologic tension bearing musculofascial closure and then a soft-tissue flap is used for the cutaneous defect. The use of the fascial component of a flap for musculofascial reconstructions can result in increased bulge or hernia. In addition, insertion of the fascial component can potentially compromise the vascularity of the soft-tissue component of the flap. Thus, for composite midline defects, myofascial reconstruction is generally performed with either synthetic or bioprosthetic mesh materials. Surgeon preference and the variables of any given clinical scenario will determine whether bioprosthetic mesh or synthetic mesh is used. Regardless of mesh type, the expectations are that the mesh will maintain the abdominal musculofascial structure, integrity, and contour, without development of a hernia or bulge. Mesh should be placed to avoid forming extensive adhesions to the intra-abdominal viscera that can lead to bowel obstruction or fistulization. Bioprosthetic and synthetic meshes can meet these expectations, and the decision to use either is based on patient comorbidities, degree of wound contamination, prior radiation, availability of greater omentum to interpose between mesh and bowel, and the quality of the overlying soft-tissue.

The reconstructive algorithm for skin coverage of full-thickness abdominal wall defects begins with local skin advancement flaps and expands to local perforator flaps, regional pedicled flap, and ultimately free-flap reconstructions. The overlapping angiosomes of the abdominal wall's cutaneous blood supply allow for wide undermining and robust skin advancement. In addition, tissue expansion (Chapter 29) can be performed in the trunk to increase the surface area and availability of local fasciocutaneous flaps as an alternative to a pedicled or free-flap donor site. In cases of prior radiation, extensive prior scars, or massive skin resection, a pedicled regional or free flap may be required to provide adequate soft-tissue coverage. Composite abdominal wall defects can involve significant loss of innervated myofascia and overlying skin in a dimension that is greater than the surrounding tissue's ability to be recruited and mobilized for closure. In such cases, regional or distant tissue flaps must be used for closure, and the resultant repair will no longer be dynamic, contractile, and coordinated with the surrounding abdominal wall musculature.

Overview of Reconstruction by Region

The anterior abdominal wall can be divided into three anatomic regions: the epigastrium, the periumbilical region and the hypogastrium. (Tables 30.1, 30.2 and 30.3) The relationship of defects

Table 30.1 Abdominal wall flap reconstruction algorithm epigastric defects

	Local	Pedicled	Free
Epigastric	Transposition IM, IC, SE	Rectus	Thigh-based (ALT, AMT, VL, TFL, RF, STF)
	Keystone	Omentum	Back-based LD, TAP, Scap/Para
	Bipedicled Fasciocutaneous		

IM internal mammary artery perforator flap, *IC* intercostal artery perforator flap, *SE* superior epigastric artery perforator flap
Thigh-based: *ALT* anterolateral thigh flap, *AMT* anteromedial thigh flap, *VL* Vastus lateralis flap, *TFL* tensor fascia lata flap, *RF* rectus femoris flap, *STF* subtotal thigh flap
Back-based: *LD* latissimus dorsi flap, *TAP* thoracodorsal artery perforator flap, *Scap/Para* scapular/parascapular flap

Table 30.2 Abdominal wall flap reconstruction algorithm periumbilical defects

	Local	Pedicled	Free
Periumbilical	Transposition DIEP, SIEP, TLP	Rectus	Thigh-based ALT, AMT, VL, TFL, RF, STF
	Keystone	Omentum	Back-based LD, TAP, Scap/Para
	Bipedicled fasciocutaneous	Thigh-based	

DIEP deep inferior artery perforator flap, *SIEP* superficial inferior epigastric artery perforator flap, *TLP* thoracolumbar perforator flap
Thigh-based: *ALT* anterolateral thigh flap, *AMT* anteromedial thigh flap, *VL* vastus lateralis flap, *TFL* tensor fascia lata flap, *RF* rectus femoris flap, *STF* subtotal thigh flap
Back-based: *LD* latissimus dorsi flap, *TAP* thoracodorsal artery perforator flap, *Scap/Para* scapular/parascapular flap

Table 30.3 Abdominal wall flap reconstruction algorithm hypogastric defects

	Local	Pedicled	Free
Hypogastric	Transposition DIEP, SIEP, TLP	Rectus	Thigh-based ALT, AMT, VL, TFL, RF, STF
	Keystone	Omentum	Back-based LD, TAP, Scap/Para
	Bipedicled Fasciocutaneous	Thigh-Based	

DIEP deep inferior artery perforator flap, *SIEP* superficial inferior epigastric artery perforator flap, *TLP* thoracolumbar perforator flap
Thigh-based: *ALT* anterolateral thigh flap, *AMT* anteromedial thigh flap, *VL* vastus lateralis flap, *TFL* tensor fascia lata flap, *RF* rectus femoris flap, *STF* subtotal thigh flap
Back-based: *LD* latissimus dorsi flap, *TAP* thoracodorsal artery perforator flap, *Scap/Para* scapular/parascapular flap

to these anatomic regions guide decision-making when regional pedicled flaps are planned for reconstruction. Options for pedicled flaps in the upper abdomen include latissimus dorsi, and omental flaps. Thigh-based flaps such as antero-lateral thigh, vastus lateralis, and tensor fascia lata flaps are generally able to reach the hypogas-trium and flank as pedicled flaps. If a pedicled flap is not available or feasible, a thoracoepigas-tric bipedicled fasciocutaneous flap may provide a local tissue alternative in patients who are not candidates for free tissue transfer.

When the volume of tissue loss or the arc of rotation needed precludes a pedicled flap trans-fer, a free flap is required for soft-tissue coverage. The thigh can serve as a source of fasciocutane-ous flaps and myocutaneous flaps that provide large skin paddles and significant muscle volume. Recipient vessels in the abdominal wall include the deep inferior epigastric, superior epigastric, internal mammary, intercostal artery, and perfo-rating thoracolumbar. When no local recipient vessels are available, vein grafts to the internal mammary or femoral vessels may be required depending on defect location.

Local Flap Options

Local flaps involve recruiting tissue adjacent to the wound defect. Well-planned incisions are critical to preserve blood supply to the local flap and avoid wound-healing complications at the donor site used to resurface the wound defect. There are various flap transposition designs available including advancement, rotation/advancement, interpolation, V-Y advancement, and bipedicled flaps. These flaps can be oriented in any dimension: vertically, obliquely, or hori-zontally. Given these flaps are perfused through random or axial blood supplies, understanding of the vascular anatomy in terms of abdominal wall angiosomes and perforator location is critical to designing robust local flaps.

It is also important to consider the impact of preexisting incisions in the abdominal wall when planning a flap design. A midline laparotomy may preclude harvesting a local flap from the contralateral abdominal wall. However, a midline defect bisected by a laparotomy scar can be divided in half and reconstructed by two local flaps, one from each hemi-abdomen. Another key factor in performing a local flap reconstruction is limiting tension across the wound closure both at the defect site and the donor site. The flap perfu-sion, especially at the most distal part of the flap, can be compromised if the flap is placed on high tension either by pushing the limits of the flap design or by creating excessive bi-axial tension across the flap when the donor site is closed.

One strategy that can be employed to mitigate excessive tension across the flap is to transpose the flap to cover the defect and then skin graft the donor site. This concept is the mainstay of the bipedicled flap in trunk reconstruction. For mid-line defects, a bipedicled fasciocutaneous flap is generally used for midline defects either unilater-ally or bilaterally. The flap is oriented vertically with a maximum of a 3:1 length/width ratio and maintains a blood supply from both the superior and inferior aspects of the flap. The flap is then directly transposed to resurface the defect and by design the donor site cannot be closed without an undue degree of tension. To offload the tension, a skin graft can be used to resurface the donor site preserving blood supply to the distal flap to maxi-mize wound healing.

Perforator flaps are based on a dominant named vessel which perfuses the entire flap through an organized vascular network. Perforator flaps present multiple options for flap design and rotation throughout the entire abdom-inal wall. Flaps based on internal mammary, superior epigastric, deep inferior epigastric, superficial inferior epigastric, and superficial cir-cumflex iliac perforators provide local flap options in all zones of the abdominal wall. The keystone flap is one strategy to reconstruct large trunk defects with perforator flaps [6]. Keystone flaps enable one stage resurfacing of both the defect and donor site. The flap is designed as a large 3:1 ellipse parallel to the long axis of the defect. The blood supply to the flap is based on cutaneous perforators that shift towards the defect when the flap is advanced. Once the lead-ing edge of the keystone flap is inset, the donor site is then closed on itself from the poles of the long axis of the flap to the side of the flap remote from the defect. The success of this flap is due to the transposition tension from the advancement and closure being distributed over the lengthy circumference of the flap skin island.

Regional Flap Options

In cases where the defect size exceeds the availability of local soft-tissue for coverage, the next line option is to consider a regional pedicled flap. Use of regional flaps is often limited as the defect is adjacent to the flap donor site, particularly if the defect is a full-thickness, or composite defect. Regional pedicled flaps are harvested from adjacent anatomic areas such as the chest, groin, thigh, or back. Pedicled flaps can be designed as fasciocutaneous flaps, myocutaneous flaps, or muscle flaps resurfaced with a skin graft. When selecting a pedicled flap it is important to factor the donor morbidity incurred. As an example, a contralateral vertical rectus abdominis myocutaneous flap can be used to reconstruct a lower lateral abdominal wall defect; however, the donor site closure may compromise the flap inset, increasing the risk of postoperative complications. In addition, not only must the pedicled flaps ability to "reach" the defect be considered, but also how the transferred flap will tolerate the rotational, flexion/extension forces placed on it in the trunk. As an example, a vastus lateralis thigh flap can be used to resurface a hypogastric defect however, as the flap's pedicled vessels remain in their site of origin in the thigh, the flap pedicle can pivot and traverse the groin and have its blood flow compromised by compression or rotation during the postoperative period.

Free Flap Options

Microsurgical free tissue transfer enables the reconstructive surgeon to provide soft-tissue coverage for abdominal wall defects that are not amenable to either local or regional flap cover-

age. Flaps of essentially any size, volume, dimension, and composition can be transferred from donor sites remote from the abdominal wall. While much more technically demanding, the evolution of microsurgical techniques enables successful free-flap transfer in excess of 98% of cases [7].

There is a multitude of free-flap donor site options available for abdominal wall reconstruction. The torso and thigh are the main areas of flap harvest for defects extending from the upper abdominal wall and epigastrium to the suprapubic region. The posterior chest wall donor site yields the latissimus dorsi myocutaneous flap, scapular/parascapular fasciocutaneous flaps, thoracodorsal artery perforator flaps, and serratus anterior muscle flaps. (Fig. 30.1a–e) In addition, these flaps can be harvested together as a chimeric flap to increase the tissue volume for flap transfer. These flaps can also be transposed to the upper epigastrium or lateral subcostal region as a pedicled flap. For defects beyond the reach of the thoracodorsal pedicle, the flap can be converted to a free flap and be transposed anywhere in the abdominal wall.

In cases where a large skin paddle is required for the abdominal wall defect, a free scapular or parascapular flap can be designed on the circumflex scapular branch of the subscapular arterial system. If a latissimus or serratus flap is harvested, the functional donor site impact must be considered as it relates to the weakened abdominal wall. Patients who have decreased core muscle strength will rely on upper extremity strength and range of motion to complete activities of daily living. The impact of impaired shoulder and upper extremity movement should be considered in these patients. In addition, in terms of logistical planning, the patient must undergo an intraoperative position change to facilitate flap dissection in the posterior chest wall. This adds complexity and additional time to the procedure and extends flap ischemia time.

The thigh represents the mainstay for flap donor sites for the abdominal wall. Both pedicled flaps for coverage of the infraumbilical abdominal wall and free flaps can be designed in several of configurations: fasciocutaneous, myocutane-

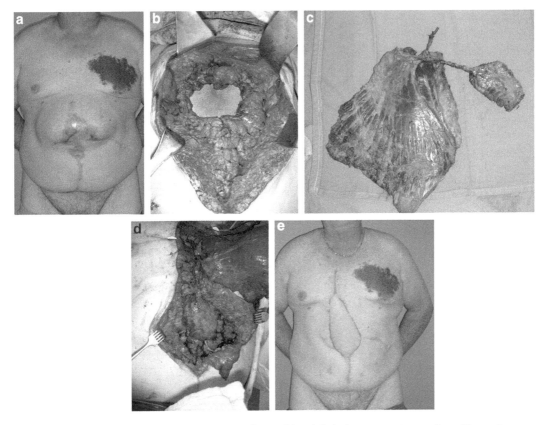

Fig. 30.1 Free chimeric latissimus myocutaneous flap with serratus muscle flap reconstruction of epigastric defect. (**a**) Preoperative view of planned composite full-thickness resection of the abdominal wall including anterior reflection of diaphragm. (**b**) Bioprosthetic mesh inlay bridging repair of the thoraco-abdominal defect. (**c**) Free chimeric latissimus myocutaneous flap with serratus muscle flap. (**d**) Serratus muscle flap inset covering the bioprosthetic mesh with the latissimus myocutaneous flap providing skin coverage. Right internal mammary vessels used as recipient vessels. (**e**) Follow-up 6 months

ous, muscle, and chimeric flaps. The descending branch of the lateral circumflex femoral system provides blood supply to the vastus lateralis, rectus femoris muscles, and anterolateral thigh skin. The transverse branch of the lateral circumflex femoral system provides blood supply to the tensor fascia lata flap. These flaps can be harvested as muscle-only flaps or as myocutaneous flaps with overlying skin paddles. The anterolateral thigh flap is designed by including a skin paddle overlying vastus lateralis muscle and can be designed as a myocutaneous or fasciocutaneous flap. The tensor fascia lata flap can be designed to include the distal fascia of the iliotibial tract and a smaller proximal skin paddle, if needed. The

anteromedial thigh flap can be designed on medial perforators from the descending branch of the lateral circumflex femoral system. The rectus femoris muscle is more commonly designed as a muscle flap; however, a skin island can be included over the central muscle when appropriate-sized cutaneous perforators are present.

These thigh-based flaps can be designed in any combination as chimeric flaps, i.e., ALT with AMT flaps, ALT with TFL, vastus lateralis with TFL. For massive abdominal wall defects, the vastus lateralis, tensor fascia lata, and the rectus femoris can be harvested with all overlying skin territory as a subtotal thigh flap for increased volume and skin coverage [8].

Recipient Vessels

The success of any free tissue transfer relies on the availability of suitable recipient vessels providing arterial inflow and venous outflow to the free flap. There are several recipient vessels available for abdominal wall reconstruction with free flaps. The main vascular axis in the central abdominal wall is the internal mammary-superior epigastric-inferior epigastric system. The internal mammary and deep inferior epigastric vessels provide large caliber 2–3 mm diameter recipient vessels for microanastomosis. However, these vessels are present at the most cephalad and caudal limits of the abdominal wall. The main challenge for identifying adequate internal mammary or epigastric recipient vessels in the periumbilical region is that they are much smaller in caliber and present more technically challenging microanastomoses. In cases where the internal mammary-epigastric vascular axis is unavailable, the thoracodorsal pedicle in the axilla can be reached by using vein grafts.

Recipient vessel options exist beyond the abdominal wall itself. There are a number of options in the groin based on the superficial femoral system. The superficial inferior epigastric artery, the superficial circumflex iliac artery, and the deep circumflex iliac artery provide reasonable caliber vessels for free flap transfer to the lower central and lateral abdominal wall. If primary anastomosis is not feasible then vein grafts or vein loops are required. Vein grafts are often harvested from the leg (greater or less saphenous vein) or arm (cephalic vein). In addition, in abdominal wall reconstructions with concurrent laparotomy intra-abdominal vessels can be used as recipients if there are no local options in the abdominal wall. The omental and gastroepiploic vessels can be mobilized to reach the undersurface of the abdominal wall. Care must be taken in insetting and supporting the flap pedicle so that there is no tension on the anastomoses when the visceral contents shift when the patient transitions from supine to sitting/standing. In addition, the morbidity of re-entering the abdominal cavity must be considered if there is a vascular thrombosis requiring flap re-exploration. In addition,

when mesh is used for the musculofascial reconstruction as an adjunct to the fascia of the flap the pedicle must traverse an aperture in the abdominal wall mesh that increases the risk of pedicle kink and vascular compromise. Moreover, defects in abdominal wall integrity increase the risk of hernia. For these reasons, local recipient options should be explored before intra-abdominal vessels are selected.

Vein grafts and arterialized vein loops can be designed to provide adequate recipient vessels in the central abdominal wall. Vein grafts can be harvested from either the upper or lower extremity as a cephalic vein graft or saphenous vein graft. For central and lower abdominal defects an arterialized saphenous vein loop can be designed. (Fig. 30.2a–e) The saphenous vein is dissected and transected distally and then anastomosed to the superficial femoral artery or a side branch. This allows delivery of the loop to the flaps recipient site where the loop is divided providing an arterialized afferent limb and a venous drainage efferent limb. One advantage of this technique is that it only requires three vascular anastomoses instead of four as in the case with direct individual arterial and venous vein grafts. The main recipient vessel sites for vein grafts or arterialized vein loops are the thoracodorsal vessels in the axilla, branches of the superficial femoral system on the groin, and the deep inferior epigastric vessels in the lateral abdominal wall, which can be used to extend the reach of vein grafts to the central abdominal wall.

Abdominal Wall Transplantation

Abdominal wall transplantation represents the zenith of abdominal wall flap reconstruction. It is generally reserved for patients undergoing single or multi-organ visceral transplants in which abdominal wall closure by autologous flaps is not technically feasible or presents significant donor morbidity. Abdominal wall closure after visceral organ transplantation is challenging in the setting of donor/recipient organ size mismatch and/or prior recipient abdominal surgery. Transplant patients can benefit from vascularized composite

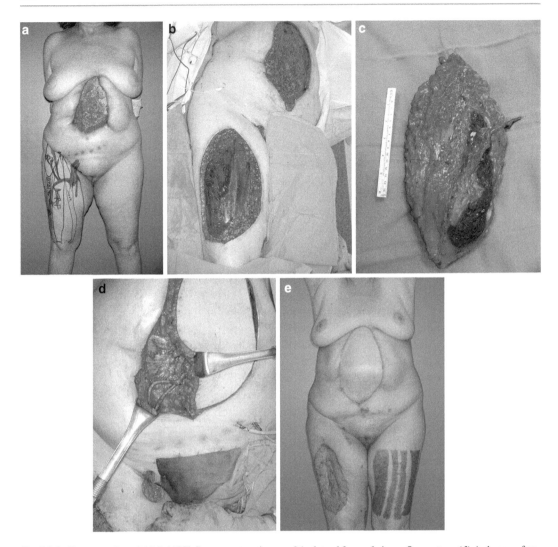

Fig. 30.2 Free anterolateral thigh (ALT) flap reconstruction of abdominal wall. (**a**) Preoperative view of open abdomen treated with NPWT. (**b, c**.) A right-sided ALT flap with vastus lateralis muscle was harvested on the descending branch of the lateral femoral circumflex system. (**d**) A shapeno-femoral A-V loop was delivered into the lower abdominal defect to serve as recipient vessels. (**e**) Patient at 12 weeks follow-up. Flap reconstruction algorithm by region

abdominal wall allotransplants as an additional strategy to expand the domain of the abdominal cavity to account for either a graft/recipient size mismatch or inability for closure in the face of extreme intestinal edema. While the risks of life-long immunosuppression potentially outweigh the potential benefits of abdominal wall transplantation in healthy non-transplant patients, transplant patients are already bound to an immunosuppressive regimen and can benefit from the addition of allograft abdominal wall musculofas-

cial tissue to reduce abdominal wall wound complication at the time of transplantation.

In the setting of transplant immunosuppression, the risk of an open abdominal wound, fascial dehiscence, septic evisceration or fistula carries significant morbidity and potential mortality. When conventional abdominal wall closure techniques are insufficient allotransplantation is performed. Extensive study of the vascular supply of the abdominal wall has allowed design of musculofasciocutaneous flaps based on the deep inferior epigastric system (DIEP). These flaps can be transferred based on either the DIEP vessels through microsurgical technique or the external iliac for a macrovascular anastomosis. Cipriani et al. describe a series of 15 abdominal wall transplants with three episodes of rejection salvage with modulating immunosuppression and two flap losses due to vascular thrombosis [9].

Abdominal wall transplantation is a field in its early stage. It has virtually eliminated the issue of donor site morbidity and future advances will likely focus on improved recipient site function. To this end, refining flap design even further to include dynamic neurotized flap transfers that can provide stable abdominal wall contour and preserved truncal core muscular stability will represent a new era in abdominal wall reconstruction.

Summary

Most abdominal wall defects do not require formal flap reconstruction since there is often redundancy in both the musculofascia and skin. When flaps are required, it is generally best to first consider local, then regional, and finally distant flaps. Regional pedicle flaps are limited by their respective arc of rotation and may not reach the defect, this is particularly true for hypogastric defects. When free flaps are required the thigh and back are generally the best donor locations. The location of recipient vessels and flap pedicle length are important to consider for these complex reconstructions. Vein grafts are often required to "extend" the length of the free flap pedicle in order to reconstruct defects, particularly in the upper abdomen. Reconstruction of composite defects that include loss of musculofascia and overlying skin require special attention. In general, we find that the musculofascia is best reconstructed with mesh and component separation

rather than with fascia from the flap. Flap reconstruction of abdominal wall defects is often complex and is best performed with a multidisciplinary approach including a plastic and reconstructive surgeon.

References

1. Fortelny RH, Hofmann A, Gruber-Blum S, Petter-Puchner AH, Glaser KS. Delayed closure of open abdomen in septic patients is facilitated by combined negative pressure wound therapy and dynamic fascial suture. Surg Endosc. 2014;28(3):735–40.
2. Deeken CR, Eliason BJ, Pichert MD, Grant SA, Frisella MM, Matthews BD. Differentiation of biologic scaffold materials through physicomechanical, thermal, and enzymatic degradation techniques. Ann Surg. 2012;255(3):595–604.
3. Glass GE, Murphy GF, Esmaeili A, Lai LM, Nanchahal J. Systematic review of molecular mechanism of action of negative-pressure wound therapy. Br J Surg. 2014;101(13):1627–36.
4. Booth JH, Garvey PB, Baumann DP, Selber JC, Nguyen AT, Clemens MW, Liu J, Butler CE. Primary fascial closure with mesh reinforcement is superior to bridged mesh repair for abdominal wall reconstruction. J Am Coll Surg. 2013;217(6):999–1009.
5. Disa JJ, Goldberg NH, Carlton JM, Robertson BC, Slezak S. Restoring abdominal wall integrity in contaminated tissue-deficient wounds using autologous fascia grafts. Plast Reconstr Surg. 1998;101(4):979–86.
6. Khouri JS, Egeland BM, Daily SD, Harake MS, Kwon S, Neligan PC, Kuzon Jr WM. The keystone island flap: use in large defects of the trunk and extremities in soft-tissue reconstruction. Plast Reconstr Surg. 2011;127(3):1212–21.
7. Selber JC, Angel Soto-Miranda M, Liu J, Robb G. The survival curve: factors impacting the outcome of free flap take-backs. Plast Reconstr Surg. 2012;130(1):105–13.
8. Lin SJ, Butler CE. Subtotal thigh flap and bioprosthetic mesh reconstruction for large, composite abdominal wall defects. Plast Reconstr Surg. 2010;125(4):1146–56.
9. Selvaggi G, Levi DM, Cipriani R, Sgarzani R, Pinna AD, Tzakis AG. Abdominal wall transplantation: surgical and immunologic aspects. Transplant Proc. 2009;41(2):521–2.

Maurice Y. Nahabedian

Introduction

Contour abnormalities of the anterior abdominal wall can present in various forms based on the specific structural anatomic deformity. The most common and notable is the abdominal wall hernia that is the result in a fascial defect with protrusion of abdominal viscera or omentum. However, contour abnormalities may also present without a fascial defect and are defined and classified as a bulge due to laxity or attenuation of the supportive layers of the anterior abdominal wall. The location of the bulge can be along the anterior rectus sheath or the linea alba. Bulges over the lateral abdominal wall or anterior rectus sheath may be due to denervation of the abdominal wall musculature or to a violation of the anterior rectus sheath. Bulges over the midline abdominal wall without a fascial defect are usually the result of attenuation of the linea alba with a separation of the rectus abdominis muscles and is referred to as diastasis recti. This chapter will focus on the etiology, diagnosis, and management of diastasis recti.

M.Y. Nahabedian, M.D., F.A.C.S. (✉)
Department of Plastic Surgery, Georgetown
University Hospital, 3800 Reservoir Rd NW,
Washington, DC 20007, USA
e-mail: DrNahabedian@aol.com

Anatomy

The aponeurotic layers of the anterior abdominal wall include the linea alba, anterior rectus sheath, posterior rectus sheath, and the external oblique fascia (Fig. 31.1). The anterior rectus sheath and the linea alba are composed of collagen fibers arranged in an interwoven lattice. The width and thickness of these structures will vary along the surface and regions of the anterior abdominal wall [1]. The width of the linea alba ranges from 11 to 21 mm between the xiphoid process and the umbilicus and decreases from 11 to 2 mm from the umbilicus to the pubic symphysis. The thickness of the linea alba ranges from 900 to 1200 μm between the xiphoid and the umbilicus and increases from 1700 to 2400 μm from the umbilicus to the pubic symphysis. The thickness of the anterior rectus sheath ranges from 370 to 500 μm from the xiphoid to the umbilicus and increases to 500–700 μm from the umbilicus to the pubic symphysis. The posterior rectus sheath is slightly thicker than the anterior rectus sheath above the umbilicus at 450–600 μm, but is thinner from the umbilicus to the arcuate line at 250–100 μm (Fig. 31.2). The vascularity of the anterior rectus sheath and linea alba is derived from the perforating branches of the deep and superior inferior epigastric vessels as well as the superficial epigastric vessels. The loose areolar fascia over the surface of the anterior sheath and linea alba is highly vascularized and important to preserve (Fig. 31.3).

© Springer International Publishing Switzerland 2016
Y.W. Novitsky (ed.), *Hernia Surgery*, DOI 10.1007/978-3-319-27470-6_31

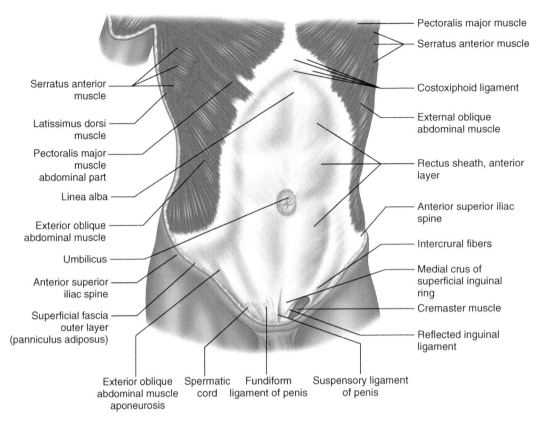

Pectoralis major muscle

Serratus anterior muscle

Costoxiphoid ligament

External oblique abdominal muscle

Rectus sheath, anterior layer

Anterior superior iliac spine

Intercrural fibers

Medial crus of superficial inguinal ring

Cremaster muscle

Reflected inguinal ligament

Serratus anterior muscle

Latissimus dorsi muscle

Pectoralis major muscle abdominal part

Linea alba

Exterior oblique abdominal muscle

Umbilicus

Anterior superior iliac spine

Superficial fascia outer layer (panniculus adiposus)

Exterior oblique abdominal muscle aponeurosis

Spermatic cord

Fundiform ligament of penis

Suspensory ligament of penis

Fig. 31.1 Illustration of the anterior abdominal wall demonstrating the anterior rectus sheath and the linea alba

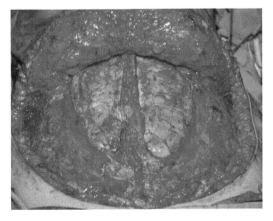

Fig. 31.2 Photograph of the anterior abdominal wall demonstrating the posterior rectus sheath and linea alba following elevation of both rectus abdominis muscles

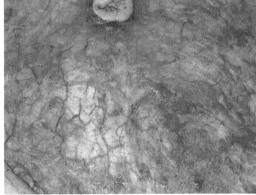

Fig. 31.3 The vascularized loose areolar fascia on the surface of the anterior rectus sheath is demonstrated

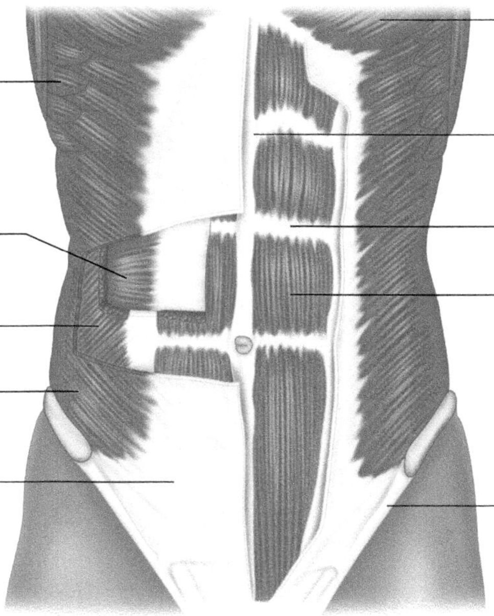

Fig. 31.4 The muscles and fascial layers of the anterior abdominal wall

The muscular layers of the anterior abdominal wall are equally important and comprised of the paired rectus abdominis muscles as well as the paired external, internal, and transverse oblique muscles (Fig. 31.4). The forces exerted by these muscles, as well as intra-abdominal pressure, can place tension on the midline linea alba and result in separation or attenuation resulting in a diastasis recti.

Etiology

The etiology of diastasis recti is typically the result of increased intra-abdominal pressure that usually occurs following pregnancy; however, obesity and prior abdominal operations can also be the cause (Fig. 31.5). It has been demonstrated that the intra-abdominal pressures associated with pregnancy will increase the distance between the rectus abdominis muscles [2] (Fig. 31.6). It has been observed that the myofascial laxity associated with diastasis recti is both vertical and horizontal and can involve the entire anterior abdominal wall and not just the linea alba [3]. Bauman has measured the inter-recti distance in

92 women and demonstrated that stretching of the linea alba is limited to 5 cm in 82% of patients and can extend up to 6 cm in 2% [3]. Abdominal laxity beyond that is usually due to attenuation of the anterior rectus sheath.

Liaw has compared the inter-rectus distance between nulliparous women and postpartum women and demonstrated a doubling of the inter-rectus distance from approximately 0.5–1.0 cm to 1.2–2.3 cm using ultrasound-assisted measurements [2]. In the postpartum group, there was a gradual decrease in the distance over time; however, baseline values were never achieved at 6-month assessments. Pregnancy also has a notable effect on the strength of the abdominal musculature with nulliparous women having 5/5 strength of the trunk flexors and rotators compared to 4/5 in women that were 6 months postpartum.

Diagnosis

The diagnosis of diastasis recti is made on physical examination and presents as a midline bulge that can occur above or below the umbilicus

Fig. 31.5 Separation of the
paired rectus abdominis
muscles associated with
pregnancy is illustrated

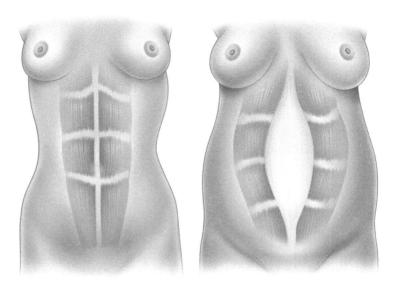

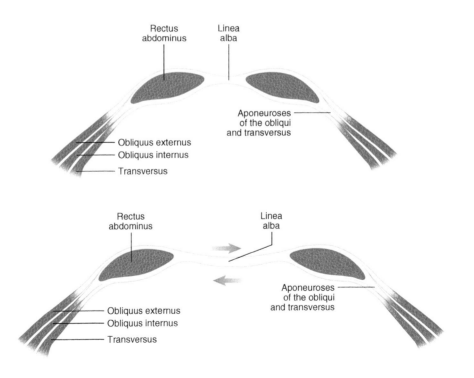

Fig. 31.6 Illustration demonstrating a normal and widened inter-rectus distance associated with a rectus diastasis

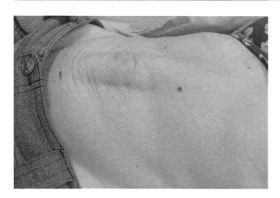

Fig. 31.7 A woman with rectus diastasis is depicted demonstrating the midline bulge

(Fig. 31.7). It is amplified by having the patient lie flat and perform a straight leg raise. Confirmation of rectus diastasis can be made using CT, MRI, or ultrasound, but these tests are usually not necessary [4–6]. All imaging modalities can be used to measure the inter-rectus distance, however, they are more often obtained to assess the success of the repair.

Classification

There are three classification systems that have been described for rectus diastasis. The Nahas classification is based on the myofascial deformity and the etiology [7] (Table 31.1). The Rath classification is based on the level of the attenuation relative to the umbilicus and the patient age [8] (Table 31.2). The Beer classification is based on the normal width of the linea alba as determined from 150 nulliparous women [9] (Table 31.3).

The Initial Consultation

During the initial consultation, it is important to obtain a thorough history and physical examination. Relevant information related to prior abdominal operations, previous pregnancies, and history of weight gain is obtained. On physical examination, abdominal scars, concomitant hernias, abdominal pannus, and extent of the diastasis are

Table 31.1 The Nahas classification based on the myofascial deformity

Deformity	Etiology	Correction
Type A	Pregnancy	Anterior sheath plication
Type B	Myoaponeurotic laxity	External oblique plication
Type C	Congenital	Rectus abdominis advancement
Type D	Obesity	Anterior sheath plication and rectus abdominis advancement

Table 31.2 The Rath classification based on the level of the attenuation relative to the umbilicus and the patient age

Level	Age <45 (mm)	Age >45 (mm)
Above umbilicus	10	15
At umbilicus	27	27
Below umbilicus	9	14

Table 31.3 The Beer classification based on the normal width of the linea alba

Normal width of the linea alba (mm)	
Level	Width
At Xiphoid	15
3 cm above umbillicus	22
2 cm below umbillicus	16

documented. Visualization of the midline diastasis is easily demonstrated with the patient supine performing a straight leg raise. Ideal candidates for a diastasis repair include patients with an isolated diastasis, low BMI, and no prior abdominal operations. Less ideal candidates include obese patients, extensive comorbidities, desire to have more children, and multiple abdominal procedures.

Indications for Surgery

Indications for diastasis repair are based on symptoms and physical findings [10]. Many patients with diastasis recti will have discomfort at the level of the defect. This is often exacerbated with movement. The appearance of the abdominal wall is often noticeably distorted in women with diastasis recti. The midline bulge is exacerbated with muscle contraction and is common in multiparous women. The pathophysiology of diastasis recti often results in the development of an umbilical hernia as well. Correction of the umbilical hernia alone without correction of the diastasis is often associated with recurrence due to the poor quality of surrounding tissue.

Not all patients will require surgery for correction. Time and conservative measures such as core strengthening are often useful. Surgery is usually indicated in women that have failed conservative measures and when the degree of rectus diastasis interferes with activities of daily living and is bothersome.

Treatment

There are several options for management of diastasis recti ranging from exercise to simple plication of the linea alba and anterior rectus sheath to more advanced excisional techniques with or without the use of mesh. Endoscopic and laparoscopic techniques can also be used in select situations where a small midline hernia is present as well. In many cases, an abdominoplasty is also indicated.

Exercise

The benefit of exercise to prevent or correct diastasis recti is somewhat controversial and has been associated with mixed results [11]. Preventative exercise protocols include walking and abdominal core strengthening. Corrective exercise protocols include core strengthening, aerobic activity, and neuromuscular re-education. Although mild benefit was noted in terms of inter-rectus distance from some studies, there was insufficient evidence to recommend exercise as a means of preventing or treating rectus diastasis.

Abdominoplasty

In most women with mild-to-severe diastasis recti, the overlying adipocutaneous component of the anterior abdominal wall has also become stretched and flaccid. An abdominoplasty is typically performed in these women to further improve the abdominal contour [12–14]. This is usually achieved using a low transverse incision incorporating the aesthetic subunits of the abdominal wall (Fig. 31.8). The anterior superior iliac crest is palpated and marked bilaterally. A curved low transverse line is drawn connecting the two points with the midpoint just above the pubic hairline. The incision extends to the anterior rectus sheath. The adipocutaneous tissues are elevated off the anterior rectus sheath preserving the vascularized loose areolar layer. The umbilicus is incised and preserved on its stalk. The undermining usually extends to the mid to upper abdomen and correlates to the length of the diastasis. The diastasis repair is commenced at this juncture utilizing a variety of techniques that will be described in the following sections. Following the repair, the patient is gently flexed at the hip and the excess skin is redraped and then excised. One or two closed suction drains are placed and the skin is sutured with a 3-layer closure.

Plication with or Without Excision

For mild-to-moderate diastasis recti, midline plication of the linea alba can be considered (Fig. 31.9). With this technique, the attenuated linea alba is delineated. Contraction of the attenuated fascia can be achieved using a low-set cautery device to create thermal contraction. Following this, a 2-layer plication can be achieved using an absorbable or nonabsorbable suture. The triangular suture technique incorporating the lateral edges of the fascia and the midline of the posterior rectus sheath is frequently used [15]. Excision of the midline fascia can also be considered when severely attenuated (Fig. 31.10).

Studies evaluating absorbable and nonabsorbable sutures have demonstrated no significant difference in the inter-recti distance as measured by CT scan 6 months following correction [16]. The first layer of sutures was usually an interrupted figure-of-8 and the second layer of suture was running continuous to reinforce the repair and to bury to suture knots from the first layer. In patients with

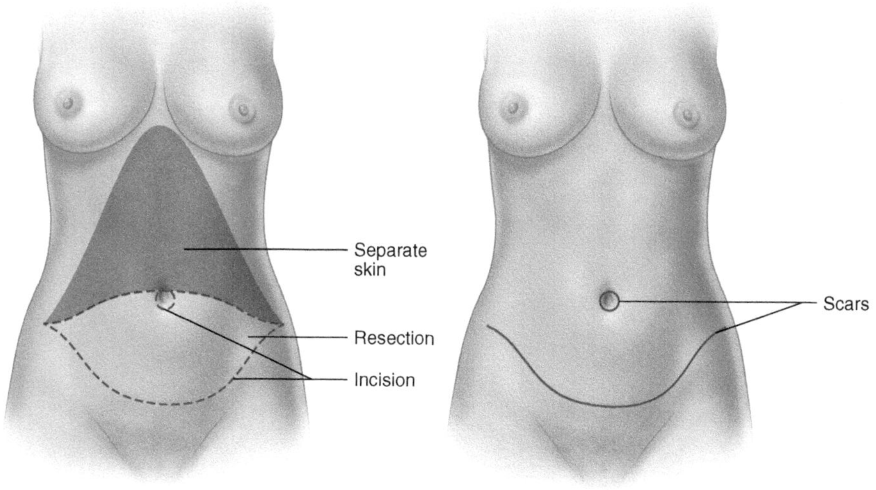

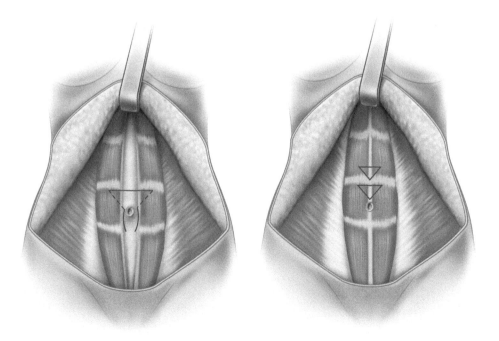

Fig. 31.8 A schematic illustration of an abdominoplasty demonstrating the location of the scar and degree of undermining

Fig. 31.9 Midline plication of the rectus abdominis muscles

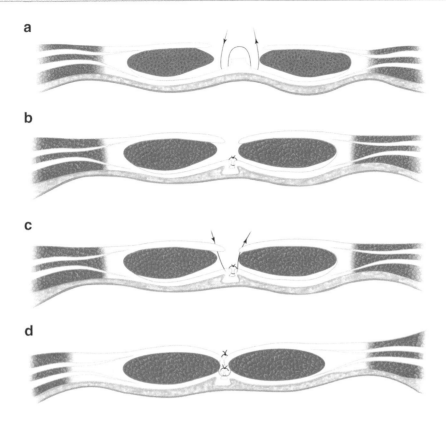

Fig. 31.10 Escision of redundant fascia and triangulation sutures to reapproximate the rectus abdominis muscles

significant laxity of the anterior rectus sheath, lateral plication can also be performed on both sides to further improve and tighten the abdominal contour. A 2-layer repair technique is usually performed using an absorbable interrupted suture followed by a running continuous suture for further reinforcement. The length of this repair can extend from approximately 2 cm below the costal margin to approximately 2 cm above the pubic bone.

Plication and Onlay Mesh

The use of a mesh can be considered in cases of extensive laxity requiring a lengthy repair [12]. Typically a resorbable or non-resorbable mesh is selected and placed over the anterior rectus sheath. It is trimmed to fit the dimensions of the anterior abdominal wall and extends from the costal margin superiorly to the pubic region infe-

riorly and also extends to the anterior axillary line bilaterally. Non-resorbable mesh is usually preferred in these cases because the patients are typically healthy with few, if any, comorbidities and are at low risk of infection or adverse outcome. The edge of the mesh is typically anchored in an interrupted manner using an absorbable suture. The central portion of the mesh is secured in a quilting pattern also using an interrupted absorbable suture. A single closed suction drain is used.

Figures 31.11, 31.12, 31.13, 31.14, 31.15, 31.16, 31.17, 31.18 and 31.19 illustrate a multiparous woman with severe rectus diastasis and skin laxity. The preoperative photographs are illustrated (Figs. 31.11 and 31.12). The plan is to plicate, reinforce with non-resorbable mesh and excise the redundant skin and fat. The lower abdominal skin is marked and incised extending from one anterior superior iliac crest to the other. Dissection proceeds

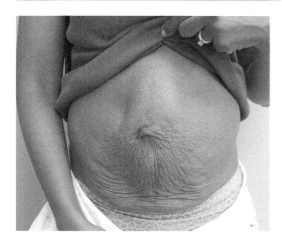

Fig. 31.11 Preoperative image of a multiparous woman with diastasis recti

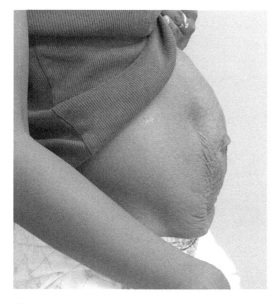

Fig. 31.12 Lateral view demonstrating significant abdominal laxity and bulge

to the anterior rectus sheath and then extends in a cephalad direction toward the xiphoid process preserving the loose areolar layer (Fig. 31.13a). The attenuated midline fascia is delineated and then plicated using the 2-layer technique. Plication lateral to the midline on both sides can also be considered in severe cases (Fig. 31.13b). The degree of abdominal tightening is demonstrated on Fig. 31.14a, b. A synthetic mesh is trimmed to fit the anterior abdominal surface and then sutured at the periphery and centrally in an interrupted technique (Fig. 31.15). The abdominoplasty is performed by first assessing

the amount of skin redundancy and then dividing it along the midline (Fig. 31.16). The excess skin is excised and the remaining skin is closed in a 3-layer fashion (Fig. 31.17). Six-month follow-up demonstrates a significant improvement in abdominal contour without recurrence (Figs. 31.18 and 31.19).

Retrorectus Repair with Mesh

In cases of moderate-to-severe diastasis recti, a retrorectus repair can be considered [17]. With this technique, an anterior paramedian incision is made adjacent to the lateral aspect of the linea alba extending from the xiphoid to the pubic bone. The medial aspect of the rectus abdominis muscle is appreciated and the muscle is undermined preserving the vascularity and laterally based innervation. The rectus abdominis muscle is completely released from the posterior rectus sheath. The degree of redundancy of the posterior rectus sheath is approximated and then plicated along its midline using a resorbable suture in an interrupted manner (Fig. 31.20). The repair can then be reinforced using a resorbable or nonresorbable mesh. The mesh is placed on the surface of the posterior rectus sheath in the retrorectus space and anchored with interrupted absorbable sutures. The purpose of the mesh is to offload the pressure placed on the midline fascial repair. The umbilical stalk is passed through an opening created in the mesh. Following the repair, the released rectus abdominis muscles are aligned in their natural location with the medial edge of both muscles positioned along the midline. The anterior rectus sheath is repaired using interrupted absorbable sutures.

Endoscopic/Laparoscopic

Luque has described using a totally endoscopic technique for diastasis repair in patients with a concomitant midline hernia [10]. The most common midline hernia associated with a diastasis is the umbilical hernia (85%) [10]. The indications for total endoscopic repair include midline/umbilical hernia measuring >2 cm, no prior hernia repair or laparotomy, and no need for abdominoplasty. The technique involves placing a trocar

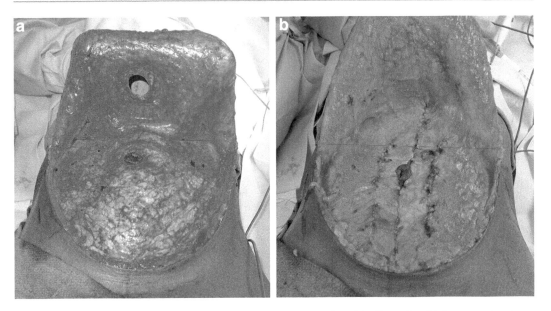

Fig. 31.13 (**a**) Intraoperative photograph demonstrating the midline bulge of the linea alba. (**b**) Intraoperative photograph following plication of the midline and lateral fascia

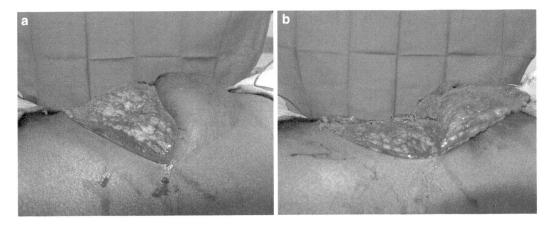

Fig. 31.14 (**a**) Intraoperative lateral photograph demonstrating the degree of abdominal protrusion prior to repair. (**b**) Intraoperative lateral photograph demonstrating the degree of abdominal protrusion following the repair

into the supra aponeurotic space and creating a dissection plane under direct vision exposing the linea alba and the anterior rectus sheath. The repair includes sheath plication and reinforcement with a synthetic mesh. A nonabsorbable barbed suture is typically used. A drain is placed and a soft-compression garment is applied.

Laparoscopic reinforcement of the anterior abdominal wall can be considered in some patients. In patients that have had plication of the attenuated linea alba and anterior rectus sheath, laparoscopic placement of an intraperitoneal mesh can be considered instead of onlay mesh placement. Huguier has applied this technique in 15 women with good-to-excellent results in 13/15 (87%) [18].

Complications

Complications following rectus diastasis repair are infrequent and include infection, mesh extrusion, recurrence, nerve injury, seroma,

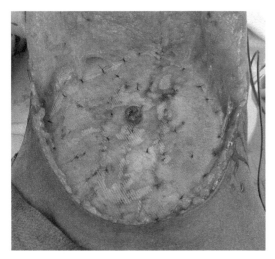

Fig. 31.15 Intraoperative photograph following place-ment of the non-resorbable mesh over the plicated anterior rectus sheath

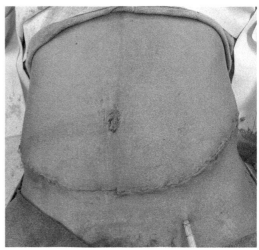

Fig. 31.17 Intraoperative photograph following comple-tion of the abdominoplasty

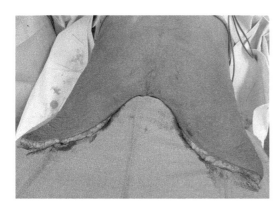

Fig. 31.16 Intraoperative photograph of the redundant skin and fat constituting the abdominoplasty

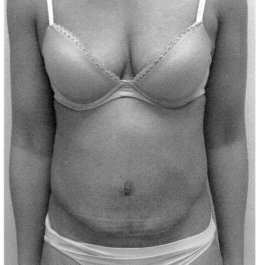

Fig. 31.18 Six-month postoperative anterior view fol-lowing successful diastasis repair and abdominoplasty

complex scar, skin necrosis, contour abnormal-ity, and visceral injury (bladder, bowel). As with most operations, caution must be exer-cised when considering this procedure in women who are active smokers, because delayed healing and tissue necrosis are more common in this population of patients [17].

Emanuelsson has performed a randomized controlled trial comparing outcomes and compli-cations in women with rectus diastasis managed with layered closure of the anterior rectus sheath or retrorectus placement of synthetic mesh [19]. Superficial wound infection occurred in 14/57 (24.5%) of which 5/57 (8.8%) were in the suture repair cohort and 9/57 (15.8%) were in the retro-rectus mesh cohort. Postoperative pain was assessed using a visual analog scale demonstrat-ing an improved reduction in pain in the retrorec-tus cohort (6.9) compared to the sheath plication cohort (4.8).

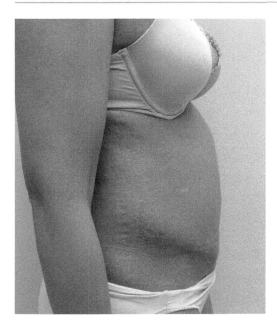

Fig. 31.19 Six-month postoperative lateral view

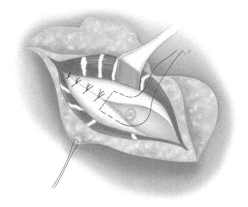

Fig. 31.20 Suture plication of the posterior rectus sheath

Outcomes

Sheath Plication

The outcomes following sheath plication for diastasis recti have been mixed and primarily related to the type of suture used for the plication.

Al-Quattan in a review of 20 women following vertical sheath plication alone using an absorbable suture demonstrated 100% recurrence after 1 year [20]. Reasons included a repair that was localized to the defect only, a repair that addressed only the horizontal component of the diastasis, and suture-related fraying of the anterior rectus sheath due to its fragile nature. Nahas using a nonabsorbable suture had positive outcomes utilizing a 2-layer plication repair [5]. Efficacy of the repair was evaluated by postoperative CT scans in 12 women at 3 weeks, 6 months, and again at a mean of 81 months postoperatively. The inter-rectus distance was measured 3 cm above and below the umbilicus. They demonstrated no recurrence of diastasis recti in any patient at all levels studied. Mestak performed a case-controlled study comparing 51 women that had diastasis recti repair via plication with an interlocking continuous absorbable suture (0-PDS) to 10 nulliparous women without a diastasis [4]. Postoperative assessment was performed via physical examination and ultrasound in all women at 12–41 months following the repair. Ultrasound measurements were obtained at the midpoint of the umbilicus and xiphoid, at the umbilicus, and at the midpoint of the umbilicus and the pubis. The mean inter-recti distance was essentially equal between the two cohorts. The authors advocated absorbable sutures because suture palpability is not a long-term issue.

The type and orientation of suture material used for diastasis repairs has also been comparatively studied. Nahas has compared diastasis repair techniques using absorbable (0-polydiaxone) sutures to nonabsorbable (2-0 nylon) sutures. CT scans obtains at 3 weeks and 6 months demonstrated no significant difference between the two suture techniques [16]. Ishida, in a cadaveric study, compared horizontal versus vertical suture repair. A dynamometer was used to determine the amount of force required to disrupt the suture repair [21]. There was significantly higher difference in the strength required for rupture for the vertical suture placement, thus vertical orientation was recommended.

Retrorectus Repair

Outcomes following the retrorectus repair have been demonstrated to be effective. Batchvarova et al. have utilized this technique in 52 women with up to 11 years of follow-up [17]. They contend that posterior plication alone may not be sufficient in all cases and for that reason have decided to place a vicryl mesh into the retrorectus space. The benefit of the mesh in that location was to redistribute the forces placed on the posterior sheath repair, reducing the risk of recurrence. According to Batchvarova, a resorbable mesh such as vicryl is preferred because it effectively relieves fascial tension, is resorbed by 6 weeks, is placed in an extraperitoneal position, and does not increase the incidence of complications.

In the Emanuelsson study, SF-36 outcomes were compared following repair via anterior sheath plication versus retrorectus mesh placement [19]. The results demonstrated improvement in both cohorts following the repair with no technique demonstrating superiority over the other. Subjective improvement in muscle strength was improved more in the retrorectus cohort compared to the suture cohort (6.9 vs. 4.5, Likert scale, 0–10, $p = 0.01$).

Endoscopic/Laparoscopic

The most frequent adverse event with the endoscopic technique is seroma (23%) [10]. In the 21 patients from the Luque study, there were no hernia or diastasis recurrences at 20-month follow-up [10]. The mean inter-rectus distance was significantly improved 1 month following the procedure with preoperative measurements ranging from 24 to 39 mm and postoperative measurements ranging from 2.1 to 2.8 mm. One- and 2-year follow-up did not change from the 1-month measurements (2.5–3.7 mm). Patient satisfaction was assessed on a visual analog scale and graded with a mean score of 8.7.

Summary

The etiology, diagnosis, and management of diastasis recti is now well understood and has demonstrated success in management. Multiparous women are at highest risk for developing diastasis recti. Diagnosis is easily made by clinical examination and symptomatology. Management options vary and will depend on the degree of separation between the rectus abdominis muscles. Simple plication has been effective for mild-to-moderate diastasis. The use of resorbable or non-resorbable mesh placed as an onlay or in the retrorectus space has been effective for moderate-to-severe diastasis.

References

1. Azer H, et al. Collagen fibers in linea alba and rectus sheath. J Surg Res. 2001;96:127–34.
2. Liaw LJ, Hsu MJ, Liao CF, Liu MF, Hsu AT. The relationships between inter-recti distance measured by ultrasound imaging and abdominal muscle function in postpartum women: a 6-month follow-up study. J Orthop Sports Phys Ther. 2011;41(6): 435–43.
3. Brauman D. Diastasis recti: clinical anatomy. Plast Reconstr Surg. 2008;122:1564.
4. Mestak O, Kullac R, Mestak J, et al. Evaluation of the long-term stability of sheath plication using absorbable sutures in 51 patients with diastasis of the recti muscles: an ultrasonographic study. Plast Reconstr Surg. 2012;130:714e.
5. Nahas FX, Ferreira LM, Augusto SM, Ghelfond C. Long-term follow-Up of correction of rectus diastasis. Plast Reconstr Surg. 2005;115:1736.
6. Elkhatib H, Buddhavarapu RS, Henna H, Kassen W. Abdominal musculoaponeuretic system: magnetic resonance imaging evaluation before and after vertical plication of rectus muscle diastasis in conjunction with lipoabdominoplasty. Plast Reconstr Surg. 2011;128:733e.
7. Nahas FX. An aesthetic classification of the abdomen based on the myoaponeurotic layer. Plast Reconstr Surg. 2001;108:1787–95.
8. Rath AM, Attali P, Dumas JL, et al. The abdominal linea alba: an anatomo-radiologic and biomechanical study. Surg Radiol Anat. 1996;18:281–8.
9. Beer GM, Schuster A, Seifert B, et al. The normal width of the linea alba in nulliparous women. Clin Anat. 2009;22:706–11.
10. Luque JB, Luque AB, Valdivia J, et al. Totally endoscopic surgery on diastasis recti associated with midline hernias.

The advantages of a minimally invasive approach. Prospective cohort study. Hernia. 2015;19(3):493–501.

11. Benjamin DR, van de Water ATM, Peiris CL. Effects of exercise on diastasis of the rectus abdominis muscle in the antenatal and postnatal periods: a systematic review. Physiotherapy. 2014;100:1–8.

12. Akram J, Matzen SH. Rectus abdominis diastasis. J Plast Surg Hand Surg. 2014;48(3):163–9.

13. Restrepo JCC, Ahmed JAM. New technique of plication for abdominoplasty. Plast Reconstr Surg. 2002;109:1170.

14. Tadiparthi S, Shokrollahi K, Doyle GS, et al. Rectus sheath plication in abdominoplasty: assessment of its longevity and a review of the literature. J Plast Reconstr Aesthet Surg. 2012;65:328–32.

15. Ferreira LM, Castilho HT, Hochberg J, et al. Triangular mattress suture in abdominal diastasis to prevent epigastric bulging. Ann Plast Surg. 2001;46:130.

16. Nahas FX, Augusto SM, Ghelfond C. Nylon versus polydioxanone in the correction of rectus diastasis. Plast Reconstr Surg. 2001;107:700.

17. Batchvarova Z, Leymarie N, Lepage C, Leyder P. Use of a Submuscular resorbable mesh for correction of severe postpregnancy musculoaponeurotic laxity: an 11-year retrospective study. Plast Reconstr Surg. 2008;121:1240.

18. Huguier V, Faure JL, Doucet C, Giot JP, Dagregorio G. Laparoscopic coupled with classical abdominoplasty in 10 cases of large rectus diastasis. Ann Chir Plast Esthet. 2012;57:350–5.

19. Emanuelsson P, Gunnarsson U, Strigard K, Stark B. Early complications, pain, and quality of life after reconstructive surgery for abdominal rectus muscle diastasis: a 3-month follow-up. J Plast Reconstr Aesthet Surg. 2014;67:1082–8.

20. Al-Qattan MM. Abdominoplasty in multiparous women with severe musculoaponeurotic laxity. Br J Plast Surg. 1997;50:450.

21. Ishida LH, Gemperli R, Longo MVL, et al. Analysis of the strength of the abdominal fascia in different sutures used in abdominoplasty. Aesthetic Plast Surg. 2011;35:435–8.

Terri A. Zomerlei and Jeffrey E. Janis

Introduction

Abdominal wall defects, whether spontaneous, traumatic or iatrogenic in origin, are a complex and heterogeneous problem and can challenge surgeons of all experience levels. One tool that that should be in the modern surgeon's armamentarium of useful adjuncts for complex abdominal wall repair is negative pressure wound therapy. Originally designed to expedite healing in chronic wounds such as diabetic foot ulcers, negative pressure wound therapy (NPWT) is a simple mechanical device that provides suction over a wound bed [1–4]. Suction is a long-established surgical practice method utilized for drainage of wounds. The advantages of formal negative pressure wound therapy devices versus simple suction are many and include the ability to tailor wound interface materials, to exchange canisters capable of removing large quantities of exudate, and the option to control both the level of suction (in millimeters of mercury) and the frequency of the suction (continuous vs. noncontinuous/intermittent). An important safety feature of all NPWT

T.A. Zomerlei, M.D., M.S. (✉)
J.E. Janis, M.D., F.A.C.S.
Department of Plastic Surgery, Ohio State University Wexner Medical Center, 915 Olentangy River Road, Suite 2100, Columbus, OH 43212, USA
e-mail: Terri.Zomerlei@osumc.edu;
Jeffrey.Janis@osumc.edu

devices is the alarm system that warns the user of loss of seal, or excessive fluid output [1]. Some specially designed NPWT units are also capable of instillation of isotonic solutions that contain antibacterial or antimicrobial agents. NPWT units vary in size and some units have been developed that are portable and even disposable. All NPWT devices share a similar basic structure with the key components of each device consisting of a suction pump capable of generating negative pressure (with power supplied by either battery or electric cord), tubing, a storage canister for effluent, a sealing apparatus and wound interface material.

Mechanism of Action

There have been many speculations regarding the mechanisms of action behind NPWT and its ability to expedite wound healing. While the exact mechanism of NPWT is largely unknown, it is generally accepted that it is likely a medley of influences that contribute to the success of NPWT in healing both acute and chronic wounds.

The theories regarding the mechanism of action of NPWT can be categorized into three broad concepts: fluid-milieu, alteration or reduction of bacterial burden, and application of mechanical stress.

Wound healing is not a simple linear process but rather a complex series of exchanges among mediators and cells [2]. The environment or milieu in which these interactions occur can have a negative or positive effect on the wound-healing process [3]. The interstitial edema that accumulates in wounds can potentially compromise the delicate microcirculation causing deleterious effects on oxygen content delivery to the end tissues. The subatmospheric pressure exerted by NPWT units efficiently draws this excess fluid out of the wound bed thus improving the healing environment of the wound. The composition of the wound extracellular matrix is determined by a dynamic balance among overall matrix synthesis, deposition, and degradation. Wound extracellular matrix itself is a key regulator of cell adhesion, migration, proliferation, and differentiation during tissue repair [1]. NPWT can improve the extracellular wound matrix by removing negative impactors on the wound-healing milieu. These factors, which can act as local tissue toxins, include acute phase proteins, proteolytic enzymes, specific cytokines, and metalloproteinases. A recently published systematic review of the molecular bases behind NPWT mechanism of action suggests that, in contrast, promotion of wound healing occurs by modulation of cytokines to an anti-inflammatory profile, and mechanoreceptor/chemoreceptor-mediated cell signaling. These interactions then culminate in angiogenesis, extracellular matrix remodeling, and deposition of granulation tissue [4].

Another hypothesized mechanism of action of NPWT is the reduction of overall bacterial burden. Controlled animal studies have demonstrated logarithmic declines in bacterial burdens with use of NPWT, though this has not been able to be reproduced in clinical studies [5, 6]. It is thought NPWT may act to decrease the overall bacterial burden of a wound in three ways. First, the closed environment acts as a physical barrier to the encroachment of adjacent skin flora. Second, the subatmospheric pressure exerted by the unit physically moves any existing bacteria away from the wound with the interstitial effluent. Lastly, as demonstrated in animal studies by Morykwas, application of subatmospheric pressure at 125 mmHg to in vivo tissues improves blood flow levels fourfold [6]. This increase in oxygen in the local tissues not only interferes with the growth of anaerobic bacteria but also

provides additional substrate for neutrophils to use for the oxidative bursts that kill bacteria.

An additional hypothesis on the mechanism of action of NPWT focuses on the biomechanical properties offered by the porous foam interface and the exerted negative pressure. There is a growing body of evidence that suggests healing tissue responds and adapts to the functional demands placed on it. These demands can be subdivided in those that exert macrostrain versus microstrain to the wound. The macrostrain theory postulates that the mechanical force from the interaction of the negative pressure with the wound interface is transmitted to the wound edges drawing them closer together [7]. In 2004, Saxena first introduced the concept that NPWT improves granulation through application of micromechanical forces or microstrain. Their tissue studies revealed that contact with the foam dressing particularly had physical effects on the tissue and noted an increase in the undulating contour of tissues corresponding to the pore geometry on the foam. The surface irregularities imposed by contact with the foam pores increased the surface area that could be subjected to negative pressure without an increase in the overall wound footprint. Specifically, the microstrain theory asserts that when more individual cells can be subjected to the application of subatmospheric pressure and the mechanical strain and deformational forces leading to cell stretch, cell proliferation and angiogenesis are stimulated leading to promotion of wound healing [8].

Foam vs. Gauze

The ability to tailor wound interface materials allows for customization of NPWT to the wound bed. By and large, there are two different dressing types that have been explored in the literature; dressing that have a gauze interface and those with a foam substrate. While studies have determined that the pressure transfer to the wound bed is similar in gauze and foam dressings, there may be particular clinical circumstances in which one product may be superior to another [9, 10]. Gauze dressings offer ease of application because they do not have to be cut and shaped to the wound bed. Some studies also report that patients experience less pain during dressing changes with gauze, which is likely related to having less tissues ingrowth with the dressing material [11]. In addition, as cost savings become an increasingly more pressing matter to our health system, gauze dressings may offer a financial advantage both in cost of materials and labor expenses. In a recent randomized trial, the daily cost of NPWT was found to be $96.51 for foam-based dressings versus $4.22 for gauze-based dressings. Likewise NPWT foam dressings were associated with increased time spent on the dressing change with the average time spent clocked at 31 min versus 19 min for the gauze group [12].

Since the inception of NPWT, foam dressings have been the more traditional wound interface material. Foam dressings are available in multiple shapes and sizes that are then cut to size to fit the wound bed during the dressing application. Several different foam contract dressings are currently employed and they are commonly known and referred to based on their color [13].

"Black" or open-cell polyurethane foam is the most traditional NPWT dressing and consists of reticulated large open pores (400–600 μm) making it particularly well suited for wounds that produce large amounts of exudate. The black foam is also hydrophobic and the large pore size allows for maximal interaction between the subatmospheric pressure provided by the NPWT and the wound bed, which results in optimizing granulation tissue formation [14].

Polyvinyl alcohol, or "white" foam, in contrast is hydrophilic and has a small, dense pore allocation (60–270 μm) making is less adherent to the wound. This composition also results in less removal of exudate and diminished ability of the NPWT to produce granulation tissue. This may be preferable in circumstances where the wound is shallow or overlying prosthetic implants or if its over/near areas that are sensitive to desiccation or pressure.

Green foam is composed of polyurethane and has an open pore structure that facilitates the monitoring of the wound bed. Green foam pore size is similar to that of black foam, but the tensile strength is superior allowing for less foam

residue in the wound bed when the foam interface material is removed [15].

Silver sponges are either polyurethane or polyvinyl sponges that have been coated in silver substrate. The silver coating on the sponges has been found to decrease the odor of infected wounds likely by decreasing the wound bacterial load. Silver-coated sponges are particularly well suited for wounds where contamination is still present (Fig. 32.1). The antimicrobial ability of silver dressing is attributed to the strong oxidative activity of the silver nanoparticle (AgNP) surfaces and the release of silver ions into the biologic environment [16]. The oxidative activity and the effects of the silver ions themselves are thought to trigger a series of negative effects on the structures and functions of cells including cytotoxicity, immunological responses, and even cell death.

Subatmospheric Pressure

An additional feature of modern NPWT units is the ability to vary the level of negative atmospheric pressure that is placed over a wound bed. Animal model blood flow studies completed by Morykwas in 1996, plotted blood flow changes measured with a Doppler needle flow probe in soft-tissue and muscle against varying levels of subatmospheric pressure. The blood flow changes in both tissues demonstrated similar bell-shaped responses. The application of 125 mmHg of negative pressure produced the optimal response in the tissues with a peak blood flow of four times baseline values. Levels of pressure above 400 mmHg were found to have deleterious effects on granulation tissue formation, likely because blood flow decreased as the capillary bed blood flow was shut down when attempting to overcome perfusion pressure. Based on in vivo studies, pressure levels in the range of 75–125 mmHg are desirable for the microdeformation and strain that produces robust granulation tissue formation [17]. Clinically, the application of pressure over a wound can produce discomfort and while a pressure of 125 mmHg is generally the "default" setting from NPWT, this level may need to be adjusted lower based on patient tolerance.

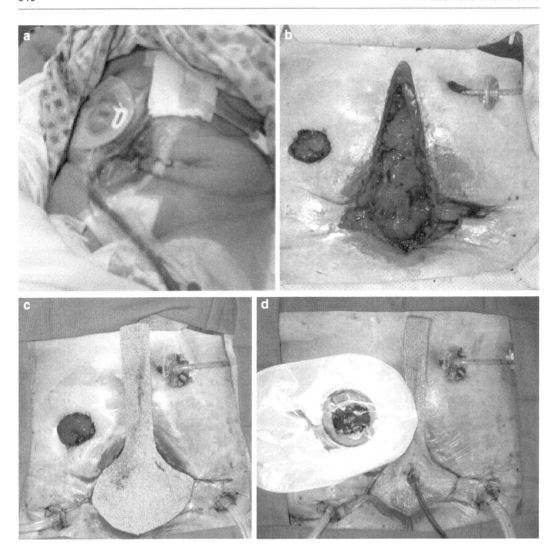

Fig. 32.1 A patient with a complex abdominal wall presented for take-down of an enterocutaneous fistula (**a, b**). Following fistula take-down, the fascial defect was repaired with a large pore biologic mesh. A silver NPWT sponge was used for treatment of the contaminated soft-tissue defect because of its antimicrobial properties (**c, d**)

In addition to demonstrating the optimal pressure to induce peak blood flow, Morykwas and his colleagues also compared constant applications of pressure to intermittent pressure application. In the intermittent studies, peak increases in local blood flow declined when "off" intervals were less than 2 min. Based on these results, a 5-min-on/2-min-off cycle for intermittent NPWT was considered optimal for maximizing blood flow and granulation formation. These settings were then used in head-to-head comparisons with continuous NPWT. The mean increase in granulation tissue formation for the wounds that received the intermittently prescribed negative pressure was significantly higher than wounds subjected to continuous pressure, specifically the intermittently treated wounds demonstrated a near 100%increased rate of granulation tissue formation versus a 60%increase in the continuous pressure-treated wounds [17].

While intermittent pressure application can achieve increased rates of granulation tissue formation there are two problems that can be encountered with its use. The first is the application of pressure can produce discomfort and, in a sensitive patient, the pain would be experienced every few minutes with the cycling of the unit. In addition, in wounds that produce a large amount of effluent, the "off" period may allow fluid to accumulate and breach the adhesive barrier resulting in loss of suction.

Instillation Therapy

A more recent development in NPWT science is the development of units that have the ability for instillation. Antimicrobials or antibiotics in an isotonic fluid delivery system can be loaded into the units and then instilled over an acutely or chronically infected wound [18]. The interval and duration of the negative pressure can be controlled as well as the type of solution instilled and the solution dwell time. Several fluids that have been explored in the literature include silver nitrate, Dakin's solution, and mixed antibiotic solution [13]. An instillation fluid that has been utilized and studied specifically with use of NPWT is Prontosan (B. Brain, Inc.; Bethlehem, Pa.). Prontosan is composed of polyhexamethylene biguanide also known as Polyhexanide, which functions as a preservative that inhibits the growth of microorganisms and Betaine, a surfactant, which serves as a cleanser and provides immediate debridement [1, 19]. The positive effect of polyhexanide-containing irrigation is thought to be from reduction of bacterial load and biofilm formation. NPWT with simultaneous irrigation has been found to further reduce bioburden over NPWT-treated wounds alone. In addition, using NPWT with installation capabilities in grossly infected wounds may have the advantage of potentially reducing trips to the operating room for washouts [20].

Negative Pressure Wound Therapy and Abdominal Wall Reconstruction

Full-Thickness Abdominal Defects

Abdominal wall defects present primarily in two varieties, partial-thickness defects and full-thickness defects and the clinical applications of NPWT differs for each.

Full-thickness defects of the abdominal wall commonly occur after surgical intervention to manage a serious insult to the abdomen. Circumstances such as, abdominal trauma, peritonitis, decompression of abdominal compartment syndrome, or ruptured aneurysm repair, commonly lead to damage control laparotomies. In those circumstances, it is not only not possible to close the abdomen, but also is usually not safe to do so. In this situation, NPWT can be used as a bridge to future more definitive closure. Application of NPWT in the situation of an "open abdomen" serves several purposes, including removing exudates and decreasing bowel edema, removing wound contamination, maintaining a closed, moist environment for abdominal viscera and minimizing loss of domain. Early adaptations of NPWT utilized to contain the abdominal contents and evacuate infectious material involved the use of an inert, fenestrated plastic sheeting in contact with the viscera, towels, or laparotomy packs placed on top of the sheeting, drains hooked up to wall suction on top of the towels or packs, and an occlusive dressing to seal the wound. Modern NPWT devices for the open abdomen come ready-made with improved function and ease of use. As visceral edema and exudate are reduced by the negative pressure, the fascia is able to be more closely approximated allowing for either primary repair of the fascia, or repair with use of mesh (Fig. 32.2). Commonly, the patient is returned to the operating room every 3–5 days to perform further washout and attempt primary fascial closure or fascial closure with the use of mesh, once contamination is minimized.

Goals with management of the open abdomen are primarily twofold—reduction of mortality rate and achievement of a high fascial closure rate. A consensus document from an expert advisory panel outlining best practices for management of the open abdomen was published in 2009 [21]. Both the expert advisory committee and a systematic review from the same year deduced that use of a NPWT unit was the superior technique for temporary abdominal closure (TAC). Closure rates were found to be highest with NPWT, ranging between 78 and 93 %. In addition, the incidence of fistulas compared to other techniques was likewise reduced with NPWT

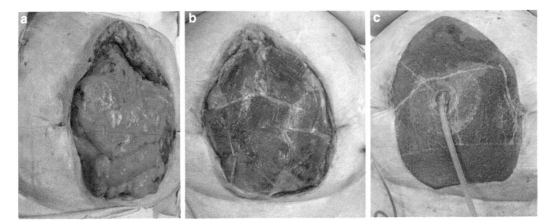

Fig. 32.2 This 67-year-old female underwent an emergent re-exploration hours after having a laparotomy with extensive lysis of adhesions, revision of her Roux-en-Y gastrojejunostomy, and duodenojejunostomy. On re-exploration she was found to have bleeding from the liver edge. Once the bleeding was addressed, the bowel wall edema was such that her abdomen was not able to be closed (**a**). She underwent placement of an ABthera device (KCI, San Antonio, TX) to decrease edema and prevent further loss of domain (**b, c**). She was returned to the OR every 3–5 days for attempts at closure

being associated with a 2.9%rate of fistula formation versus other techniques such as zipper, silo, and loose packing with resultant 5.7 to 28%occurrence of fistula formation [22].

Partial-Thickness Abdominal Defects

Partial-thickness abdominal wall defects indicate that there is some component of the native musculofascial abdominal wall or a mesh that is preventing the evisceration of the abdominal contents. In this situation, depending on the size of the defect and the situation in which it is being addressed, NPWT can serve as a primary treatment, a bridge to more definitive treatment, or as a mitigator of postsurgical complications. As a primary treatment, NPWT can be applied to an open soft-tissue wound to enhance granulation tissue formation. Once granulation of the wound is complete and the wound size has contracted, the device can be removed allowing for re-epithelialization of the wound. For particularly large defects, the NPWT can be used to temporize the defect and provide an optimal wound-healing environment, so that the wound footprint can be reduced by granulation and contraction until it is determined that coverage with a skin graft is feasible. In those cases, the NPWT device may also be used to help promote graft take. If a large defect is relatively clean, black foam can be used as the interface with the pressure set to 125 or 150 mmHg, if there is significant effluent. The continuous mode initially will aid in the evacuation of edema and promotion of blood flow. In the case of a contaminated wound bed, silver foam can be used initially in a similar fashion to help reduce bioburden until the first or second dressing change, at which time the black foam can be substituted. More frequent initial dressing changes may be necessary as well depending on the degree of wound contamination that is present. When the amount of effluent from the wound begins to stabilize or lessen, the NPWT can be prescribed in an intermittent mode as described above (5-min-on/2-min-off) in order to stimulate granulation tissue formation, provided the patient will tolerate it.

Negative Pressure Wound Therapy and Special Circumstances

Closed Incisions

Recently, the application of a short duration of NPWT on closed surgical wounds in order to prevent the morbidity of postsurgical complications has been publicized [23–25]. This technique, which was first appraised in the trauma and orthopedic literature, is aimed predominantly at reducing seroma formation, infections, and wound dehiscence. Seromas, in particular, have long been a frustrating complication following ventral hernia repair with the prevalence proven to be as high as 100%on routine ultrasound exams and 35%with clinical assessments [26]. In addition to seromas being a bothersome postoperative problem, they can also be a harbinger for more worrisome complications. Seromas can lead to wound complications because they can prevent the ingrowth of mesh, and can become seeded with bacteria either from seepage from the incision or iatrogenically from repeat fluid aspirations.

Studies across many surgical fields have all demonstrated increased surgical complications including wound infections in the obese population [24, 27, 28]. Wound infections in the obese may originate because of traction and shear forces on wounds closed with suture, thereby permitting seepage of bacteria into deeper layers of tissue. In addition, as previously described in the cardiothoracic literature, skin incisions in the obese can present specific problems from a mechanical standpoint. In the supine position, the weight of the obese tissue on either side of the incision pulls the skin edges apart, this is especially problematic in the areas of skin folds where bacterial colonization can be ample [23]. Likewise, when the obese patient is in the sitting position, any areas of skin folding are subjected to increased traction pulling the skin edges apart. If mesh has been utilized to help facilitate primary closure of the abdomen, the avoidance of bacterial colonization of the wound becomes even more imperative. A recent retrospective study suggests that incisional NPWT following abdominal wall reconstruction, in particular, significantly improves rates of wound complications (22%vs. 63%) and skin dehiscence (9%vs. 39%) when compared with conventional dressings. Regardless of the surgical technique employed, in order to prevail over the specific obstacles that the repair of complex abdominal wall defects can present, the prophylactic use of NPWT in a continuous suction mode of 125 mmHg for 7 days duration over a closed incision has been shown to improve outcomes [29] (Fig. 32.3).

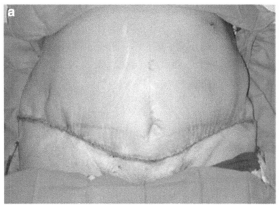
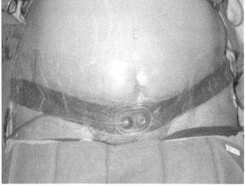

Fig. 32.3 A transverse incision was employed to repair the recurrent ventral hernia in this patient so that that a concomitant panniculectomy could also be performed (**a**). An incisional NPWT device (Prevena, KCI, San Antonio, TX) was placed over the closed surgical wound to splint the incision and prevent seroma accumulation (**b**)

Mesh Salvage

Infection is a formidable opponent of ventral hernia repair with the reported incidence of prosthetic mesh infection being as high as 8%[30, 31]. Previously, mesh that was colonized with bacteria causing infection left the surgeon with few options for definitive treatment other than the unsavory task of explanting the mesh entirely and frequently relegating the patient back to having a ventral hernia and an abdominal wall defect. As described previously, the application of subatmospheric pressure on a wound bed both increases blood flow and may decrease bacterial colonization. These biologic properties as well as the power to remove large quantities of fluid while still providing a closed, moist wound environment has gained NPWT a place in the treatment and salvage of infected large pore monofilament mesh. In 2013, a prospective study by Berrevoet et al. demonstrated effective salvage of large pore meshes composed of equal parts polypropylene and absorbable poliglecaprone 25 monofilaments with application of NPWT. In this monocentric study that spanned a 6-year period, 724 open ventral and incisional hernia repairs were performed. A total of 63 patients developed wound infections and had NPWT applied. With the exception of 4 patients who required operative debridement, all large pore monofilament meshes were able to be salvaged [31].

Incisional NPWT along with a methylene blue tracking system can be employed to salvage more focal mesh infections. On occasion, a patient who is several months to years status post ventral/incisional hernia repair will present with a complaint of chronically draining sinuses from their repair. In the operating suite, these tracts are gently probed with a blunt needle and diluted methylene blue is instilled into the tract. An incision is then performed and the methylene blue tracts can be followed through the tissue to the infectious nidus, usually knots of permanent suture. The sutures and tracts are then removed and any focal granuloma or abscess is debrided. After all the tracts have been addressed, a skin ellipse that encompasses all the sinus tracts is excised, the wound is irrigated thoroughly and closed primarily in a layered fashion. An incisional VAC is then placed over the closed incision and stays in place for a week (Fig. 32.4).

Skin Grafts for Abdominal Wall Reconstruction

Negative pressure wound therapy can be employed for two different indications in some patients with partial-thickness abdominal wall defects. The NPWT unit is first used to granulate the base of the wound bed in order to provide an optimal surface for skin grafting. A split-thickness skin graft can then be harvested and placed on the wound bed and NPWT can again be applied over the skin graft for 5 days to improve skin graft take [32]. Maintaining contact between the wound bed and a skin graft, especially if the wound surface is uneven or concave/convex as is commonly the case on the abdomen, can be especially daunting. The advantages of NPWT versus traditional bolster dressings are many and include uniform compression of the wound bed, and prevention and minimization of dead space, including the very concave areas. NPWT also drains the exudate or blood and avoids the shear phenomenon [33]. Seroma, hematoma, and shear are adversaries of skin graft take and, if these are present, plasmatic imbibition, inosculation, and revascularization will not take place and the graft will slough. Several studies have observed that with the use of negative-pressure wound therapy, the split-thickness skin graft take rate is significantly higher approaching 100%, compared with 87–89%for conventional graft bolstering [34, 35].

Complex Abdominal Wall Defect Reconstruction

A multipronged approach to the problem of abdominal wall defects is vital to achieve the goal of re-establishing continuity of the abdominal wall with one surgery. Appropriate patient selection for abdominal wall reconstruction procedures

Fig. 32.4 This patient presented nearly a year after recurrent ventral hernia repair with complaints of "draining holes" in the abdomen (**a**). Each sinus tract was filled with methylene blue (**b**) and after incision; a probe was used to locate the base of the tract (**c**). Knots of polypropylene suture with associated stitch abscess were found at the base of each sinus tract. The sutures were removed, the focal abscesses debrided, and the sinus tracts were excised. The patient underwent primary closure with placement of incisional NPWT

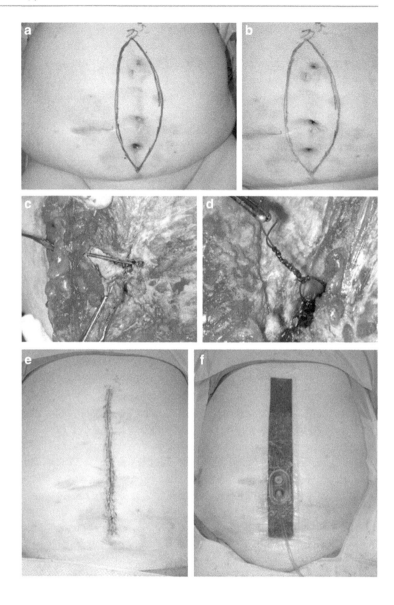

is essential and its importance cannot be overstated. There are several patient factors that can quickly undermine even the most well-devised surgical plan if they are not addressed or controlled for. These patient factors include tobacco abuse, chronic obstructive pulmonary disease, glucose control, history of wound infection, and high body mass index (BMI) [36]. In 2010, the Ventral Hernia Working Group proposed a grading system from Grade 1 (low risk) to Grade 4 (infected) to stratify hernias based on wound classification as well as patient-risk factors for surgi-

cal site infection [37]. This grading system was recently further modified by Kanters et al. to include three grades with statistically significant differences in surgical site occurrences serving as the separation criteria for the grades [38].

A clinical algorithm for deciding which patients would be best served by NPWT is based in part on the Modified Hernia Grading system. In the high-risk abdominal wall reconstruction patients (high Grade 2 or Grade 3 with clean-contaminated wounds), who have obesity and *plus* one of more additional comorbidities, as outlined by the Modified Hernia Grading System, we have employed a novel technique, as described below, of NPWT application method following hernia repair that gives this population a "best chance" at healing by controlling the risk of dehiscence and seroma.

Prior to repair of the hernia, the abdominal contents are freed from aberrant attachments, lysis of adhesions is performed, scar and devitalized tissue is debrided and mesh is explanted if needed. As previously described by Butler, and as subsequently modified by Janis, a minimally invasive component separation is then performed [39, 40]. Repair of the native musculofascia is the gold standard in ventral hernia surgery and all surgical efforts should be geared toward this goal. As is commonly the case though, mesh is frequently employed to provide additional structure and support to the musculofascial repair as a retrorectus sublay mesh. This placement is preferred as it is associated with lower ventral hernia reoccurrence rates [41]. The minimally invasive component separation technique uses tunneled incisions for external oblique aponeurosis release and thus preserves both the connection between the subcutaneous fat and the anterior rectus sheath and the myocutaneous perforator vessels originating from the rectus abdominis. This accomplishes two goals:

1. Reduction of subcutaneous dead space thereby reducing seroma formation
2. Improved vascularity to the skin flaps

Following the minimally invasive components separation, NPWT can be incorporated into the sutured skin closure in order to mitigate the risk of dehiscence, which is almost preordained in this population (Fig. 32.5).

1. The Scarpa's fascia is approximated in an interrupted fashion with a 2-0 absorbable suture with each suture being placed about 3 finger breadths apart.
2. Interrupted sutures or staples are placed in the deep dermis along the entire length of the incision. These are again placed about 3 fingerbreadths apart.

3. Following placement of the deep dermal sutures, the midline closure should have a "string of pearls" appearance with areas that are closed (the string) and area that are an open ellipse (pearls).
4. A piece of "extra large" black, polyurethane foam that is already pre-perforated is separated into strips, or alternatively, silver foam is cut into strips. These strips are then placed into each opening between the interrupted closures ("French fries").
5. The foam strips are inserted into the openings in the incision, ensuring that each strip traverses the entire thickness of the abdominal flap and rests against the myofascial closure. The foam strips should protrude from the incision a few centimeters.
6. The closed sections of the incision between with foam strips are covered with a nonadherent contact layer such as Xeroform (Covidien, Mansfield, MA) or Adaptic (Johnson & Johnson, New Brunswick, NJ) to prevent desiccation.
7. A rectangular strip of black foam is then cut to size that will allow it to act as a "crossbar" and traverse the entire length of the incision over the tops of the previously placed black foam strips.
8. The occlusive dressing is then applied over the foam, allowing for a considerable area of contact with the skin. A skin adhesive can be applied to the skin to promote adhesion. The suction tubing is applied to the dressing and the suction device is set to a continuous suction mode at 125 mmHg.

The negative atmospheric pressure distributed within the closed wound environment allows for removal of exudate from the thick abdominal flaps. The blacks foam "French fries" also eliminate any potential dead space within the abdominal flap closure thus preemptively thwarting seroma formation. In addition, the uniform negative pressure essentially holds the tissues in gentle static compression thus offering a significant reduction in mechanical tractive forces and shearing forces between the skin flaps. Placing a negative pressure wound dressing on clean skin

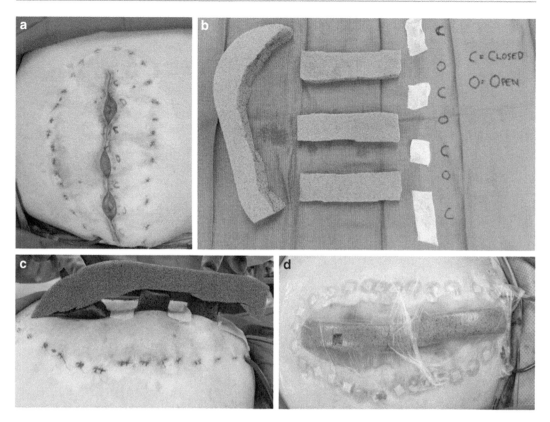

Fig. 32.5 This high-risk obese patient with a recurrent ventral hernia had removal of an old mesh and placement of a new widely placed retrorectus mesh (**a**). Foam strips and occlusive dressings were laid out in a template fash-ion with "C" representing the closed areas of the incisions and "O" representing the open areas (**b**). The NPWT was then incorporated into the closure (**c**) and the sealing apparatus applied (**d**)

immediately after suturing also provides a closed environment that discourages the seepage of encroaching skin flora as the suction provides a one way egress from the incision. In essence, this "French fry, string of pearls" technique is a com-bination of open NPWT to reduce fluid build-up, improve local blood flow, and apply macro- and microstrain advantages combined with the bene-fits of incisional NPWT along the intermittent areas of primary closure.

The final group of hernia patients are those with either open abdomens or enterocutaneous fistula (Grade 3). These patients are commonly treated with a two-step approach with the affected bowel addressed first and NPWT utilized as a bridge to address contamination and infection and decrease bowel edema, if abdomen is left open. In those with open abdomens, reoperation with washout and attempted definitive abdominal repair should be staged at 3–5-day intervals after the initial surgery with intra-abdominal NPWT applied between closure attempts.

Conclusion

NPWT is an easy-to-use versatile treatment with a broad range of clinical indications. Understanding the use and application of vari-ables such as wound interface material, level of subatmospheric applied, mode of pressure appli-cation, and use of instillation allows the practitio-ner to prescribe NPWT that is customized to the patient's specific needs.

While NPWT is not a panacea for defects of the abdominal wall, its ability to expedite wound healing, improve skin graft take, salvage mesh infections, and mitigate surgical complications such as wound infections and dehiscence makes NPWT a valuable implement for the modern surgeon.

References

1. Argenta LC, Morykwas MJ, Marks MW, DeFranzo AJ, Molnar JA, David LR. Vacuum-assisted closure: state of clinic art. Plast Reconstr Surg. 2006;117(7 Suppl):127S–42.
2. Broughton 2nd G, Janis JE, Attinger CE. The basic science of wound healing. Plast Reconstr Surg. 2006;117(7 Suppl):12S–34.
3. Moues CM, van den Bemd GJCM, Heule F, Hovius SER. Comparing conventional gauze therapy to vacuum-assisted closure wound therapy: a prospective randomised trial. J Plast Reconstr Aesthet Surg. 2007;60(6):672–81.
4. Glass GE, Murphy GF, Esmaeili A, Lai LM, Nanchahal J. Systematic review of molecular mechanism of action of negative-pressure wound therapy. Br J Surg. 2014;101(13):1627–36.
5. Assadian O, Assadian A, Stadler M, Diab-Elschahawi M, Kramer A. Bacterial growth kinetic without the influence of the immune system using vacuum-assisted closure dressing with and without negative pressure in an in vitro wound model. Int Wound J. 2010;7(4):283–9.
6. Morykwas MJ, Argenta LC, Shelton-Brown EI, McGuirt W. Vacuum-assisted closure: a new method for wound control and treatment: animal studies and basic foundation. Ann Plast Surg. 1997;38(6): 553–62.
7. Urschel JD, Scott PG, Williams HT. The effect of mechanical stress on soft and hard tissue repair; a review. Br J Plast Surg. 1988;41(2):182–6.
8. Saxena V, Hwang CW, Huang S, Eichbaum Q, Ingber D, Orgill DP. Vacuum-assisted closure: microdeformations of wounds and cell proliferation. Plast Reconstr Surg. 2004;114(5):1086–96; discussion 97–8.
9. Campbell PE, Smith GS, Smith JM. Retrospective clinical evaluation of gauze-based negative pressure wound therapy. Int Wound J. 2008;5(2):280–6.
10. Malmsjo M, Ingemansson R, Martin R, Huddleston E. Negative-pressure wound therapy using gauze or open-cell polyurethane foam: similar early effects on pressure transduction and tissue contraction in an experimental porcine wound model. Wound Repair Regen. 2009;17(2):200–5.
11. Borgquist O, Gustafson L, Ingemansson R, Malmsjo M. Tissue ingrowth into foam but not into gauze during negative pressure wound therapy. Wounds. 2009;21(11):302–9.
12. Dorafshar AH, Franczyk M, Gottlieb LJ, Wroblewski KE, Lohman RF. A prospective randomized trial comparing subatmospheric wound therapy with a sealed gauze dressing and the standard vacuum-assisted closure device. Ann Plast Surg. 2012;69(1):79–84.
13. Kim PJ, Attinger CE, Steinberg JS, Evans KK, Lehner B, Willy C, et al. Negative-pressure wound therapy with instillation: international consensus guidelines. Plast Reconstr Surg. 2013;132(6):1569–79.
14. Malmsjo M, Ingemansson R. Green foam, black foam or gauze for NWPT: effects on granulation tissue formation. J Wound Care. 2011;20(6):294–9.
15. Malmsjo M, Ingemansson R. Effects of green foam, black foam and gauze on contraction, blood flow and pressure delivery to the wound bed in negative pressure wound therapy. J Plast Reconstr Aesthet Surg. 2011;64(12):e289–96.
16. Jones S, Bowler PG, Walker M. Antimicrobial activity of silver-containing dressings is influenced by dressing conformability with a wound surface. Wounds. 2005;17(9):263–70.
17. Morykwas MJ, Faler BJ, Pearce DJ, Argenta LC. Effects of varying levels of subatmospheric pressure on the rate of granulation tissue formation in experimental wounds in swine. Ann Plast Surg. 2001;47(5):547–51.
18. Gabriel A. Integrated negative pressure wound therapy system with volumetric automated fluid instillation in wounds at risk for compromised healing. Int Wound J. 2012;9 Suppl 1:25–31.
19. Kim PJ, Attinger CE, Steinberg JS, Evans KK, Powers KA, Hung RW, et al. The impact of negative- pressure wound therapy with instillation compared with standard negative- pressure wound therapy: a retrospective, historical, cohort, controlled study. Plast Reconstr Surg. 2014;133(3):709–16.
20. Gabriel A, Kahn K, Karmy-Jones R. Use of negative pressure wound therapy with automated, volumetric instillation for the treatment of extremity and trunk wounds: clinical outcomes and potential cost-effectiveness. Eplasty. 2014;14, e41.
21. Kaplan M, Banwell P, Orgill DP, Ivatury RR, Demetriades D, Moore FA, et al. Guidelines for the management of the open abdomen. Wounds-a Compendium of Clinical Research and Practice. 2005;1–24.
22. Boele van Hensbroek P, Wind J, Dijkgraaf MG, Busch OR, Goslings JC. Temporary closure of the open abdomen: a systematic review on delayed primary fascial closure in patients with an open abdomen. World J Surg. 2009;33(2):199–207.
23. Grauhan O, Navasardyan A, Hofmann M, Muller P, Stein J, Hetzer R. Prevention of poststernotomy wound infections in obese patients by negative pressure wound therapy. J Thorac Cardiovasc Surg. 2013;145(5):1387–92.
24. Matatov T, Reddy KN, Doucet LD, Zhao CX, Zhang WW. Experience with a new negative pressure incision management system in prevention of groin wound infection in vascular surgery patients. J Vasc Surg. 2013;57(3):791–5.
25. Lopez-Cano M, Armengol-Carrasco M. Use of vacuum-assisted closure in open incisional hernia

repair: a novel approach to prevent seroma formation. Hernia. 2013;17(1):129–31.

26. Susmallian S, Gewurtz G, Ezri T, Charuzi I. Seroma after laparoscopic repair of hernia with PTFE patch: is it really a complication? Hernia. 2001;5(3): 139–41.

27. Fleck TM, Fleck M, Moidl R, Czerny M, Koller R, Giovanoli P, et al. The vacuum-assisted closure system for the treatment of deep sternal wound infections after cardiac surgery. Ann Thorac Surg. 2002;74(5): 1596–600.

28. Stannard JP, Volgas DA, McGwin 3rd G, Stewart RL, Obremskey W, Moore T, et al. Incisional negative pressure wound therapy after high-risk lower extremity fractures. J Orthop Trauma. 2012;26(1):37–42.

29. Conde-Green A, Chung TL, Holton 3rd LH, Hui-Chou HG, Zhu Y, Wang H, et al. Incisional negative-pressure wound therapy versus conventional dressings following abdominal wall reconstruction: a comparative study. Ann Plast Surg. 2013;71(4):394–7.

30. Meagher H, Clarke Moloney M, Grace PA. Conservative management of mesh-site infection in hernia repair surgery: a case series. Hernia. 2013;20(3):249–52.

31. Berrevoet F, Vanlander A, Sainz-Barriga M, Rogiers X, Troisi R. Infected large pore meshes may be salvaged by topical negative pressure therapy. Hernia. 2013;17(1):67–73.

32. Birke-Sorensen H, Malmsjo M, Rome P, Hudson D, Krug E, Berg L, et al. Evidence-based recommendations for negative pressure wound therapy: treatment variables (pressure levels, wound filler and contact layer)—steps towards an international consensus. J Plast Reconstr Aesthet Surg. 2011;64(Suppl):S1–16.

33. Blackburn JH, Boemi L, Hall WW, Jeffords K, Hauck RM, Banducci DR, et al. Negative-pressure dressings as a bolster for skin grafts. Ann Plast Surg. 1998;40(5):453–7.

34. Petkar KS, Dhanraj P, Kingsly PM, Sreekar H, Lakshmanarao A, Lamba S, et al. A prospective randomized controlled trial comparing negative pressure dressing and conventional dressing methods on split-thickness skin grafts in burned patients. Burns. 2011;37(6):925–9.

35. Llanos S, Danilla S, Barraza C, Armijo E, Pineros JL, Quintas M, et al. Effectiveness of negative pressure closure in the integration of split thickness skin grafts: a randomized, double-masked, controlled trial. Ann Surg. 2006;244(5):700–5.

36. Attinger CE, Janis JE, Steinberg J, Schwartz J, Al-Attar A, Couch KA. Clinical approach to wounds: debridement and wound bed preparation including the use of dressings and wound-healing adjuvants. Plast Reconstr Surg. 2006;117(7):72S–109.

37. Ventral Hernia Working G, Breuing K, Butler CE, Ferzoco S, Franz M, Hultman CS, et al. Incisional ventral hernias: review of the literature and recommendations regarding the grading and technique of repair. Surgery. 2010;148(3):544–58.

38. Kanters AE, Krpata DM, Blatnik JA, Novitsky YM, Rosen MJ. Modified hernia grading scale to stratify surgical site occurrence after open ventral hernia repairs. J Am Coll Surg. 2012;215(6):787–93.

39. Butler CE, Campbell KT. Minimally invasive component separation with inlay bioprosthetic mesh (MICSIB) for complex abdominal wall reconstruction. Plast Reconstr Surg. 2011;128(3):698–709.

40. Janis JE, Khansa I. Evidence-based abdominal wall reconstruction: The maxi-mini approach. Plast Reconstr Surg. 2015;136(6):1312–23.

41. Albino FP, Patel KM, Nahabedian MY, Sosin M, Attinger CE, Bhanot P. Does mesh location matter in abdominal wall reconstruction? A systematic review of the literature and a summary of recommendations. Plast Reconstr Surg. 2013;132(5):1295–304.

Sarah Sher and Karen Evans

Introduction

In this chapter we introduce our approach to management of abdominal wounds, both acute and chronic. We will begin the chapter with an overview of general wound healing, and then transition to various methods of wound care, followed by our approach to managing abdominal wounds. Our goal is to help practitioners in identifying different stages of wound healing and how to manage each respectively.

A thorough understanding of the etiology of the wound is paramount, along with identifying other sources of contamination that may impede wound healing, such as fistulae, contamination from stoma, and malnutrition. It is important to recreate a dynamic, functional abdominal wall, which is a much more complex scenario than healing a wound. Our general approach is early surgical debridement of abdominal wounds. Our experience has shown that this approach allows us to ultimately heal the wounds in less time and preserve more tissue. In addition, early aggressive intervention in failed skin closure after primary laparotomies may prevent later development of incisional hernia.

S. Sher, M.D. (✉) • K. Evans, M.D.
Department of Plastic Surgery, Georgetown
University Hospital, Washington, DC, USA
e-mail: sarah.sher@gmail.com

Overview of Wound Healing

Wound closure is established by primary, secondary, or tertiary intention. Secondary and tertiary techniques are frequently used in management of abdominal wounds. Primary closure of a wound occurs when all layers of tissue including the skin are closed at the completion of the operation with suture material. Secondary intention occurs when some or all of the tissues are left open and allowed to close naturally over time. Tertiary intention or staged closure occurs when the wound is initially left open for a short amount of time (days) and then closed [1]. This technique is often used in the traumatic setting.

The wound healing process is an elegant cascade of cellular interactions, which involve balanced feedback loops of inflammatory mediators in response to signals from the wound and surrounding environment. A healed wound will only achieve at most 80% of the original tissue's tensile strength. There are three phases of wound healing: the inflammatory phase, fibroproliferative phase, and the remodeling phase. The inflammatory phase takes place once the skin barrier is broken until approximately 7 days later [2]. This phase is predominated by the initial vasoconstriction and then cell migration to the wound, which occurs via cell signaling from the wound environment and damaged epithelium. Neutrophils are initially recruited to the wound bed, however, by day 3, macrophages are the predominant inflammatory cells within the wound. The fibroproliferative phase overlaps with the inflammatory phase; the fibroproliferative phase begins at day 4 and continues through day 21. During this phase, a matrix is established with recruitment of fibroblasts and the production of glycosaminoglycans. Early angiogenesis and neoepithelialization also occurs during this phase and granulation tissue can be seen in healthy wounds. The third stage, wound contraction, occurs from day 21 until 1 year. Type 1 collagen replaces type 3 collagen during this phase, the peak wound tensile strength is achieved by day 60 under normal conditions [2, 3].

Acute vs. Chronic Wounds

Patients often present to surgeons with abdominal wounds in the acute setting, after a traumatic episode or postsurgical event. In the acute setting the etiology of the abdominal wound is due to failed primary closure. The level of contamination can be variable, however, it is usually low. Superficial dehiscence of primary closure can be managed non-operatively with appropriate dressings. However, if the dehiscence extends to the fascia level, we recommend surgical debridement and delayed primary closure to expedite healing and prevent fascia separation. Drainage in a closed incision is a sign that underlying tissue planes are not healing well and should be examined closely to make sure that there is not deeper separation or fluid collection [4]. This is especially true for obese patients if the deeper layers become devascularized, infected, or were not closed primarily. Poorly healing adipose tissue commonly presents as fat necrosis and drainage [5].

In the traumatic setting, the level of contamination is also variable due to the etiology of the wound. In the setting of a traumatic abdominal wound there is often a loss of soft tissue, fascia, or both. The intra-abdominal process should be controlled, and attempts to decrease visceral edema, and contamination should be the focus of patient care after the patient is stabilized [6]. These steps are critical to achieving a stable abdominal wound that then can be suitable for reconstruction. The overall health of the patient will dictate how aggressive one can be with wound care and reconstructive options.

Chronic wounds of the abdominal wall are more likely to be contaminated. These patients have likely failed primary and possibly secondary attempts at closure. The wounds become halted in the inflammatory stage of wound healing secondary to a prolonged inflammatory response due to bacterial contamination and senescent cells at the periphery of the wound. The contamination must be controlled and debridement of the biofilm and non-viable tissue must occur [4–6]. Chronic wounds of the abdominal wall should be measured every week to ensure that proper wound healing is occurring. Wound healing trajectories should be assessed for each patient. Depending on the patient's comorbidities, wound surface area, depth and tunneling should be decreasing at a steady rate. Dressings can be tailored to the type of wound that is present. Patients can either be managed conservatively with dressing changes or with surgical closure, depending on the nutritional and medical status of the patient.

There are many factors that predispose patients to difficulties with healing abdominal wounds. Obese patients (BMI >30 kg/m^2) have higher rates of complications after both emergent and elective procedures. Excess abdominal skin and tissue results in functional and hygienic challenges. In the obese patient with a large pannus, a panniculectomy might be necessary to improve healing. In all closures, we recommend closing the scarpa's fascia layer with an absorbable suture (2-0 PDS), the skin should then be closed as indicated in either a staged fashion with negative pressure wound therapy, staples, interrupted sutures, or multilayer closure. Abdominal wound dehiscence following surgery of the abdominal wall is not uncommon, and can predispose patients to an incisional hernia. Other associated risk factors for abdominal wall complications are male sex, chronic obstructive pulmonary disease, anemia, cough, infection, and smoking. These comorbidities should be optimized when possible prior to definitive closure or elective operations.

When we are faced with chronic wounds of the abdominal wall, our goal is to preserve as much tissue as possible to maintain a functional and dynamic abdominal wall. We prefer to debride these wounds early to help convert a chronic wound to an acute one. In the following section we describe how we use the appearance of normal tissue and methylene blue to thoroughly and equally debride the entire wound.

Surgical Debridement

Our goal in surgical treatment of abdominal wounds is to debride any senescent cells and remove any contamination from the wound. Our role in wound debridement occurs once the intra-abdominal process is controlled. The bacterial load of a chronic wound can promote the prolonged inflammatory response, which halts the wound-healing process (Fig. 33.1). Previous

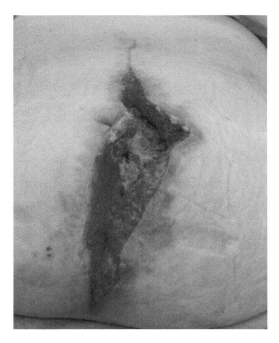

Fig. 33.1 Chronic abdominal wound. Please note the biofilm burden at the base of the wound. The rolled edges and fibrinogranular tissue at the superior and lateral wound edges

studies have shown that the majority of chronic wounds (90%) contain biofilm on the wound surface. The biofilm downregulates cell turnover, prevents antibiotic delivery, and prevents the chronic wound from proceeding through the normal stages of wound healing [7–9]. In efforts to decrease the bacterial burden and remove the biofilm from an abdominal wound, the patient should undergo surgical debridement in an operative setting. Deep tissue cultures of the wound should be taken prior to applying surgical prep to the wound site; this will determine the presence of bacteria, fungus, or yeast in the wound prior to debridement (Fig. 33.2). A thin confluent layer of methylene blue is then painted along all surfaces of the wound. This will help guide the surgeon in removing all biofilm and senescent cells from the wound bed, it is also pertinent to remove a 2–4 mm rim of tissue from the wound edges [10] (Figs. 33.3, 33.4, and 33.5). All foreign bodies, including sutures, should be removed (Fig. 33.5). Colonized fascial sutures must be removed if the fascia has healed. If infected biologic or synthetic mesh exists, it should be removed. If a sinus tract is present in the wound, methylene blue can gently be injected using an 18-gauge angiocatheter inserted gently into the tract. Debridement should then proceed using one or a combination of the following modalities: scalpel, curette, rongeur, or Versajet. The purpose of using methylene blue during the debridement is to remove all biofilm from the wound bed and to note "normal" tissue colors: red muscle, yellow fat, white fascia. Fascia should be debrided until clean healthy tissue remains (see Fig. 33.6, Case 1) [10]. The surgeon should be aware of what lies at the base of an abdominal wound, and to proceed carefully so that the intra-abdominal contents are not violated. In an acute necrotizing infection, we do not recommend using methylene blue for the initial debridement; normal tissue colors and vascularized tissue should guide your debridement in this setting. After the debridement is complete, a sterile occlusive dressing or negative pressure wound therapy should be applied. If viscera is exposed, we recommend using a silastic pouch or Bogota bag

Fig. 33.2 Surgical debridement of an abdominal wound using a Versajet® (Smith and Nephew.) Note the normal colors of tissue throughout the wound: red muscle, white fascia, and crisp wound edges

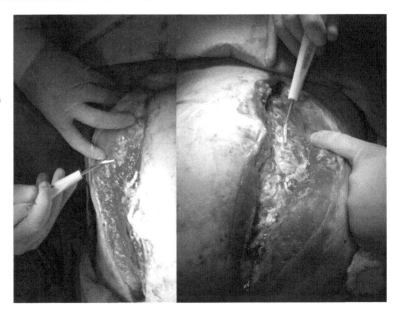

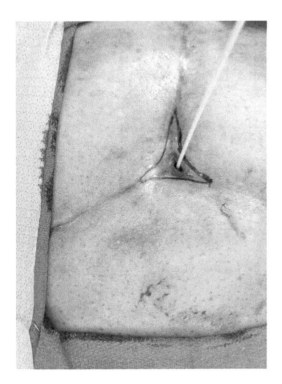

Fig. 33.3 Abdominal wound with a sinus tract at the base Skin surrounding the tract is comprised of unstable scar with a central non-healing area. This figure depicts the surgeon gently probing the wound with a sterile cotton tip applicator to evaluate the depth of the tract

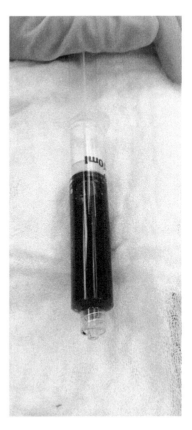

Fig. 33.4 A syringe with methylene blue that will be used to gently inject into the fistula tract

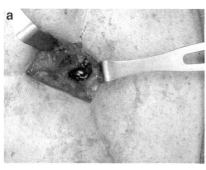
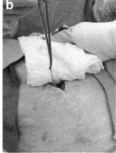
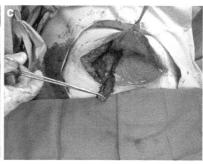

Fig. 33.5 (**a**) Abdominal wound with chronic edges excised, the tract has been injected with methylene blue. The area that is stained blue should be debrided until the normal appearance of tissue is seen. Sinus tracts usually lead to foreign bodies such as mesh or sutures. (**b**) Colonized sutures and all foreign bodies including mesh must be removed if the wound is infected. (**c**) Patient presented with small sinus tract, non-healing wound for many months s/p TRAM flap for breast reconstruction. Picture shows infected overlay synthetic mesh being removed

over the bowel, negative pressure wound therapy can then be applied. In addition, post-debridement tissue cultures are obtained which guide antibiotic regimen as well as whether the wound is ready to be closed. Closure options include primary closure, skin grafting, local flap, or free-flap reconstruction.

There is some debate over the use of negative pressure wound therapy in the setting of abdominal wounds, and if the use of negative pressure wound therapy increases the rate of enterocutaneous or enteroatmospheric fistula. The highest rate of fistula was seen after mesh placement alone (17.2%) while negative pressure wound therapy had a fistula rate of 5.7% [16]. We have not seen this to be a problem in our treatment algorithm, which can likely be attributed to early frequent debridements, the use of biologic mesh to support fascial closure, and motivation to achieve soft-tissue closure using local flaps over secondary healing.

Wound Care Adjuncts and Dressings

There are numerous factors that help guide clinicians to select appropriate strategies to care for wounds of the abdominal wall. The size of the wound, level of contamination, healthcare setting, comfort level and exposed structures are only a few factors that determine what products will be used. If an abdominal wound has exposed viscera, it is treated in the inpatient setting, usually with a silo, absorbable mesh, dynamic methods, or inert dressing over the viscera. Most clinicians will then elect to cover this with a negative pressure dressing until the patient can be returned to the operating room. The temporary abdominal wall closure should protect the intra-abdominal contents, prevent evisceration, assist in eliminating infection, attempt to preserve domain, and prevent enterocutaneous fistula [11].

Miller et al. has shown that use of negative pressure wound therapy alone in the acute open abdomen has been shown to prevent visceral adherence to the abdominal wall and to maintain traction on the medial fascial edge [12]. Several studies have shown that adding negative pressure wound therapy to the treatment regimen for an acute abdominal wound does decrease the overall number of operations and decreases the time to closure. If negative pressure therapy is not available, other temporary closure devices such as the Bogota Bag or Wittman patch can be used in the acute setting. A non-adherent layer such as Mepitel, Adaptic, or the white KCI VAC sponge should be applied directly over the bowel [13, 14].

When negative pressure wound therapy is used in abdominal wounds, some wound centers are able to use negative pressure alone or negative pressure with instillation. When instillation is

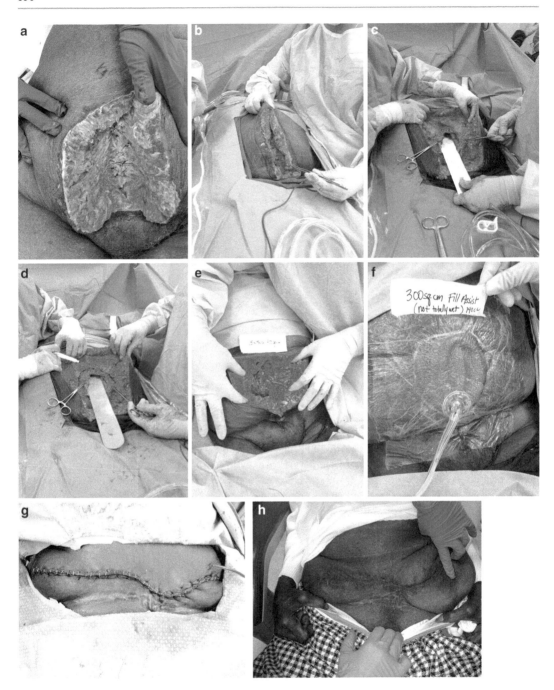

Fig. 33.6 (a) Details of a 74-year-old patient s/p TAH/ BSO for uterine cancer who presented with a draining wound 7 days after surgery. Note the fat necrosis and fascial separation. (b) Marked skin for excisional debridement. All dead and necrotic tissue must be removed. (c) All sutures and dead fascia must be removed. (d) Fascia is marked for resection based on color and viability. (e) Fascia has been resected and re-closed. (f) VAC with instillation will be used and secondary skin closure will be considered after deep culture-directed antibiotics have been started. (g) Serial debridements continue until the wound and fascia look clean and closure can be achieved. (h) Two-month postoperative view with healed wound

added to negative pressure wound therapy, it has been shown to decrease the number of debridements and decrease the length of hospital stay. There is early evidence to show that instillation with polyhexadine solution is more effective than saline alone when used with negative pressure wound therapy to combat biofilm and to decrease the bacterial burden of wounds. Currently, negative pressure wound therapy with instillation is only available to inpatients. As a result, if the patient is being transitioned from the inpatient setting they would need to use a negative pressure wound therapy device without instillation [11]. Negative pressure wound therapy should only be applied to clean healthy wounds which have been debrided [13–16] (Fig. 33.7.) In our practice, if there is concern for infection or biofilm we will initiate negative pressure wound therapy with instillation between debridements. When the wound bed appears to be granulating and the cultures are negative we switch to traditional negative pressure wound therapy. We are currently using Prontosan as our irrigation; the amount of infiltrate is determined during the "fill" phase when the sponge begins to appear moistened [11].

Traditionally, wet to dry dressings were used to assist in secondary healing of open wounds. Studies involving lower extremity wound sites demonstrate a 55% rate of healing by secondary intention when wet to dry dressings are used alone, compared to 82.7% rate of healing when negative pressure wound therapy is used. Wet to dry dressings can be used between treatment regimens, if the patient does not have access to negative pressure wound therapy or if the patient is unable to tolerate wound therapy or dressing changes.

Wound Dressings

There are options for local wound care if there is a soft-tissue defect. However, prior to selecting a wound dressing one should determine why the wound is not healing, address any mechanical or structural issues with the wound bed (biofilm, senescent cells), and the wound bed should be optimized. There has yet to be a single "ideal" dressing, and no dressing has achieved level I evidence to be the superior dressing for a given wound [17] (see Table 33.1).

In general, to promote epithelialization, dressings should: create a moist wound environment, have factors to promote wound healing, provide mechanical protection, absorb exudate, allow gaseous exchange, inhibit microorganisms, and be cost effective [4, 17]. The ideal dressing should not adhere to the wound, and it should be able to be changed without pain or trauma to the patient.

Normal Saline wet to dry dressings can be applied using gauze or foam. When the two dressings are compared, foam dressings are preferred to gauze dressings. Foam dressings are less painful, easier to apply, and have higher rates of patient satisfaction. If there is surface contamination or

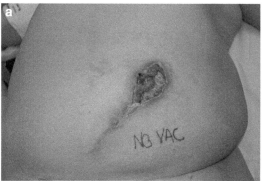 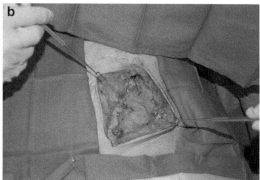

Fig. 33.7 (a) An example of surgical dehiscence should not be managed with negative pressure. There is significant undermining, drainage, and fat necrosis. We recommend surgical debridement prior to placing negative pressure wound therapy. (b) Entire wound has been debrided and negative pressure can now be used for wound management

Table 33.1 Choosing wound dressing types

Wound characteristic	Goal	Wound dressing type
Heavily draining wound	Control moisture and effluent	Absorptive dressings such as alginates
Superficial Bacterial colonization with odor	Control bacterial load	Bacteriostatic dressings such as Dakins or Acetic Acid wet to dry dressings
Superficial wound with granulation tissue	Promote epithelialization	Collagen matrix dressing

odor, ¼ strength Dakin's or Acetic Acid is recommended. These dressings should be changed twice per day.

Alginate dressings are another category of dressings that are helpful in abdominal wall wounds. This class of dressings is extremely absorptive; they can help prevent maceration of surrounding normal skin. Alginates are historically fabricated from seaweed products. However, modern dressings are calcium or sodium salts of alginic acid. These dressings are easily removed and can absorb up to 40 times their weight in fluid. They do require a secondary dressing as an overlay and they must be changed daily. Some Alginate dressings have silver impregnated into the fiber that is anti-microbial. Alginate dressings can be useful in tunneling and undermining wounds, and this is a therapy that we often use in the outpatient setting for smaller wounds that do produce an exudate [18].

The initial goal of wound care is to promote a healthy wound base with granulation tissue and to prevent undermining and tunneling. Once granulation tissue is present, collagen matrix dressings such as Prisma® can be used to promote neo-epithelialization and final wound healing [19, 20].

Any patient with an abdominal wound should be closely monitored for fluid and electrolyte imbalances, especially if the abdomen is open.

The patient should also be closely managed by a nutritionist to ensure they are able to meet the metabolic demands of wound healing. It is also pertinent that during this period the patients abstain from smoking to improve oxygen delivery to tissues. If the patient has other comorbidities prior to acquiring the abdominal wound, specifically diabetes or hypertension, these should be optimized in order to decrease potential complications [6].

The majority of abdominal wall wounds can be closed primarily. When abdominal wall wounds are closed, our practice often utilizes incisional negative pressure wound therapy. The efficacy in incisional NPWT has been debated in the literature as to whether it improves healing time, however in our practice its use has been shown to limit contamination when an ostomy or fistulae are in proximity to the incision [13, 14].

If a large soft-tissue defect exists, we recommend closure with local or free-flap reconstruction. Some patients are not candidates for a flap or a skin graft, in these rare instances, wound-healing adjuncts can be used. The common biosynthetic dressings which are used in our practice are Integra® or a xenograft. These can be placed over intact fascia, muscle, or partial soft-tissue defects (Fig. 33.8). Both dressings require that

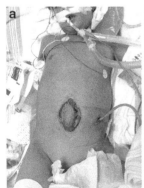 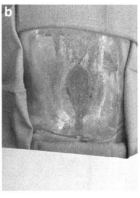 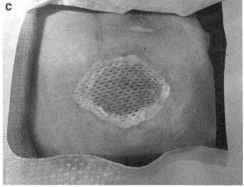

Fig. 33.8 (**a**) Five-year-old patient with metastatic neuroblastoma with history of abdominal compartment syndrome. Negative pressure wound therapy with a non-adherent sponge or interface was started to create granulation tissue over bowel. (**b**) After several weeks of negative pressure wound therapy, significant granulation tissue formed over the bowel. He is now ready for skin grafting, however due to comorbidities, xenograft will be used as an indicator if a skin graft has a high chance of success. (**c**) Xenograft was used as a temporary dressing and as an indicator if a skin graft has a high chance of success. The xenograft is left on the wound for 5–7 days, if it is adherent, then a skin graft can be preformed

the bacterial burden of the wound is below 10^3 colony forming units/gram and that the wound bed is well vascularized. Integra® will incorporate into the wound bed, which allows for future placement of a skin graft. Xenograft is usually placed in the operating room on a clean wound. Xenograft adherence to a wound bed is a good indicator that a skin graft will take. If Integra® is used, we will then cover the incorporated dermal substitute with a split thickness skin graft (STSG). The use of STSG in this setting will give a more stable closure, and when it is healed will not require wound care. In our practice, we offer STSG to patients who are not smoking, have good glycemic control, and have a wound bed ready to accept a skin graft. We use a Zimmer® dermatome to harvest a skin graft which is traditionally 0.012 in. thick. The skin graft is sewn into place using 5-0 chromic. A layer of mepitel is then applied followed by negative pressure wound therapy for 5–7 days. This is commonly performed on an outpatient basis in our practice.

In conclusion, our approach to wound healing in abdominal wall defects focuses on early operative debridement and delayed primary closure to achieve strong fascial and skin healing. Operative closure can usually be achieved with careful dissection of the abdominal skin flaps, taking care to spare perforators to ensure the abdominal skin flaps are well perfused. If fascial closure cannot be achieved, temporary bridges with biologic mesh and components separation can be employed with local or free-flap skin closure. However, if the wound cannot be closed, appropriate dressings and careful follow-up of the progress of the wound will help achieve expeditious wound healing.

References

1. Broughton G, Janis J, Attinger C. A brief history of wound care. Plast Reconstr Surg. 2006;117:6S–11.
2. Eming S, Krieg T, Davidson J. Inflammation in wound repair: molecular and cellular mechanisms. J Invest Dermatol. 2007;127:514–25.
3. DiPietro L. Wound healing: the role of the macrophage and other immune cells. Shock. 1995;4: 233–40.
4. Field C, Kerstein M. Overview of wound-healing in a moist environment. Am J Surg. 1994;167:S2–6.
5. Singer A, Clark R. Cutaneous wound healing. N Engl J Med. 1999;341:738–46.
6. Diaz J, Cullianane D, Khwaja K. Eastern Association for the Surgery of Trauma: management of the open abdomen, part III—review of abdominal wall reconstruction. J Trauma Acute Care Surg. 2013;75:376–86.
7. Gillespie D, Kistner B, Glass C, et al. Venous ulcer diagnosis, treatment, and prevention of recurrences. J Vasc Surg. 2010;52:8S–14.
8. Koolen PG, et al. Patient selection optimization following combined abdominal procedures; analysis of 4925 Patients undergoing panniculectomy/abdominoplasty with or without concurrent hernia repair. Plast Reconstr Surg. 2014;134:539e–50.
9. James G, Swogger E, Wolcott R, et al. Biofilms in chronic wounds. Wound Repair Regen. 2008;16:37–44.
10. Endara M, Attinger C. Using color to guide debridement. Adv Skin Wound Care. 2012;25:549–55.
11. Atema J, Gans S, Boermeester MA. Systemic review and meta-analysis of the open abdomen and temporary abdominal closure techniques in non trauma patients. World J Surg. 2015;39(4):912–25.
12. Miller M, Whinney R, McDaniel C. Treating a non-healing wound with negative pressure wound therapy. Adv Skin Wound Care. 2008;19:204–5.
13. Roberts D, Zygun D, Grendar M, et al. Negative-pressure wound therapy for critically ill adults with open abdominal wounds; a systemic review. J Trauma Acute Care Surg. 2012;73:629–40.
14. Kim P, Attinger C, Steinberg J, et al. The impact of negative-pressure wound therapy with instillation compared with standard negative-pressure wound therapy; a retrospective, historical, cohort, controlled study. Plast Reconstr Surg. 2014;133:709–16.
15. Davis K, Bills J, Barker J, et al. Simultaneous irrigation and negative pressure wound therapy enhances wound healing and reduces wound bioburden in a porcine model. Wound Repair Regen. 2013;21:869–75.
16. Zannis J, Angobaldo J, Marks M. Comparison of fasciotomy wound closures using traditional dressing changes and the vacuum assisted closure device. Ann Plast Surg. 2009;62:407–9.
17. Vermeulen H, Ubbink D, Goossens A, et al. Dressings and topical agents for surgical wounds healing by secondary intention. Cochrane Database Syst Rev. 2004;2:CD003554.
18. Gove J, Hampton S, Smith G. Using the exudate decision algorithm to evaluate wound dressings. Br J Nurs. 2014;23:S26–9.
19. Ding X, Shi L, Liu C. A randomized comparison study of Aquacel Ag and Alginate Silver as skin graft donor site dressings. Burns. 2013;39:1547–50.
20. Durnville J, Deshpande S, O'Meara S. Hydrocolloid dressings for healing diabetic foot ulcers. Cochrane Database Syst Rev. 2013;8:CD009099.

Gregory J. Mancini and Hien N. Le

Definition

"Loss of domain" is not well defined in the literature. It is most commonly described as a large abdominal wall hernia with a significant amount of abdominal content herniated through the abdominal wall into a hernia sac that forms a secondary abdominal cavity. Some define loss of domain by the amount of abdominal content outside the abdominal cavity, with as little as 15–50% or greater. Chevrel described it in 1987 as abdominal ventral hernias whose contents were held in place by adhesions and not reducible, thus losing their "right of domain." Figure 34.1 is a cross-sectional image of an abdominal CT scan demonstrating a loss of domain hernia. Regardless, the primary abdominal cavity is unable to accommodate the viscera without prohibitively high intra-abdominal pressures. If herniated contents are difficult to reduce below the level of the fascia when the patient is in supine position during physical exam, loss of domain should be suspected. We routinely use Computed Tomography (CT) to further evaluate

and define the anatomy. Most experts agree that loss of domain requires specialized strategies for successful repair.

Physics of LOD

Cylinder Concept

The abdomen can be described as a cylinder with a fairly uniform internal pressure. The anterior abdominal wall is made up of the rectus muscles that connect in the midline at the linea alba. The lateral abdominal wall is formed by the external oblique, internal oblique, transversus abdominis, and their aponeuroses fuse at the lateral border of the rectus abdominis to form the semilunar line. The posterior abdominal wall is relatively rigid, formed by the spine and erector spinae muscles. The rectus abdominis muscles are the principal flexors of the anterior abdominal wall and stabilize the pelvis while walking. The lateral abdominal wall muscles, all with different vectors of movement, work in conjunction to rotate and laterally flex the spine. Their overall direction of pull is to distract from the midline. The erector spinae muscles extend the vertebral column. Together, the abdominal muscles work through coupling to stabilize the torso and allow coordinated movement and weight shifts [1]. The top of the cylinder is the diaphragm muscle and the bottom of the cylinder is the pelvic floor. When

G.J. Mancini, M.D., F.A.C.S. (✉) • H.N. Le, M.D.
University of Tennessee Graduate School of
Medicine, University of Tennessee Medical Center,
Knoxville, 1924 Alcoa Highway, Box U-11,
Knoxville, TN 37290, USA
e-mail: gmancini@mc.utmck.edu;
hlei@mc.utmck.edu

© Springer International Publishing Switzerland 2016
Y.W. Novitsky (ed.), *Hernia Surgery*, DOI 10.1007/978-3-319-27470-6_34

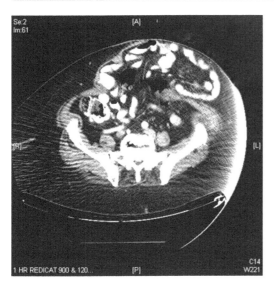

Fig. 34.1 A cross-sectional image of an abdominal CT scan demonstrating a loss of domain hernia

simultaneously contracted, they function to increase abdominal pressure, which facilitates expiration, micturition, defecation, and even parturition.

Broken Cylinder Concept

When a hernia develops, and in particular a loss of domain exists, there is lack of confinement of the intra-abdominal contents within the cylinder, resulting in significant viscera outside the abdominal domain and low intra-abdominal pressure. The linea alba is no longer connecting the rectus abdominis muscles in the midline, breaking the cylinder. The lateral abdominal muscles are no longer mechanically coupled, altering their functionality. As the lateral abdominal muscles foreshorten, they retract the rectus muscles rendering them ineffective in increasing intra-abdominal pressure. The pressure normally generated with the action instead decompresses into the low-pressure hernia sac. CT scans often demonstrate a foreshortening of the oblique muscles. This broken cylinder results in many morbid conditions, as described next.

Morbidity of Loss of Domain

Loss of domain is often a morbid condition. Patients usually have poor overall quality of life with many complaints, including postural musculoskeletal dysfunction, chronic gastrointestinal and genitourinary pathology, pulmonary dysfunction, and psychosocial issues. As described previously, the abdominal musculature is vital for upper and lower body activity, allowing coordinated movement, weight shifts, and stabilization during physical activity. Normally, torso stability is maintained by two columns, the erector spinae muscles posteriorly and the rectus abdominis muscles anteriorly. When the linea alba is disrupted, the rectus abdominis muscles become dysfunctional, and the columns are mechanically uncoupled. This results in greater pressure on the posterior column, leading to chronic back pain and spine curvature disorders.

Chronic gastrointestinal and genitourinary pathology can develop due to the inability to increase intra-abdominal pressures. Simple bodily functions such as defecation and micturition can become much more difficult leading to constipation and overflow urinary incontinence. Chronic intestinal incarceration is also common due to the usual complicated surgical history with formation of adhesions, causing pain and other obstructive symptoms.

Pulmonary dysfunction is also a major problem because the abdominal wall plays an accessory role to the intercostal muscles, thorax, and diaphragm in respiration. The abdominal wall primarily functions in forced expiration with the lateral abdominal muscles to raise intra-abdominal pressure during exercise to meet increased demands of breathing. The increased pressure is transmitted through the diaphragm to the thorax and forces air from the lungs. With a dysfunctional abdominal wall, forced expiration is decreased. This will not only affect exercise tolerance, but also simple functions as coughing and clearing secretions.

These problems often combine leading to decreased mobility and increased obesity. This usually only worsens the existing issues, increasing the hernia size, and in turn causing more strain on the musculoskeletal, gastrointestinal, genitourinary, and pulmonary systems. This unfortunate cycle leads to psychosocial issues with overall poor quality of life that may only be restored with surgical repair.

Complications of Repair

When repairing loss of domain, the challenge is to restore physiologic, mechanical, and functional capacity of the abdominal wall. Repairing the cylinder forces and bringing abdominal contents back into the abdominal cavity can increase intra-abdominal tension which can lead to abdominal compartment syndrome (ACS). It also results in elevation of the diaphragm which can lead to respiratory insufficiency. Component separation, a commonly used method of repair, increases the size of the cylinder allowing a decrease in intra-abdominal tension.

Presentation

Introduction

Loss of domain hernias seem to be is an increasingly frequent problem. This is a function of the high-quality trauma critical care that saves lives, but may yield more complex chronic open abdominal wounds. Also recurrent hernia and mesh complications lead to attenuated, distorted, or destroyed anatomy. Finally, obesity makes a significant contribution to the incidence and prevalence of the loss of domain hernia.

Emergency Surgery's Role

Current trauma and critical care techniques and protocols have improved survival from acute traumatic and surgical emergencies. The use of open abdomen techniques for repeated abdominal washouts has saved lives, but resulted in emergence of unintended challenging consequences. Based on the individual injury pattern, there may be a basic mismatch between abdominal content volume and abdominal wall circumference, preventing primary closure of the midline fascia. This

usually results from crystalloid volume expansion in the acute phase of injury that leads to bowel edema and increased intra-abdominal volume. Third-spacing of fluids also produces myofascial wall edema that results in a non-compliant abdominal wall that interferes with midline closure. These patients are often closed with an absorbable mesh material with either a skin flap advancement closure or skin grafted after a granulation bed is established. A more complicated open abdomen scenario is when a prior midline closure dehisces, a midline wound infection develops, or traumatic injury occurs that mandates abdominal wall debridement. In this situation, there is loss of anterior rectus fascia and rectus muscle. This problem leads to both an increase of the width of the hernia defect and less healthy anatomy for a future abdominal wall reconstruction. Most of these patients present 8–24 months after hospital discharge with a skin graft over the midline hernia defect. Figure 34.2 demonstrates a loss-of-domain hernia that has a skin graft closure of a traumatic abdominal injury.

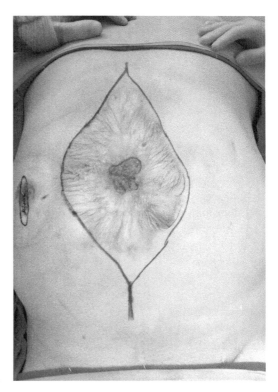

Fig. 34.2 Loss of domain hernia that has a skin graft closure of a traumatic abdominal injury

Recurrent Hernia's Role

Recurrent hernia and mesh complications can also contribute to the development of a loss of domain hernia. Multiple prior surgical procedures with mesh implantation and subsequent explantation can lead to loss of tissue integrity. This can be prior motor nerve damage that leads to muscle atrophy. Conversely, fully integrated and rigid mesh implants from prior repairs can reduce body wall compliance that limits myofascial advancement for midline closure. Damage done by recurrent hernia surgery can create tissue loss and compromise tissue plans similar to those of the emergency or traumatic type.

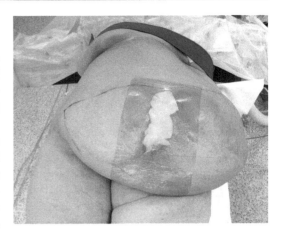

Fig. 34.3 Loss of domain hernia in the setting of severe morbid obesity

Obesity's Role

Obesity is highly prevalent and is both a cause and an effect of hernias. Patients with hernias gain weight due to physical limitations, and patients who become obese develop hernias more frequently. Central obesity is a major contributor to loss of domain hernias due to increased tensile forces loaded on the abdominal wall musculature. It is well documented that obesity by definition is a state of chronic intra-abdominal hypertension. Freeze et al. estimated that for every 1 kg/mm^2 increase in BMI, there was on average a 0.07 mmHg increase in intra-abdominal pressure [2]. Similarly, obesity is a major limitation to proper hernia repair, due to the volume mismatch between the abdominal viscera and the abdominal domain. Even though a component separation technique may increase the volume of the abdominal domain, it may not be enough to allow visceral return into the abdominal cavity with facial closure. Figure 34.3 demonstrates a loss of domain hernia related to morbid obesity.

Optimization for Surgery

Introduction

Preoperative preparation of both the surgeon and the patient is absolutely mandatory to treat loss of domain hernias. This concept will be addressed more broadly in other chapters. Here I will focus on preoperative steps specific to cases of loss of domain.

The Surgeon's Preparation

Surgeon preparation focuses on three areas: old chart review, a physical exam, and a radiographic assessment. Most patients with loss of domain have a complicated surgical history. Obtaining and reviewing those notes will help the surgeon to understand the distorted surgical anatomy that will be encountered at the time of the planned hernia repair. Details about the type of sutures placed, implanted mesh material type, location and size, as well as any prior facial component layers that may have been released, are all important facts to know prior to surgery. The second important step is a thorough physical exam. Generally, a functional capacity and readiness for surgery can be assessed during an office exam. Focusing on the abdomen, matching the abdominal scars with the past surgical history can build a continuity to the case. Assessing for open wounds, broad scars, skin grafts, and stomas provides more data that will be factored into the surgical plan. A functional exam of the abdomen can quantify the size of the hernia defect and assess for the relative compliance of the abdominal wall. While the patient is supine and relaxed, I often try to palpate the medial rectus edges and try to pull them toward the midline. If there is laxity in the abdominal wall, this is a good predictor of potential midline closure. Also, if a skin graft is present, the "pinch test" can be performed to assess if the underlying bowel will separate from the graft. The third preoperative step is obtaining and reviewing an abdominal Computed Tomography (CT) scan. Again, building congruency between the history, exam, and imaging is very important to mitigate the chances of intraoperative surprises. I assess the CT for old mesh, metal tacks, surgical staples, the hernia width and length, volume of the abdominal contents outside the abdominal wall, and the quality of the abdominal wall anatomy available for reconstruction.

Once the medical records, physical exam findings, and CT scan are reviewed and correlated, the surgical technique planning can occur. Preoperative patient goals for risk reduction, prehabilitation, and recovery timeline can be set in cooperation with the patient and family.

The Patient's Preparation

Most loss of domain hernias are not emergency cases, such as an acute bowel obstruction or mesh-related sepsis. As elective cases, these hernia repairs allow for maximal preoperative preparation of the patient. I have five main parameters that must be met prior to surgery. The patient must be tobacco-free for at least 1 month prior to surgery and must agree to stay tobacco-free for a minimum of 2 months after surgery. This will reduce pulmonary and wound complications that are frequent enough in complex hernia repairs without a smoking history. Nutritionally, the patient must have an albumin greater than 3.5 g/dL. Dozens of studies since the late 1990s across all medical specialties have demonstrated worse surgical outcomes and higher mortality rates in patients who are chronically hypoalbuminemic. For patients who are nutritionally deficient, a nutrition consultation and focused plan is developed to correct the problem before surgery. For diabetics, proper glucose control is critical. A hemoglobin A1c (HgA1c) of 7% correlates to an average blood glucose level of 150 mg/dL, and 8% correlated to 200 mg/dL. A serum HgA1c greater than 7% is associated with a increased wound infections and overall poor wound healing. Collaboration with the primary care provider or endocrinologist can greatly improve this metric. For patients with a poor baseline functional status, a pre-habilitation plan is established. Though a loss of domain hernia can greatly reduce a patient's ability to exercise, I place no limitations on their ability to ambulate. The cardiopulmonary physiologic strain which will be created after re-establishing a functional abdominal wall requires patients to build a physiologic reserve prior to elective surgery. I ask that patients progress to walking a minimum of 30 min per day. Weight loss is a common point of preoperative discussion with patients. In loss of domain hernias, the ability to close the fascia is directly related to the volume of the abdominal viscera. Preoperative weight loss can reduce the volume of the liver, omentum, and retroperitoneal adiposity. Typically, a body mass index (BMI) above 40 kg/m^2 will trigger a weight loss discussion. This is particularly important for patients with central obesity and high BMI. No myofascial advancement surgical technique can compensate for inadequate preoperative weight loss. The reality is that many of our patients present with one or more of the above-described risk factors. Once again, we require smoking cessation, weight control, diabetes optimization, healthy eating, and daily exercise, to ensure the best possible results. It is the surgeon's responsibility to counsel the patient on the complexity of a loss of domain hernia and the life-treating risks of surgery done under suboptimal circumstances. The patient as an advocate is more likely to prepare than the patient as an adversary.

Surgical Strategies for Loss of Domain

Introduction

When approaching a patient with a loss of domain hernia, several questions need to be answered. First can the hernia be technically fixed. This means that if the patient is fully optimized, is the proper functional anatomy available to obtain primary fascial closure of the abdomen with mesh implant reinforcement? If the answer is yes, then the question whether it should be fixed needs to be answered. This means that if the operation is done, will the patient be functionally better off? If the answer is yes, the question of how technically should the repair be done can be approached. Finally, who is the surgeon to undertake the repair?

There are many techniques that have been applied to the treatment of complex hernias. The loss of domain hernia is one of the most challenging hernia scenarios. Often, multiple advanced hernia techniques will need to be woven together in order for the repair to be successful. It is important to remember that the core principles of hernia repair, such as primary fascial closure under physiologic mention, wide mesh overlap, aseptic technique, and proper soft-tissue debridement and closure, must be maintained for the repair to have durability.

Component Separation Techniques

Component separation is a commonly used term for multiple different surgical techniques applied to closing abdominal wall defects. At its roots, component separation is the dismantling of the individual layers of the abdominal wall in order to advance innervated and vascularized myofascial tissue across a defect. There are multiple different techniques that will be more thoroughly covered in other chapters. In cases of loss of domain hernias, the two most commonly used are the external oblique release and the transversus abdominis release (TAR).

The Ramirez technique is the most widely adopted component separation technique, utilized by both plastic and general surgeons [3]. It is highly reproducible and provides 4–10 cm of advancement on each side, allowing closures of midline defects up to 20 cm wide. An important benefit to this technique is the flexibility of potential locations to implant the mesh. Ramirez affords the option of placing the mesh intra-abdominally, retro-rectus or as an onlay, to best fit the repair. In contrast, a downside to the external oblique

release is the need to mobilize adipocutaneous flaps to access the lateral abdominal wall. Skin flap creation can reduce perfusion to the overlying skin, increasing the risk for flap necrosis and postoperative wound complications.

I typically select the Ramirez technique to repair a loss of domain hernia in two distinct scenarios. The first scenario is when creation of skin flaps is adventageous, such a performing a concomient panniculectomy or when removing a prior large skin graft. In this situation the skin will be excised, necessitating the adipocutaneous layer advancement to obtain skin closure over the fascial closure. Figure 34.4 demonstrates how a panniculectomy exposes the external oblique aponeurosis. The second scenario is when the hernia sac extends laterally past the semilunar line. In this case, the hernia sac has essentially dissected the skin flaps, so when the hernia sac is mobilized, the external oblique aponeurosis will be exposed, allowing easy division for myofascial advancement.

The Novitsky technique, also called posterior component separation or TAR, is a myofascial release of the transversus abdominis muscle [4]. Access to the release point is made by entering the posterior sheath in the retro-rectus location. By releasing the transversus abdominis muscle, the lateral pre-peritoneal location can be accessed all the way to the paraspinal muscles. This affords wide area from the diaphragm to the pelvis in the vertical axis and from paraspinal muscles to paraspinal muscles in the transverse axis in which to implant the mesh. Since the mesh will lay in the pre-peritoneal location, an inexpensive, non-barrier, macroporous mesh can be used. A major benefit of the TAR approach is that no skin flaps are raised for the reduction of the hernia, the myofascial advancement, or for mesh implantation. This may yield lower postoperative wound complications when compared to other component separation techniques. Conversely, the TAR is technically more difficult and makes the peritoneal layer of prime importance in the repair. The peritoneum is of variable thickness and can easily tear requiring suture repair or absorbable mesh interposition.

I apply the TAR technique in two distict settings. First is in the setting of atypical hernias such as

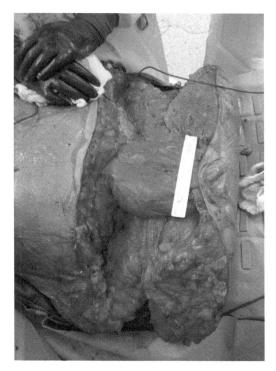

Fig. 34.4 Demonstration of how a lower abdominal panniculectomy will expose the lateral abdominal wall facilitating external oblique fascial release

flank, paramedian, subcostal, or subxyphoid hernias. The TAR affords access to the preperitoneal lateral abdominal and subdiaphragmatic spaces for wide mesh overlap in these notoriously difficult hernias. Second, Novitsky's technique is ideal in settings where skin flap creation would cause excessive wound complication risk to the patient. This may be an obese, smoking, diabetic patient undergoing abdominal wall reconstruction, but without a need for a panniculectomy. These two patient situations are common within my practice and, therefore, the TAR technique has served as a powerful tool to help treat loss of domain hernias.

Mesh Location and Choice

In loss of domain situations, there are two main mesh characteristics that dictate mesh selection. The prosthetic needs to be both strong in tensile strength and large in size. Mesh choice for patients with loss of domain hernias runs coun-

ter to the current trends toward light-weight mesh. The large hernia size, in both length and width, mandates large-sized mesh to gain proper mesh overlap. This may even require quilting two or more large off-the-self meshes to accomplish this task. If I sew mesh together, I use a #1 suture, that most mimics the mesh material (polypropylene, polyester, or gore-tex). Additionally, the increased vector forces of a loss of domain hernia mandate a mesh with high tensile strength. For loss of domain hernia repairs, I often choose a mid-weight, monofilament, polypropylene or polyester mesh. This is particularly critical in obese patients, for whom I avoid light-weight or ultralight meshes all together. For intra-abdominal placement, the mesh must have a microporous layer against the viscera. For retro-rectus or pre-peritoneal placement, a non-barrier polypropylene or polyester mesh will suffice. For the rare onlay mesh, I trend toward using monofilament polypropylene. I have used ePTFE mesh in rare cases where I have intra-abdominal mesh placement over a stoma, during the Sugarbaker repairs. The marginal results reported with biologic and absorbable meshes have reduced their current use in cases of loss of domain hernia repair.

Drain Placement and Management

Drains in open abdominal wall reconstruction are a necessity and a nuisance to both the patient and the surgical care team. Drains require patient education about care and complications that can challenge the hygiene, aptitude, and coping skills of the patient and family. In loss of domain hernias, the number and location of the drains greatly depends on the reconstruction technique used. For the Ramirez technique, I place at least one drain subcutaneously for each skin flap raised. These drains stay until the drainage approaches zero. Figure 34.5 demonstrates the placement of subcutaneous flap drain. If the mesh is retro-rectus, I place a drain between the mesh and the rectus muscle, and this drain is removed prior to hospital discharge. I place no drain for

Fig. 34.5 Placement of subcutaneous flap
drain

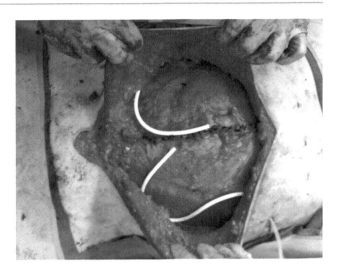

intra-abdominal mesh, and the onlay mesh will
be drained by the subcutaneous drains.

Preoperative Pneumoperitoneum

The main concern about repairing a hernia with
a loss of domain is figuring out if the fascia can
be closed primarily. Preoperative progressive
pneumoperitoneum has been described as a
technique that could help increase abdominal
wall compliance to aid fascial closure [5]. Like
a tissue expander, progressive pneumoperitoneum may place a pressure load on the abdominal wall to stretch the abdominal wall
musculature. This is done over a 5–14-day preoperative period by placing a tunneled catheter
into the abdomen and adding a volume of air
each day as the patient tolerates. I have not
been an advocate of this technique for the following reasons. First, a 5–14-day hospital stay
prior to abdominal wall reconstruction elevated
the patient's risk for wound infections, pulmonary complications, deep vein thrombosis, and
pulmonary embolus. Second, in loss of domain
patients, I believe the giant hernia sac is where
the instilled air will decompress, applying little
pressure to stretch the abdominal wall. Finally,
the patient rarely tolerates the progressive
instillation of air due to the sensation of being
short of breath. Therefore, for me, progressive
preoperative pneumoperitoneum is a method of

discouraging patients from undergoing repair
of a loss of domain hernia.

Postoperative Care and Complications

Complications of repair are common and include
respiratory compromise, ACS, and wound complications, in addition to the usual surgical
complications.

ACS and Pulmonary Complications

As discussed earlier, repairing the cylinder can
cause respiratory compromise and ACS. The
abdominal contents are forced back into the
abdominal cavity and this results in increased
intra-abdominal tension with elevation of the diaphragm. Component separation increases the size
of the cylinder, allowing a decrease in
intra-abdominal tension and prevention of
ACS. Typical signs of ACS, including high peak
pressures on the ventilator, a hard distended
abdomen, increased bladder pressures, and
decreased urine output, should alert the surgeon
of the possible diagnosis [6]. Respiratory compromise can result in difficulty with extubation
immediately postoperatively and pneumonia due
to the inability to cough and clear secretions well.
Ventral hernia repair has been shown to increase

intra-abdominal pressures that negatively impact pulmonary function [7]. Aggressive pulmonary toilet must be stressed perioperatively for optimal results.

Wound Complications

Wound complications are common in the short term, reaching up to 40%, and even higher in the obese population. This includes surgical site infections, seroma, hematoma, and skin flap necrosis. Surgical site infections can be minimized with appropriate preoperative antibiotics, sound surgical technique, and optimizing the patient preoperatively, as discussed above. Seroma or hematoma can develop due to the extensive flap dissection and the cavity left behind from repair. Most of those collections are sterile, usually do not require drainage, and resorb spontaneously. Suction drains can be useful, but if left too long can result in infection of the prosthesis. Skin flap necrosis causes much of the morbidity associated with the component separation repair. It is related to ischemia of the skin flaps after division of the perforators arising within the rectus sheath and supplying the anterior abdominal wall skin. Minimizing skin flap dissection may reduce rates of necrosis. Figure 34.6 demonstrates skin necrosis and wound infection after abdominal wall reconstruction.

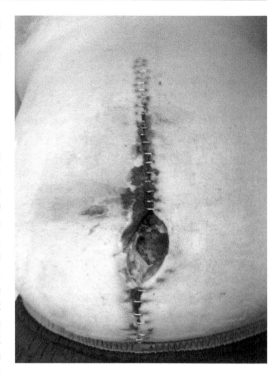

Fig. 34.6 Skin necrosis and wound infection after skin abdominal wall reconstruction

Intestinal Complications

As most patients undergoing repair in the setting of a loss of domain usually require extensive adhesiolysis, they are at risk for postoperative obstruction and leak/fistula. Careful tissue handling and meticulous dissection can reduce bowel injuries. It is also imperative to assure that all layers are satisfactorily re-approximated, as a breakdown of the posterior sheath with exposure of mesh can lead to recurrence of herniation or bowel erosion. Incomplete adhesiolysis may lead to unresolved obstruction with failure to progress in the postoperative period. It may benefit the patient to maximize all conservative treatments, as re-operation is almost prohibitive in these patients.

Summary

In summary, loss of domain hernias represent the highest complexity defects to repair. The impairment caused by this condition makes a hernia repair an important surgical option to help alleviate patient suffering. The complexity of the disease and the morbidity that accompanies the surgical risks places tremendous pressure on the surgeon to get it right. With proper patient selection, surgeon preparation, preoperative patient optimization, advanced hernia repair techniques, and solid general surgery postoperative care protocols, loss of domain hernias can be repaired with reasonable results. It is up to the surgeon, who wants to take care of this disease, to create and maintain a high-quality system to ensure good patient outcomes.

References

1. Stokes IA, Gardner-Morse MG, Henry SM. Intra-abdominal pressure and abdominal wall muscular function: spinal unloading mechanism. Clin Biomech. 2010;25(9):859–66.
2. Frezza EE, Shebani KO, Robertson J, Wachtel MS. Morbid obesity causes chronic increase of intraabdominal pressure. Dig Dis Sci. 2007;52(4): 1038–41.
3. Ramirez OM, Ko MJ, Dellon AL. "Components separation" method for closure of abdominal wall defects: an anatomic and clinical study. Plast Reconstr Surg. 1990;86:519–26.
4. Novitsky YW, Elliott HL, Orenstein SB, Rosen MJ. Transversus abdominis muscle release: a novel approach to posterior component separation during complex abdominal wall reconstruction. Am J Surg. 2012;204(5):709–16.
5. Mcadory RS, Cobb WS, Carbonell AM. Progressive preoperative pneumoperitoneum for hernias with loss of domain. Am Surg. 2009;75(6):504–8.
6. Agnew SP, Small W, Wang E, Smith LJ, Hadad I, Dumanian GA. Prospective measurements of intra-abdominal volume and pulmonary function after repair of massive ventral hernias with the components separation technique. Ann Surg. 2010;251(5):981–8.
7. Gaidukov KM, Raibuzhis EN, Hussain A, Teterin AY, Smetkin AA, Kuzkov VV, Malbrain ML, Kirov MY. Effect of intra-abdominal pressure on respiratory function in patients undergoing ventral hernia repair. World J Crit Care Med. 2013;2(2):9–16.

Brent D. Matthews

Challenges of Adhesiolysis

The most common risk factor for enterotomy is a previous laparotomy. The risk increases with subsequent laparotomies. In fact, patients with three or more previous laparotomies have a tenfold increase in experiencing an enterotomy compared with patients with one or two previous laparotomies [1] (Fig. 35.1). An enterotomy alters the wound classification from Clean (Class I) to Clean/Contaminated (Class II) or Contaminated (Class III). Higher rates of surgical site infection (SSI) are observed when progressing from clean to clean/contaminated to contaminated wounds. The consequence of a wound and/or mesh infection is a recurrence after ventral hernia repair [2]. Adjuncts placed at the time of surgery to minimize adhesiolysis-related complications during subsequent surgery have been disappointing. In a clinical trial of loop ileostomy closure, sodium hyaluronate and carboxymethyl cellulose membrane (Seprafilm®, Genzyme Biosurgery, Framingham, MA, USA) signifi-

cantly reduced postoperative adhesions at the site of application, but did not have an effect on the rate of enterotomy [3]. This was confirmed in a Cochrane Analysis evaluating intraperitoneal prophylactic agents for preventing adhesions and adhesive intestinal obstruction after non-gynecological abdominal surgery [4].

The rate of enterotomy during abdominal surgery is perhaps underreported. A recent audit of operative notes revealed that only 1 in 7 enterotomies was dictated in the operative report [5]. This underreporting could also have a significant influence on risk-adjusted outcomes as the accountability of value-based care becomes central to reimbursement. Risk factors for an enterotomy in abdominal wall hernia patients have been well-documented. In a prospective study of 133 patients undergoing an abdominal wall hernia repair, ten Broek et al. reported 33 enterotomies in 17 patients (12.8%) [6]. Predictors of enterotomy were adhesiolysis time, mesh in situ and hernia wider than 10 cm. An extended adhesiolysis time and increasing ventral hernia size are likely surrogates of a more complex ventral hernia. The impact on patient outcomes in this study of an enterotomy was an increased incidence of sepsis, reinterventions, need for parenteral nutrition, prolonged intensive care unit and hospital stay as well as increased medication cost. In another study over a 5-year period in 16 tertiary Veterans Affairs medical centers, Gray et al. reported an overall incidence of 7.3% for an enterotomy or unplanned bowel resection during

B.D. Matthews, M.D. (✉)
Surgery Care Division, Carolinas HealthCare System Medical Group, Department of Surgery, Carolinas Medical Center and University of North Carolina—Charlotte Campus,
1000 Blythe Boulevard, 2nd Floor Administrative Suites, Charlotte, NC 28203, USA
e-mail: brent.matthews@carolinashealthcare.org

© Springer International Publishing Switzerland 2016
Y.W. Novitsky (ed.), *Hernia Surgery*, DOI 10.1007/978-3-319-27470-6_35

Fig. 35.1 Relationship between the percentage of reoperation with and without enterotomy and the number of previous enterotomies. Reprinted from van der Krabben AA, Dijkstra FR, Nieuwenhuijzen M et al. (2000) Morbidity and mortality of inadvertent enterotomy during adhesiolysis. Br J Surg 87:467–71

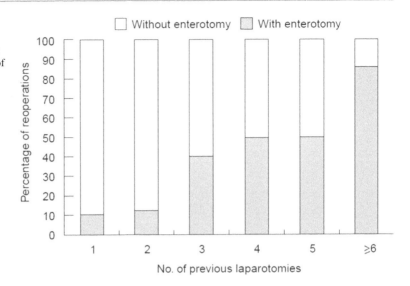

elective incisional hernia repair [7]. The incidence of enterotomy or unplanned bowel resection was significantly greater in patients after a previous mesh-based repair (20.3%) versus prior suture repair (5.7%) (Fig. 35.2). In a study more specifically defining the risk of enterotomy after mesh placement, Halm et al. reported a small bowel resection rate of 20.5% and a fivefold increase in SSI as a consequence of reoperation after intraperitoneal polypropylene mesh [8]. A recent presentation at the 1st World Conference on Abdominal Wall Hernia Surgery in Milan, Italy, described the consequences of an inadvertent enterotomy that occurred in 46 of 1842 patients who underwent open ventral hernia repair [9]. Risk factors for an enterotomy were previous abdominal surgery, prior hernia repair, mesh placement in a prior hernia repair and an infection present at the time of open ventral hernia repair. A higher rate of wound infections, mesh infections (12-fold), and hernia recurrences (6-fold) were reported in the enterotomy group compared to patients not experiencing this event, even when controlling for the use of synthetic mesh in clean/contaminated and contaminated wounds.

Absorbable and nonabsorbable barrier-coated meshes were designed for intraperitoneal placement during both laparoscopic and open ventral hernia repair in order to minimize visceral adhesions to mesh. There is a paucity of outcomes studies evaluating the effectiveness of these barriers in clinical trials. Jenkins et al. reported on 69 patients who underwent laparoscopic surgery after prior intraperitoneal mesh placement for ventral hernia repair [10]. Characterization of adhesions and complexity of adhesiolysis were measured as adhesion tenacity, adhesion surface area percentage over the mesh, and the ratio of adhesiolysis time to mesh surface area. An enterotomy was avoided in all patients with intraperitoneal absorbable and nonabsorbable barrier-coated meshes. However, adhesion characteristics and the complexity of adhesiolysis appeared to be associated with the unique properties of the barrier and/or mesh (Table 35.1). Two of 12 patients with intraperitoneal bare polypropylene mesh suffered injuries to the bladder and small intestine, respectively. Thus, the hollow viscus injury rate was similar to previously published studies. The study was underpowered to allow for definitive conclusions, but provocative nonetheless. A multicentered, prospective clinical trial of comparative effectiveness of barrier-coated meshes (*Comparative Effectiveness Multicenter Trial for Adhesion Characteristics of Ventral Hernia Repair Mesh*, ClinicalTrials.gov Identifier: NCT01355939) is ongoing.

A survey to assess practices and opinions regarding incisional hernia repair queried surgeons about enterotomy risk and management

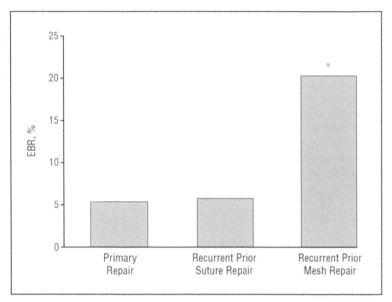

Fig. 35.2 Incidence of enterotomy or bowel resection (EBR) by the type of hernia repair. Reprinted from Gray SH, Vick CC, Graham LA et al. (2008) Risk of Complications From Enterotomy or Unplanned Bowel Resection During Elective Hernia Repair. Arch Surg 143(6):582–586

Figure. Incidence of enterotomy or bowel resection (EBR) by type of hernia repair. * $P < .001$ vs the other types of repair.

[11]. Eighty-one percent of surgeons responding to the survey who were not performing laparoscopic ventral hernia repair did not anticipate performing this procedure in the future. The second most common reason that the surgeons did not anticipate performing this procedure in the future was the perceived risk of enterotomy during laparoscopic ventral hernia repair. Nevertheless, the reported incidence of enterotomy in laparoscopic ventral hernia repair has been comparable to open ventral hernia repair in independent, prospective, longitudinal noncomparative studies. In a series of 850 consecutive patients undergoing laparoscopic ventral hernia repair repairs, Heniford et al. reported 10 (1.2%) enterotomies [12]. This is comparable to the rate of 1.4% reported by Sharma et al. in 2346 patients over a 17-year period [13]. However, in a meta-analysis of randomized, controlled trials of laparoscopic versus open ventral hernia repair, Awaiz et al. revealed a statistically significant increase in "bowel complications" in the laparoscopic group [14]. However, enterotomies, serosal tears, and postoperative small bowel obstruction were pooled and reported as "bowel complications," confounding the actual incidence of enterotomy.

One of the most devastating situations after laparoscopic ventral hernia repair is an unrecognized enterotomy or one that occurs in a delayed fashion. It should be noted that this is not exclusive to laparoscopic ventral hernia repair. The mortality rate for an unrecognized enterotomy after laparoscopic ventral hernia repair approaches 8% [15]. An enterotomy most frequently happens during adhesiolysis, although a trocar or access injuries can occur, especially in the re-operative abdomen. The trocar placement strategy is critical in the re-operative abdomen to avoid bowel injury. An ideal location for the initial trocar is in an abdominal quadrant remote from previous surgery. An open (Hasson) or closed (Veress) technique is appropriate and the method for placement should be based on the surgeon's experience. If the optical trocar without Veress insufflation is chosen, the access point should be right off the costal margin at the mid-clavicular or anterior axillary lines, away from previous scars/operations. The overwhelming majority of iatrogenic enterotomies occur in the small intestine. An unrec-

Table 35.1 Adhesion characteristics defined by tenacity, surface area, and ratio of adhesiolysis time to mesh surface area

Adhesion characteristics	Score		
No adhesion	0		
Filmy adhesions: viscera/omentum not attached to mesh, disrupted manually	1		
Dense adhesion: viscera/omentum attached to mesh requiring blunt dissection to separate viscera/omentum from mesh	2		
Dense adhesion: viscera/omentum attached to mesh requiring sharp dissection to separate viscera/omentum from mesh	3		
Dense adhesion: viscera/omentum entwined to mesh requiring sharp dissection to separate mesh from abdominal wall, leaving mesh attached to viscera/omentum	4		

Intraperitoneal mesh	Adhesion tenacity	Adhesion surface area (0–10)	Adhesiolysis time per mesh surface area (min/cm^2)
DualMesh ($n=14$)	2.4±0.6	5.9±1.8	0.14±0.1
Composix ($n=17$)	3.5±0.6	8.6±1.1	0.36±0.1
Absorbable-barrier-coated mesh ($n=18$)	3.2±0.5	6.9±2.0	0.21±0.1
Uncoated macroporous mesh ($n=12$)	3.5±0.9	8.4±1.1	0.38±0.4
Biologic mesh ($n=8$)	2.9±0.4	6.6±1.8	0.33±0.1

Reprinted from Jenkins ED, Yom V, Melman L et al. (2010) Prospective evaluation of adhesion characteristics to intraperitoneal mesh and adhesiolysis-related complications during laparoscopic re-exploration after prior ventral hernia repair. Surg Endosc 24(12):3002–7

ognized enterotomy can occur due to the inherent difficulty with examining the intestine laparoscopically if it has moved out of the field of vision. As such, vigilance is paramount. Inspection of the bowel is recommended after initial trocar entry, during adhesiolysis and at the conclusion of adhesiolysis or the end of the procedure. A delayed enterotomy may be the result of a partial thickness injury at the time of laparoscopic adhesiolysis or the consequences of a thermal injury to the intestine. Electrosurgery or ultrasonic coagulation should be employed judiciously for adhesiolysis and minimized or avoided when the intestine is in close proximity. Maneuvers to enable adhesiolysis and minimize the risk of enterotomy are described in the *Guidelines for Laparoscopic Ventral Hernia Repair* from the Society of American Gastrointestinal and Endoscopic Surgeons [16]. These maneuvers, many fundamental to laparoscopic surgery, include traction/counter-traction technique, use of an angled or flexible laparoscope, alternating the laparoscope among the various ports, improved exposure utilizing outside pressure on the abdominal wall for "inline" dissection, meticulous sharp dissection under direct vision, limited use of an energy source, particularly near the hollow viscera, repositioning/adding ports to maintain appropriate ergonomic position and access to the operative field, use of instruments with appropriate length (as longer instruments are occasionally required to maintain the fulcrum near the middle of the instrument shaft), avoiding too much torque on access ports during critical aspects of the adhesiolysis, keeping a clear camera image, maintaining a conscious vigilance for the mucosa of the gastrointestinal tract (as an enterotomy may only be visible for a fleeting moment), and mandatory final inspection of the bowel to identify enterotomies.

Management of Enterotomies

There is a general debate about the most appropriate management strategy for an enterotomy during laparoscopic and open ventral hernia repair. This highlights the paucity of evidence-based data to support a preferred approach. In a survey of practicing general surgeons, Adler et al. asked "if you encounter an enterotomy, how would you proceed?" [11]. Only 3% of respondents would place mesh regardless of the amount of spillage from the gastrointestinal tract while 41% would place mesh only if "minimal" spillage occurred. The majority, 56% of respondents, would not place mesh. If the respondents were to delay the ventral hernia repair, the mean time from the enterotomy would be 4 weeks (range, 3 days–6 months). Regardless of the treatment strategy, the patient should be knowledgeable preoperatively, as part of the informed consent process, of the procedural options and basic decision algorithm for management of an enterotomy. Typically, the hernia sac has not been violated during laparoscopic adhesiolysis; therefore options exist for staging the ventral hernia repair in 3 months or beyond to avoid a ventral hernia repair in a clean/contaminated or contaminatied field. This is the most conservative approach and preferable if the enterotomy can be repaired without conversion to open. Nonetheless, this is considered Level 4 evidence (expert committee opinions, or clinical experience of respected authorities, or both) in published guidelines for the management of bowel injury during laparoscopic ventral incisional hernia repair. In the *Guidelines for Laparoscopic Treatment of Ventral and Incisional Abdominal Wall Hernias*, the International Endohernia Society gives Grade C (low-quality evidence) recommendations for enterotomy management [17]. The recommendations from the International Endohernia Society include:

1. Conversion to laparotomy is advisable if the surgeon is not proficient with laparoscopic bowel repair techniques.
2. A primary open repair is advisable in the presence of gross spillage. An open prosthetic repair may be undertaken if conditions remain sterile.
3. A small laparotomy away from the hernia defect may be used to repair a bowel injury and may be followed by continuation of laparoscopic ventral hernia repair.
4. If a bowel injury is repaired laparoscopically, laparoscopic ventral hernia repair may be performed after an observation period of 3–7 days on intravenous antibiotic therapy if no evidence of infection is observed.

5. A laparoscopic ventral hernia repair may be performed in the event of a bowel injury repaired immediately with minimal spillage, but this option requires experience with laparoscopic repair of bowel injury.

A staged repair during the index hospitalization with a period of observation (3–7 days) on broad spectrum intravenous antibiotics, and return to the operating room for a laparoscopic ventral hernia repair has been described as a successful approach [18]. The unpredictability of infection-related complications after the 7-day period presents additional risk versus a 3 month or greater interval. Recent published data would support a more conservative management algorithm. In 33 patients who had an inadvertent enterotomy during laparoscopic ventral hernia repair, Sharma et al. reported 6-month follow-up in 31 patients [13, 19]. The additional 2 patients died postoperative due to sepsis and multisystem organ failure for a mortality rate of 6% in this cohort. The overall complication rate was 49%. The most common complications were wound infection (27%), ileus (24%), hernia recurrence (24%), mesh infection (18%), unplanned readmission (18%), and fistula formation (6%). Additional surgical procedures were required in 55% of these patients within 6 months of the index procedure. As expected, outcomes were worse in patients who had an enterotomy recognized postoperatively.

In the event the enterotomy occurs during an open ventral hernia repair or conversion to open is required to repair the intestinal injury or perform a bowel resection and the hernia sac is violated, several options exist for management of the ventral hernia. If possible, primary repair is a simple option, although the majority of patients will develop a recurrent ventral hernia. More commonly, surgeons are repairing the hernia using a biologic (allograft or xenograft) or absorbable synthetic mesh [20]. Depending on the complexity of the hernia and the degree of contamination, a retrorectus (Rives-Stoppa) repair, transversus abdominis release (TAR), anterior component release or external oblique aponeurosis release, may be required for re-approximation of the linea alba.

Outcomes studies describing single-stage repairs utilizing biologics or absorbable synthetic mesh for clean-contaminated, contaminated and infected wounds are limited. The RICH (Repair of Infected and Contaminated Hernias) trial is the only long-term multicentered, prospective trial to evaluate biologic mesh in CDC Class II–IV wounds [21]. This prospective trial reported a 66% surgical site occurrence rate and 37% hernia recurrence rate (intention-to-treat) after 2 years follow-up in patients who underwent ventral hernia repair with a non-crosslinked porcine dermis. The recurrence rate in "bridged" ventral hernia repairs was 45%. In addition, location of mesh placement appeared to influence recurrence rates with a higher rate of recurrence when the biologic mesh was placed intraperitoneal compared to the retrorectus position. In a similar multicentered prospective, longitudinal clinical trial, an absorbable synthetic mesh was evaluated in single-staged ventral hernia repair in Class II–III wounds [22]. The primary endpoint in the COBRA (Complex Open Bioabsorbable Reconstruction of the Abdominal Wall) trial was ventral hernia recurrence. Based on Kaplan-Meier analysis, the overall hernia recurrence rate was 17% at 24 months, almost 20% less than in the RICH trial. Similar to the RICH trial, hernias repaired with intraperitoneal mesh in the COBRA trial had a higher recurrence rate (3.41-fold increase). Although the RICH and COBRA trials describe ventral hernia repair in clean-contaminated and contaminated wounds, the clinical scenario is different from an unanticipated enterotomy during elective ventral hernia repair in a patient with an initial clean wound. Extrapolating data from these trials to an enterotomy during elective ventral hernia repair may not be representative of actual clinical outcomes.

There is an increasing amount of experience with synthetic mesh in clean-contaminated and contaminated wounds. Specifically, clinical studies evaluating large pore, reduced weight synthetic mesh in clean-contaminated and contaminated ventral hernia repairs have been published. Carbonell et al. reported primary outcomes of SSI, surgical site occurrence, need for mesh removal, and hernia recurrence in 100 patients with Class II–III wounds undergoing ventral hernia repair with retrorectus mesh placement [23]. The overall incidence of surgical site occurrence was 31%, higher in the contaminated then clean-contaminated cases. The 30-day SSI rate was 14%. The recurrence rate was 7% (intention-to-treat) at mean follow-up of 10.8 ± 9.9 months (range 1–63 months). Mesh removal was required in 4 patients, all due to unrelated explorations for anastomotic leaks. The impetus for permanent synthetic mesh is to reduce the recurrence rate witnessed for biologic and absorbable synthetic mesh and reduce the cost primarily associated with biologic meshes. Carbonell et al. calculated that the overall cost for the 100 pieces of 30×30 cm large pore, reduced weight synthetic mesh (15 cents/cm^2) to repair the ventral hernias was equivalent to the cost of one single piece or biologic mesh ($10,000). Despite the significant potential for reduction in healthcare expenditures with the use of synthetic mesh in these patients, it is off-label to use synthetic mesh in clean-contaminated, contaminated, or infected wounds. In addition, extrapolating data from this clinical trial to an enterotomy during elective ventral hernia repair in initially clean wounds may not be representative of actual clinical outcomes.

Conclusions

An inadvertent enterotomy during a laparoscopic or open ventral hernia repair is unavoidable. An enterotomy is associated with an increased risk of wound infections, mesh infections, enterocutaneous fistulas, and hernia recurrences. Multiple options exist for management of the ventral hernia when an enterotomy occurs; however, the management of the enterotomy takes priority. A postoperatively recognized enterotomy increases the mortality rate after ventral hernia repair so attentiveness is paramount throughout the entire procedure. Although certain risk factors associated with an increased risk of enterotomy during ventral hernia repair, such as previous surgical history, previous ventral hernia repair with mesh and in situ intraperitoneal mesh, are identifiable preoperatively, all patients should be advised of the risk of enterotomy and instructed of the basic decision algorithm for management of an enterotomy during the informed consent process.

References

1. van der Krabben AA, Dijkstra FR, Nieuwenhuijzen M, et al. Morbidity and mortality of inadvertent enterotomy during adhesiolysis. Br J Surg. 2000;87:467–71.
2. Igbal CW, Phar TH, Jospeh A, et al. Long-term outcome of 254 complex incisional hernia repairs using the modified Rives-Stoppa technique. World J Surg. 2007;31(12):2398–404.
3. Salum M, Wexner SD, Nogueras JJ, et al. Does sodium hyaluronate- and carboxymethylcellulose-based bioresorbable membrane (Seprafilm) decrease operative time for loop ileostomy closure? Tech Coloproctol. 2006;10(3):187–91.
4. Kumar S, Wong PF, Leaper DJ. Intra-peritoneal prophylactic agents for preventing adhesions and adhesive intestinal obstruction after non-gynaecological abdominal surgery. Cochrane Database Syst Rev. 2009;21(1):1–34.
5. ten Broek RPG, van den Beukel BAW, vn Goor H. Comparison of operative notes with real-time observation of adhesiolysis-related complications during surgery. Br J Surg. 2013;100:426–32.
6. ten Broek R, Schreinemacher M, Jilesen A, et al. Enterotomy risk in abdominal wall repair: a prospective study. Ann Surg. 2012;256:280–7.
7. Gray SH, Vick CC, Graham LA, et al. Risk of complications from enterotomy or unplanned bowel resection during elective hernia repair. Arch Surg. 2008;143(6):582–6.
8. Halm JA, de Wall LL, Steyerberg EW, et al. Intraperitoneal polypropylene mesh hernia repair complicates subsequent abdominal surgery. World J Surg. 2007;31:423–9.
9. Huntington CR, Augenstein VA, Blair LJ et al. (2015) Inadvertent enterotomy: significant consequences for the open ventral hernia patient. Paper presented at the 1st world conference on abdominal wall hernia surgery, Milan, Italy, April 25–29, 2015.
10. Jenkins ED, Yom V, Melman L, et al. Prospective evaluation of adhesion characteristics to intraperitoneal mesh and adhesiolysis-related complications during laparoscopic re-exploration after prior ventral hernia repair. Surg Endosc. 2010;24(12):3002–7.
11. Adler AC, Adler SC, Livingston EH, et al. Current opinions about laparoscopic incisional hernia repair: a survey of practicing surgeons. Am J Surg. 2007;194(5):659–62.
12. Heniford BT, Park A, Ramshaw BJ, et al. Laparoscopic repair of ventral hernias nine years' experience with 850 consecutive hernias. Ann Surg. 2003;238:391–400.
13. Sharma A, Khullar R, Soni V, et al. Iatrogenic enterotomy in laparoscopic ventral/incisional hernia repair: a single center experience of 2,346 patients over 17 years. Hernia. 2013;17:581–7.
14. Awaiz A, Rahman F, Hossain MB, et al. Meta-analysis and systematic review of laparoscopic versus open mesh repair for elective incisional hernia. Hernia. 2015.
15. LeBlanc KA, Elieson MJ, Corder JM. Enterotomy and mortality rates of laparoscopic incisional and ventral hernia repair: a review of the literature. JSLS. 2007;11:408–14.
16. Earle D, Roth S, Saber A et al (2014) Guidelines for laparoscopic ventral hernia repair. http://www.sages.org/publications/guidelines/guidelines-for-laparoscopic-ventral-hernia-repair.
17. Bittner R, Bingener-Casey J, Dietz U, et al. Guidelines for laparoscopic treatment of ventral and incisional abdominal wall hernias (International Endohernia Society [IEHS])—Part 2. Surg Endosc. 2014;28(2):353–79.
18. Tintinu AJ, Asonganyi W, Turner PL. Staged laparoscopic ventral and incisional hernia repair when faced with enterotomy or suspicion of an enterotomy. J Natl Med Assoc. 2012;104(3–4):202–10.
19. Lederman AB, Ramshaw BJ. A short-term delayed approach to laparoscopic ventral hernia when injury is suspected. Surg Innov. 2005;12(1):31–5.
20. Harth KC, Krpata DM, Chawla A, et al. Biologic mesh use practice patterns in abdominal wall reconstruction: a lack of consensus among surgeons. Hernia. 2013;17:13–20.
21. Itani KM, Rosen M, Vargo D, et al. Prospective study of single-stage repair of contaminated hernias using a biologic porcine tissue matrix: the RICH Study. Surgery. 2012;152(3):498–505.
22. Rosen MJ, Carbonell AM, Cobb WS et al. Multicenter, prospective, longitudinal trial evaluating recurrence, surgical site infection and quality of life after contaminated ventral hernia repair using biosynthetic absorbable mesh. Paper presented at the 1st world conference on abdominal wall hernia surgery, Milan, Italy, April 25–29, 2015.
23. Carbonell AM, Criss CN, Cobb WS, et al. Outcomes of synthetic mesh in contaminated ventral hernia repairs. J Am Coll Surg. 2013;217:991–8.

Abdominal Wall Surgery in the Setting of an Enterocutaneous Fistula: Combined Versus Staged Definitive Repair

Michael G. Sarr

Enterocutaneous fistulas are usually the consequence of an intra-abdominal operation gone bad and, as such, are all-too-often accompanied by an incisional hernia, further complicating an already unpleasant situation for both the patient and surgeon. Both parties (patient and surgeon) want the fistula and the hernia fixed as soon as possible, raising the questions of "How soon can it be done?" and "Please, can we fix both at the same time?" However, it is important to remember that the basic principles of the management of enterocutaneous fistulae, as well as the basic principles of repair of incisional hernias, must be followed and each considered individually. Level 1 evidence for the latter topic is absent, as is Level 2 evidence, and much of the discussion on this topic is filled with bravado, opinion, and lack of appropriate follow-up [1]. Just because something *can* be done (simultaneous repair of both fistula and hernia) does not mean it *should* be done. Failed hernia repairs in this setting will have major consequences. This chapter will address briefly the preoperative considerations of preparing for the repair of the fistula and then will address whether a simultaneous or staged DEFINITIVE repair is prudent.

M.G. Sarr, M.D. (✉)
James C. Masson Professor of Surgery, Department of Surgery, Subspecialty General Surgery, Mayo Clinic, 200 1st St SW, Rochester, MN 55902, USA
e-mail: sarr.michael@mayo.edu

Preoperative Considerations in the Patient with an Enterocutaneous Fistula

Most often, an enterocutaneous or colocutaneous fistula occurs from a complication of an intraperitoneal procedure (enteric or colonic anastomosis or unappreciated enterotomy) and is complicated initially by some element of abdominal wall sepsis that disrupts the fascial closure leading to the hernia. Thus, the clinical situation is often complicated by sepsis, nutritional challenges, and abdominal wall infection, colonization, and/or an open wound such as an enteroatmospheric fistula, each of which will challenge the option of any definitive repair of the hernia.

The Basics First

Initially, the focus must be directed at the fistula from the aspect of a GI surgeon, and not from that of a "herniologist." One of the best overall discussions of the evaluation and approach to the management of enterocutaneous fistulas was by Visschers and colleagues [2] who proposed the SOWATS approach: S-sepsis; O-optimization of nutrition; W-wound care; A-anatomy; T-timing of operation; and S-surgical strategy. This approach should be utilized during the three phases of the clinical course of an enterocutaneous fistula: development, the early phase, and the late phase [3, 4].

© Springer International Publishing Switzerland 2016
Y.W. Novitsky (ed.), *Hernia Surgery*, DOI 10.1007/978-3-319-27470-6_36

Development: If the fistula occurs early postoperatively, immediate reoperation in the first week to 10 days (before the hernia forms) should be considered, provided there was not an extensive adhesiolysis, because if there was an extensive adhesiolysis, then after the second or third postoperative day, the bowel will be agglutinated. Most fistulas, however, become evident later, and reoperation is not necessarily a consideration.

Early phase: This phase requires the focus to be directed on control of sepsis, nutritional resuscitation, and control of the fistula; reoperation during this phase is contraindicated.

Late phase: Here the focus should be on the planning for operative repair after adequate maturation and resolution of the acute inflammatory phase, maximizing nutritional resuscitation, and definition of all the relevant anatomy.

The GI surgical approach should involve the following points during the early phase (Table 36.1). Read all prior operative notes; you will want no surprises in the operating room. Exclude any areas of sepsis; persistent undrained collections can prevent fistula closure and nutritional

Table 36.1 Surgical principles of evaluation and repair of an enterocutaneous fistula

Early phase
Read and understand all operative notes
Exclude undrained sepsis
Maximize nutrition
Feed the gut whenever possible; re-feed pancreatobiliary secretions distal to the fistula
Multidisciplinary approach (in addition to surgeon)
• Nutritionist/dietician
• Psychiatrist—situational depression helped by antidepressant(s)?
• Physical therapist—reverse deconditioned state
• Family support
• Social worker
Bag/control the fistula—consult a trained enterostomal therapist if any difficulty
Late phase
Image all the pertinent gut
Define the anatomy—no surprises in the OR!
Allow acute/subacute inflammation to resolve; do not be bullied into operating too soon
Plan the operation; recruit the potential help of a reconstructive plastic surgeon

resuscitation. Maximize nutrition possibly by feeding (or re-feeding enteric content) distal to the fistula; enteric feeding is more effective than parenteral feeding and maintains the health, integrity, and function of the distal gut. Involve a multidisciplinary team, including a nutritionist (dietitian or physician), physical therapist, psychologist if necessary (patients are often situationally depressed), family/social supports, and, very importantly, an enterostomal therapist if you are having *any* difficulty bagging the fistula [1]. For the patient, there is nothing worse than an uncontrolled fistula. And, finally, remember TPN can be cycled and given via a backpack to allow increased patient mobility.

The GI approach to the late phase requires experience and a resolute surgeon. Everyone will be pressuring you to operate—the patient, the family, and all the other physicians who are not surgeons [4]! Your goal is to allow the acute/subacute inflammation to subside. Most fistulas require 3 months to mature, some 6 months, and some maybe even 12 months. A good barometer of resolution of the inflammation is the ability to "pinch" a skin graft if present or the redness of the primary incision. Remember, many fistulas occur/reoccur from too early a reoperation. Other considerations involve the nutritional state of the patient, as shown by Visschers et al. [2]. Optimal outcomes, occur when the patient's serum albumin is ≥3.0 g/dL. Operative planning requires imaging of all parts of the involved gut, especially excluding any distal obstruction. Likewise, the goals of a successful fistula repair are careful technique, full mobilization, and coverage of the repair with autogenous tissue; the latter may require assistance of a reconstructive plastic surgeon.

Should You Fix the Hernia Concurrently?

Your operative plan should be FIRST to fix the fistula—that is the patient's primary concern! The fistula takes precedence, while the repair of the hernia should be a somewhat distant second precedence. The decision to repair the abdominal wall hernia should not be influenced by emotion, but rather by good, sound, surgical judgment based on several considerations: patient factors/ nutritional state, local conditions/tissues/risk of infection, confidence in your repair of the fistula, size of the defect/need for tissue advancement (components separation), and, in this author's opinion, whether the patient is a hernia-former which goes hand-in-hand with the latter consideration of the need for tissue advancement, because use of a permanent, alloplastic prosthesis classically is contraindicated (although see below—"Use of Permanent Prosthetic Material").

Definitive Herniorrhaphy at Time of Fistula Repair

Obviously, the worries of any operation involving takedown of an enterocutaneous fistula are anastomotic leak and surgical site infection, both of which jeopardize markedly any abdominal wall hernia repair. Takedown of a traumatic enterocutaneous fistula in an otherwise healthy, non-malnourished, non-obese, 22-year-old male is completely different from an enterocutaneous fistula in an obese, elderly patient in whom the fistula developed secondary to an unrecognized enterotomy that occurred during an extensive adhesiolysis while attempting to repair an abdominal wall hernia or in a patient who is immunosuppressed either from chronic disease/malnutrition, malignancy, or because of a prior organ transplantation. The spectrum of clinical presentation of enterocutaneous fistulas complicated by concomitant abdominal wall hernias is very broad.

Who are the best candidates for a *definitive* repair concurrently (Table 36.2) Note: Just because a definitive repair *can* be done does not mean it *should* be done. This decision requires non-emotional, good, mature surgical judgment. In addition, there are some senior surgeons who feel that many (perhaps most) abdominal wall hernias complicating an enterocutaneous fistula should not undergo any complicated *definitive* repair other than a simple autogenous fascia reapproximation. Ideal patients are those lacking any of the underlying risk factors for incisional hernia—obesity, malnutrition, prior incisional

Table 36.2 Who can be considered for simultaneous repair of the abdominal wall hernia?

Small defect allowing primary fascial reapproximation
None of the following underlying risk factors for incisional hernia
• Marked obesity
• Large open wound
• Malnutrition
• Immunosuppressed patient
• Concomitant infected mesh
• Prior incisional hernia
• Smoking
Larger defect able to be repaired by components separation in the ideal patient[a]
• The patient who is not a hernia-former
• Has no malnutrition
• Has good local tissues

[a]Taken at a calculated risk, because wound infection will probably lead to fascial breakdown, hernia formation, and a very difficult subsequent hernia to repair

hernia (i.e., a hernia-former), or signs of local abdominal wall infection, cellulitis, or a large surface area of open wound (that contains bacterial colonization). Small defects able to be closed with a primary, autogenous tissue repair are dealt with quite easily by simple reapproximation of the fascia and, should a wound infection occur and develop into another hernia, no loss of abdominal wall tissue has occurred; equally important, a later definitive repair has not been jeopardized by lateral dissection. In contrast, when the defect is large, unable to be reapproximated by primary repair, and will require some form of tissue transfer/myocutaneous advancement (components separation) to obtain midline myofascial approximation, very serious pause should be taken. A wound infection would lead to a subsequent hernia that will be very difficult to repair. Two large series [5, 6] of combined takedown of fistulas and components separation techniques describe what in this author's opinion are unsatisfactory outcomes with rates of recurrent hernias of 21% and 32%, respectively, and recurrent fistulas of 26% and 20%. Thus, only the low-risk, ideal patients should be considered for takedown of an enterocutaneous fistula with simultaneous abdominal wall reconstruction. In this author's opinion, consideration of definitive repair by a so-called "tension-free" components separation in a hernia-former should be reconsidered; remember, this repair is an autogenous tissue repair, and the "tension-free" situation is only when the patient is anesthetized and paralyzed–not when the patient coughs, sits up, or strains to have a bowel movement. Use of permanent prosthetic material to reinforce the repair is classically contraindicated (see below, "Use of Permanent Prosthetic Material"). The recurrence rate will be very high, and should a surgical site infection occur, the resultant hernia will be extremely difficult to repair, because your best option in this high-risk group of patients has already been used—and you have burned your bridges. This group of patients gets one good chance at definitive hernia repair (abdominal wall reconstruction), and a staged repair seems most prudent.

Who should not have a definitive repair? (Table 36.3) By "definitive" repair, I mean either a permanent, prosthetic-based incisional herniorraphy or a true abdominal wall reconstruction requiring myofascial advancement/transfer. Inappropriate candidates include the markedly obese, malnourished, or immunosuppressed patients, those with dirty or open wounds, the chronically ill or markedly deconditioned, those with infected/colonized mesh from a prior abdominal wall herniorrhaphy, or those with a history of a prior incisional hernia (the "hernia-former"). It should go without saying that a definitive repair should not be entertained seriously in someone still smoking and especially any form of tissue transfer!

Table 36.3 Who should not have a simultaneous DEFINITIVE hernia repair?

Dirty wound (subjective observation)
Large open area
Poor nutrition
Large defect "able to be closed" by components separation in patients with risk factors
• Obesity
• Prior incisional hernia (hernia-formers)
• Concomitant mesh infection?

How to Deal with the Hernia Defect

After takedown of the enterocutaneous fistula, every attempt should be used to provide two important principles: (1) autogenous, vascularized tissue coverage of all anastomoses, and (2) abdominal wall stability, even if only temporary (several weeks to several months). Ideally, primary fascial closure is best and will provide abdominal wall stability; although recurrence of the hernia may be quite high and should be expected in the high-risk patient (hernia-former, malnourished, immunosuppressed, etc.), you provide autogenous coverage and at least temporary abdominal wall stability.

The larger defects unable to be reapproximated present major challenges that are more difficult. Again, autogenous coverage of the anastomoses is paramount. Input and options from a reconstructive plastic surgeon can really help [7]. Techniques include omental coverage, mesenteric or serosal coverage from adjacent bowel, or use of the hernia "sac." On rare occasions, a vascularized tissue transfer from the thigh (rectus femoris or gracilis grafts) or back (latissimus dorsi grafts) can provide vascularized tissue cover, but these types of "flaps" do not provide abdominal wall stability and cannot reach the areas of the abdominal wall cranial to the umbilicus.

Some form of abdominal wall stability is usually necessary to prevent evisceration. In the very unusual patient with a frozen abdomen in whom you can repair the fistula and provide viable, vascularized coverage of exposed bowel but cannot provide coverage of adhesed bowel not at risk for evisceration, no attempt at spanning the hernia defect may actually be the best choice. The open wound can then be managed with a wound vac (not directly on bowel, however) or simple dressings with the future aim of placing a skin graft and delaying the hernia repair to the future under ideal conditions (closed epithelialized wound, full nutritional resuscitation, and a planned elective abdominal wall reconstruction) [8].

Unfortunately, the more common situation is the patient in whom a more extensive adhesiolysis for fistula repair results in mobile bowel that demands provision of some form of abdominal wall stability. In this situation, the possible solutions involve performing a components separation (in the appropriate patient) with a primary autogenous fascial closure, possibly reinforced with a bioprosthesis or synthetic *absorbable* prosthesis placed as either a sublay or an onlay [5, 6]. The concept of performing a components separation, knowing that fascial re-approximation will not be possible but planning on spanning the fascial defect with a bioprosthesis, is not a good option in my opinion, because the likelihood of such bioprosthesis providing a definitive repair is highly unlikely [9, 10]. Similarly, spanning such a defect with a permanent prosthesis in this type of "contaminated" wound would not be considered standard of care, and also result in violating spaces that may preclude the use of a technique that would be best for a future abdominal wall reconstruction.

In most patients, a better solution would be to accept the idea of not being able to provide a definitive repair of the hernia, plan for a staged repair, and to span (patch) the hernia defect with either a bioprosthesis or a synthetic *absorbable* prosthesis [1, 3]. Although adding a components separation would decrease the size of the hernia defect, it will essentially prevent the ability to use this technique of abdominal wall reconstruction to perform a much better, definitive repair in the future under elective conditions. Therefore, the goal should be to fix the *primary* indication for operation and the major complaints of the patient—i.e., THE FISTULA—and to address the *secondary* concern—i.e., THE HERNIA—at a later date under elective, non-bacterially contaminated conditions in a stable, nutritionally optimized patient.

Choice of "temporary," absorbable prostheses vary considerably with their characteristics [3]. These bioprostheses are usually constructed from proprietary processes that remove most cells and immunologic epitopes that could cause a true immune response when implanted in humans. The tissues from which these bioprostheses are commonly derived include human cadaveric or porcine dermis, porcine intestinal submucosa, or bovine pericardium. Most of the bioprostheses are designed biochemically to encourage vascular ingrowth and deposition of native host connective tissue. While proprietary claims allege the reproduction of a "functional neo-abdominal wall," the extent to which this really happens is questionable. These bioprostheses, however, do provide stable, albeit temporary, abdominal wall support (coverage of the intra-abdominal viscera) for 6–12 months before being broken down by host tissues or "stretching." This time frame allows healing of the fistula, closure of any skin wounds, nutritional repletion, and reversal of physical deconditioning.

Another option involves the absorbable synthetic prostheses, which also provide temporary abdominal wall stability, but generally for a shorter duration than the bioprostheses. The polyglactin meshes are initially permeable (they are meshed) and allow drainage of peritoneal fluid/transudate for the first 4–7 days, which may be an advantage in selected patients; the bioprostheses are generally considered watertight. The disadvantage of these prostheses is that they are degraded more rapidly and become less stable as an abdominal wall support after 6–8 weeks; thus, these more rapidly absorbed prostheses are used in selected patients who may not need a prolonged abdominal wall support. When these more rapidly absorbable prosthetics are used, the eventual goal is often to skin graft the subsequent wound in 1–2 months. This concept of split-thickness skin grafting [8] should be evaluated carefully, because although the skin graft will "cover" the wound, the skin graft will also stop further medial wound contracture and will usually delay eventual abdominal wall reconstruction for about 6 months. This 6-month time interval allows the skin graft to mature such that safe excision of the graft is possible (i.e., when the skin graft is "pinchable" meaning that the inflammatory vascularization response has largely abated).

Several newer synthetic, absorbable prostheses have been developed to last longer and for up to 6–18 months. Again, the manufacturing details of how they are constructed are proprietary, but these prostheses do have their place in selected patients, although long-term clinical experience is still lacking.

Finally, several systems for providing passive tension to help to encourage fascial or skin approximation exist. Similar in principle to the "wound vac" systems and the Wittmann patch [11], these devices are fixed to either the fascial edges or the skin bilaterally to provide a force to pull together the edges of the wound. These various devices allow readjustment as the width of the wound decreases. Their use for skin closure over open wounds is well supported in preliminary studies [12]. Their efficacy in leading to fascial reapproximation is unproven.

Whichever form of "patching" of the defect is utilized, coverage of the prosthetic with autologous vascularized tissue should be sought aggressively. Local skin/subcutaneous advancement or rotational flaps are the most readily available options and will prevent desiccation and help to promote vascularization into or through the prosthetic material. Sometimes, pedicled myocutaneous flaps might be indicated for deep, high-risk wounds in the lower or upper abdomen. Such vascularized pedicle flaps usually do not reach the periumbilical region, and considerable thought should be given in conjunction with a reconstructive plastic surgeon before using a rectus abdominus rotational flap across the midline. Those additional considerations are necessary since this approach will disrupt abdominal wall integrity and may lead to major problems when considering a future definitive abdominal wall reconstruction.

Use of Permanent Prosthetic Material

Is there a precedent for use of a nonabsorbable, synthetic prosthesis to repair a concomitant abdominal wall hernia at the time of takedown of an enterocutaneous fistula? Classically, the answer would be a NO, as contaminated wound has traditionally been viewed as a contraindication. Recently, however, with the introduction of the large-pore, lightweight polypropylene prosthetics, this contraindication has been challenged. Work by Israelsson and colleagues [13, 14] has

shown that placement of an intraabdominal, lightweight, large-pore polypropylene mesh is safe at the time of construction of an enterostoma. While this type of clean-contaminated procedure is not necessarily comparable to takedown of an enterocutaneous fistula in most patients, there are selected patients with a fistula who have a fully controlled fistula and are in excellent physical and nutritional shape, making them acceptable candidates for a definitive repair in contaminated environment. In addition, Carbonell and colleagues [15] have collected a series of 100 patients with clean-contaminated and contaminated wounds in whom a hernia repair was carried out using a large-pore, reduced-weight polypropylene prosthetic placed in the highly vascular retrorectus space. Wound infections occurred in 8 patients (8%), and 4 patients developed a recurrent hernia in the first year postoperatively. Obviously, these were selected patients, and this type of study requires confirmation. Nevertheless, as herniologists, we need to keep an open mind. In addition, several authorities have claimed that when exposed, the large-pore, lightweight permanent prosthetic meshes (non-ePTFE materials) will granulate successfully and allow healing without sinus formation. In this author's limited experience, similar findings have occurred in contrast to the small-pore, heavyweight polypropylene materials or ePTFE. Some surgeons have suggested that this propensity for healing, even after a wound infection, supports the use of macroporous prosthetics and onlay grafts as hernia repairs [16].

Summary

Remember, your first goal is to repair the enterocutaneous fistula. Your second goal, IF SAFE, is to repair the hernia. Just because "repair" of the hernia can be done, it does not mean it should be done. A failed concomitant hernia repair, especially involving a major abdominal wall reconstruction involving either the classic anterior

Ramirez type [17] or posterior transversus abdominis release, popularized by Novitsky [18] creates a significant challenge for the surgeon managing the recurrence. The primary concerns for concomitant hernia repair are the risk of infection which will breakdown the hernia repair, the inability to utilize a permanent prosthetic, and the possibility (or in many instances, probability) that the patient is a "hernia-former" and any form of autogenous repair or "repair" with a bridging bioprosthesis will likely fail. Patients as well as their families and physicians should understand that recovery from an enterocutaneous fistula complicated by a ventral hernia might very likely require a two-staged approach.

References

1. Johnson EK, Tushoski PL. Abdominal wall reconstruction in patients with digestive tract fistulas. Clin Colon Rectal Surg. 2010;23(3):195–208.
2. Visschers RG, Olde Damink SW, Winkens B, Soeters PB, van Gemert WG. Treatment strategies in 135 consecutive patients with enterocutaneous fistulas. World J Surg. 2008;32(3):445–53.
3. Slade DA, Carlson GL. Takedown of enterocutaneous fistula and complex abdominal wall reconstruction. Surg Clin North Am. 2013;93(5):1163–83.
4. Schecter WP, Hirshberg A, Chang DS, Harris HW, Napolitano LM, Wexner SD, et al. Enteric fistulas: principles of management. J Am Coll Surg. 2009;209(4):484–91.
5. Wind J, van Koperen PJ, Slors JF, Bemelman WA. Single-stage closure of enterocutaneous fistula and stomas in the presence of large abdominal wall defects using the components separation technique. Am J Surg. 2009;197(1):24–9.
6. Krpata DM, Stein SL, Eston M, Ermlich B, Blatnik JA, Novitsky YW, et al. Outcomes of simultaneous large complex abdominal wall reconstruction and enterocutaneous fistula takedown. Am J Surg. 2013;205(3):354–8. Discussion 8–9.
7. de Vries Reilingh TS, Bodegom ME, van Goor H, Hartman EH, van der Wilt GJ, Bleichrodt RP. Autologous tissue repair of large abdominal wall defects. Br J Surg. 2007;94(7):791–803.
8. Cheesborough JE, Park E, Souza JM, Dumanian GA. Staged management of the open abdomen and enteroatmospheric fistulae using split-thickness skin grafts. Am J Surg. 2014;207(4):504–11.
9. Blatnik J, Jin J, Rosen M. Abdominal hernia repair with bridging acellular dermal matrix—an expensive hernia sac. Am J Surg. 2008;196(1):47–50.
10. Abdelfatah MM, Rostambeigi N, Podgaetz E, Sarr MG. Long-term outcomes (>5-year follow-up) with porcine acellular dermal matrix (Permacol) in incisional hernias at risk for infection. Hernia. 2015;19(1):135–40.
11. Wittmann DH, Aprahamian C, Bergstein JM. Etappenlavage: advanced diffuse peritonitis managed by planned multiple laparotomies utilizing zippers, slide fastener, and Velcro analogue for temporary abdominal closure. World J Surg. 1990;14(2): 218–26.
12. Quyn AJ, Johnston C, Hall D, Chambers A, Arapova N, Ogston S, et al. The open abdomen and temporary abdominal closure systems—historical evolution and systematic review. Colorectal Dis. 2012;14(8): e429–38.
13. Israelsson LA. Preventing and treating parastomal hernia. World J Surg. 2005;29(8):1086–9.
14. Israelsson LA. Parastomal hernias. Surg Clin North Am. 2008;88(1):113–25. ix.
15. Carbonell AM, Criss CN, Cobb WS, Novitsky YW, Rosen MJ. Outcomes of synthetic mesh in contaminated ventral hernia repairs. J Am Coll Surg. 2013;217(6):991–8.
16. Kingsnorth AN, Shahid MK, Valliattu AJ, Hadden RA, Porter CS. Open onlay mesh repair for major abdominal wall hernias with selective use of components separation and fibrin sealant. World J Surg. 2008;32(1):26–30.
17. Ramirez OM, Ruas E, Dellon AL. "Components separation" method for closure of abdominal-wall defects: an anatomic and clinical study. Plast Reconstr Surg. 1990;86(3):519–26.
18. Novitsky YW, Elliott HL, Orenstein SB, Rosen MJ. Transversus abdominis muscle release: a novel approach to posterior component separation during complex abdominal wall reconstruction. Am J Surg. 2012;204(5):709–16.

Kamal M.F. Itani and C. Jeff Siegert

Overview and Costs

Ventral hernia is one of the most common surgical problems addressed by general surgeons. The introduction of synthetic mesh improved hernia recurrence rates but resulted in potentially serious complications with mesh infection being one of the most feared among those complications. Treatment of an infected mesh requires tremendous time and patience from both patient and surgeon. It is estimated that 3–10% of meshes will become infected after ventral hernia repair, and that 5% of all meshes will be partially removed or totally explanted at some point after surgery. Mesh infection places the patient at higher risk for subsequent infections after re-repair and higher risks for recurrence of the hernia.

Placing a prosthetic mesh in either a clean-contaminated or contaminated field increases the hospital length of stay to 7 and 15 days, respectively. It is estimated that the average inpatient cost of a ventral hernia repair averages $15,899 in

non-governmental hospitals in the United States. In 2006, ventral hernia repair accounted for 3.2 billion dollars. Each case of open ventral hernia repair with component separation and biologic mesh reinforcement costs over $20,000. Mesh infection results in additional operative procedures, loss of ability to work, chronically draining wounds requiring outpatient care, occasional sepsis, and even death. The non-financial toll a mesh infection takes on the patients, their families, and overall life is hard to quantify [1].

The goal of this chapter is to review various management strategies and techniques in order to tackle this serious problem, minimize impact on patients, and improve outcome. The methods of treatment range from oral antibiotics to radical abdominal wall reconstruction. There is no tried-and-true algorithm, and the remainder of the chapter's discussion on treatment of ventral hernia mesh infection is arranged from least invasive to most invasive. The surgeon must tailor therapy to the individual patient depending on health status, microbiologic data, nature of previous hernia operations, and the mesh that was implanted. The immediate goal of treatment is control of the infection. The endpoint of therapy is a durable repair of the abdominal wall and prevention of another infection and recurrence of the hernia. Ultimate success is measured by the prevention of hernia recurrence, subsequent surgical site infection (SSI) in the new prosthesis, and other wound-related complications. The data on the treatment of mesh infection is mostly anecdotal

K.M.F. Itani, M.D. (✉)
Veterans Affairs Boston Health Care System, Boston University and Harvard Medical School,
(112A), 1400 VFW Pkwy, West Roxbury, MA 02132, USA
e-mail: kitani@va.gov

C.J. Siegert, M.D.
Veterans Affairs Boston Health Care System,
1400 VFW Pkwy, West Roxbury, MA 02132, USA
e-mail: jeffsiegert@gmail.com

© Springer International Publishing Switzerland 2016
Y.W. Novitsky (ed.), *Hernia Surgery*, DOI 10.1007/978-3-319-27470-6_37

from small series, single institution, or single-author experience. Most of the data on handling wounds and recurrences after a mesh infection is extrapolated from data available on ventral hernia repairs in clean-contaminated and contaminated fields.

Mesh Selection and Wound Classification

Since the 1960s, many innovations in biomaterial design have taken place in order to create an optimal mesh for abdominal wall reconstruction and ventral hernia repair. Bacteria have also evolved to use the prosthetic material as a platform for colonization. Mesh attributes such as pore size, hydrophilicity, and filament engineering can select for or against bacteria. The most common bacterial pathogens are the gram-positive skin flora such as *Staphylococcus* species including methicillin-resistant *Staphylococcus aureus* (MRSA) and Streptococcus species. Gram-negative organisms such as *E. coli* are also capable of colonizing mesh. Certain bacteria such as Staphylococcal species produce slime on synthetic material that decreases the ability of antibiotics and phagocytic cells to reach bacteria.

Synthetic meshes can broadly be classified into monofilament Polypropylene (PP), multifilament polyester, expanded polytetrafluroethylene (ePTFE), and composite meshes. PP has a high tensile strength but forms stout adhesions to bowel if placed intraperitoneally. Multifilament polyester meshes have similar strength to polypropylene meshes but a tendency to result in less inflammation and connective tissue formation if low weight. They still are not recommended for placement intraperitoneally and behave similar to PP in the face of infection. ePTFE was developed to counteract these enteric adhesions but seems to be less salvageable in the case of infection. Composite meshes usually combine polypropylene on one side to promote fibrous in growth and a smooth surface of another material such as PTFE on the other side to prevent enteric adhesions. Clearance of bacteria from composite mesh has been shown to be poor compared to clearance from monofilament polypropylene mesh [2].

Bioprosthetic matrices have been introduced as an alternative to synthetic mesh and are used by surgeons in contaminated fields. These products were not approved by the FDA for this specific indication but remain an appealing option for surgeons when faced with contamination. The ingrowth of fibroblasts within the collagen scaffold and neovascularization allow for incorporation of the bioprosthesis within native tissues and clearance of microorganisms. Outcomes with these meshes in contaminated fields have been less than optimal in small prospective studies (Fig. 37.1).

Wounds are classified as clean, clean-contaminated, contaminated and dirty. In the abdominal cavity, a clean-contaminated case is the result of entry into the gastrointestinal (GI) tract but no spillage of enteric contents. In a contaminated field, there is usually spillage from the GI tract or bowel ischemia/necrosis.

The majority of mesh infections occur in ventral hernia repairs undertaken in clean-contaminated and contaminated fields. Surgeons have to often make a decision on whether to perform a single-stage repair in these instances or the more traditional multi-stage repair. In a single-stage repair a bioprosthetic matrix is favored [3]. In a multi-stage repair, infection is controlled in the first operation with drainage of abscesses, debridement of necrotic tissue, and takedown of an enterocutaneous fistula if it exists. Repair of the ventral hernia or abdominal

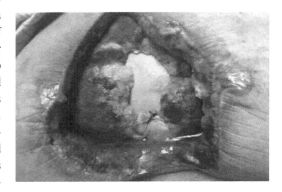

Fig. 37.1 Biologic mesh in an infected field after multiple debridements

wall reconstruction is performed at a later time when the patient is fully recovered from the infection and the wound is healed.

The combination of wound classification and mesh selection is crucial in preventing a mesh infection after ventral hernia repair. The Ventral Hernia Working Group (VHWG) introduced a classification system to help the surgeon in the decision making when selecting a mesh repair (Table 37.1). In grades 3 and 4, synthetic meshes should be avoided and consideration given for either a single-stage bioprosthetic matrix or a multi-stage repair. In small prospective trials, a single-stage repair in these complex patients, demonstrate that recurrence rates and wound occurrences remain high.

Mesh Salvage

Salvage refers to a conservative approach of treating mesh infections and leaving it in place. The first step in salvaging a mesh is timely treatment of any wound occurrence and the long-term assessment of the patient, as a mesh involved with infection might not manifest until 6–12 months after surgery. A SSI, wound separation, or skin edge necrosis usually present in the immediate postoperative period. The first thought is whether the mesh is infected and if it needs to be removed. If the mesh is deep to the wound with an overlying healthy tissue layer, a bacterial infection could potentially be eradicated and a colonization of the mesh be prevented. Superficial wound occurrences happen earlier in the postoperative period. When detected, the goal is to prevent extension to the level of the mesh by aggressive local wound care and broad-spectrum antibiotics. In cases of cellulitis alone, antibiotics should be administered until resolution of the local symptoms and systemic symptoms, if present. If local symptoms progress or systemic symptoms do not resolve within 24–48 hours, a deeper infection should be suspected and a CT scan performed to rule out a deep abscess (Fig. 37.2).

Most fluid collections in the subcutaneous tissues or around the mesh are seromas or hematomas. It is crucial to avoid tapping these collections unless they are symptomatic or suspicious for an ongoing infection. The presence of a fluid collection associated with systemic signs and symptoms of infection mandate aspiration and culture of the fluid in question. In the case of infected fluid around the mesh, recent anecdotes of total mesh salvage with locally guided treatment using systemic antibiotics coupled with a percutaneous drain and gentamycin drain flushes have been reported. Typically the drain is placed under radiographic guidance and gentamycin flushes are initiated after drainage drops to a manageable daily amount. This may be a reasonable step to avoid explantation of the mesh and abdominal wall reconstruction in a patient with a contained infection, and no systemic compromise [4]. However, the surgeon must determine when this approach has failed, and avoid delaying more definitive treatment.

Table 37.1 Ventral hernia working group grading system (reproduced from Breuing et al. Incisional ventral hernias: Review of the literature and recommendations regarding the grading and technique of repair. Surgery. 2010;148:544–58)

Grade 1	Grade 2	Grade 3	Grade 4
Low risk	Comorbid	Potentially contaminated	Infected
Low risk of complications	Smoker	Previous wound infection	Infected mesh
No history of wound infections	Obese	Stoma present	Septic dehiscence
	Diabetic	Violation of the gastrointestinal tract	
	Immunosuppressed		
	COPD		

Adapted from: Ventral hernia working group grading system (reproduced from Breuing et al. Incisional ventral hernias: Review of the literature and recommendations regarding the grading and technique of repair. Surgery. 2010;148:544–58)

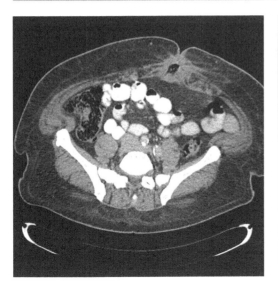

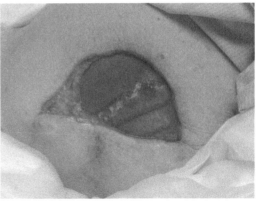

Fig. 37.3 Granulation tissue within a macroporous polypropylene mesh after multiple debridements and wet-to-dry dressing changes

Fig. 37.2 CT scan depicting a deep-seated abscess after mesh repair of a ventral hernia

A fluid collection in the spaces accessed during surgery, should raise suspicion to bowel injury or leak and should be aggressively pursued. Mesh salvage can still be undertaken if the organ/space infection is separate from the mesh by percutaneously tapping or draining the abscess. An enteric leak can be converted to controlled fistula through the drain. Should the mesh be totally exposed as a result of a deep SSI after subcutaneous tissue debridement, one can consider few options that are available to salvage the mesh. Negative pressure wound therapy (NPWT) could be used after achieving control of the infection. The negative pressure therapy accelerates the granulation tissue incorporation throughout the mesh. If NPWT is not available, aggressive wet-to-dry dressing changes are also suitable. Macropore polypropylene mesh is associated with the best outcome in this situation (Fig. 37.3) while ePTFE usually fails to incorporate and has to be explanted entirely (Fig. 37.4) [5].

Partial Salvage

Partial salvage of the mesh is the next step among available surgical options. In many instances, a patient will present with a chronically draining

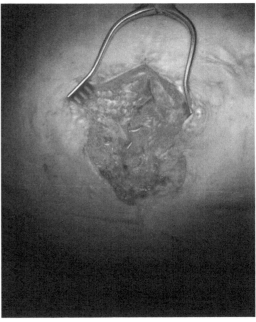

Fig. 37.4 Infected ePTFE mesh floating in purulent fluid

sinus track after ventral hernia repair with mesh without any systemic signs or symptoms of infection. Sometimes there may be exposure or extrusion of synthetic mesh, evident at the base of the wound or with minor exploration in clinic. In order to assess the extent of tissue and mesh involvement, methylene blue can be injected through the sinus track. Under local anesthesia, with or without light sedation, the sinus is removed along with the exposed mesh at the base of the track. The tissue and any excised prosthesis are sent for culture/sensitivities, and the patient is placed on long-term antibiotics targeting the cultured organisms. Once clean, the wound can be treated with NPWT or wet-to-dry dressings [6].

All salvage techniques do spare the patient a major explantation procedure, but may require several additional operations to control the infection and remove non-incorporated and/or infected mesh. The patient may also end up with chronically draining wounds, which would adversely affect their quality of life. All patients undergoing partial salvage are at increased risk for hernia recurrence.

Mesh Explantation

If the mesh cannot be salvaged using the above techniques, then explantation is necessary. Explantation is usually the only solution with ePTFE mesh, as ePTFE fails to integrate in the presence of infection. This is also true to some extent with low-weight multifilament polyester meshes (Fig. 37.4). The dilemma for the surgeon is whether to plan a staged procedure in which the infected mesh is removed and the patient is left with a large fascial defect or undergo a one-stage procedure with explanting the mesh and performing a primary repair or placing a new prosthesis in a contaminated field. In a staged procedure, the time frame between infected mesh explantation and placement of new mesh ranges from 6 months to 2 years. Obviously, the patient may develop a loss of domain between explantation and abdominal wall reconstruction. Patients with signs and symptoms of sepsis should be taken immediately to the operating room for removal and debridement of mesh and any associated necrotic tissue and to control spillage of bowel contents, if present. A temporary closure strategy would be reasonable in these patients using skin only, an abdominal wound vacuum system, Bogotá bag or other available techniques. Explantation should include the removal of any fixation sutures or tacks in addition to the mesh itself as they can cause chronic cutaneous sinuses. Reconstruction should be undertaken at a later time in these patients.

A one-stage operation should be selected only if the amount of contamination is minimal and all necrotic tissues are satisfactorily debrided. In this situation, a primary fascial closure with or without component separation can be chosen. Alternatively, reconstruction with a biologic matrix can be performed. Great caution should be applied when deciding on a one-stage repair after mesh explantation as new dissection planes within the abdominal wall can be placed at risk for additional infections. Component separations without a mesh or a biologic mesh reconstruction in this situation have a hernia recurrence rates above 20% at 2 years [7, 8].

Risk Factors and Prevention

Efforts in the prevention of a mesh infection are paramount and outweigh any efforts expanded in the care of patients with a subsequent mesh infection. There are important patient and operative risk factors that increase the likelihood of a ventral hernia mesh infection. Some of these factors are more easily addressed than others. Smoking, diabetes, chronic obstructive pulmonary disease, nutritional status, immunosuppression, chronic steroid use, obesity, advanced age, large hernia defects, prolonged operative time, and postoperative wound infections have all been shown to be risk factors for mesh explantation. Strategies to address these risk factors and optimize the patient should be in place prior to any elective ventral hernia surgery. Additionally, a properly dosed and re-dosed intravenous prophylactic antibiotics, normothermia, and normoglycemia in the perioperative period are evidence-based measures that should be observed. Smoking cessation and weight loss should be part of the care plan in these patients. The use of ePTFE mesh or concomitant procedures during hernia repair has been shown to result in a higher rate of mesh explantation in one large cohort of patients. Regarding the prevention of ventral hernia mesh infection during initial repair, there is no good data in the literature to support topical or embedded antibacterial agents within the mesh in addition to prophylactic IV antibiotics [9].

Conclusion

Preventing a mesh infection in ventral hernia repair should be the main goal of every surgeon caring for those patients. Once it occurs, the treatment is a complicated and costly process. Many treatment options are described and the choice of one over the other should be individualized based on patient's condition and presentation.

The key principle in caring for those patients is to first control the infection. Salvaging a mesh is a secondary goal and should only be attempted if the patient's condition allows. The type of mesh implanted and the technique used will often dictate whether a mesh can be salvaged. Partial salvage and explantation of a mesh are associated with hernia recurrence and additional surgeries.

References

1. Poulose BK, Shelton J, Phillips S, Moore D, Nealon W, Penson D, Beck W, Holzman MD. Epidemiology and cost of ventral hernia repair: making the case for hernia research. Hernia. 2012;16(2):179–83.
2. Carbonell AM, Cris CN, Cobb WS, Novitsky YW, Rosen MJ. Outcomes of synthetic mesh in contaminated ventral hernia repairs. J Am Coll Surg. 2013;217(6):991–8.
3. Itani KMF, Rosen M, Vargo D, Awad SS, Denoto III G, Butler CE. Prospective study of single-stage repair of contaminated hernias using a biologic porcine tissue matrix: the RICH study. Surgery. 2012;152(3):498–505.
4. Trunzo JA, Ponsky JL, Jin J, Williams CP, Rosen MJ. A novel approach for salvaging infected prosthetic mesh after ventral hernia repair. Hernia. 2009;13(5):545–9.
5. Stremitzer S, Bachleitner-Hofmann T, Gradl B, Gruenbeck M, Bachleitner-Hoffman B, Mittlboeck M, Bergmann M. Mesh graft infection following abdominal hernia repair: risk factor evaluation and strategies of mesh graft preservation. A retrospective analysis of 476 operations. World J Surg. 2010;34(7):1702–9.
6. Sabbagh C, Verhaeghe P, Brehant O, Browet F, Garriot B, Regimbeau JM. Partial removal of infected parietal meshes is a safe procedure. Hernia. 2012;16(4):445–9.
7. Sanchez V, Abi-Haidar YE, Itani KMF. Mesh infection in ventral incisional hernia repair: incidence, contributing factors, and treatment. Surg Infect. 2011;12(3):205–10.
8. Cevasco M, Itani KMF. Ventral hernia repair with synthetic, composite and biologic mesh: characteristics, indications and infection profile. Surg Infect. 2012;13(4):209–15.
9. Hawn MT, Gray SH, Snyder CW, Graham LA, Finan KR, Vick CC. Predictors of mesh explantation after incisional hernia repair. Am J Surg. 2011;202(1):28–33.

Management of Ventral Hernia in the Morbidly Obese Patient

Jeffrey A. Blatnik and Ajita S. Prabhu

Introduction

Ventral hernia repair in the United States is estimated to occur up to 365,000 times a year, with an estimated healthcare cost of $3.2 billion [1]. The development of a ventral hernia itself is one of the most frequent complications following abdominal surgery. As the prevalence of morbid obesity and ventral hernias continues to increase, this remains an ongoing challenge for the practicing general surgeon who is faced with repairing hernias in this complicated population [1, 2]. Additionally, while the specific role of obesity in hernia recurrence is difficult to define, it seems clear that morbid obesity may indeed be a contributing factor [3], and thereby also places these patients in a different risk category of patients undergoing hernia repair [4]. In fact, morbidly obese patients are nearly four times more likely to develop recurrence after both open and laparoscopic ventral hernia repair than their non-obese counterparts [5, 6]. This may be related to higher intra-abdominal pressure in obese patients [7], and/or to an increased risk of surgical site infection associated with these patients [8]. Numerous concerns have led surgeons to resist offering elective hernia operations to the morbidly obese population which include increased wound morbidity as well as higher rate of other systemic complications such as thromboembolic or cardiac events, increased hernia recurrence rate, and finally technical challenges of the operation specifically related to the patient's size.

While it is clear that there is a higher incidence of complication and hernia recurrence associated with morbid obesity, to date there is still no working consensus for how to approach these patients from the standpoint of patient selection. Additionally, there is a lack of an accepted classification or staging system to help describe the disease entity specific to each patient. It follows that when we are unable to define the disease process and differentiate between varying levels of complexity, then it becomes difficult to standardize algorithms to the approach of these patients. The objectives of this chapter are to detail different obese patients' variable and how they factor into our surgical decision-making. Additionally, we will provide a suggested algorithm (Fig. 38.1) for the management of the obese patients.

J.A. Blatnik, M.D. (✉)
Department of Surgery, Section of Minimally Invasive Surgery, Washington University School of Medicine, St. Louis, MO, USA
e-mail: BlatnikJ@wudosis.wustl.edu

A.S. Prabhu, M.D., F.A.C.S.
Department of Surgery, University Hospitals Case Medical Center, Cleveland, OH, USA
e-mail: Ajita.Prabhu@UHhospitals.org

© Springer International Publishing Switzerland 2016
Y.W. Novitsky (ed.), *Hernia Surgery*, DOI 10.1007/978-3-319-27470-6_38

Body Mass Index

Body Mass Index (BMI) was originally described by Adolphe Quetelet in 1832, but owes its popularity to a study by Keys in 1972 which found BMI to be the best proxy for calculating body fat percentage based on weight and height [9, 10]. It has found use in everything from calculating life expectancy to determine insurance premiums. BMI as a data point alone is insufficient to determine an operative approach for a morbidly obese patient, and should be considered only as one of the factors in decision-making, as opposed to the only factor. Despite the fact that BMI has limited use as an index of obesity, because it does not take into account the ratio of fat mass to fat-free mass, it is nevertheless frequently used as a surrogate for the designation of obesity. This phenomenon is well described in athletes [11]. In addition to BMI, other patient-specific characteristics that should be considered include those listed in Table 38.1. Previous attempts at creation of an algorithm have failed to take into account the heterogeneous patient population and therefore are not widely applicable [12].

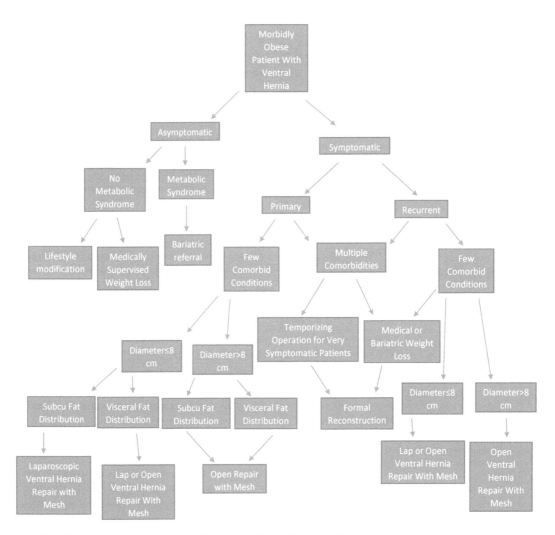

Fig. 38.1 Proposed algorithm for a morbidly obese patient with a ventral hernia.

Table 38.1 Factors in determining operative approach to morbidly obese patients with hernias

Absolute diameter of defect ($\leq$8 cm; >8 cm)
Surface area of defect compared to surface area of abdominal wall
Body morphology of patient (android vs. gynoid vs. ovoid)
Distribution of fat (visceral vs. subcutaneous)
Number of previous recurrences/intended technique
Mesh location/history of contamination
Mesh choice

Size of the Defect

The size of the hernia defect relative to the depth of the abdominal wall is a relevant factor in helping to determine the ultimate operative approach, whether it will be minimally invasive or open. In the case of a morbidly obese patient with a relatively small defect size, an open approach may become unmanageable or unreasonable based on the thickness of the subcutaneous tissue. For instance, a laparotomy incision for a 9 cm^2 defect may be considered excessive in a patient with abdominal wall thickness greater than 5 cm and BMI of 70, whereas the same sized defect in a patient with a normal BMI may be approached in an open fashion without reservation, while using one relatively small incision, and possibly even avoiding general anesthesia. In the former case, the challenge lies in gaining appropriate exposure to place the mesh, and subsequently also determining the appropriate plane in which to place the mesh and, finally, how to fixate it. In the author's own practice, relatively small hernias (<8 cm width) in patients fitting this description (thick layer of subcutaneous fat/thick abdominal wall or BMI>40) would undergo minimally invasive repair. With the abdomen insufflated, there is relatively good visualization of the defect, giving the surgeon the ability to achieve adequate mesh overlap while avoiding a large incision which could potentially result in significant wound morbidity and lengthened recovery times. Additionally, defects of small to medium size (up to 8 cm greatest diameter in the author's personal practice) may still be closed laparoscopically using the so-called laparo-

scopic "shoelace technique" (Chapter 23) by which a suture passer device is used under direct laparoscopic vision to place a series of interrupted figure-of-eight sutures to close the defect primarily before placing a prosthetic reinforcement. This provides the benefit of closing the tissue defect in addition to mesh placement which may restore some function of the abdominal wall and reduce seroma formation by closing the dead space above the mesh.

As the defect size becomes larger and its relative surface area as compared to the surface area of the abdominal wall increases, mesh eventration may occur with laparoscopic repair over time if the fascia is not reapproximated. This is likely due to excessive intra-abdominal pressure against the mesh, resulting in an undesirable outcome. Strong consideration should be given to open repair in these patients, with myofascial release and wide prosthetic reinforcement of the visceral sac in order to restore the natural contour of the abdominal wall and avoid "pseudohernia" formation which is when the laparoscopically placed mesh takes on the contour of the original hernia and appears as a recurrence.

Body Morphology of the Patient

Distribution of fat is another factor that should be considered when determining operative approach. Fat may be distributed in an apple-shaped or android distribution, a pear-shaped or gynoid distribution, or an ovoid distribution, which is a hybrid or intermediate shape where fat may be more evenly distributed throughout the body. While the term "android" implies "male" and the term "gynoid" implies "female," body morphologies are not restricted to sex, and either fat distribution may be seen in both males or females. Android obesity refers to distribution of fat around the central portion of the body, or the abdomen. In addition, android fat distribution may be further categorized as either visceral (also known as intra-abdominal fat) or subcutaneous fat as the predominant distribution type. Gynoid obesity refers to the greatest distribution of fat around the hips and buttocks as opposed to the abdomen, and may be the most preferable body type in the morbidly obese population in terms of operative candidacy for hernia repair. Android obesity represents the least preferable fat distribution for hernia repair as this places the largest amount of stress on the abdominal wall. A primarily subcutaneous fat distribution leads to increased wound morbidity, difficulty in gaining exposure for open operations, excessive torque on minimally invasive ports, and ergonomic difficulty for the surgeon. In contrast, visceral fat confers a greater issue in terms of volume and occasionally domain, therefore making open repair technically challenging. While a large volume of visceral fat may be more manageable laparoscopically, the presumably greater intra-abdominal pressure may still put excessive outward force on the prosthetic repair and confer a greater risk of long-term repair failure.

For patients with android and visceral type fat distribution both open and laparoscopic approach may be considered. In general, our approach to those patients favors minimally invasive repair, especially when the defect is ≤8 cm wide. Notably, visceral obesity (as opposed to other fat distribution types) is associated with insulin resistance, dyslipidemia, hypertension, and coronary artery disease, all of which may contribute to perioperative morbidity. It remains to be further elucidated whether visceral fat distribution should affect the decision to operate on the patient prior to weight loss and if so, if one should utilize a laparoscopic or open technique. Gynoid fat distribution may lend itself to either operative approach as the hip, thigh, and buttock are relatively uninvolved in ventral hernia repair. Android fat distribution may be challenging for either open or laparoscopic approach due to the fact that excess fat is centered around the abdomen. With this type of distribution, the decision to operate is more dependent upon the severity of obesity than with other types of fat distribution.

Number of Previous Repairs

Morbidly obese patients who have had multiple hernia recurrences represent a different level of complexity than the same patients with new hernias. Factors to consider in these patients include prior use of mesh, reason for failure, and location of prior mesh, if present. For instance, a morbidly obese patient with a failed onlay mesh repair of a small to moderate sized defect may still remain a candidate for laparoscopy because there is no mesh in the abdomen. In contrast, a patient with a failed prior laparoscopic repair and retained intraperitoneal mesh may necessitate open operation if the mesh cannot be removed laparoscopically. Additionally, for multiply recurrent hernias, even if laparoscopic approach is considered feasible, the surgeon should consider a possibility of conversion to open repair during preoperative planning. This speaks to the variable nature of reoperative surgery in a complex group of patients and may suggest that such patients are best managed at specialty centers.

For very symptomatic patients who have multiple recurrences in the setting of multiple comorbidities, consideration should be given to a temporizing or non-reconstructive approach. This is especially true if it is felt that the degree of obesity precludes a good definitive outcome at the time of the original operation. Options for temporizing approach include intraperitoneal biologic mesh with transfascial suture fixation, or intraperitoneal onlay mesh (IPOM) through a laparoscopic approach, depending on the size of the hernia and distribution of fat. At that point, the patient would be referred for either medical or surgical weight loss, with delay of formal reconstruction until the patient reached a goal weight as decided between the patient and surgeon.

Mesh Location

It is generally agreed upon that morbid obesity is an indication to repair ventral hernia defects with prosthetic reinforcement. For laparoscopic ventral hernia repair, mesh (typically with an anti-adhesive barrier on the visceral-facing surface) is placed into the intraperitoneal position. Despite the presence of anti-adhesive barriers, intraperitoneal onlay mesh (IPOM) is arguably a less desirable location for prosthetic reinforcement due to increased risk of adhesions, fistula formation, and fixation-related complications such as chronic pain or tack-related bowel injury. The relationship of IPOM to these complications has been studied but is difficult to define, and the efficacy of anti-adhesive barriers remains unclear. Still, in morbidly obese patients, as mentioned above, the body habitus of the patient may dictate laparoscopic repair in order to decrease perioperative morbidity. If one is operating under the assumption that IPOM is less desirable than preperitoneal, retrorectus, or onlay mesh position due to these potential complications, it can be argued that morbidly obese patients undergoing laparoscopic repair of ventral hernias may not receive the optimum repair. As minimally invasive techniques continue to evolve and priorities of hernia repair change, it remains to be seen if modalities such as robotics may lend themselves to preperitoneal placement of mesh through small incisions, thereby avoiding some of the potential complications of intraperitoneal mesh with minimal wound morbidity.

When considering open hernia repair, choice of mesh location may differ based upon the patient's obesity. For open repair, we typically avoid intraperitoneal mesh placement as more desirable options for location are made feasible by the open approach. Other options for mesh location include onlay or retrorectus sublay mesh placement. While there is some good evidence to support the use of onlay mesh reinforcement in certain patients, the already-increased risk of wound morbidity owing to excessive adipose tissue, poor vascularity, large potential subcutaneous space, and insulin resistance may subsequently result in increased wound morbidity and resultant mesh infection. As a result, we prefer to avoid onlay repairs in morbidly obese patients. Other options for open repair include retrorectus mesh placement, which has become our preferred approach to open hernia repair in morbidly obese patients. Limitations to this approach may include technical and physical challenge to the surgeon, particularly in the case of visceral obesity. Benefits of this approach include finer control of tension on the mesh, potential ease of reapproximating the midline, avoidance of a large subcutaneous space, and avoidance of intraperitoneal or subcutaneous mesh. Importantly, wound infections in patients with sublay mesh reinforcement rarely progress to mesh infections and need for explantation.

Mesh Choice

Choice of prosthetic reinforcement is an additional consideration. Broad mesh categories include synthetic mesh, biologic mesh, hybrid mesh, and absorbable mesh. Rapidly absorbable meshes (half-life of <6 months) are indicated for contaminated fields or staged operations, and essentially serve no role in the elective repair of hernia in morbidly obese patients. Newer iterations of slowly absorbing meshes have come to market, however their role is not yet well defined. Similarly, hybrid meshes typically consist of a biologic element as well as a permanent synthetic element, but to date have not been well studied. Biologic mesh, while widely utilized in plastic surgery literature for elective hernia repair, is associated with a significant rate of eventration or recurrence and is also significantly more expensive than synthetic meshes. Its best use may be in contaminated fields or emergency settings where staged repair may be anticipated. An additional indication for biologic mesh use may be intraperitoneal positioning for patients in whom weight precludes a definitive operation.

For elective clean cases, the preferred mesh material remains permanent polypropylene synthetic mesh. There are many different configurations of these mesh materials, and consideration should be given to the porosity and weight of the mesh material making a selection for use in a morbidly obese patient. While higher porosity/lower weight meshes may be advantageous in terms of better ability to clear infection, they are not currently available in large enough sizes for certain situations to cover the necessary surface area without sewing multiple pieces of mesh together. Moreover, it remains unclear at which point the reduced-weight meshes are unable to withstand intra-abdominal forces and yield to central mesh failures and recurrences. For this reason, when given large hernia defects in morbidly obese patients, in absence of active infection, it is our preferred approach to use a mid-to-heavy weight polypropylene mesh for most open repairs.

Preoperative Planning and Weight Loss

Preoperative preparation and planning for elective hernia repair in the morbidly obese patient population is generally similar to that of other general surgery procedures, perhaps with some additional caveats. When evaluating patients in the office, we find it helpful to obtain a CT scan of the abdomen and pelvis, especially since physical exam can be very challenging in the obese. This helps to assess the size of the defect, the depth of the subcutaneous tissue in the abdominal wall, the extent of visceral fat, the width of the specific abdominal wall muscles (hence potential for myofascial release if indicated), and loss of domain if present. All of these variables weigh into the selection of the optimal operative approach.

Depending on the severity of symptoms from the hernia, the surgeon may choose to delay surgery in order to allow the patient time to lose weight. The importance of weight loss in terms of overall health and potential reduction of hernia recurrence risk is discussed in the office with each patient, and potential strategies for weight loss are offered. Initial discussion for all patients should begin with lifestyle modification. Additional strategies may include referral for evaluation for bariatric surgery or referral to a medical weight loss clinic for guided weight loss planning. Here it is important to note that in our own center it remains unclear what percentage of our patients who are given referrals are ever evaluated by weight loss specialists. In our experience, those patients who are able to undergo medical weight loss treatment under the care of a physician have significant success at losing weight. However the majority of them have regained at least some portion of the lost weight over the next 18 months. Additionally, very few of our patients follow through with referrals to our bariatric center, and the reason for this remains uncertain. The benefits of preoperative weight loss may include reduction of risks of recurrence, wound morbidity, and perioperative events as well as decrease in the technical challenges of the operation for the surgeon; however, this has not been well studied or

described in hernia literature. Also, as obesity in and of itself has not been identified as an independent risk factor for hernia recurrence, the ultimate impact of weight loss in the perioperative period remains unclear. In support of the relationship between BMI and postoperative morbidity, Sanni et al. reported that in the bariatric surgical patient for every point increase in BMI, there was a 2% increase in the risk of postoperative complications [13]. Finally, as patients may struggle with keeping weight off once it is lost, the ultimate consequence of regaining weight after hernia repair is also unknown. While it seems intuitive that preoperative weight loss should result in a better overall outcome, this remains difficult to prove. The ultimate decision of timing of an operation then falls to the surgeon and may depend on the surgeon's comfort level and skill set.

All morbidly obese patients undergoing major abdominal surgery at our institution are also sent to the Center for Perioperative Medicine, where they are evaluated for cardiac and pulmonary issues. Many patients with morbid obesity also undergo preoperative sleep study to rule out obstructive sleep apnea, and if found to be positive will be placed on continuous positive airway pressure for their postoperative care in order to reduce perioperative respiratory events. They are also monitored continuously for oxygen saturation levels during the postoperative period. Diabetic patients have a preoperative hemoglobin A1C tested and surgery is delayed until the level is ≤ 8 to minimize potential wound morbidity.

Concomitant Bariatric Surgery with Ventral Hernia Repair

The question regarding the safety of a combined bariatric surgery and ventral hernia repair is a recent area of discussion. The potential of saving the patient an additional operation is an obvious benefit. However, there is some concern regarding the risk for mesh infection when combining with a sleeve gastrectomy or roux-en-y gastric bypass. Cozacov et al. evaluated intraoperative cultures in patients undergoing bariatric surgery and found the positive culture rate following sleeve gastrectomy to be zero; in contrast, the positive culture rate was 15% in patients undergoing roux-en-y gastric bypass [14]. Recently, several authors have reviewed their series and have found that a combined procedure can be performed with good success and a low risk of perioperative morbidity [15–17].

Conclusion

In conclusion, morbidly obese patients who present for hernia repair represent a challenge for surgeons. For the surgeon, preoperative and intraoperative decision-making remains complex. In addition, stratifying a patient's risk for complications remains nearly impossible due to the variability of factors. One certainty is that the incidence of morbid obesity in the United States appears to be increasing, and it stands to reason that the percentage of morbidly obese patients with hernias will continue to rise as well. While patients should be encouraged to lose weight preoperatively, the authors recognize that this is largely unsuccessful, and even when weight loss is successfully achieved, keeping the weight off becomes another challenge. Regardless, it is incumbent upon the surgeon to address the care of these patients and to consider the variables which may affect the possible outcome and postoperative morbidity. It is therefore crucial to employ some strategy and consistent approach to these patients despite the lack of a standard algorithm.

References

1. Poulose BK, Shelton J, Phillips S, Moore D, Nealon W, Penson D, et al. Epidemiology and cost of ventral hernia repair: making the case for hernia research. Hernia. 2012;16(2):179–83.
2. Ogden CL, Carroll MD, Kit BK, Flegal KM. Prevalence of childhood and adult obesity in the United States, 2011–2012. JAMA. 2014;311(8): 806–14.
3. Sugerman HJ, Kellum JM, Reines HD, Demaria EJ, Newsome HH, Lowry JW. Greater risk of incisional hernia with morbidly obese than steroid-dependent

patients and low recurrence with prefascial polypropylene mesh. Am J Surg. 1995;171:80–4.
4. Breuing K, Butler CE, Ferzoco S, Franz M, Hultman CS, Kilbridge JF, et al. Incisional ventral hernias: review of the literature and recommendations regarding the grading and technique of repair. Surgery. 2010; 148(3):544–58.
5. Heniford BT, Park A, Ramshaw BJ, Voeller G. Laparoscopic repair of ventral hernias: nine years' experience with 850 consecutive hernias. Ann Surg. 2003;238(3):391–9. discussion 399–400.
6. Sauerland S, Korenkov M, Kleinen T, Arndt M, Paul A. Obesity is a risk factor for recurrence after incisional hernia repair. Hernia. 2004;8(1):42–6.
7. Cobb WS, Burns JM, Kercher KW, Matthews BD, James Norton H, Todd Heniford B. Normal intraabdominal pressure in healthy adults. J Surg Res. 2005;129(2):231–5.
8. Pessaux P, Lermite E, Blezel E, Msika S, Hay J-M, Flamant Y, et al. Predictive risk score for infection after inguinal hernia repair. Am J Surg. 2006;192(2):165–71.
9. Eknoyan G. Adolphe Quetelet (1796–1874)—the average man and indices of obesity. Nephrol Dial Transplant. 2008;23(1):47–51.
10. Keys A, Fidanza F, Karvonen MJ, Kimura N, Taylor HL. Indices of relative weight and obesity. J Chronic Dis. 1972;25(6):329–43.
11. Mathews EM, Wagner DR. Prevalence of overweight and obesity in collegiate American football players, by position. J Am Coll Health. 2008;57:33–8.
12. Eid GM, Wikiel KJ, Entabi F, Saleem M. Ventral hernias in morbidly obese patients: a suggested algorithm for operative repair. Obes Surg. 2013;23:703–9.
13. Sanni A, Perez S, Medbery R, Urrego HD, McCready C, Toro JP, et al. Postoperative complications in bariatric surgery using age and BMI stratification: a study using ACS-NSQIP data. Surg Endosc. 2014; 28(12):3302–9.
14. Cozacov Y, Szomstein S, Safdie FM, Lo Menzo E, Rosenthal R. Is the use of prosthetic mesh recommended in severely obese patients undergoing concomitant abdominal wall hernia repair and sleeve gastrectomy? J Am Coll Surg. 2014;218(3):358–62.
15. Praveen Raj P, Senthilnathan P, Kumaravel R, Rajpandian S, Rajan PS, Anand Vijay N, et al. Concomitant laparoscopic ventral hernia mesh repair and bariatric surgery: a retrospective study from a tertiary care center. Obes Surg. 2012;22(5):685–9.
16. Spaniolas K, Kasten KR, Mozer AB, Sippey ME, Chapman WHH, Pories WJ, et al. Synchronous ventral hernia repair in patients undergoing bariatric surgery. Obes Surg. 2015;25(10):1864–8.
17. Raziel A, Sakran N, Szold A, Goitein D. Concomitant bariatric and ventral/incisional hernia surgery in morbidly obese patients. Surg Endosc. 2013;28(4): 1209–12.

Emergent Surgical Management of Ventral Hernias

Phillip Chang and Levi D. Procter

Introduction

Presentation of incarcerated or strangulated hernias is one of the most common reasons for consultation from the emergency room a general surgeon receives. For clinical and/or socioeconomic reasons, many of these hernias have progressed over time to reach "emergency" status. In addition to the emergent nature, the patient's underlying physiology predisposes these patients to higher perioperative risks. Morbidity and mortality are significantly increased in this patient population [1–4]; and likewise, the durability of these repairs is significantly lower than elective repairs. These patients can be complex and the surgical options are diverse. Risks and benefits for both the immediate and long term time frames have to be considered to achieve the best outcome.

The most common emergent abdominal wall hernias are comprised of ventral and groin hernias. Ventral hernias include incisional, parastomal, spigelian, epigastric, and umbilical. Groin hernias include inguinal and femoral hernias. The clinical characteristics of these hernias include reducible, incarcerated, and strangulated. The crux of the clinical decision is operating early on incarcerated hernias prior to the transition to strangulation. This decreases the likelihood of bowel ischemia, perforation, and need for resection. Strangulated hernias have a much greater likelihood of mortality and morbidity and significantly limit the choices for repair [3, 5–15].

The workup of these complex hernias can be cumbersome and is often performed by non-surgeons. These patients have often been relegated to minimal resuscitation and aggressive imaging that is often unnecessary. A good surgical history, especially timing and techniques used in prior repair, is always important. On physical examination, an immediate operation is indicated when there is significant tenderness, peritonitis, or severe pain out of proportion to exam. In addition, hard signs on imaging, such as free air and pneumatosis, as well as physiologic derangement are also indications for an urgent exploration.

In addition to the patients' physiology, the surgical considerations are different as well. Specifically, in addition to the abdominal wall defect, the surgeon's first consideration is now the content of the hernia sac and assessing for presence of transition point and viability of bowel. Furthermore, the hernia itself takes on a new dimension of complexity that includes soft tissue swelling, potential loss of domain, and presence of prior mesh and whether the mesh itself may be contaminated.

In this chapter we will describe how to approach the workup, imaging, and surgical management of common hernia emergencies.

The original version of this chapter was revised.
An erratum to this chapter can be found at
DOI 10.1007/978-3-319-27470-6_51

P. Chang, M.D. (✉) • L.D. Procter
University of Kentucky, Lexington, KY, USA
e-mail: phillipkchang@gmail.com

Inguinal Hernia

Inguinal hernias are the most common hernias in males and females. Asymptomatic reducible inguinal hernias can be watched safely in select patients and these patients do not require emergent operations [16, 17]. The remainder of inguinal hernia "emergencies" falls into three categories. First category includes those patients that present with pain and their hernias are difficult to reduce. Once reduced either with conscious sedation or the surgeon's skilled hands, these patients should be considered for early elective repair or admitted for urgent repair. The second category includes those who have acutely incarcerated inguinal hernias that are irreducible despite sedation. The timing of this operation depends on whether the surgeon believes this represents a strangulated hernia or if the hernia is the cause of bowel obstruction. The third category of patients includes those with strangulated inguinal hernias. The risk for acute strangulation is 3/1000 patients [7]. Clinical exam findings that suggest need for operative repair are skin discoloration, such as dark red or blue-black. Other findings include pain out of proportion to exam, evidence of severe sepsis or shock, and lactate associated acidemia.

As expected, emergent groin hernia repairs have increased morbidity and mortality compared to elective repairs [7, 14, 18–20]. The pathology that contributes to this increased morbidity and mortality is often the presence of necrotic or ischemic bowel causing intra-abdominal sepsis. Bowel resections are not uncommon in this disease process. Additionally, vascular supply to the testicle could be compromised during the repair of the most complex inguinal hernias, such as recurrent hernias. These are important discussion points with the patient during the informed consent process.

Patients undergoing emergent inguinal hernia repair in the absence of bowel resection, ischemia, or peritonitis have no increased risk of mesh-related morbidity [6, 8, 13, 21–24].

The two approaches to consider are either open or laparoscopic. Laparoscopic hernia repair has merit in selected patients. Diagnostic laparoscopy can be performed with attempted manual extracorporeal reduction and/or laparoscopic reduction. Aside from the minimally invasive approach for reduction, bowel viability can be easily inspected; and laparoscopic hernia repair could be followed. Mesh selection deserves special consideration if the operative field is deemed contaminated. The surgeon may also choose to convert to an open, tissue-based repair.

Open repair can proceed in one of two ways, supra inguinal or via laparotomy. If bowel is unable to be reduced safely, or resection and anastomosis will be technically challenging, then laparotomy should be performed to facilitate resection and anastomosis. The hernia is often constricted by the internal inguinal ring therefore sharply incising the internal inguinal ring can allow reduction and/or evaluation of the hernia contents. Once performed, it is key to prevent the hernia from reducing into the abdominal cavity until the hernia sac has been opened and contents identified. If the hernia content was reduced, laparoscopy is a useful adjunct to evaluate for bowel viability.

Strangulated bowel can be addressed via the groin incision, laparotomy, or laparoscopy. If the bowel is not grossly ischemic or infarcted, then reduction into the abdominal cavity is appropriate. It is prudent to ascertain return of blood supply prior to the definitive repair.

Repair of the hernia can be tissue or prosthetic repair. If gross contamination occurs or if a surgeon feels that the risk of mesh infection is high, there are some options:

- Tissue repairs commonly employed are the Bassini and McVay repairs
- Lichtenstein with biologic mesh—options are acellular dermal matrix, porcine dermal matrix, and other "bio-synthetic" mesh
- Absorbable mesh plug such as polyglactin

Femoral Hernia

Watchful waiting cannot be applied in the majority of patients with femoral hernias, especially if they are symptomatic. There is a very high risk of incarceration and strangulation [25–27] and femoral hernias are more commonly present in women [28]. Emergency surgery for incarcerated or strangulated hernia has increased morbidity and mortality. Pain is typically pinpointed in the area of femoral canal and the patients can also complain of paraesthesias in the leg in this region.

Typically this hernia is diagnosed based on physical exam, but it's not uncommon to be diagnosed on imaging modalities, such as a CT scan. Femoral hernias can move cranially near or above the inguinal ligament making them difficult to palpate.

Operative management can be laparoscopic or open. In the laparoscopic approach, one can identify size and extent of hernia, presence of bowel ischemia, or infarction and concomitant hernias. Reduction can be successful; however, one must consider opening hernia defect sharply to allow reduction. Repair of hernia has many options after reduction:

1. Suture repair intra-corporally
2. Ligation of hernia sac intra-corporally
3. Peel down peritoneum with placement of mesh prosthesis or mesh plug placement

Open repair can be performed via different approaches:

1. Supra-inguinal
2. Infra-inguinal
3. Laparotomy

Supra-inguinal approach is the most common approach to the femoral hernia. The type of repair depends on hernia contents and viability. If the contents are ischemic/necrotic or there is a concern for bacterial translocation, most surgeons would consider a tissue repair (Bassini or McVay) and/or Vicryl plug of the femoral canal. Mesh prosthesis in a Lichtenstein repair is considered safe in a clean-contaminated case; however, gross contamination comes with exceedingly high risk for mesh infection and, therefore mesh should be avoided. The inguinal and/or lacunar ligament can be divided if the hernia contents cannot be reduced.

If the hernia contents spontaneously reduce during induction of anesthesia, a diagnostic laparoscopy should be performed to evaluate the reduced contents. If no ischemia or necrosis is seen, then proceeding with an open or laparoscopic mesh repair is logical.

Umbilical Hernia

True umbilical hernias are quite common and are typically reducible in the non-obese patient. Problematic umbilical hernias that can present emergently are often in the obese and/or patient with cirrhosis. Obesity profoundly impacts the ability to reduce all hernias, even umbilical hernias. The thick abdominal wall adipose tissue often prevents the clinician from appreciating the hernia orifice; therefore, reduction is difficult. Also, complete reduction can be hard to confirm secondary to thickness of abdominal wall.

The decision-making becomes complex in the presence of cirrhosis. Classically, surgeons are trained to never operate on these hernias; however, evisceration from an umbilical hernia in a cirrhotic patient has an extremely high mortality rate [29, 30]. Ultimately, cirrhotic patients with large and/or problematic umbilical hernias are best treated by liver transplantation, if possible. If an emergent repair is needed, cirrhotic patients with umbilical hernias are best suited to undergo repair at a tertiary care facility. These patients benefit from having access to surgical intensive care units, interventional radiologists (for trans-hepatic porto-systemic shunts), hepatologists and acute care general surgeons for preoperative optimization and postoperative management [31]. The literature now favors elective repair of the umbilical hernia in a cirrhotic patient, provided that preoperative optimization of their liver function and ascites is undertaken [32–34]. This is achieved largely through salt and fluid restriction and diuresis. These are not always reasonable options in the patient presenting with acute incarceration and/or strangulation. Reduction with sedation can be attempted as well. The goal for reduction is to address the emergent problem to allow for optimization of liver function in preparation for a surgical repair. Large-volume paracentesis can help achieve easier reduction secondary to increased abdominal domain and decreased intra-abdominal pressure. Placement of a drain should be considered; but the volume of drainage needs to be controlled and the patient's intravascular volume should be monitored closely and managed appropriately. Otherwise, the surgical technique for a hernia repair is not unlike that of an elective repair.

Ventral Incisional Hernia

An incisional hernia is typically an elective operation. In the emergent situations, there are two parts to the operation that can be considered independently:

1. Bowel viability and/or bowel obstruction related to the hernia
2. Hernia itself

On examination, the patients requiring emergency surgery will often be in excruciating pain, can have nausea, vomiting, skin changes over the hernia, as well as focal and generalized peritonitis. Attempts at reduction are appropriate; however, recurrence is highly likely. The hernia sac is often fused to the previous mesh prosthesis and will never allow for complete reduction. This creates a lead point to re-herniate. Also, true reduction in the obese patient with a large defect is typically unlikely. Recurrent admissions for these patients should warrant serious consideration for inpatient repair after optimization.

These are often the most difficult hernia to deal with in an urgent or emergent scenario. Complicating factors are typically:

1. Presence of mesh(es)
2. Large hernia sac
3. Swiss-cheese defects
4. Large hernia components
5. Morbid obesity
6. Decreased abdominal domain

CT scans should be obtained as it gives valuable information about the dimensions of the defect as well as associated intestines. Plain films demonstrating a bowel obstruction with the presence of a ventral incisional hernia is helpful, but does not provide other anatomic information such as:

1. Location of hernia
2. Size of hernia
3. Abdominal domain available
4. Multiple defects
5. Bowel appearance, transition point in the hernia, hernia contents
6. Presence of mesh (not always able to visualize on CT)

Finally, for many of these patients, comparison to the prior CT scan can provide a sense of progression of the disease.

Small bowel obstruction (SBO) in the setting of a ventral incisional hernia is not straightforward. The initial management should always be nil per os (NPO), fluid resuscitation, correction of electrolyte abnormalities, and a nasogastric tube at the discretion of the surgeon. Then, one should define the obstruction with CT imaging and/or contrast enterography. Nonoperative management can be successful; however, the patient with frequently recurrent SBO in the setting of ventral incisional hernia often lends itself to the need for repair in the nonelective setting. Other characteristics that would predict failure of nonoperative management of an SBO in the presence of a ventral incisional hernia are:

1. Large defect
2. Large volume of viscera in the hernia sac
3. Obstruction at hernia edge

Contrast that easily passes without reproduction of symptoms can warrant non-operative therapy. Imaging findings warranting emergency surgery typically include pneumoperitoneum, significant bowel wall thickening, and lack of contrast opacification of bowel wall, significant free fluid, and pneumatosis.

The approach to repair can be open or laparoscopic. Laparoscopic repair is best suited for relatively small defects. Laparoscopic approaches could be complicated by the presence of dilated loops of bowel that are often present due to some degree of bowel obstruction. The surgeon must exercise extreme caution in order to avoid bowel injury during entry, reduction of bowel, and closure of port sites. If a laparoscopic approach is attempted, the surgeon must have a plan for closing or covering the hernia orifice. This can be done primarily with transfascial suturing or intra-corporeal suturing. More commonly, mesh is used to cover the defect in an underlay fashion with adequate tissue overlap. Leaving the defect present will increase risk of early re-incarceration and/or strangulation. If bowel resection is needed, use of biologic mesh or tissue-only closure is recommended.

Open surgery for incarcerated or strangulated ventral incisional hernias remains the mainstay of emergent hernia repair. It is often initiated directly over the hernia sac. If a patient is in extremis, going through hernia sac will identify the source of sepsis, and the necrotic bowel can be relatively quickly resected. Often, the hernia defect has to be extended in order to reduce the hernia content. Once the viscera are free and obstruction(s) are relieved, the contents of the hernia sac can be reduced into the abdominal cavity. Decision for the "damage control" option should be made early in the operative course, and the anastomosis could be completed in the subsequent operations. It is completely acceptable to resect the ischemic or necrotic viscera, reduce it into the abdominal cavity, and apply a temporary abdominal closure device, such as negative pressure wound dressing. After physiology has been restored, the patient can return to the operating room in 24–48 hours for anastomosis or diversion, and hernia management.

The management of the hernia itself is not straightforward. For patients in septic shock from a ventral incisional hernia, the primary objective becomes effective source control and resuscitation. The standard repair of a ventral incisional hernia requires a mesh prosthesis with about 5 cm overlap circumferentially. The concern of mesh infection with gross contamination is legitimate and can be highly morbid and potentially mortal for the patient. Primary repair in critically

ill patients with a defect that can be primarily closed is most reasonable. Although recurrence rates of this strategy are nearly 100%, the goal in these cases is patient survival through this critical time period and bringing them back electively for a more definitive repair remains is the safest and most appropriate option.

If the defect is too large and there is a fear of mesh infection, the surgeon has the options of using biologic or absorbable mesh and skin-only closure. Ideally, all of these repairs should have mesh in an underlay fashion. The bridge technique has a very high rate of failure (regardless of mesh); however, for some patients, this may be all that can be done. Very large defects can be considered for skin only closure. Formal abdominal wall reconstructions in critically ill patients are not well tolerated and compromises future elective abdominal wall reconstruction and therefore should be avoided. As evidenced by the recent publication by the World Society of Emergency Surgery, the literature on this issue is limited to observational series or case series [35].

Understanding of mesh prosthesis aids in decision-making. Macroporous lightweight polypropylene mesh is highly resistant to infection [36]. If it becomes infected, these mesh prosthesis can typically be salvaged with local wound care and a short course of antibiotics. Polytetrafluoroethylene (PTFE) or expanded PTFE (ePTFE) mesh prosthesis are very durable and will not adhere to viscera or other adjacent tissue. However, its lack of ingrowth prohibits mesh salvage if it becomes infected and antimicrobial therapy is not reasonably expected to sterilize the actual prosthesis because there is not blood flow within the mesh prosthesis [37]. Therefore, PTFE or ePTFE has little or no place in emergent hernia repair, particularly in the contaminated field.

Conclusion

Emergent hernia repairs are one of the most challenging cases for the general surgeon. However, the surgeon must arm him or herself with a thorough understanding of various surgical techniques and available meshes. Furthermore, managing expectations and setting realistic treatment goals in these difficulty situations will allow the surgeon to achieve optional outcomes for this difficult cohort of patients.

References

1. Alvarez JA, Baldonedo RF, Bear IG, Solis JA, Alvarez P, Jorge JI. Incarcerated groin hernias in adults: presentation and outcome. Hernia. 2004;8(2):121–6.
2. Derici H, Unalp HR, Bozdag AD, Nazli O, Tansug T, Kamer E. Factors affecting morbidity and mortality in incarcerated abdominal wall hernias. Hernia. 2007;11(4):341–6.
3. Nilsson H, Nilsson E, Angeras U, Nordin P. Mortality after groin hernia surgery: delay of treatment and cause of death. Hernia. 2011;15(3):301–7.
4. Nilsson H, Stylianidis G, Haapamaki M, Nilsson E, Nordin P. Mortality after groin hernia surgery. Ann Surg. 2007;245(4):656–60.
5. Martinez-Serrano MA, Pereira JA, Sancho JJ, Lopez-Cano M, Bombuy E, Hidalgo J. Risk of death after emergency repair of abdominal wall hernias. Still waiting for improvement. Langenbecks Arch Surg. 2010;395(5):551–6.
6. Nieuwenhuizen J, van Ramshorst GH, ten Brinke JG, de Wit T, van der Harst E, Hop WC, et al. The use of mesh in acute hernia: frequency and outcome in 99 cases. Hernia. 2011;15(3):297–300.
7. Hernandez-Irizarry R, Zendejas B, Ramirez T, Moreno M, Ali SM, Lohse CM, et al. Trends in emergent inguinal hernia surgery in Olmsted County, MN: a population-based study. Hernia. 2012;16(4): 397–403.
8. Panagiotopoulou IG, Richardson C, Gurunathan-Mani S, Lagattolla NR. Infection of laparoscopically inserted inguinal hernia repair mesh following subsequent emergency open surgery: a report of two cases. Ann R Coll Surg Engl. 2012;94(1):e3–4.
9. Romain B, Chemaly R, Meyer N, Brigand C, Steinmetz JP, Rohr S. Prognostic factors of postoperative morbidity and mortality in strangulated groin hernia. Hernia. 2012;16(4):405–10.
10. Compagna R, Rossi R, Fappiano F, Bianco T, Accurso A, Danzi M, et al. Emergency groin hernia repair: implications in elderly. BMC Surg. 2013; 13(2):S29.
11. Lohsiriwat D, Lohsiriwat V. Long-term outcomes of emergency Lichtenstein hernioplasty for incarcerated inguinal hernia. Surg Today. 2013;43(9):990–4.
12. Primus FE, Harris HW. A critical review of biologic mesh use in ventral hernia repairs under contaminated conditions. Hernia. 2013;17(1):21–30.
13. Argudo N, Pereira JA, Sancho JJ, Membrilla E, Pons MJ, Grande L. Prophylactic synthetic mesh can be safely used to close emergency laparotomies, even in peritonitis. Surgery. 2014;156(5):1238–44.
14. Huerta S, Pham T, Foster S, Livingston EH, Dineen S. Outcomes of emergent inguinal hernia repair in veteran octogenarians. Am Surg. 2014;80(5):479–83.
15. Koizumi M, Sata N, Kaneda Y, Endo K, Sasanuma H, Sakuma Y, et al. Optimal timeline for emergency surgery in patients with strangulated groin hernias. Hernia. 2014;18(6):845–8.
16. Fitzgibbons Jr RJ, Giobbie-Harder A, Gibbs JO, Dunlop DD, Reda DJ, McCarthy Jr M, et al. Watchful waiting vs repair of inguinal hernia in minimally symptomatic men: a randomized clinical trial. JAMA. 2006;295(3):285–92.
17. Stroupe KT, Manheim LM, Luo P, Giobbie-Harder A, Hynes DM, Jonasson O, et al. Tension-free repair versus watchful waiting for men with asymptomatic or minimally symptomatic inguinal hernias: a cost-effectiveness analysis. J Am Coll Surg. 2006;203(4):458–68.
18. Altom LK, Snyder CW, Gray SH, Graham LA, Vick CC, Hawn MT. Outcomes of emergent incisional hernia repair. Am Surg. 2011;77(8):971–6.
19. Beadles CA, Meagher AD, Charles AG. Trends in emergent hernia repair in the United States. JAMA Surg. 2015;150(3):194–200.
20. Samuel JC, Tyson AF, Mabedi C, Mulima G, Cairns BA, Varela C, et al. Development of a ratio of emergent to total hernia repairs as a surgical capacity metric. Int J Surg. 2014;12(9):906–11.
21. Chan G, Chan CK. Long-term results of a prospective study of 225 femoral hernia repairs: indications for tissue and mesh repair. J Am Coll Surg. 2008;207(3):360–7.
22. Sawayama H, Kanemitsu K, Okuma T, Inoue K, Yamamoto K, Baba H. Safety of polypropylene mesh for incarcerated groin and obturator hernias: a retrospective study of 110 patients. Hernia. 2014;18(3):399–406.
23. Venara A, Hubner M, Le Naoures P, Hamel JF, Hamy A, Demartines N. Surgery for incarcerated hernia: short-term outcome with or without mesh. Langenbecks Arch Surg. 2014;399(5):571–7.
24. Carbonell AM, Cobb WS. Safety of prosthetic mesh hernia repair in contaminated fields. Surg Clin North Am. 2013;93(5):1227–39.
25. Gallegos NC, Dawson J, Jarvis M, Hobsley M. Risk of strangulation in groin hernias. Br J Surg. 1991;78(10):1171–3.
26. Oishi SN, Page CP, Schwesinger WH. Complicated presentations of groin hernias. Am J Surg. 1991;162(6):568–70. discussion 71.
27. Hachisuka T. Femoral hernia repair. Surg Clin North Am. 2003;83(5):1189–205.
28. Naude GP, Ocon S, Bongard F. Femoral hernia: the dire consequences of a missed diagnosis. Am J Emerg Med. 1997;15(7):680–2.
29. Kirkpatrick S, Schubert T. Umbilical hernia rupture in cirrhotics with ascites. Dig Dis Sci. 1988;33(6):762–5.

30. McKay A, Dixon E, Bathe O, Sutherland F. Umbilical hernia repair in the presence of cirrhosis and ascites: results of a survey and review of the literature. Hernia. 2009;13(5):461–8.
31. Triantos CK, Kehagias I, Nikolopoulou V, Burroughs AK. Surgical repair of umbilical hernias in cirrhosis with ascites. Am J Med Sci. 2011;341(3):222–6.
32. Eker HH, van Ramshorst GH, de Goede B, Tilanus HW, Metselaar HJ, de Man RA, et al. A prospective study on elective umbilical hernia repair in patients with liver cirrhosis and ascites. Surgery. 2011;150(3):542–6.
33. Ecker BL, Bartlett EK, Hoffman RL, Karakousis GC, Roses RE, Morris JB, et al. Hernia repair in the presence of ascites. J Surg Res. 2014;190(2):471–7.
34. Choi SB, Hong KD, Lee JS, Han HJ, Kim WB, Song TJ, et al. Management of umbilical hernia compli-
cated with liver cirrhosis: an advocate of early and elective herniorrhaphy. Dig Liver Dis. 2011;43(12): 991–5.
35. Sartelli M, Coccolini F, van Ramshorst GH, Campanelli G, Mandala V, Ansaloni L, et al. WSES guidelines for emergency repair of complicated abdominal wall hernias. World J Emerg Surg. 2013;8(1):50.
36. Bury K, Smietanski M, Justyna B, Gumiela P, Smietanska AI, Owczuk R, et al. Effects of macroporous monofilament mesh on infection in a contaminated field. Langenbecks Arch Surg. 2014;399(7): 873–7.
37. Grevious MA, Cohen M, Jean-Pierre F, Herrmann GE. The use of prosthetics in abdominal wall reconstruction. Clin Plast Surg. 2006;33(2):181–97.

William W. Hope and William F. Powers IV

Introduction

With the increased use of damage control surgery and the improved knowledge related to abdominal compartment syndrome, surgeons are increasingly faced with the problem of how to manage the open abdomen. Primary closure, when appropriate, remains the repair of choice. This is not always feasible due to the need for future surgery, the physiologic nature of the patient, or for technical reasons. Treatments range from simple to quite complex procedures to facilitate planned hernia repairs or delayed primary closure, depending on the clinical situation. Mastering temporary abdominal closure is essential to surgeons successfully treating patients with open abdomens and complex abdominal wall pathology.

Abdominal Compartment Syndrome/Damage Control Surgery

History

Since its first description by Stone et al. [1], the concept of damage control surgery has gained widespread acceptance in trauma surgery patients

W.W. Hope, M.D. (✉) • W.F. Powers IV, M.D.
Department of Surgery, New Hanover Regional
Medical Center, Wilmington, NC, USA
e-mail: William.Hope@nhrmc.org;
William.Powers@nhrm.org

and even in complex abdominal operations and procedures. The recognition and understanding of the physiology of abdominal compartment syndrome has also improved the outcome of acutely ill trauma and complex general surgery patients. Although the concept of damage control surgery and abdominal compartment syndrome has improved outcomes, this has left surgeons with the novel and daunting task of abdominal wall management in acutely ill patients. This presents the unique challenge of trying to obtain both temporary and ultimately definitive abdominal closure for patients.

Rationale for the Open Abdomen

In general, damage control principles are applied to multiply injured patients with what has been referred to as the lethal triad of death, which includes acidosis, coagulopathy, and hypothermia. These damage control principles can also be applied in general surgery operations when patients have severe systemic disease, instability, and the lethal triad. The rationale related to damage control surgery is to perform a focused, timely surgical operation to help address the immediate surgical problem (e.g., bleeding or contamination). Following this, the patient can be resuscitated, coagulopathies can be addressed, the patient can be warmed, and acidosis managed in the intensive care unit. In these cases, the abdomen can be left open with methods described in this chapter. When the patient's condition improves, more definitive surgeries, and, if needed, multiple reoperations can be undertaken.

Physiologic Consequences of Intra-abdominal Hypertension and Abdominal Compartment Syndrome

The physiologic understanding of intra-abdominal hypertension and abdominal compartment syndrome leading to multi-system organ dysfunction has greatly increased over the last two decades. The initial physiologic insult or critical illness leads to systemic inflammatory response, inflammation, and cytokine release with resulting capillary leak. This in turn often requires ongoing fluid resuscitation that will cause more tissue edema (including bowel and mesenteric edema) and can increase intra-abdominal hypertension and start a lethal chain of events if no intervention is undertaken.

Abdominal compartment syndrome can affect many organ systems often due to direct compression. Cardiac effects include decreased cardiac output, decreased venous return due to compression of the vena cava, and elevated intrathoracic pressures. Increased intra-abdominal pressures can also affect the pulmonary system by elevating the diaphragm, reducing lung volume, decreasing functional residual capacity, and increasing peak airway pressures. Gastrointestinal manifestations are related to decreased cardiac output and compression on the mesenteric veins, which can lead to decreased intestinal perfusion, increased bowel edema, and possibly intestinal ischemia. The effects of abdominal compartment syndrome on the renal system are also related to decreased cardiac output and direct compression of the renal veins and parenchyma, which can cause reduced blood flow to the kidney, congestion and edema, and in some cases renal failure. Increased intra-abdominal pressures also can affect the central nervous system by causing increases in central venous and intracranial pressures and decreased cerebral perfusion pressure

related to increased intrathoracic and superior vena caval pressures.

The recognition of intra-abdominal hypertension and abdominal compartment syndrome in the early stages is critical because the cascading effect can ultimately end in organ failure and death. Knowledge of the effects on the different organ systems and accurate diagnosis, which usually require bladder pressure monitoring, are a key feature for positive outcomes for these complex patients.

Options for Temporary Abdominal Closure

Open Packing/Planned Ventral Hernia

One of the earliest and perhaps the simplest methods of managing the open abdomen is open packing with a plan for future skin grafting and ventral hernia repair. Various techniques on how to pack the abdomen have been described, and many "home-made" devices have been used at different institutions. The majority of techniques described used dressings placed on the abdomen without causing trauma or fistula formation. Before the commercially available vacuum-assisted wound closure device, many surgeons devised a vacuum device by placing towels, chest tubes or other drains, and an occlusive dressing that facilitated suction.

Despite the different descriptions and techniques, the goal in many of these initial cases was for the viscera to granulate in the midline of the open abdomen and then to undertake split thickness skin grafting. After skin grafting is completed and the abdominal viscera are properly covered, surgeons might wait up to 1 year before excising the skin graft and repairing the incisional hernia (Fig. 40.1a–f). One way to help with the timing of the hernia surgery is to use a "pinch" test. For this test, the skin graft overlying the viscera is pinched. If it is soft and pliable when rubbed between the fingers, there should be an adequate plane for dissection without enterotomies.

Although open packing and planned ventral hernia repair is a safe and effective method that is

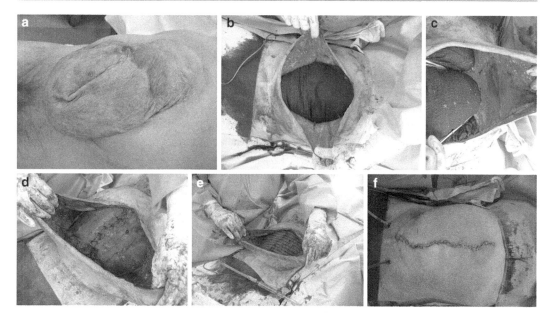

Fig. 40.1 (**a**) Patient with previous open abdomen treated with split thickness skin grafting now ready for abdominal wall reconstruction. (**b**) Large fascial defect once adhesiolysis has been performed. Skin graft was easily resected from abdominal contents. (**c**) Abdominal wall reconstruction using an external oblique component separation to allow for midline closure. (**d**) Primary midline closure obtained by using bilateral external oblique component separation. (**e**) Hernia repair with buttressing of midline closure with onlay large pore polypropylene. (**f**) Abdominal wall reconstruction with skin closure and two drains used in subcutaneous space

reproducible by most surgeons, there are many downsides to this technique, which limit its current widespread use. Perhaps the biggest drawback of this technique is the large ventral hernia with significant soft tissue deficit that is created and the very difficult operation that is required to repair it. During the initial era of damage control laparotomy and abdominal compartment syndrome, patient survival was considered a successful outcome. The large hernia was often considered a minor point and, in some cases, was left untreated. Because of extreme complexity of resultant hernias, researchers investigated different options to treat the open abdomen during the acute phase to avoid this planned hernia repair or at least minimize the defects that were created.

Towel Clip Closure/Skin Closure

Towel clip closure is perhaps one of the simplest and fastest ways to achieve temporary abdominal closure. It involves placing penetrating towel clips approximately 1 cm off the skin edge and 1 cm apart (Fig. 40.2). Many clips are required. An adherent plastic drape can be added to minimize the manipulation of the clips and possibly provide improved sterility. The benefit of this technique is that it is rapid and cost-effective. Unfortunately, it does not provide a long-term solution to abdominal closure and is typically used when a patient will need reoperation or multiple reoperations with the ultimate plan for either primary closure or alternative open abdomen treatment techniques depending on the clinical scenario.

Another rapid method in patients requiring a reoperation is simple skin closure with a large suture. This is usually done in a running fashion and allows closure of the skin but not the fascia. It is slightly easier to manage for nurses and ancillary staff than the towel clips, as this is a more familiar scenario.

While these two techniques have the benefits of low cost, simplicity, and speed of closure, they must be monitored closely in patients who are at risk for abdominal compartment syndrome because there is some compression caused by skin closure alone. Both of these techniques can be quickly reversed in patients that develop abdominal compartment syndrome by removing the clips or cutting the sutures and placing the appropriate dressing for an open abdomen per the surgeon's discretion. With the introduction of other techniques, many surgeons have abandoned the towel clip and simple skin closure techniques.

Silastic Closure/Bogota Bag

A resident in a hospital in Bogotá, Colombia (Oswaldo Borraez) first described the use of a silastic bag for closure of the abdomen, commonly referred to as the Bogota bag. This technique involves suturing of a 3 L sterile intravenous fluid bag to the fascial or skin edges. The benefits of this type of closure are that it is readily available, is easy to accomplish, facilitates visualization of the abdominal contents through the clear bag, and it protects the abdominal viscera (Fig. 40.3a–b). The limitations of this technique are that it can be difficult in patients with large volume of fluid loss, it provides only a small amount of fascial or skin retraction, it does not allow for removal of fluid that may be infectious or may precipitate an ongoing SIRS response, and it is not a definitive abdominal closure.

Zipper-Based Repairs

Zipper-based closures were popularized by Stone et al. [1] and may be used with conventional or commercially based zippers that are sutured to the skin or fascia. This technique allows easy access to the abdominal cavity if

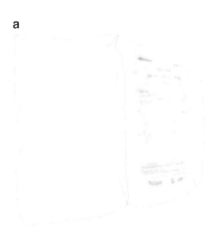

Fig. 40.2 Towel clip closure showing multiple towel clips used to reapproximate the skin

a

b

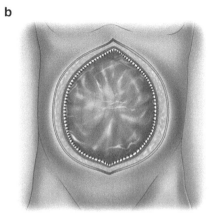

Fig. 40.3 (**a**) A 3-L intravenous fluid bag used for a Bogota bag closure. (**b**) Suturing the sterile bag to the fascial edges is rapid and allows visualization of the bowel

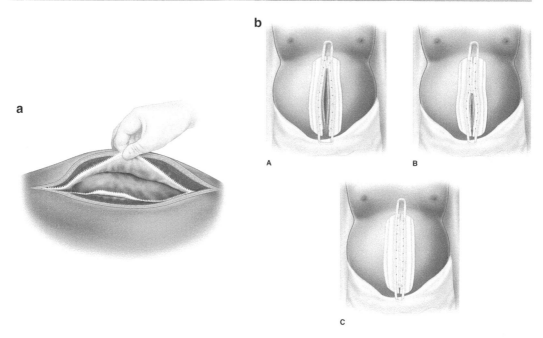

Fig. 40.4 (**a**) Zipper sutured to fascial edges to allow easy access to abdominal cavity in patients that will need multiple reoperations. (**b**) Zippers can also be sutured to the skin to allow easy access to the abdominal cavity

reoperations are needed and prevents some lateral retraction of the fascia if sewn to the fascia. Although a novel approach at the initial time of development, this technique has been replaced by some alternatives based on similar principles and is not widely used nowadays (Fig. 40.4).

Wittmann Patch

One of the problems associated with many forms of temporary abdominal closure is that retraction of the fascia makes delayed primary closure or future hernia repair more difficult. The use of the Wittmann Patch™ (Starsurgical, Inc., Burlington, WI), first reported by Teichman et al. [2], Wittmann et al. [3, 4], and Aprahamian et al. [5], involves suturing two Velcro®-like materials to the midline fascia. The Velcro-like material can be fastened together as overlapping sheets (Fig. 40.5a–c). This device can be used alone or in combination with other open abdomen techniques such as the ABThera™ (Kinetic Concepts, Inc., San Antonio, TX). As bowel and intra-abdominal edema improve, the Velcro material can be tightened to bring the fascial edges closer to the midline to ultimately achieve primary closure. If the patient requires several surgeries, the Velcro material can be unfastened and the intra-abdominal cavity can be easily entered.

The potential advantages of this technique are that it allows easy access to the abdominal cavity in patients that require future operations and that it places tension on the midline fascia that helps prevent later retraction. The disadvantages of a Wittmann Patch include potential ischemic and tension damage to the fascia, as well as the inability to remove fluid that may be infectious or may precipitate an ongoing SIRS response when used alone.

Mesh Based Techniques

The use of mesh has been reported as an adjunct for temporary abdominal closure and also when attempting primary closure. The use of synthetic meshes such as polytetrafluoroethylene (PTFE)

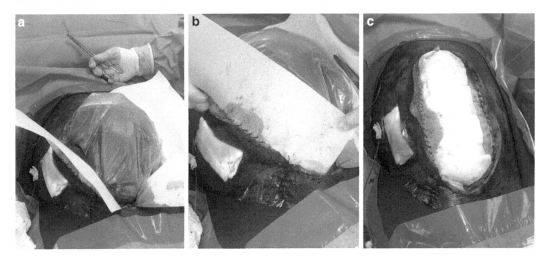

Fig. 40.5 (a) The Wittmann Patch™ being sutured to the edge of the fascia and being used in conjunction with an ABThera™ (Kinetic Concepts, Inc., San Antonio, TX). (b) Suturing of the Wittmann Patch™ to the right fascial edge of the open abdomen. (c) Wittmann Patch™ once it has been sutured to both fascial edges and overlapped in the midline. These Velcro like patches can be gradually brought closer and closer together and ultimately help achieve primary fascial closure

and polypropylene, and bioabsorbable meshes such as Vicryl® (Ethicon, Cincinnati, OH) and Dexon™ (Covidien, Mansfield, MA) have been reported. As initially described, the mesh was sutured to the fascial edges to allow granulation tissue to develop and to support a split-thickness skin graft. With concern for infection risk associated with permanent synthetic meshes, the bioabsorbable synthetic meshes became the mainstay mesh for temporary abdominal closure, although hernias would often develop long term due to the resorption of the mesh.

In recent years, there has been increasing research related to mesh, and new categories of mesh such as biologic and synthetic absorbable meshes have evolved. Despite limited literature describing efficacy and the true role of these products in the management of the open abdomen and hernia repair, the use of these products has increased substantially. Due to the low risk of infection and good granulation tissue associated with the biologic meshes and likely the synthetic absorbable meshes, the use of these products in temporary abdominal closure has increased. Suturing of a biologic mesh to the midline fascia and placing a wound V.A.C. has become an efficacious and easy, although very expensive, means

of temporary abdominal closure. Despite the ease and low risk of side effects, this type of closure will likely result in future hernia formation and is recommended when the surgeon does not believe that primary closure will be possible.

As surgeons gain more experience with temporary abdominal closure, the ultimate goal is primary fascial closure. To this end, another technique related to the use of mesh for temporary closure is serial mesh excision. In this technique, a mesh is sutured to the midline fascia and as bowel wall and intra-abdominal edema decrease, an elliptical piece of the mesh is excised and sutured back together bringing more tension on and medializing the fascial edges (Fig. 40.6a–g).

Negative Pressure Therapy/ Wound Vac

Perhaps the most commonly used method for temporary abdominal closure involves the use of the Vacuum Assisted Closure® device (V.A.C®; Kinetic Concepts, Inc., San Antonio, TX). The components of the commercially available ABThera™ (Kinetic Concepts, Inc., San Antonio,

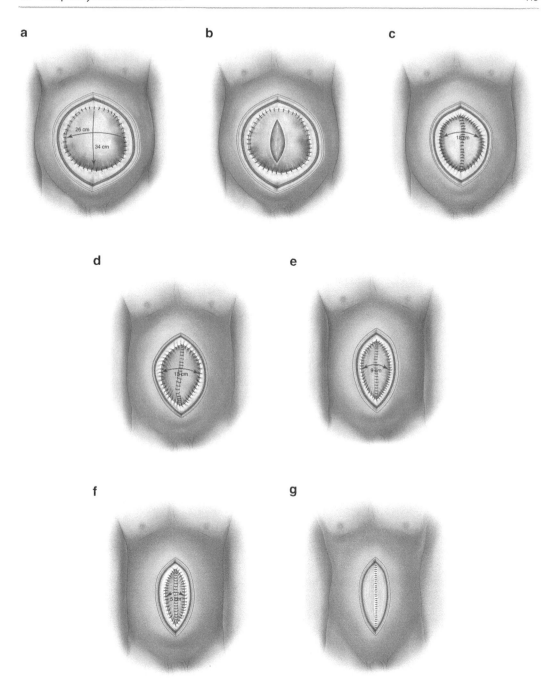

Fig. 40.6 (**a**) Open abdomen with large defect. ePTFE mesh sutured to fascial edges with plan for serial mesh excision. (**b**) Center portion of the ePTFE mesh is cut in an elliptical fashion and then sutured back to bring fascial edges closer together. (**c**) Large ePTFE mesh has been excised and fascial edges are now brought closer together decreasing the defect. (**d**) With further mesh excision, the fascial edges are brought closer together. (**e**) Further mesh excision with now a much smaller fascial defect. (**f**) Fascial defect with small, only 5 cm defect and ready for primary fascial closure. (**g**) Ultimate primary fascial closure achieved by serial mesh excision

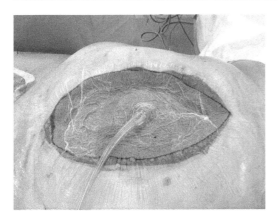

Fig. 40.7 The commercially available ABThera™ (Kinetic Concepts, Inc., San Antonio, TX) is placed into an open abdomen. This technique is rapid and easy to learn especially for surgeons who are familiar with the wound vac

TX) open abdomen negative pressure therapy unit include a polyethylene sheet that acts as a visceral retractor, a polyurethane sponge that is placed above the sheet in the abdominal wound, and an adherent dressing that is placed over the sponge with suction tubing that can be attached to a suction apparatus to apply vacuum pressure (Fig. 40.7). This is a relatively simple technique that can be done quickly and prevents retraction of the fascia by the suction and vacuum that is applied in the wound. The V.A.C. can be easily changed at the bedside in the intensive care unit or in the operating room.

The potential and reported benefits of the ABThera are that it facilitates easy access to the abdominal cavity in patients requiring reoperation, provides medial tension, limits fascial retraction, reduces edema, helps remove fluid and infected material from the abdominal cavity, and helps protect the viscera from the external environment. Because of its ease of use and efficacy, the ABThera has become a mainstay in the treatment of open abdomens and temporary abdominal closure.

Dynamic Fascial Closure Systems

One main evolution in the care of patients with open abdomens is an emphasis on providing temporary abdominal closure when needed. The goal is still achieving primary fascial closure when reoperations are no longer needed, and the edema related to the initial insult has subsided. Currently, the philosophy of accepting an open abdomen and planned ventral hernia repair, although still a necessity in some patients, has evolved to using techniques that can help achieve delayed primary fascial closure.

Dynamic fascial closure systems were designed to allow abdominal components to expand with resulting edema to prevent abdominal compartment syndromes and allow gradual, adjustable tension that can be placed on the fascia as the clinical scenario improves.

The ABRA® abdominal wall closure system (Canica Designs, Almonte, ON, Canada) is indicated for use in patients with abdominal compartment syndrome or other complex abdominal conditions when there is an open abdomen. The system components include a perforated silicone sheet that acts as a visceral retractor, silicone elastomers that are placed full thickness through the abdominal wall and provide continuous dynamic force to help close the wound, and button tails with pads that help distribute the compression force over a wide area of skin to allow easy tightening of the elastomers. This device is also used in conjunction with negative pressure wound therapy (Fig. 40.8a–d).

The ABRA abdominal wall closure system is indicated for full-thickness, retracted midline abdominal defects with the goal of primary closure. This dynamic wound closure system works by allowing elastomers to provide graduated tension to different parts of the wound at different times. Over the course of the patient's illness, the elastomers can be tightened at the bedside, and abdominal massage can help to redistribute the tension in the abdominal cavity. After the edema has resolved and the patient's clinical course improves, the ABRA device can be removed and primary fascial closure completed, obviating the need for mesh, skin grafting, or planned ventral hernia repair (Fig. 40.9). The proposed benefits of the ABRA are that it allows primary fascial closure, alleviates the need for mesh, preserves fascia margins, restores normal physiology, and allows bedside dressing changes.

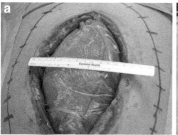
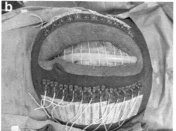
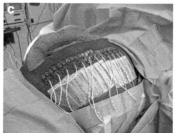

Fig. 40.8 (**a**) Open abdomen with large defect. Markings on the abdominal wall of 5 cm away from wound edge and 3 cm apart to illustrate where elastomers should be placed. Stab incisions with a knife or bovie may be made at these points. (**b**) Open abdomen with ABRA® abdominal wall closure system (Canica Designs, Almonte, ON, Canada). The perforated silicone sheet has been placed to protect the viscera. The elastomers have been placed 5 cm away from the wound and 3 cm apart. A spacer is placed in the wound to coordinate the elastomers. The button pads and tails have been placed. (**c**) Side view of the button pads and tails that are placed to help hold the elastomers. Placement of a surgical drape such as Ioban™ (3M, Saint Paul, MN) (not shown in picture) may help minimize skin trauma from the button pads and tails. (**d**) View of abdomen once ABRA® abdominal wall closure system (Canica Designs, Almonte, ON, Canada) has been placed with wound vac

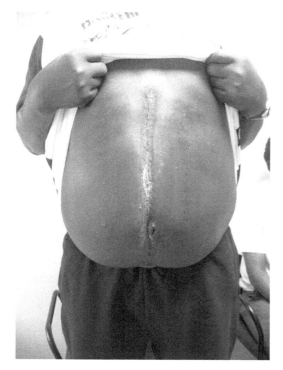

Fig. 40.9 A patient with open abdomen who had ABRA® (Canica Designs, Almonte, ON, Canada) placed and has undergone primary fascial closure with no evidence of recurrent hernia at 1-year follow-up

Enteroatmospheric Fistulas

Patients who develop an enteroatmospheric fistula during treatment for an open abdomen are another clinical challenge. Source control is essential and is often difficult to achieve without reoperations and application of multiple techniques. The abdomen that is open for more than 5–7 days is at greatest risk of developing this complication. It is difficult to contain a fistula's output because an ostomy appliance is usually not effective. The effluent continues to drive the inflammatory response and can precipitate the formation of more fistulas and prevent healing.

Foley catheter placement through the fistula should not be attempted, because it will result in limited effluent control and an increase in fistula size. Porous, petroleum-based, non-adherent dressing can be laid on the bowel surrounding the fistula with white foam placed over the fistula. GranuFoam™ (Kinetic Concepts, Inc., San Antonio, TX) can then be cut to the size of the wound (not covering the white foam) and a transparent adherent dressing applied. A superficial

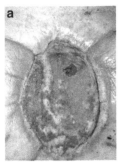 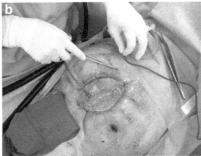 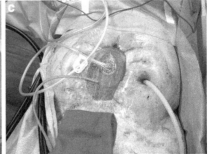

Fig. 40.10 (**a**) Open abdomen with enteroatmospheric fistula. There is a good bed of granulation tissue that would be amenable to split thickness skin grafting. (**b**) Split thickness skin grafting of open wound. Foley cathe- ter is placed in fistula in attempts to drain and patient also has left lower quadrant colostomy. (**c**) Wound vac placed over split thickness skin graft with drains in fistula as well as colostomy

portion of the white foam can then be excised and the V.A.C. tubing system applied. The pressure should be adjusted to the lowest pressure that prevents leakage around the stoma. A standard baby bottle nipple can also be used for effluent control. A small hole is cut in the nipple to allow placement of a Foley with its balloon slightly inflated. The bowel is covered with a non-adherent, petroleum-based dressing as described previously. A standard V.A.C. is applied to the remainder of the wound leaving the fistula uncovered by foam. The nipple can be placed over the fistula and isolated with stoma paste or an Eakin ring with GranuFoam™ placed around the nipple. The adherent drape can then be applied and the V.A.C. set to a standard setting with the Foley placed to gravity drainage. These two techniques often work well for proximal fistulas when effluent is mostly liquid.

The fistula ring can be instituted for distal fistulas when the effluent is thicker. This requires a round piece of GranuFoam to be sandwiched between adherent VAC tapes. An Eakin ring is then applied to the base of the fistula ring. A small hole is created in the center of the ring the size of the fistula. Non-adherent, petroleum-based dressing is applied to exposed bowel, excluding the fistula, and a standard V.A.C. is applied. The suction device is placed away from the site of the fistula, and an ostomy appliance is placed over the fistula ring. Certainly, there are surgical techniques that can be used to facilitate fistula closure, but these are beyond the scope of

this chapter. Standard tenants of fistula management including TPN therapy, nutritional optimization, and delayed (up to 6 months) definitive surgical procedures to decrease inflammation in the abdomen should all be applied on a case by case basis. In patients with enteroatmospheric fistulas, attention is often placed on fistula management and control, and abdominal closure techniques are often not employed. These patients often require open abdomen management, and the goals of therapy are shifted to closing and controlling the fistula rather than abdominal wall closure. Early skin grafting can help manage these fistulas and convert them from an enteroatmospheric fistula into a standard fistula (Fig. 40.10a–c). Definitive abdominal wall reconstruction and closure are often delayed until the fistula is healed. When the fistula doesn't heal, single-stage or double-stage abdominal wall reconstructions with fistula takedowns can be undertaken depending on the clinical condition.

Outcomes

There are few prospective or comparative studies on which to base decision-making regarding temporary abdominal closure, since this is a heterogeneous population and involves many different strategies, techniques, and outcome measures.

Several reports from single centers using one technique or protocol to manage open abdomens show good success rates and achievement of primary fascial closure; however, few are comparative studies. Meta-analyses and systemic reviews have shown improvements in primary fascial closure rates and lower mortality rates using the Wittmann patch, VAC systems, and dynamic retention sutures [6, 7]; however, firm conclusions cannot be made due to the limited nature of the data.

How to Choose

With limited data to guide treatment of the open abdomen, the surgeon is left with several options. The treatment used is often based on previous experience, comfort level, and patient outcomes. Certain centers may have treatment protocols for patients with open abdomens, and often these result in high rates of fascial closure.

When evaluating a patient with an open abdomen requiring temporary abdominal closure, the clinical picture must first be evaluated, and desired outcomes must be established. In some patients, primary abdominal closure is likely not possible, so the main priority is patient survival. In these cases, many of the techniques described in this chapter will suffice, and, often if the patient survives, skin grafting and planned ventral hernia repair can be used. In these cases, the V.A.C. works quite well since it is easy to apply and facilitates superb fluid management.

In other cases, the patient's clinical status improves substantially, and primary fascial closure should be attempted. In these cases, it is important to use one of the techniques for temporary abdominal closure that prevents fascial retraction. These techniques are at the surgeon's discretion and include the V.A.C., Wittmann patch, and dynamic fascial closure systems. Surgeons must also use sound clinical judgment regarding how difficult the abdomen will be to close.

Patients who are not obese, have minimal abdominal edema, and do not require multiple reoperations, are often easy to close. In this situation, a V.A.C. is a good option that provides adequate coverage, fluid management, and limits fascial retraction until the patient's abdomen can be closed in a few days. In patients that are more challenging (e.g., morbidly obese patients, patients with existing hernias, patients requiring multiple reoperations with large amounts of edema), the Wittmann patch or dynamic fascial closure system are good options that allow for graduating levels of tension that can be adjusted to prevent fascial retraction. We have begun to use the dynamic fascial closure systems in these cases due to our belief that that the fascia is perhaps healthier and stronger after primary closure, since no sutures are placed in the midline fascia (elastomers are placed several centimeters off the midline fascia). This is not supported by known data at this time.

In most circumstances, techniques used to treat an open abdomen should rely on some mechanism to prevent fascial retraction, split thickness skin grafting, and planned ventral hernia repair. Due to the lack of objective data on what techniques to use and when to attempt closure, surgeons must rely on their clinical judgment and experience. We are currently studying objective abdominal tension measurements to help establish guidelines to determine the appropriate time to close an abdomen and the best closure techniques to use.

Conclusions

Knowledge and experience with temporary abdominal closure is increasingly important, as damage control surgery and open abdomens are more commonplace. Several different techniques can be used for primary closure, and their use depends on the patient's clinical status and the desired treatment goals. In most cases, primary fascial closure can be achieved using sound surgical techniques and attentiveness to the patient. Achieving primary fascial closure has evolved from simple packing methods and planned ventral hernia repair to more dynamic means of closure. Additional study is needed to evaluate these new methods and outcomes.

References

1. Stone HH, Strom PR, Mullins RJ. Management of the major coagulopathy with onset during laparotomy. Ann Surg. 1983;197(5):532–5.

2. Teichmann W, Eggert A, Wittmann DH, Bocker W. Zipper as a new method of temporary abdominal wall closure in abdominal surgery. Chirurg. 1985; 56(3):173–8.

3. Wittmann DH, Aprahamian C, Bergstein JM. Etappenlavage: advanced diffuse peritonitis managed by planned multiple laparotomies utilizing zippers, slide fastener, and velcro analogue for temporary abdominal closure. World J Surg. 1990;14(2): 218–26.

4. Wittmann DH, Aprahamian C, Bergstein JM, Edmiston CE, Frantzides CT, Quebbeman EJ, et al. A burr-like device to facilitate temporary abdominal closure in planned multiple laparotomies. Eur J Surg. 1993;159(2):75–9.

5. Aprahamian C, Wittmann DH, Bergstein JM, Quebbeman EJ. Temporary abdominal closure (TAC) for planned relaparotomy (etappenlavage) in trauma. J Trauma. 1990;30(6):719–23.

6. Quyn AJ, Johnston C, Hall D, Chambers A, Arapova N, Ogston S, et al. The open abdomen and temporary abdominal closure systems—historical evolution and systematic review. Colorectal Dis. 2012;14(8): e429–38.

7. Boele van Hensbroek P, Wind J, Dijkgraaf MG, Busch OR, Goslings JC. Temporary closure of the open abdomen: a systematic review on delayed primary fascial closure in patients with an open abdomen. World J Surg. 2009;33(2):199–207.

Manuel López-Cano
and Manuel Armengol-Carrasco

"The accuracy not necessarily leads to truth,
speculation is not incompatible with the rigor"
Thomas S. Kuhn
The Structure of Scientific Revolutions, 1962

Introduction

Nowadays evidence-based medicine is widely used across many, if not all, medical disciplines. In 1996, David Sackett [1], a pioneer in evidence-based medicine, wrote: *"Evidence-based medicine is the conscientious, explicit, and judicious use of current best evidence in making decisions about the care of individual patients. The practice of evidence-based medicine means integrating individual clinical expertise with the best available external clinical evidence from systematic research. By individual clinical expertise we mean the proficiency and judgment that individual clinicians acquire through clinical experience and clinical practice"*. Karl Popper [2] perhaps summarized this best in an accurate commentary: *"Evidence is information that is used to approach truth, whereas truth is an infallible, unequivocal, immutable fact. The definition of knowledge … is typically used as a representation of a person's comprehension of a particular subject"*. Evidence-based medicine acquires special importance when new diagnostic and/or therapeutic indications for a particular pathologic process become available in clinical practice.

We have made remarkable progress and innovation over the last few decades in the field of abdominal wall surgery not only in the technical aspects of procedures, but also in the preoperative preparation for operation [3]. The recent development of the so-called *Chemical Component Separation* (CCS) [4] is an example of such innovation. CCS consists of the application of botulinum neurotoxin type A (BoNT-A) [5] for abdominal muscular relaxation as an aid to repairing ventral and incisional hernias and for facilitating closure of midline abdominal wall defects [4, 6, 7]. BoNT-A is a potent muscle-paralyzing agent commonly used for various medical and cosmetic indications. The objective of this chapter is to present current data on CCS from a three different perspectives: (1) a general overview of botulinum neurotoxins (BoNTs); (2) the evidence available for the use of BoNT in abdominal wall surgery, and (3) a comprehensive summary from a personal point of view.

Electronic supplementary material: The online version of this chapter (doi:10.1007/978-3-319-27470-6_41) contains supplementary material, which is available to authorized users.

M. López-Cano, M.D. (✉)
Abdominal Wall Surgery Unit, General and Digestive Surgery, Hospital Universitario Vall d'Hebron, Universitat Autònoma de Barcelona, Barcelona, Spain
e-mail: mlpezcano@gmail.com

M. Armengol-Carrasco, M.D.
Department of Surgery, Hospital Universitario Vall d'Hebron, Barcelona, Spain

Background: Botulinum Toxin and Therapeutic Use

BoNTs are produced by *Clostridium botulinum*, a Gram-positive, rod-shaped, anaerobic, spore-forming bacterium. BoNTs bind to specific receptors at nerve terminals and inhibit the release of acetylcholine. According to the different tissues, BoNTs may cause inactivity of muscles or glands by blocking the release of acetylcholine in nerve terminals of the neuromuscular junction, exocrine glands, and smooth muscle [8]. BoNTs have been used in the treatment of neurological conditions, such as blepharospasm, cervical dystonia, and other forms of dystonia or spasticity when painful and even incapacitating spasms are present. The indications, however, have been widened and BoNTs are also used for treating axillary or palmar hyperhidrosis and other hypersecretory disorders, as well as a variety of gastrointestinal, urological, dermatological, cosmetic, and painful disorders [9].

The exact mechanism of action of the nociceptive effects of BoNTs remains unclear, although it seems to be related to a direct action-inhibiting release of pain-related neurotransmitters (pain-modulating molecules calcitonin gene-related peptide and substance P) from the presynaptic motor nerve terminal, as well as an indirect action by reducing muscle contractions/spasms [10]. The toxin requires 24–72 hours to take effect, and the maximum paralysis is achieved between the first- and second-week post-injection. The affected nerve terminals do not degenerate, but the blockage of neurotransmitter release is irreversible. Function can be recovered by formation of new synaptic contacts; this usually takes 2–7 months in humans [11].

C. botulinum elaborates seven antigenically and serologically distinguishable exotoxins (A, B, C [C_1, C_2], D, E, F, and G) with a similar structure [12]. Botulinum toxin types A (BoNT-A) and B (BoNT-B) are used in clinical practice [13]. Doses of all commercially available botulinum toxins are expressed in terms of units of biologic activity. One unit of botulinum toxin corresponds to the calculated median intraperitoneal lethal dose (LD_{50}) in female Swiss-Webster mice [14]. However, commercial products are different and

unit doses are not interchangeable because there are differences in the strains of C. botulinum used in the manufacturing, formulation, and purification processes [15]. To reduce potential dosing errors and to highlight the non-interchangeability characteristics of BoNTs, the US Food and Drug Administration (FDA) established a single generic name for each botulinum toxin product [16] (Table 41.1). In practice, BoNT-B has very specific indications [11] and BoNT-A is the most commonly used due to the multifunctional activity and long-lasting duration of effect [17, 18].

Administration, Immunological Considerations, and Formulation

BoNTs are administered intramuscularly with the adequate aseptic measures [19]. The number of injections and characteristics of the needle are tailored to the mass of the muscle or muscle groups being injected [19, 20]. Recommended techniques to guide botulinum toxin injection include electromyography, electric nerve stimulation, ultrasound, and anatomical localization (anatomical landmarks) [20]. Localization of injection, availability of technical equipment, and the clinician's experience are important factors for the choice of the guidance procedure.

Injection of BoNT-A may lead to the development of neutralizing antibodies and secondary non-responsiveness [11, 21]. Although development of neutralizing antibodies occur in a small percentage of patients, especially in cosmetic indications, patients who receive higher individual doses or frequent booster injections seem to have a higher risk of developing antibodies [22, 23]. Therefore, using the lowest dose of toxin necessary to achieve the desired clinical effect and avoiding reinjection within 1 month appear prudent in an effort to keep antibody formation as low and unlikely as possible [11].

There are three commercially available serotype A formulations (Table 41.1): onabotulinum toxin A (Botox®, Allergan Inc., Irvine, CA, USA), abobotulinum toxin A (Dysport®, Ipsen Ltd., Slough, Berkshire, UK), and incobotulinum toxin A (Xeomin®, Marz Pharmaceuticals, Frankfurt, Germany).

Table 41.1 Generic name for each botulinum toxin by the U.S. Food and Drug Administration (FDA)

Generic name	Commercial name (manufacturer)	Distribution licence	Indications
OnaBotulinumtoxin A	Botox® (Allergan, Inc.)	Worldwide	Cervical dystonia, strabismus, blepharospasm, hemifacial spasm, hyperhidrosis, post-stroke spasticity, overactive bladder, improved appearance of glabellar lines
AboBotulinumtoxin A	Dysport® (Ipsen Pharmaceuticals)	USA, UK, and Europe	Cervical dystonia. In clinical trials in USA for other conditions
Incobotulinumtoxin A	Xeomin® (Merz)	Europe, USA	Cervical dystonia, blepharospasm, glabellar lines
RimaBotulinumtoxin B	Myobloc®/NeuroBloc®a (Solstice Neurosciences)	USA, Europe, and Japan	Cervical dystonia

aBrand name in Europe

Onabotulinum toxin A (Botox®) is available in 100 or 200 unit vials. One 100 unit vial is diluted with 1, 2, 4, or 8 mL of preservative-free 0.9% saline, yielding preparations of 10.0, 5.0, 2.5, or 1.25 units/0.1 mL, respectively. However the final dilution of BOTOX® is mostly a matter of personal preference [11]. Botox® is denatured easily by bubbling or agitation; gently inject the diluent onto the inside wall of the vial and discard the vial if a vacuum does not pull the diluent in. Reconstituted Botox® should be stored in a refrigerator 2–8 °C and used within 24 hours [24].

Abobotulinum toxin A (Dysport®) is available in 300 or 500 unit vials. For the treatment of some neurological disorders, such as cervical dystonia, one 500 unit vial is diluted with 1 mL preservative-free 0.9% saline, yielding a preparation of 500 units/mL. Reconstituted Dysport® should be used within 4 hours and should be stored in a refrigerator at 2–8 °C.

Incobotulinum toxin A (Xeomin®) is available in 50 and 100 unit vials and reconstituted with 0.9% saline. Reconstituted Xeomin® should be used within 24 hours and should be stored at 2–8 °C. Unopened vials can be stored at room temperature, refrigerated or frozen.

Reconstituted products should be clear and free from suspended particles. All vials, including expired vials, or equipment used with the drug should be disposed of carefully as is done with all medical waste.

Manufacturers of botulinum toxin produce their product as 150 kDa protein (incobotulinum toxin A), 500–700 kDa (abobotulinum toxin A), and 900 kDa (onabotulinum toxin A). This protein includes both the primary active component as well as complexing proteins. Although it has been suggested that these proteins are responsible for the development of anti-toxin antibodies, it is unclear whether clinically there is a significant effect of these molecular differences in terms of both antigenicity and efficacy [21]. Presumed clinical effects of 1 unit are not interchangeable between formulations, and the dose ratio between onabotulinum and abobotulinum is 1:3 [25–27].

In both dermatocosmetological and neurological applications, BoNT-A doses vary according to the muscle mass to be treated, degree of spasticity or the patient's body weight. In successive sessions, doses and injection points are usually individualized according to results obtained with the starting dose [21, 28]. Doses of Botox® should not exceed 400–600 units per session but maximum absolute doses of Dysport® are unknown, although a maximum dose should probably not exceed 2000 units. Maximum doses of Xeomin® have not been established [20]. Also, different formulations of BoNT-A are not identical and may behave differently in clinical practice, partly due to differences in the degree of migration of the neurotoxin–protein complex from its injection site [29, 30]. The lower potential of onabotulinum to migrate promotes more precise localization of clinical effects, thereby helping to optimize the risk/benefit ration [31].

Tolerability and Contraindications

Injections of BoNT-A are generally well tolerated [11]. Side effects are rare, but adverse effects may be both local or systemic [9, 11]. Local unwanted weakness/paralysis is commonly related to spread of the botulinum toxin from the injection site to nearby muscles or other secretion and sensory systems. It usually resolves in several months depending on the site, strength of the injections, and the muscles made excessively weak [11]. Occasionally autonomic effects (e.g., dry mouth) and local effects at the injection site, such as pain, bruising, infection, or rash may occur. In some cases, local effects are related to an enhanced response of the injected muscles. Most of these local side effects may be prevented using the lowest effective dose and accurately selecting the site of injection in the selected muscle.

Systemic adverse events may include a transient generalized reaction with headache, discomfort, or mild nauseas. Direct intravascular puncture should be avoided and the presence of botulinum toxin in the bloodstream may cause a generalized botulism-like syndrome [32]. Other side effects, such as brachial plexopathy [33], gallbladder dysfunction [34] or necrotizing fasciitis [35] have been reported as a complication of botulinum toxin treatment.

Satisfactory results are generally obtained with the use of BoNT-A in cosmetic and/or neurological indications [36], but applicability to abdominal wall surgery remains to be established. However, lack of response can be observed in 10% of patients [37]. In contrast to primary non-responders, development of secondary resistance after an initial response has also been reported in up to 10% of patients [38]. Technical factors such as incorrect storage or reconstitution of the toxin may be responsible for isolated secondary treatment failures. Sustained late failure of response include underdosing, injection of

inappropriate muscles, a worsening or change in the pattern of dystonia or underlying disorder, muscular atrophy, altered perception of atrophy, and development of immunity [39]. Risk factors for the development of antibodies seem to be higher frequency of injections, the use of "booster" injections, and higher doses of Botox® per treatment [40].

Absolute contraindications to the use of BoNTs include known hypersensitivity to components of the product formulation, neuromuscular diseases, myasthenia gravis, Lambert-Eaton syndrome, neuropathies, brain tumors, aneurysms, heart, renal or liver failure, psychiatric disorders, pregnancy, lactation, and drugs affecting the muscle tone, and infections in the site of injection. The relative contraindications include concurrent treatment with aminoglycosides (may increase the effect), penicillamine, quinine, chloroquine and hydroxychloroquine (may reduce the effect), calcium channel blockers, and platelet antiaggregants or anticoagulants (which may increase the risk of hematoma) [11]. Treatment with BoNTs seems to be contraindicated in patients with severe chronic obstructive pulmonary disease [4, 43] for the possibility of botulinum toxin to affect respiratory dynamics.

The preceding paragraphs present relevant information that, in our opinion, should be known by a general surgeon interested in the use of botulinum toxin for the repair of abdominal wall defects rather than to provide an exhaustive description of the clinical application of BoNTs. Most of the aforementioned data have been obtained from a large clinical experience with the use of BoNTs in cosmetics and motor disorders, although there are limitations in the consistence of the evidence.

Botulinum Toxin in Abdominal Wall Hernia: Evidence and Outcome

The application of BoNTs in abdominal wall surgery is a special field of increasing interest. However, at the time of writing this chapter, information on the use of BoNTs in this particular context is limited [4–7, 41–48]. Two references are comments to clinical studies [44, 45] and two publications were experimental studies [41, 46]. The first experimental study [41] assessed the effect of botulinum A toxin-induced paralysis of abdominal muscles on intra-abdominal volume and pressure at 3 days after injection of 2 mL (5 U/mL) of onabotulinum toxin A (BOTOX®) into the abdominal muscles at 16 different points (right, left, upper and lower quadrants, and rectus muscles) in Sprague–Dawley rats. It was found that botulinum A toxin injection to abdominal muscles of the rats increased intra-abdominal volume which therefore decreased the pressure. According to these findings it was suggested that this application may be used as an adjunct in abdominal wall closure in selective cases. In the second experimental study carried out in a porcine model [46], advance of the abdominal wall toward the midline was analyzed after randomly-assigned injections of 150–200 U of onabotulinum toxin A (the brand name was not specified) in the external oblique muscle in one side and placebo in the contralateral side. Botulinum A injection achieved 68% advance of the abdominal wall as a result of open component separation.

Clinical studies are mainly based on (a) the paralyzing effects of BoNTs on the abdominal wall lateral muscles (oblique and transverse) to facilitate repair of ventral defects, and (b) the direct (inhibition of pain-related neurotransmitters) and indirect (reduction of muscular contraction) antinociceptive effects of BoNTs as an adjuvant technique for the relief of pain after surgery.

Paralyzing Effects of BoNTs

The first clinical study to propose botulinum toxin type A before abdominal Hernia repair to reduce muscle tension and lateral retraction was published in 2009 [7]. In this study, 12 patients with midline incisional hernias secondary to intentional open abdomen [49] were treated with injections of abobotulinum toxin A (Dysport®) in five different points of the lateral abdominal wall (two over the mid-axillary line, between the costal border and the superior iliac crest, and three

over the external oblique muscle). Bilateral application of abobotulinum toxin A was performed under electromyographic guidance. A total of 500 units were injected (250 units for each hemi-abdomen, 5 units per point). Transverse abdominal wall defect measurement was practiced at weekly intervals (clinically in 2 patients and with computed tomography scan [CT] in 10). At 4 weeks after treatment, a significant overall mean reduction of the transverse defect was observed, and hernia repair was successfully performed with no recurrence after a mean follow-up of 9 months. This first report of botulinum A toxin application before abdominal wall hernia reconstruction showed that the lateral muscles paralysis can be achieved and transverse hernia defect reduction can subsequently be accomplished with minimal tension closure.

In 2013, Zielinski et al. [4] developed the novel technique of CCS which incorporates injection of botulinum toxin A (Botox®) into the lateral abdominal wall musculature to avoid extensive dissection in critically ill patients with extensive infected/contaminated abdominal domains. The study was a retrospective review of 18 patients with open abdomen who underwent ultrasound-guided Botox® injections into six separate injection sites (right/left subcostal, right/left anterior axillary, and right/left lower quadrants) of the external oblique, internal oblique, and transversus abdominis muscles (50 units per point, 150 units for each hemiabdomen, total 300 units). The primary fascial closure rate was 83% with a fascial dehiscence rate of 11%. The technique of CCS described by the authors was safe and feasible, and created less tension at the midline throughout the duration of the open abdomen surgery.

In 2014, the results of a clinical trial in 17 male trauma patients with abdominal wall hernia secondary to open abdomen management were reported [6]. The aim of the study was to evaluate if botulinum toxin type A application in the lateral abdominal wall muscles could modify its thickness and length. An injection of 50 units of Dysport® between the external and internal oblique muscles was performed under ultrasonographic guidance at five application sites (two at the middle axillary line between costal margin and iliac crest level, and three between anterior axillary line and middle clavicular line between costal margin and iliac crest level) in both sides of the abdomen (250 units for each hemiabdomen, total 500 units). Four weeks after NoBT-A injection, a CT scan was performed and the thickness and length of the lateral abdominal wall muscles were compared with previous measures. The abdominal wall reconstruction surgery was scheduled afterwards. In all patients, a statistically significant reduction of left and right muscle thickness and length was achieved.

Botulinum toxin A has recently been used in patients with incisional hernia. In one study [47], 14 patients with giant incisional hernias were infiltrated with 10 units of botulinum toxin A (Botox®) in five points of each side of the abdominal wall under electromyographic guidance (50 units per side, total 100 units). Four weeks later they were submitted to surgery. A reduction in the hernia diameter was found in 50% of the patients. The authors concluded that the use of preoperative botulinum toxin A markedly reduces tension during surgical repair and increases the rate of primary closure. Moreover, in a single patient with bilateral inguinoscrotal hernia with loss of domain, and remaining abdominal wall intact, the use of 55.55 units of abobotulinum toxin A (Dysport®) injected into five different points of the lateral abdominal wall and four points of the ipsilateral rectus abdominus muscle under anatomic guidance (499.95 units per each abdominal side, total 999.9 units) was useful to relax the abdominal wall muscles and facilitated performing the surgery [48]. Although the evidence is still anecdotal, the authors concluded that this adjunct treatment should be considered as a new alternative for hernias with loss of domain.

Antinociceptive Effects of BoNTs

In 2011, Botox® was used for the first time for postoperative pain control after laparoscopic ventral hernia repair [42]. Three injection sites (right/left subcostal, right/left anterior axillary, right/left lower quadrants) were chosen on each side of the abdominal wall. All three muscles (external oblique, internal oblique, and transversus) were identified by ultrasound. A total of 300 units of Botox® were utilized (50 units per point, 150 units for each abdominal side). Pain scores improved from 10/10 to 2/10 and were durable at 3-month follow-up.

In 2013, Zendejas et al. [43] evaluated the usefulness of botulinum toxin A injection to reduce postoperative pain and the consumption of opioid analgesia in 22 patients undergoing elective incisional hernia repair compared to concurrent matched controls. The primary outcome measure was in-hospital mean morphine equivalents (MEs) on hospital day (HD) 2, considering the operative day to be HD1. Secondary outcome measures included in-hospital ME per day for HD3 through HD7, in-hospital daily patient reported pain scores (visual analogue scale [VAS] 1-10), duration of hospital stay, perioperative complications, opioid-related adverse effects, surgical-site occurrences, and hernia recurrence. The technique of Botox® injection also included three injection sites (right/left subcostal, right/left anterior axillary, right/left lower quadrants) on each side of the abdominal wall, with ultrasound identification of the external oblique, internal oblique, and transversus muscles, with a dose of 50 units per injection (150 units for each hemiabdomen, total 300 units). Patients in the active treatment group used significantly less opioid analgesia on HD2 and 5, and reported significantly less pain on HD2 and 4, as compared to controls. Differences in secondary outcome measures were not observed. The authors concluded that, patients who underwent chemical component paralysis reported less pain and required significantly less opioid analgesia.

A summary of these studies is shown in Table 41.2.

Personal Comprehension

The terms CCS [4] or chemical myotomy [46] should be abandoned because they may cause confusion with results obtained from surgical

Table 41.2 Clinical studies of the use of BoNTs in abdominal wall surgery

	Paralyzing effects					Antinociceptive effects
Author (year) [reference]	Ibarra-Hurtado [7]	Zielinski [4]	Ibarra-Hurtado [6]	Chávez-Tostado [47]	Ibarra-Hurtado [48]	Zendejas [43]
Study design	Observational	Observational	Observational	Observational	Case report	Observational
Abdominal wall defect	Midline	Midline	Midline	Midline + flanks	Inguinoscrotal hernia	Midline and laterals
Initial transverse mean diameter (cm)	13.85	?	14.65	14.6	–	?
Indication	IH after OA	OA	IH after OA	IH	Bilateral inguinal hernia	Postoperative pain (IHR)
Number of patients	12	18	17	14	1	22
Objective	IH repair	Fascial closure after OA	Modification of length and thickness of lateral abdominal muscles	IH repair	Reintroduction into the abdominal cavity after loss of domain	Postoperative decrease of pain and use of opioids
Botulinum toxin	Dysport®	Botox®	Dysport®	Botox®	Dysport®	Botox®
Injection points				or at each side of the defect		
Guidance technique	EMG. Point of maximal activity	US. Selective injection transversus, external, internal	US. Injection between the external and internal oblique muscles	EMG. Point of maximal activity TC	Anatomic landmarks	US. Selective injection transversus, external, internal oblique muscles
Hemiabdomen dose (total dose), units	250 (500)	150 (300)	250 (500)	50 (100)	499.95U (999.9U)	150 (300)
Timing of administration	Preoperative (definition unknown)	<24 hours of OA / >24 hours of OA	Preoperative (definition unknown)	Preoperative (definition unknown)	Preoperative (definition unknown)	During surgery (59%). Prior to surgery 41% (mean 6 days before)

(continued)

Table 41.2 (continued)

	Paralyzing effects					Antinociceptive effects
Timing intervention/measurement	1 week=2 patients 4 weeks=10 patients	NR	4 weeks after injection	4 weeks after injection	45 days after injection	2nd to 7th postoperative day
Definition of positive effect	Decrease transverse diameter wall defect	Fascial closure after OA	Reduction of length and thickness of lateral abdominal muscles	Decrease transverse diameter wall defect	Changes in abdominal muscles and abdominal cavity measured by CT	Morphine equivalents administered and pain relief (VAS)
Assessment of efficacy	Clinical, 2 patients CT, 10 patients	Clinical (fascial closure)	CT	CT	CT	Clinical (decrease of morphine equivalents administered and pain relief [VAS])
Assessment of duration of action	NR	NR	NR	NR	NR	NR
Primary midline closure (%)	50	83	23.5	78	–	–
Closure by abdominoplasty (%)	50	–	76.5	22	–	–
Total complications (%)	16.6	67	41	28.5	0	–
Complication toxin A	0	0	0	0	0	0
Mean follow-up (months)	9	?	49	15	46	18
Overall mortality (%)	0	11	0	7	0	0
Toxin-related mortality	0	0	0	0	0	0
Conclusions	Decrease of transverse diameter of the abdominal wall defect	Botulinum toxic relaxes but combined with TAC techniques	Botulinum toxin reduces thickness and increases length of abdominal wall	Botulinum toxin is effective in the treatment of giant IH. Studies are needed to standardize the technique	Botulinum toxic relaxes increasing the volume of abdominal cavity	Botulinum toxic reduces postoperative pain and use of opioids

HI incisional hernia, OA open abdomen, IHR incisional hernia repair, NR not reported, CT computed tomography, VAS visual analogue scale, TAC temporary abdominal closure procedures of similar names. In our opinion, the use of BoNTs in abdominal wall surgery is a technique for primarily preparing the patient, not for repairing patient's defect. "Chemical component paralysis" [43], or even better "chemodenervation of abdominal wall musculature" seems more appropriate designations.

Although BoNTs have shown a favorable clinical profile in cosmetic/dermatological applications for decades, some important aspects are still pending to be clarified [21]. It is interesting to note that uncertainties on some of these clinical questions are still present when BoNTs are used in the field of abdominal wall surgery. In this respect, assessment of the efficacy of botulinum toxin across studies is heterogeneous, ranging from a clinical evaluation (potential bias related to subjectivity of the examiner) to indirect techniques, such as an abdominal CT. Therefore, a clear criterion to define a positive clinical effect of the application of botulinum toxin in the abdominal wall is lacking. Injection strategies, including timing, which is important to determine the onset of action, duration of effect and, ultimately, the impact of BoNTs on the abdominal wall muscular function, remain unclear. A better definition of these aspects would contribute to our understanding of which type of botulinum toxin may be the most appropriate for its application in different scenarios of abdominal wall surgery, given the characteristics of abdominal muscles and formulations. Formulations are not interchangeable and differ in relation to their molecular structure, mode of action, dosing, migration characteristics, and potential adverse effects.

Clinical studies of the application of BoNTs in abdominal wall surgery are still preliminary experiences based on observational designs and carried out in small study populations. Therefore, results of these studies should be interpreted taking into account these limitations. At the present time, there is only one ongoing registered clinical trial (NCT01495962) aimed to determine whether botulinum toxin A (Botox®) will facilitate fascial closure after damage control laparotomy (DCL) [50]. The primary endpoint is the rate of delayed primary fascial closure. Delayed primary fascial closure will be considered when the rectus abdominus fascia is directly approximated in the midline during the same hospitalization as the initial DCL without the use of mesh.

Potential applications of the paralyzing and antinociceptive effects of BoNTs in the abdominal wall in adult patients may include complex and non-complex midline incisional hernias, open abdomen, or reconstructions when the abdominal wall is intact. Although a clear definition of "complex" abdominal hernia is missing, recently, consensus on criteria used to define a patient with complex hernia was reached [51]. Such consensus includes 22 patients and hernia variables for "complex" hernia criteria inclusion which were grouped under four categories: "Size and location," "Contamination/soft tissue condition," "Patient history/risk factors," and "Clinical scenario." These variables were further divided into three patient severity classes ("Minor," "Moderate," and "Major") to provide guidance for perioperative planning and measures, the risk of a complicated postoperative course, and the extent of financial costs associated with treatment of these hernia patients [51].

On the basis of previous considerations and taking into account that each case treatment should be individualized, the paralyzing effect of BoNT-A could be indicated, with or without preoperative progressive pneumoperitoneum (PPP), in patients with complex midline incisional hernia with a loss of domain (hernia sac can form a second abdominal cavity), small or large defects and minor or moderate severity class. Our group has a short experience with excellent results in a small clinical series of five patients with complex midline incisional hernia and loss of domain (large/small defects, minor/moderate severity class), which have been treated with a combination of onabotulinum toxin A (Botox®) and PPP. Two weeks prior to starting PPP, botulinum toxin A is injected. The injection technique used in our patients is based on the method described by Ibarra-Hurtado et al. [7], in 2009, with the difference that we use onabotulinum toxin A (Botox®). Briefly, after preparing the sterile material (gloves, gauzes, syringes, etc.,) and a mioject needle of 75 mm length (TECANeedles, MyoJect Disposable Hypodermic Needle Electrode, VIASYS Healthcare, Madison, WI, USA), 100 units of BoNT-A (Botox®) are diluted with 5 cm³ of preservative-free 0.9% saline and a total of five syringes of 1 cm³ is obtained (20 units of BoNT-A). Five points are identified at each side of lateral abdominal wall. Two points over the mid-axillary line (between the costal border and the superior iliac crest) and three points over the external oblique muscle. The skin is cleaned with alcohol and no local anesthesia is used. The mioject needle is applied and under electromyographic guidance, the needle is used to identify the maximal electromyographic recording points in the five points of the lateral abdominal wall. The depth of injection

will depend on the anthropometric characteristics of the individual and the location of the point of maximum electromyographic activity. Then, 20 units (1 cm³) per point (100 units for each hemiabdomen) are injected. The procedure is performed in the outpatient setting. The purpose of this combined approach was to increase elongation of the lateral abdominal wall muscles (i.e., increase of the abdominal cavity/capacity) adding the effect of BoNT-A with the effect of PPP. Alternatively, the injections may be performed under ultrasound guidance, with each of the lateral abdominal muscles injected separately.

The algorithm for the management of midline incisional hernias with suspicion of loss of domain currently used by our group is shown in Fig. 41.1. Details of our technique of BoNT-A injection are presented in the video supplement. Our strategy to measure BoNT-A effects is based on radiological evidence of a reduction of muscle thickness on post-injection CT and a shorter time of pneumoperitoneum (usually without BoNT-A

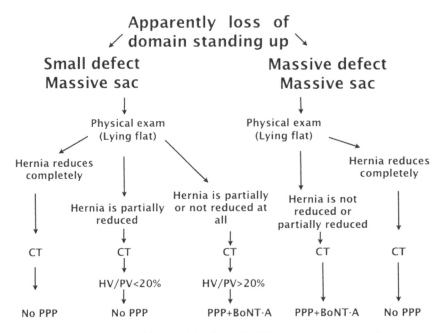

Fig. 41.1 Management algorithm of midline incisional hernias with potential loss of domain *CT* computed tomography, *HV/PV* hernia volume/peritoneal volume ratio, *PPP* preoperative progressive pneumoperitoneum, *BoNT-A* botulinum neurotoxin A, in our experience Botox®)

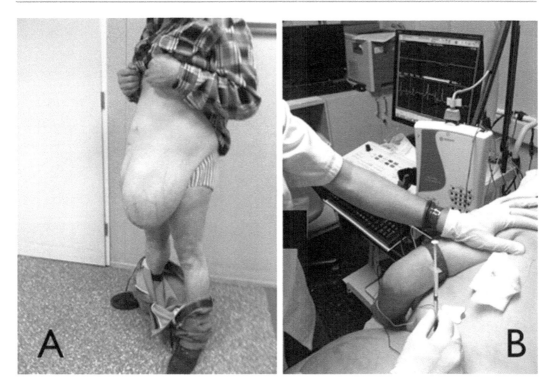

Fig. 41.2 (a) Complex midline incisional hernia with loss of domain, (b) Botox® injection with electromyographic guidance

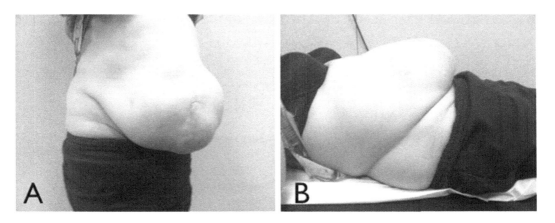

Fig. 41.3 (a) Complex midline incisional hernia with loss of domain standing up, (b) Lying flat (hernia is not reduced)

it takes between 2 and 3 weeks and with BoNT-A is reduced to 1–2 weeks). Illustrative cases of the combined use of BoNT-A and PPP are presented in Figs. 41.2, 41.3, and 41.4.

Patients with a complex midline incisional hernia without loss of domain (large/small defects, minor/moderate severity class) may be candidates for BoNT-A application (Fig. 41.5). In these cases, the laparoscopic approach together with BoNT-A injection would be only considered in the absence of trophic cutaneous lesions, when defects are small and closed with or without asso-

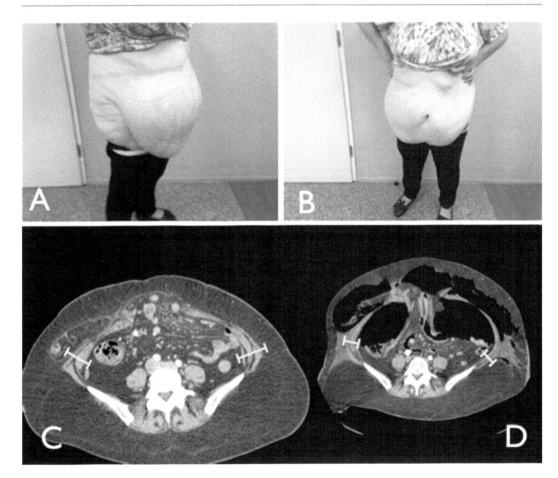

Fig. 41.4 (**a**, **b**) Complex midline incisional hernia with loss of domain standing up. This patient may be candidate for combined preoperative progressive pneumoperitoneum and botulinum toxin A application. (**c**) CT previous to BoNT-A + PPP, highlighted in yellow wide lateral abdominal wall muscles. (**d**) CT after BoNT-A + PPP, highlighted in yellow narrow lateral abdominal wall muscles

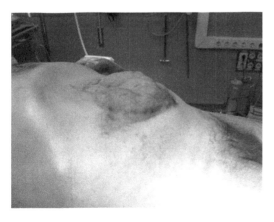

Fig. 41.5 Complex midline incisional hernia without loss of domain and large defect

ciated endoscopic component separation (ECS). The use of BoNT-A should not be indicated as a preoperative preparation of a non-complex midline incisional hernia (5–10 cm of transverse diameter), unless a laparoscopic approach with closure of the defect, with or without ECS would be chosen.

The open abdomen may be a reasonable indication for BoNT-A in patients with an abdominal temporal closure technique with vacuum-assisted negative pressure [52] (Fig. 41.6).

In cases of abdominal defects with intact abdominal wall, BoNT-A application could be used in inguinal hernia with loss of domain, with

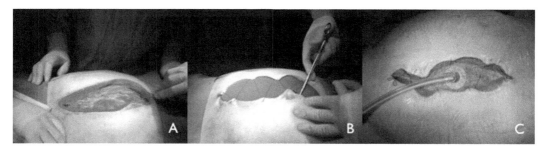

Fig. 41.6 Temporary abdominal closure of open abdomen with non-absorbable synthetic mesh traction (pleating or serial excision of the mesh as the fascial edges are re-approximated) (**a**) with combined negative pressure wound therapy (**b**, **c**)

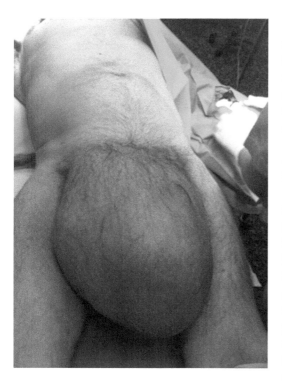

Fig. 41.7 Inguinal hernia with loss of domain

or without associated PPP (Fig. 41.7). Other rare cases may be treated with BoNT-A without PPP, such as a giant diaphragmatic hernia.

Potential separation of the paralyzing and antinociceptive effects of BoNTs is artificial and, theoretically, indications related to one effect may favor the other, and vice versa. For this reason, potential indications of the antinociceptive effects of BoNTs are the same than those previously described (Table 41.3).

Concluding Remarks

Potential applications of BoNT-A here described to achieve tension- and retraction-free conditions in abdominal wall reconstruction are exclusively based on the author's opinion and experience. Further studies (preferably randomized-controlled designs) are necessary to clarify a number of relevant clinical questions, including patient's eligibility, dosing of the different botulinum toxin A formulations, optimal administration technique, or benefits of potential association with other procedures (such as PPP or ECS). Injections of BoNT-A into the abdominal wall muscles to facilitate complex hernia repair is a promising technique, but the evidence available at the present time is still weak and a clear role of BoNT-A in abdominal wall surgery remains to be defined.

Table 41.3 Potential indications of botulinum toxins in abdominal wall surgery

			Potential indication paralyzing affect (preparation for surgery)			Potential indication antinociceptive effect		
			Open surgery	Laparoscopic surgery		Open surgery	Laparoscopic surgery	
				Closing defect	Without closing defect		Closing defect	Without closing defect
Complex midline incisional hernias	With loss of domain	Small defect	Yes (with or without PPP)	Noᵃ		Yes	Noᵃ	
Risk minor/moderate		Large defect	Yes (with or without PPP)	Noᵃ		Yes	Noᵃ	
	Without loss of domain	Small defect	Yes	Yes (with or without ECS)	No	Yes		
		Large defect	Yes	Noᵃ		Yes		
Non-complex midline incisional hernias			No	Yes (with or without ECS)	No	Yes		
Open abdomen			Yes	Noᵃ		Yes		
Intact abdominal wall	With loss of domain	Inguinal hernia	Yes (with or without PPP)	Noᵃ		Yes		
		Other†	Yes	Noᵃ		Yes		
	Without loss of domain	Inguinal hernia	No			No		
		Other†	No			No		

ᵃNo indication for laparoscopic surgery; †Diaphragmatic hernias; *PPP* preoperative progressive pneumoperitoneum, *ECS* endoscopic component separation

Acknowledgment The authors thank Marta Pulido, MD, for editing the manuscript and editorial assistance.

References

1. Sackett DL, Rosenberg WM, Gray JA, Haynes RB, Richardson WS. Evidence based medicine: what it is and what it isn't. BMJ. 1996;312:71–2.
2. Glasser SP, Duval S. Meta-analysis, evidence-based medicine, and clinical guidelines. In: Glasser SP, editor. Essentials of clinical research. 2nd ed. Berlin: Springer International; 2014. p. 203–32.
3. López-Cano M. Evidence-based surgery and incisional hernia. Rev Hispanoamer Hernia. 2013;1:18–26.
4. Zielinski MD, Goussous N, Schiller HJ, Jenkins D. Chemical component separation with botulinum toxin A: a novel technique to improve primary fascial closure rates of the open abdomen. Hernia. 2013;17:101–7.
5. Aoki KR. Botulinum toxin: a successful therapeutic protein. Curr Med Chem. 2004;11:3085–92.
6. Ibarra-Hurtado TR, Nuño-Guzmán CM, Miranda-Díaz AG, Troyo-Sanromán R, Navarro-Ibarra R, Bravo-Cuéllar L. Effect of botulinum toxin type A in lateral abdominal wall muscles thickness and length of patients with midline incisional hernia secondary to open abdomen management. Hernia. 2014;18:647–52.
7. Ibarra-Hurtado TR, Nuño-Guzmán CM, Echeagaray-Herrera JE, Robles-Vélez E, de Jesús González-Jaime J. Use of botulinum toxin type A before abdominal wall hernia reconstruction. World J Surg. 2009;33: 2553–6.
8. Erbguth FJ. Historical notes on botulism, Clostridium botulinum, botulinum toxin, and the idea of the therapeutic use of the toxin. Mov Disord. 2004;19 Suppl 8:S2–6.
9. Bigalke H, Dressler D, Jankovic J. Basic and therapeutic aspects of neurotonins. Mov Disord. 2004;19 Suppl 8:S1.
10. Chaddock JA, Purkiss JR, Alexander FC, Doward S, Fooks SJ, Friis LM, et al. Retargeted clostridial endopeptidases: inhibition of nociceptive neurotransmitter release in vitro, and antinociceptive activity in in vivo models of pain. Mov Disord. 2004;19 Suppl 8:S42–7.
11. Nigam PK, Nigam A. Botulinum toxin. Indian J Dermatol. 2010;55:8–14.
12. Dolly JO, Aoki KR. The structure and mode of action of different botulinum toxins. Eur J Neurol. 2006;13 Suppl 4:1–9.
13. Klein AW, Carruthers A, Fagien S, Lowe NJ. Comparisons among botulinum toxins: an evidence-based review. Plast Reconstr Surg. 2008;121:413–22.
14. Hoffman RO, Helveston EM. Botulinum in the treatment of adult motility disorders. Int Ophthalmol Clin. 1986;26:241–50.
15. Aoki KR, Guyer B. Botulinum toxin type A and other botulinum toxin serotypes: a comparative review of biochemical and pharmacological actions. Eur J Neurol. 2001;8 Suppl 5:21–9.
16. U.S. Food and Drug Administration.
17. Aoki KR, Ranoux D, Wissel J. Using translational medicine to understand clinical differences between botulinum toxin formulations. Eur J Neurol. 2006;13: 10–9.
18. Kranz G, Paul A, Voller B, Posch M, Windischberger C, Auff E, Sycha T. Long-term efficacy and respective potencies of botulinum toxin A and B: a randomized, double-blind study. Br J Dermatol. 2011;164:176–81.
19. Esquenazi A, Mayer N. Botulinum toxin for the management of muscle overactivity and spasticity after stroke. Curr Atheroscler Rep. 2001;3:295–8.
20. Pathak MS, Nguyen HT, Graham HK, Moore AP. Management of spasticity in adults: practical application of botulinum toxin. Eur J Neurol. 2006;13 Suppl 1:42–50.
21. Bonaparte JP, Ellis D, Quinn JG, Ansari MT, Rabski J, Kilty SJ. A comparative assessment of three formulations of botulinum toxin A for facial rhytides: a systematic review and meta-analyses. Syst Rev. 2013;2:40.
22. Borodic G. Immunologic resistance after repeated botulinum toxin type A injections for facial rhytides. Ophthal Plast Reconstr Surg. 2006;22:239–40.
23. Dressler D, Wohlfahrt K, Meyer-Rogge E, Wiest L, Bigalke H. Antibody-induced failure of botulinum toxin: a therapy in cosmetic indications. Dermatol Surg. 2010;36 Suppl 4:2182–7.
24. Ranoux D, Gury C, Fondarai J, Mas JL, Zuber M. Therapy with botulinum toxin. J Neurol Neurosurg Psychiatry. 2002;72:459–62.
25. Panjwani N, O'Keeffe R, Pickett A. Biochemical, functional and potency characteristics of type A botulinum toxin in clinical use. Botulinum J. 2008;1:153–66.
26. Kranz G, Haubenberger D, Voller B, Posch M, Schnider P, Auff E, et al. Respective potencies of Botox and Dysport in a human skin model: a randomized, double-blind study. Mov Disord. 2009;24:231–6.
27. Jandhyala R. Relative potency of incobotulinum toxin A vs onabotulinum toxin A: a meta-analysis of key evidence. J Drugs Dermatol. 2012;11:731–6.
28. Persaud R, Garas G, Silva S, Stamatoglou C, Chatrath P, Patel K. An evidence-based review of botulinum toxin (Botox) applications in non-cosmetic head and neck conditions. JRSM Short Rep. 2013;4:10.
29. Borodic GE, Ferrante R, Pearce LB, Smith K. Histologic assessment of dose-related diffusion and muscle fiber response after therapeutic botulinum A toxin injections. Mov Disord. 1994;9:31–9.
30. Hsu TS, Dover JS, Arndt KA. Effect of volume and concentration on the diffusion of botulinum exotoxin A. Arch Dermatol. 2004;140:1351–4.
31. Cliff SH, Judodihardjo H, Eltringham E. Different formulations of botulinum toxin type A have different migration characteristics: a double-blind, randomized study. J Cosmet Dermatol. 2008;7:50–4.
32. Bakheit AM, Ward CD, McLellan DL. Generalised botulism-like syndrome after intramuscular injections of botulinum toxin type A: a report of two cases. J Neurol Neurosurg Psychiatry. 1997;62:198.

33. Glanzman RL, Gelb DJ, Drury I, Bromberg MB, Truong DD. Brachial plexopathy after botulinum toxin injections. Neurology. 1990;40:1143.

34. Schnider P, Brichta A, Schmied M, Auff E. Gallbladder dysfunction induced by botulinum A toxin. Lancet. 1993;342:811–2.

35. Latimer PR, Hodgkins PR, Vakalis BRE, Evans AR, Zaki GA. Necrotising fasciitis as a complication of botulinum toxin treatment. Eye. 1998; 12:51–3.

36. Dressler D. Clinical presentation and management of antibody-induced failure of botulinum toxin therapy. Mov Disord. 2004;19 Suppl 8:S92–100.

37. Greene P, Fahn S, Diamond B. Development of resistance to botulinum toxin type A in patients with torticollis. Mov Disord. 1994;9:213–7.

38. Jankovic J, Schwartz KS. Clinical correlates of response to botulinum toxin injections. Arch Neurol. 1991;48:1253–6.

39. Sheean GL, Lees AJ. Botulinum toxin F in the treatment of torticollis clinically resistant to botulinum toxin A. J Neurol Neurosurg Psychiatry. 1995;59: 601–7.

40. Dressler D, Dirnberger G. Botulinum toxin therapy: risk factors for therapy failure. Mov Disord. 2000;15 Suppl 2:51.

41. Cakmak M, Caglayan F, Somuncu S, Leventoglu A, Ulusoy S, Akman H, et al. Effect of paralysis of the abdominal wall muscles by botulinum A toxin to intraabdominal pressure: an experimental study. J Pediatr Surg. 2006;4:821–5.

42. Smoot D, Zielinski M, Jenkins D, Schiller H. Botox A injection for pain after laparoscopic ventral hernia: a case report. Pain Med. 2011;12:1121–3.

43. Zendejas B, Khasawneh MA, Srvantstyan B, Jenkins DH, Schiller HJ, Zielinski MD. Outcomes of chemical component paralysis using botulinum toxin for incisional hernia repairs. World J Surg. 2013;37: 2830–7.

44. Rosin D. Outcomes of chemical component paralysis using botulinum toxin for incisional hernia repairs. World J Surg. 2013;37:2838.

45. Ibarra-Hurtado TR, Nuño-Guzmán CM. Comment to: chemical components separation with botulinum toxin A: a novel technique to improve primary fascial closure rates of the open abdomen by Zielinski et al. Hernia. 2013;17:109–10.

46. Harth K, Rosen M, Blatnik J, Schomisch S, Cash A, Soltanian H. Chemical myotomy with botulinum toxin for abdominal wall reconstruction: results of a porcine pilot study. Plast Reconstruct Surg. 2011;127 Suppl 5:S99.

47. Chávez-Tostado KV, Cárdenas-Lailsonb LE, Pérez-Trigosb H. Results of preoperative application of botulinum toxin type A in treatment of giant incisional hernias. Rev Hispanoam Hernia. 2014;2:145–51.

48. Ibarra Hurtado TR, Negrete Ramosa GI, Preciado Hernández F, Nuño Guzmán CM, Tapia Alcalá E, Bravo CL. Botulinum toxin type A as an adjuvant in bilateral inguinoscrotal hernia with loss of domain. First case report and literature review. Rev Hispanoam Hernia. 2014;2:139–44.

49. López-Cano M, Pereira JA, Armengol-Carrasco M. "Acute postoperative open abdominal wall": Nosological concept and treatment implications. World J Gastrointest Surg. 2013;5:314–20.

50. ClinicalTrials.gov [NCT01495962]. https://clinical-trials.gov/ct2/show/study/NCT01495962?term=botulinum+toxin+and+abdominal+wall+reconstruction&rank=1.

51. Slater NJ, Montgomery A, Berrevoet F, Carbonell AM, Chang A, Franklin M, et al. Criteria for definition of a complex abdominal wall hernia. Hernia. 2014;18:7–17.

52. Petersson U, Acosta S, Björck M. Vacuum-assisted wound closure and mesh-mediated fascial traction—a novel technique for late closure of the open abdomen. World J Surg. 2007;31:2133–7.

Sean M. O'Neill, David C. Chen, and Parviz K. Amid

Introduction

Inguinal hernia repairs comprise both open and laparoscopic techniques. This chapter discusses open techniques, which are further divided into tissue- and prosthetic-based repairs. Introduced in 1887, Bassini's technique of restoring the integrity of the inguinal floor using native tissue layers resulted in fewer recurrences and less morbidity than its predecessors, which relied on simple closure of the internal ring. The Shouldice and McVay repairs are variations on the Bassini technique, as is a more recent repair introduced by Desarda in 2001. Prosthetic-based repairs are predicated upon restoring the integrity of the inguinal floor by placing synthetic mesh either anteriorly or posteriorly to the transversalis fascia. Three key scientific advancements contributed to the widespread adoption of mesh repairs:

Electronic supplementary material: The online version of this chapter (doi:10.1007/978-3-319-27470-6_42) contains supplementary material, which is available to authorized users.

S.M. O'Neill, M.D., Ph.D. • D.C. Chen, M.D. (✉)
P.K. Amid, M.D.
Department of Surgery, Lichtenstein Amid Hernia Clinic at UCLA, Santa Monica, CA, USA

David Geffen School of Medicine at UCLA, Los Angeles, CA 90095, USA
e-mail: soneil@mednet.ucla.edu;
dcchen@mednet.ucla.edu

the recognition that impaired collagen synthesis contributes to hernia formation, the realization that suture line tension contributes to recurrence, and the refinement of prosthetic materials to be lightweight, flexible, strong, and biologically inert.

In the 1980s, Lichtenstein popularized the tension-free anterior mesh repair that now bears his name. Variations on the Lichtenstein technique include mesh plug and patch repairs and the Prolene Hernia System (PHS) repair. In 1973, Stoppa developed an open tension-free hernia repair with mesh placed posteriorly to the transversalis fascia in the preperitoneal space addressing all potential defects in the myopectineal orifice of Fruchaud. This operation is the precursor for modern open and laparoscopic preperitoneal repairs. The transinguinal preperitoneal (TIPP) repair, a modified Rives operation described by Schumpelick, and transrectus sheath preperitoneal (TREPP) repair, a modified unilateral Stoppa operation described by Wantz, are examples of open posterior approaches used today.

Thus, the current methods of open hernia repair can be categorized as: (1) tissue approximation repair (Bassini, Shouldice, McVay, Desarda) and (2) open tension-free prosthetic repair, in which mesh is placed in front of the transversalis fascia (Lichtenstein), behind it (Rives, Wantz, Kugel, Stoppa, TIPP, TREPP), or both (Plug and Patch, Prolene Hernia System).

Tissue Approximation Repairs

More than 70 types of different tissue repairs have been reported in the surgical literature; those commonly in use today are the Bassini, Shouldice, McVay, and Desarda repairs. Among these, the European Hernia Society guidelines recommend the Shouldice technique as the best option among tissue repairs [1]. Numerous randomized comparative trials, however, have clearly demonstrated the superiority of tension-free mesh repair over the traditional tissue approximation methods [2–4]. Therefore, indications for tissue repairs include operative field contamination, emergency surgery, and when the viability of hernia contents is uncertain.

Bassini Repair

The original repair includes dissection of the spermatic cord, dissection of the hernia sac with high ligation, and extensive reconstruction of the floor of the inguinal canal. In a "proper" Bassini repair, the entire spermatic cord is dissected and

isolated along with any indirect hernia sac, excising the cremasteric muscle. The inguinal floor is then exposed and the transversalis fascia is incised from the pubic tubercle to the internal inguinal ring. This step is often left out in modern interpretations of Bassini's repair. After the fascia is sufficiently mobilized, a triple-layer repair is performed. The internal oblique, transversus abdominis, and transversalis fascia are fixed to the shelving edge of the inguinal ligament and pubic periosteum with 6–8 nonabsorbable interrupted sutures (Fig. 42.1a). The lateral aspect of the repair reinforces the medial border of the internal inguinal ring.

Shouldice Repair

The Shouldice repair distributes the suture line tension over several layers, resulting in lower recurrence rates compared to the Bassini technique. The genital branch of the genitofemoral nerve is routinely divided during cord dissection. The operator incises the transversalis fascia between the pubic tubercle and internal ring, and

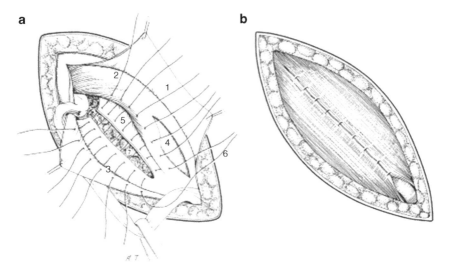

Fig. 42.1 Bassini repair (Reproduced from [5]). (**a**) Note the correct method of performing this procedure: the fascia transversalis is incised widely to allow suturing to the deep layer. The sutures take up the inguinal ligament and the fascia transversalis below, and the fascia transversalis and falx inguinalis above. (*1*) Aponeurosis of the external oblique; (*2*) internal oblique; (*3*) inguinal ligament; (*4*) relaxing incision of the falx inguinalis; (*5*) fascia transversalis; (*6*) repair with 00 gauge nonabsorbable suture; (*7*) subperitoneal fat. (**b**) The aponeurosis of the external oblique is repaired in front of the conjoint tendon

bluntly dissects the preperitoneum to mobilize the upper and lower fascial flaps. The tissue reapproximation then proceeds as follows. Starting at the pubic tubercle, the iliopubic tract is sutured in a running fashion to the lateral edge of the rectus sheath using a synthetic, non-absorbable, monofilament suture. This suture line approximates the edge of the inferior transversalis flap (or "iliopubic tract") to the posterior aspect of the superior flap (or "triple layer") (Fig. 42.2a). At the internal inguinal ring, the suture incorporates the lateral cremasteric stump and reverses back in the medial direction and approximates the edge of the superior transversalis fascia flap (or "triple layer") to the shelving edge of the inguinal ligament (Fig. 42.2b). This is then tied down at the pubic tubercle. The next stitch begins at the internal ring and proceeds medially, approximating the aponeuroses of the internal oblique and transversus abdominis to that of the inguinal ligament (Fig. 42.2c). At the tubercle, this suture line then reverses through the same structures medially, and through the inner aspect of the lower end of the external oblique aponeurosis laterally, and is tied down at the internal ring (Fig. 42.2d). The aponeurosis of the external oblique is then closed over the repair

with the spermatic cord replaced into its anatomic bed. The Shouldice repair has demonstrated the best outcomes of tissue-based repairs approaching those seen with mesh repairs in specialized centers. It requires inguinal anatomy to be properly understood and carried out, which accounts for its limited use. As a technique, it effectively addresses all inguinal hernias and is our preferred option for tissue repair when mesh is not feasible or contraindicated.

McVay Repair

The McVay repair addresses both inguinal and femoral ring defects. After isolation of the spermatic cord, the operator incises the transversalis fascia to enter the preperitoneal space. Gentle blunt dissection mobilizes the upper flap and exposes the surface of Cooper's ligament. A 2–4 cm vertical relaxing incision is made in the anterior rectus sheath at the pubic tubercle (Fig. 42.3a, b). This is essential to reduce tension on the repair, but may increase the risk of postoperative pain and ventral abdominal herniation. The superior transversalis flap is then sutured medially to Cooper's ligament, and the repair is

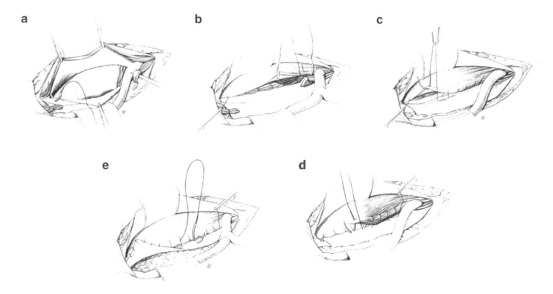

Fig. 42.2   Shouldice repair (Reproduced from [5])

Fig. 42.3 McVay repair
(Reproduced from [5])

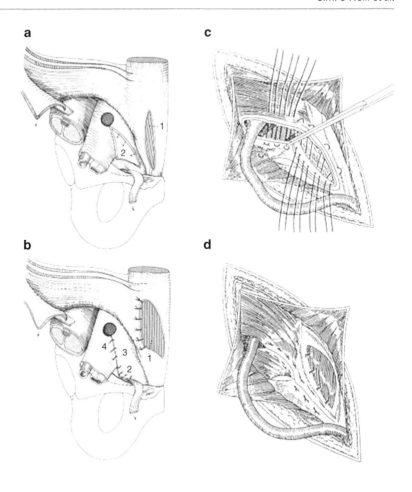

continued laterally along Cooper's ligament to cover the femoral ring. Lateral to the femoral ring, a transition stitch affixes the transversalis fascia to the femoral sheath and inguinal ligament, and the suture line approximating these layers is then continued laterally out to the internal ring (Fig. 42.3c). Again, an essential step in McVay repair is the relaxing incision of the anterior lamina of the rectus sheath prior to repair of the external oblique (Fig. 42.3d).

Desarda Repair

The tissue-based technique introduced by Desarda in 2001 [7, 8] involves reinforcing the floor of the inguinal canal with a medially based strip of undetached external oblique aponeurosis.

The operation itself is not novel as case reports from Halsted and colleagues at Johns Hopkins in the 1890s describe similar techniques using the rectus aponeurosis or external oblique aponeurosis to reinforce the floor [9]. Madden, Koontz, Calman, Halsted, Goodblood, McArthur, Andrews, and Zimmermann have all described similar inguinal floor-based repairs that have fallen out of popular use [8–10]. However, the Desarda operation has gained recent interest especially in resource poor countries in which mesh is not readily available and in cases where mesh is not desired. In this operation, the undetached aponeurotic strip is used to reconstruct the inguinal floor by moving it to the posterior wall of the canal. It is secured to the internal oblique muscle superiorly and the inguinal ligament inferiorly with interrupted sutures (Fig. 42.4).

Fig. 42.4 Desarda technique (from Szopinski et al. [6])

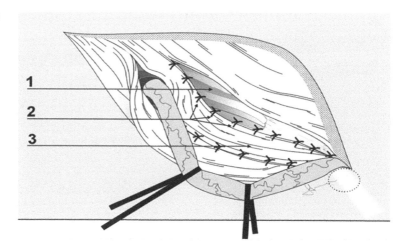

Prosthetic Repairs

The widespread adoption of tension-free prosthetic mesh repairs represented a paradigm shift in inguinal hernia surgery. Mesh-based hernioplasty is the most commonly performed general surgical procedure, due to its efficacy and superior outcomes. The next section describes techniques for the Lichtenstein, Plug and Patch, Prolene Hernia System, and open preperitoneal repairs.

Concerns over the validity of outcomes associated with this technique arise from the claims of superiority over mesh-based techniques with no recurrences and no pain with all data from a single center [10]. Physiologically, the use of intrinsic tissue as a tension-free based flap has been questioned due to the metabolic connective tissue derangements known to exist in patients with hernias [8, 10]. Results from a randomized controlled trial comparing the Desarda and Lichtenstein techniques through 3 years of follow-up appear to demonstrate similar results [8], although broader employment of this technique in general practice has yet to be studied. Furthermore, the duration of these studies is inadequate to detect the later recurrences expected with tissue-based repairs. Five- and ten-year data from well-controlled studies will help to elucidate if this repair will achieve similar outcomes to Shouldice, the current gold standard tissue-based repair.

Lichtenstein Tension-Free Repair

The open tension-free mesh hernioplasty was pioneered by the Lichtenstein group in 1984. As is often the case, the root of most new developments in surgery can be traced back to the old. A tension-free anterior hernioplasty using nylon mesh similar to the Lichtenstein repair had been previously described in the French literature in 1944 by Don Acquaviva and in 1959 by Zagdoun and Sordinas [11]. The inguinal canal is dissected to expose the shelving edge of the inguinal ligament, the pubic tubercle, and sufficient area for mesh (Fig. 42.5a). The mesh is a 7×15 cm rectangle with a rounded medial edge, and it must be large enough to extend 2–3 cm superior to Hesselbach's Triangle. The lateral portion of the mesh is split into two tails such that the superior tail comprises 2/3 its width, and the inferior tail comprises the remaining 1/3. The medial edge of the mesh is affixed to the anterior rectus sheath such that it overlaps the pubic tubercle by 1.5–2 cm, in order to prevent medial recurrence. A non-absorbable synthetic monofilament suture is used to fix the inferior edge of the mesh to the shelving edge of the inguinal ligament (Fig. 42.5b). The upper edge of the mesh is then fixed to the internal oblique aponeurosis laterally and to the rectus sheath medially using a synthetic, absorbable suture (Fig. 42.5c). The lateral tails of the mesh are placed snugly around the cord at the internal ring, but not too tight to strangulate it. The tails are then sutured to the inguinal ligament with an interrupted stitch

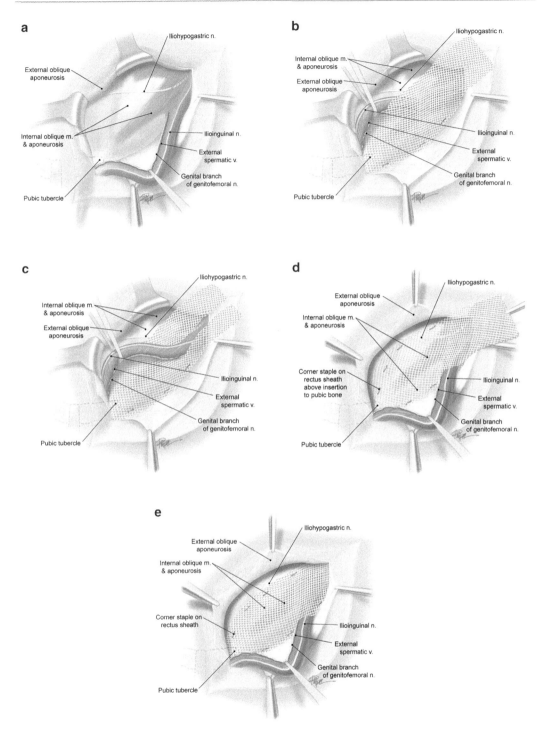

Fig. 42.5 (**a**) Modified Lichtenstein repair: anatomy of the inguinal canal. (**b**) Modified Lichtenstein repair: lateral fixation of mesh with 1–2 cm of overlap over the pubic tubercle. (**c**) Modified Lichtenstein repair: slit made in mesh. (**d**) Modified Lichtenstein repair: medial fixation of the mesh and recreation of the mesh internal ring. (**e**) Modified Lichtenstein repair: mesh tails placed below the external oblique aponeurosis

(Fig. 42.5d) and placed beneath the external oblique aponeurosis (Fig. 42.5e).

As described previously [11], five concepts are fundamental to the Lichtenstein repair:

1. Using a large sheet of mesh that extends 2 cm medially beyond the pubic tubercle, 3–4 cm above Hesselbach's triangle, and 5–6 cm lateral to the internal ring.
2. Crossing the tails of the mesh to avoid lateral recurrence.
3. Securing the upper edge of the mesh to the rectus sheath and internal oblique aponeurosis (avoiding the internal oblique muscle to prevent injury to the intramuscular segment of the iliohypogastric nerve) with two interrupted sutures, and the lower edge of the mesh to the inguinal ligament with one continuous suture. This prevents folding, wadding, and movement of the mesh in the mobile area of the groin.
4. Keeping the mesh in a slightly relaxed, tented up, or sagitated configuration [12] to counteract the forward protrusion of the transversalis fascia when the patient stands up and, more importantly, to compensate for contraction of the mesh.
5. Visualizing and protecting the ilioinguinal, iliohypogastric, and genital nerves [13]. The iliohypogastric nerve is identified during separation of the external oblique aponeurosis from the internal oblique layer. The most vulnerable portion of the iliohypogastric is the intramuscular segment, which courses along the lower edge of the internal oblique muscle [13]. This portion is most likely to be injured or entrapped by suture, and may happen if the upper edge of the mesh is sutured to the internal oblique muscle instead of internal oblique aponeurosis. The genital branch of the genitofemoral nerve is protected by not removing the cremasteric sheath, and keeping the easily visible blue external spermatic vein [13] en bloc with the spermatic cord when it is being lifted from the inguinal floor under direct vision using blunt dissection instead of encircling and elevating the cord with blunt finger dissection. The ilioinguinal nerve can be easily located as it passes

over the spermatic cord. Manipulating and lifting the nerve from its natural bed increases the risk of perineural fibrosis and chronic postherniorrhaphy inguinodynia, so ideal technique minimizes the mobilization and disruption of the nerves from their investing fascia during dissection [13].

Plug and Patch Technique

The use of a mesh plug was first described by Lichtenstein in 1974 for the repair of femoral hernias and for selected recurrent inguinal hernias [14]. Gilbert expanded this to include the repair of primary indirect inguinal hernias, with an added small sheet of flat mesh placed over the inguinal floor [15]. Rutkow and Robbins then applied the concept to direct inguinal hernias [16].

Prior to placing a mesh patch over the inguinal floor as in the Lichtenstein repair, a cone-shaped prosthetic mesh plug is first placed in the hernia defect. For an indirect hernia, the plug is placed alongside the spermatic cord through the internal ring and sutured to the edges of the ring. For a direct hernia, the transversalis fascia at the base of the direct bulge is incised, the sac is reduced, and the plug is sutured to the margin of the defect which could include Cooper's ligament, the inguinal ligament, and the internal oblique muscle or aponeurosis. A mesh onlay patch is then placed according to the Lichtenstein technique.

From the perspective of hernia repair, plug as well as plug and patch techniques are effective, with similar low recurrence rates to other mesh-based techniques. The ease of this repair and comfort that a plug gives surgeons at the time of operation has led to widespread adoption. However, the three-dimensional nature of the plug may lead to greater issues with mesh sensation, meshoma, as well as migration and erosion. We have not used the mesh plug in our practice since the 1990s. Rare but severe complications caused by migration of the mesh were well documented at the time and continue to be reported in the literature at a steady rate. These include small and large bowel obstruction, perforation,

Fig. 42.6 The Prolene hernia System. Image Copyright Ethicon, Inc.

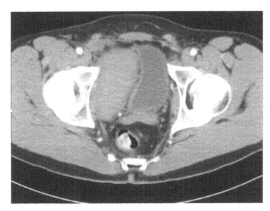

Fig. 42.7 Large hematoma compresses the bladder after inguinal hernia repair with bilayer mesh (Reproduced from [9])

and fistula [17–25], bladder erosion [26], and scrotal migration [24, 27]. Additionally, in 6% of cases, chronic pain required explantation of the plug [28]. In our extensive experience with post-herniorrhaphy complications, plug-related problems remain a common theme and often require removal. While no technique is without issue or potential for complications, it is our opinion that the three-dimensional component of a plug is unnecessary with several other available options for open and laparoscopic inguinal hernia repairs.

Prolene Hernia System

The Prolene Hernia System (PHS) repair was developed by Gilbert in 1999 and is a two-layer mesh that allows prosthetic reinforcement both posterior and anterior to the transversalis fascia (Fig. 42.6). In case of an indirect hernia, the sac is dissected from the cord and the preperitoneal space accessed through the internal ring. For a direct hernia, the transversalis fascia is opened at the defect, providing access to the preperitoneal space. The preperitoneal space is then bluntly dissected to create space for the underlay portion of the bilayer mesh, which is then placed through the defect. The spermatic cord is placed through a slit in the onlay portion of the mesh, which functions similarly to the onlay mesh in a

Lichtenstein repair. Three to four circumferential interrupted sutures anchor the anterior layer of the mesh to the inguinal canal floor.

Because deployment of the PHS mesh requires blunt, blind dissection of the vascular preperitoneal space, these cases have a higher risk of bleeding and hematoma formation than traditional anterior repairs. Furthermore, because the deep layer of the device is not fixed in place, it may lead to folding, wrinkling, and meshoma formation (Fig. 42.7). Mesh migration and bowel-related complications have also been reported [29]. When properly executed, PHS repair is cost-effective, minimally invasive, and results are similarly favorable as compared to other mesh-based techniques. The deployment of the posterior fold of the mesh remains the challenge to obtain a good outcome and prevent complication, folding, or meshoma.

Open Preperitoneal Repairs

Open preperitoneal repair, initially referred to as giant prosthetic reinforcement of the visceral sac or GPRVS, was pioneered by Stoppa in 1973 [30] and has served as the anatomic basis for open and laparoscopic posterior repairs. Multiple open approaches to the preperitoneal space have been developed, including those described by Rives [31] and Kugel [32]. Variations such as the transinguinal preperitoneal (TIPP) approach and transrectus sheath preperitoneal repair have also recently been studied [33], and are discussed below. Preperitoneal repairs are ideally suited to address all defects of the myopectineal orifice including direct, indirect, and femoral hernias. However, the preperitoneal space is more challenging with potentially greater morbidity, and meticulous technique is crucial to ensure good outcomes and minimize complications. Adequate dissection can be attained through an open approach, but visualization may be limited by small incisions and minimally invasive "keyhole" approaches. While several open preperitoneal repair techniques have demonstrated good outcomes, safety, and efficacy in multiple studies, laparoscopy provides the greatest visualization to this space, leading to the popularity and wide adoption of TEP and TAPP over open preperitoneal repairs. This allows for adequate dissection and placement of the mesh over the entire myopectineal orifice with less risk of folding or improper positioning. Open preperitoneal techniques, however, can be performed under local anesthesia with lower cost, a lower learning curve, low morbidity, and comparable outcomes in experienced centers (Fig 42.8).

It should be noted that the placement of mesh posterior to the transversalis fascia, as occurs in these repairs and in all laparoscopic repairs, obliterates the spaces of Retzius and Bogros, and can complicate future urologic or vascular procedures, specifically radical prostatectomy (RP). Multiple series [34, 35] have shown that RP per-

formed following preperitoneal hernia repair is technically more difficult to perform, increases operative time, increases length of stay, and results in less adequate lymph node sampling. However, preperitoneal inguinal repair performed concurrently with RP has been shown to be safe and expeditious and is recommended [36–38].

Transinguinal Preperitoneal Repair

The TIPP repair, named by Schumpelick, is a recent modification to the Rives operation. The repair utilizes a self-expanding soft mesh and was first described by Pelissier in 2006 [33, 39, 40]. The TIPP technique begins with a standard open approach and isolation of the spermatic cord. The cremaster muscle is divided around the internal ring. For indirect hernias, high dissection of the sac is performed and the sac is reduced. For direct hernias, the transversalis fascia is divided circularly around the hernia bulge and the sac is reduced. The preperitoneal space is then bluntly dissected through the corresponding defect, medially in the direction of the pubic spine and laterally behind the epigastric vessels in direction of the iliac spine. The mesh is introduced through the defect into the preperitoneal space and then spread to cover all areas of weakness. Under local or regional anesthesia, the patient can be asked to cough or strain, which facilitates correct anatomical spreading of the mesh. A prospective randomized trial in two hospitals [41] found no significant differences in recurrence between Lichtenstein and TIPP repair at 1-year follow-up. A systematic review of three trials comparing Lichtenstein and TIPP likewise suggested similar results [42]. Because this approach invades both the inguinal canal and preperitoneal space with the attendant complications previously discussed, it is our preference to utilize a laparoscopic approach (TEP or TAPP) when performing a repair in the preperitoneal space. However, in dedicated, experienced centers, this technique is safe, cost-effective, and demonstrates excellent outcomes.

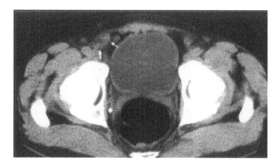

Fig. 42.8 CT Scan of a meshoma formed by wrinkling of the deep layer of a Bilayer PHS (Reproduced from [9])

Transrectus Sheath Preperitoneal Repair

Another variation of the aforementioned open preperitoneal techniques is the TREPP repair, a modification of a technique originally described in 1993 by Wantz as a unilateral Stoppa operation [43] which approaches the preperitoneal space through the anterior rectus sheath. This approach is begun with a 5-cm horizontal incision 1 cm superior to the pubic bone. The anterior rectus sheath (below the arcuate line) and transversalis fascia are opened and retracted medially. The inferior epigastric vessels are identified and retracted medially. The preperitoneal space is then dissected bluntly. Using three long, thin retractors, the preperitoneal space can be adequately visualized with views of the direct, indirect, and femoral areas. The iliac vessels, internal ring, spermatic cord, and testicular vessels are identified, and any hernias are reduced. A self-expandable mesh (Polysoft® "Large" BARD Benelux, Belgium) is then placed to cover the entire myopectineal orifice. Abdominal pressure and placement in this plane obviates the need for fixation. The anterior rectus sheath is closed with absorbable suture. The TREPP approach is compelling due to the avoidance of inguinal canal dissection and mesh fixation, but has yet to be widely studied [44]. The ENTREPPMENT trial [45] is a prospective RCT that will compare TREPP to TIPP. Similar to TIPP, it is our preference to approach the preperitoneal space laparoscopically to avoid blind dissection, ensure wide clearance of the myopectineal orifice, and optimize mesh placement. However, of the open preperitoneal repairs, this technique has the distinct advantage of minimizing nerve injury by avoiding the inguinal canal, and results in specialized centers have been excellent with regard to recurrence, pain, costs, and efficiency.

Discussion

While it is important for all practicing hernia surgeons to be familiar with how to execute the techniques described in this chapter, it is equally important to know and recognize the advantages and disadvantages of each as well. In terms of navigating the multitude of approaches available to the operating surgeon at large, we would point first to the most current consensus guidelines for hernia repair. The European Hernia Society (EHS) Guidelines state that "The Lichtenstein technique, introduced in 1984, is currently the best evaluated and most popular of the different open-mesh techniques: it is reproducible with minimal perioperative morbidity, it can be performed in day care (under local anesthesia) and has low recurrence rates (<4%) in the long term." [1] For this reason, all open approaches are compared relative to this gold standard technique. Our practice is comprised predominantly by the Lichtenstein approach for patients preferring an open operation or surgery under local anesthesia. The Lichtenstein is, furthermore, the most widely applicable and reproducible by surgeons at all levels of training.

In regard to open versus laparoscopic repairs, the EHS guidelines maintain that for primary unilateral and bilateral hernias both open and laparoscopic approaches are indicated, but with the significant caveat that the laparoscopic surgeon must be sufficiently experienced and have demonstrated a record of expertise with the technique. Both open and laparoscopic approaches using mesh have shown similar efficacy and are considered standard of care for primary unilateral or bilateral hernias [1]. In relation to laparoscopic repairs, open mesh repairs maintain several distinct advantages, the first of which is the option of performing the repair under regional or local anesthesia. For patients in whom the risks of general anesthesia are elevated, a repair under local anesthesia is ideal. Open repairs are much easier to learn and teach, as the learning curve for achieving proficiency with laparoscopic repairs is 50–100 cases [1]. Therefore, the European Hernia Society guidelines consider prosthetic open and laparoscopic approaches equally acceptable for primary repairs, contingent upon the operator having acquired sufficient experience. Both approaches have been demonstrated to be safe, but laparoscopic repairs have a small potential for visceral and major vessel injury. On the other hand, open techniques allow for direct visualization of all three nerves. This important technical consideration is unfortunately not uniformly practiced but minimizes the risk of chronic pain and injury. Studies have suggested that postoperative chronic pain is improved with laparoscopic repairs compared to open, but long-term data suggest the chronic pain rates are the same. What is known is that pain consequent to a posterior mesh placement can be more difficult to manage.

Among the open repairs, mesh is preferred to tissue, and Lichtenstein repair remains the gold standard, performing reliably in the hands of surgeons at large, in all settings. RCTs have been conducted or are ongoing to compare alternative open approaches to Lichtenstein, and all of those mentioned in this chapter have demonstrated their effectiveness [33, 39, 40]. Additionally, several of the open repairs discussed above have shown equivalent or improved outcomes in terms of chronic pain, recurrence, and ease of implementation.

In our own practice, we concur with the EHS recommendations and offer either an open Lichtenstein approach or laparoscopic total extraperitoneal repair for primary inguinal hernias. Patients are routinely counseled that both of these techniques have similar excellent outcomes without superiority of one technique over the other, especially with regard to the two primary outcomes of recurrence and chronic pain. Rather, each has different considerations and limitations. For patients that wish to avoid general anesthesia, those with increased cardiopulmonary risk, or prior lower abdominal surgery/prostatectomy, the open Lichtenstein approach minimizes the operative risk and has excellent outcomes for both unilateral and bilateral primary hernias. It is effective for all variations of inguinal hernia, but may be more challenging or require modification for femoral hernias or recurrence after prior anterior mesh repair. For primary bilateral hernias, recurrences after prior anterior repair, females, and known femoral hernias, the relative advantages of a laparoscopic approach (TEP/TAPP) are discussed and commonly accepted. In cases where mesh is either contraindicated or refused, we perform a Shouldice operation.

From our extensive experience with chronic pain and mesh complications, we are partial to the avoidance of three-dimensional meshes and those that cross both the anterior and posterior planes (plug, plug and patch, PHS). While they are effective techniques for the repair of hernia, remediation of complications is more problematic than those with the standard flat mesh used in Lichtenstein, TIPP, TREPP, and laparoscopic (TEP, TAPP) approaches. After treating thousands of patients with inguinodynia, recurrence, and mesh-based complications, it is important to clearly assert that all techniques (tissue, open, and laparoscopic) have complications and problems. That being said, everything that the individual surgeon can do to perfect his or her preferred technique will optimize personal results and patient outcomes. Regardless of the approach chosen, the fundamental principles underlying every successful hernia repair, that avoids both recurrence and chronic pain, are a profound understanding of the neuroanatomy of the inguinal canal and the use of a technique that results in the lowest possible amount of tension on native tissues.

References

1. Simons MP, Aufenacker T, Bay-Nielsen M, et al. European Hernia Society guidelines on the treatment of inguinal hernia in adult patients. Hernia. 2009;13(4):343–403.
2. McGillicuddy JE. Prospective randomized comparison of the Shouldice and Lichtenstein hernia repair procedures. Arch Surg. 1998;133:974–8.
3. Danielsson P, Isacson S, Hansen MV. Randomized study of Lichtenstein compared with Shouldice inguinal hernia repair by surgeons in training. Eur J Surg. 1999;165:49–53.
4. Nordin P, Bartelmess P, Jansson C, et al. Randomized trial of Lichtenstein versus Shouldice hernia repair general surgical practice. Br J Surg. 2002;89:45–9.
5. Stoppa R, Chevrel JP. Hernias and surgery of the abdominal wall. 2nd ed. New York: Springer; 1997.
6. Bendavid R, Chevrel JP. Hernias and surgery of the abdominal wall. 2nd ed. New York: Springer; 1997.
7. Desarda MP. Inguinal herniorrhaphy with an undetached strip of external oblique aponeurosis: new approach used in 400 patients. Eur J Surg. 2001;167:443–8.
8. Szopinski J, Dabrowiecki S, Pierscinski S, Jackowski M, Jaworski M, Szuflet Z. Desarda versus Lichtenstein

technique for primary inguinal hernia treatment: 3-year results of a randomized clinical trial. World J Surg. 2012;36(5):984–92.

9. Bloodgood JC. Operations on 459 cases of hernia in the Johns Hopkins Hospital from, June, 1889 to January, 1899. Baltimore: Friedenwald Co; 1899.

10. Losanoff JE, Millis JM. Aponeurosis instead of prosthetic mesh for inguinal hernia repair: neither physiological nor new. Hernia. 2006;10(2):198–9; author reply 200–2002.

11. Amid PK. Groin hernia repair: open techniques. World J Surg. 2005;29(8):1046–51.

12. Amid PK, Shulman AG, Lichtenstein IL. Critical scrutiny of the open tension-free hernioplasty. Am J Surg. 1993;165:369–71.

13. Amid PK. Causes, prevention, and surgical treatment of post- herniorrhaphy neuropathic inguinodynia: triple neurectomy with proximal end implantation. Hernia. 2004;8:343–9.

14. Lichtenstein IL, Shore JM. Simplified repair of femoral and recurrent inguinal hernias by a "plug" technic. Am J Surg. 1976;132:121.

15. Gilbert AI. Sutureless repair of inguinal hernia. Am J Surg. 1992;163:331–5.

16. Rutkow IM, Robbins AW. "Tension-free" inguinal herniorrhaphy: a preliminary report on the "mesh plug" technique. Surgery. 1993;114:3–8.

17. Chuback JA, Singh RS, Sills C, et al. Small bowel obstruction resulting from mesh plug migration after open inguinal hernia repair. Surgery. 2000;127:475–6.

18. Tokunaga Y, Tokuka A, Oshumi K. Sigmoid colon diverticulosis adherent to mesh plug migration after open inguinal hernia repair. Curr Surg. 2001;58:493–4.

19. Benedetti M, Albertario S, Niebel T, et al. Intestinal perforation as a long-term complication of plug and mesh inguinal hernioplasty: case report. Hernia. 2005;9:93–5.

20. Murphy JW, Misra DC, Silverglide B. Sigmoid colonic fistula secondary to Perfix plug left inguinal hernia repair. Hernia. 2006;10:436–8.

21. Zubaidi A, Al Saghier M, Kabbani M, Abdo A. Colocutaneous fistula after mesh plug inguinal hernia repair—a delayed complication. Ann Saudi Med. 2006;26:385–7.

22. Stout CL, Foret A, Christie DB, Mullis E. Small bowel volvulus caused by migrating mesh plug. Am Surg. 2007;73:796–7.

23. Ishiguro Y, Horie H, Satih H, Miyakura Y, Yasuda Y, Lefor AT. Colocutaneous fistula after left inguinal hernia repair using the mesh plug technique. Surgery. 2009;145:120–1.

24. Moorman ML, Price PD. Migrating mesh plug: complication of well-established hernia repair technique. Am Surg. 2004;70:298–9.

25. Yamamoto S, Kubota T, Abe T. A rare case of mechanical bowel obstruction caused by mesh plug migration. Hernia. 2014;19(6):983–5.

26. Amid PK. Classification of biomaterials and their related complications in abdominal wall hernia surgery. Hernia. 1997;1:12–9.

27. Dieter RA. Mesh plug migration into scrotum: a new complication of hernia repair. Int Surg. 1999;84:57–9.

28. Kingsnorth AN, Hyland ME, Porter CA, et al. Prospective double- blind randomized study comparing Perfix plug-and-patch with Lichtenstein patch in inguinal hernia repair: one year quality of life results. Hernia. 2000;4:255–8.

29. Lo DJ, Bilimoria KY, Pugh CM. Bowel complication after prolene hernia system (PHS) repair: a case report and review of the literature. Hernia. 2008;12:437–40.

30. Stoppa R, Petit J, Abourachid H, Henry X, Duclaye C, Monchaux G, Hillebrant JP. Original procedure of groin hernia repair: interposition without fixation of Dacron tulle prosthesis by subperitoneal median approach. Chirurgie. 1973;99:119–23.

31. Rives J, Lardennois B, Flament JB, Convers G. The Dacron mesh sheet, treatment of choice of inguinal hernias in adults. Apropos of 183 cases. Chirurgie. 1973;99:564–75.

32. Kugel RD. Minimally invasive, nonlaparoscopic, preperitoneal, and sutureless, inguinal herniorrhaphy. Am J Surg. 1999;178:298–302.

33. Pélissier EP, Blum D, Ngo P, Monek O. Transinguinal preperitoneal repair with the Polysoft patch: prospective evaluation of recurrence and chronic pain. Hernia. 2008;12:51–6.

34. Peeters E, Joniau S, Van Poppel H, Miserez M. Case-matched analysis of outcome after open retropubic radical prostatectomy in patients with previous preperitoneal inguinal hernia repair. Br J Surg. 2012;99(3):431–5.

35. Haifler M, Benjamin B, Ghinea R, Avital S. The impact of previous laparoscopic inguinal hernia repair on radical prostatectomy. J Endourol. 2012;26(11):1458–62.

36. Brunocilla E, Vece E, Lupo S, et al. Preperitoneal prosthetic mesh hernioplasty for the simultaneous repair of inguinal hernia during prostatic surgery: experience with 172 patients. Urol Int. 2005;75(1):38–42.

37. Antunes AA, Dall'oglio M, Crippa A, Srougi M. Inguinal hernia repair with polypropylene mesh during radical retropubic prostatectomy: an easy and practical approach. BJU Int. 2005;96(3):330–3.

38. Savetsky IL, Rabbani F, Singh K, Brady MS. Preperitoneal repair of inguinal hernia at open radical prostatectomy. Hernia. 2009;13(5):517–22.

39. Pélissier E, Ngo P. Subperitoneal inguinal hernioplasty by anterior approach, using a memory-ring patch. Preliminary results. Ann Chir. 2006;131:590–4.

40. Koning GG, de Schipper HJ, Oostvogel HJ, Verhofstad MH, Gerritsen PG, van Laarhoven KC, et al. The Tilburg double blind randomised controlled trial comparing inguinal hernia repair according to Lichtenstein and the transinguinal preperitoneal technique. Trials. 2009;10:89.

41. Koning GG, Keus F, Koeslag L, Cheung CL, Avçi M, van Laarhoven CJHM, Vriens PWHE. Randomized clinical trial of chronic pain after the transinguinal preperitoneal technique compared with Lichtenstein's method for inguinal hernia repair. Br J Surg. 2012;99:1365–73.

42. Willaert W, De Bacquer D, Rogiers X, Troisi R, Berrevoet F. Open preperitoneal techniques versus Lichtenstein repair for elective inguinal hernias. Cochrane Database Syst Rev. 2012;7:CD008034.

43. Wantz GE. Technique of properitoneal hernioplasty. Unilateral reinforcement of the visceral sac with Mersilene giant prosthesis. Chirurgie. 1994;119(6–7): 321–6.

44. Koning GG, Andeweg CS, Keus F, van Tilburg MWA, van Laarhoven CJHM, Akkersdijk WL. The transrectus sheath preperitoneal mesh repair for inguinal hernia: technique, rationale, and results of the first 50 cases. Hernia. 2012;16(3):295–9.

45. Prins MW, Koning GG, Keus EF, et al. Study protocol for a randomized controlled trial for anterior inguinal hernia repair: transrectus sheath preperitoneal mesh repair compared to transinguinal preperitoneal procedure. Trials. 2013;14:65.

Sergio Roll and James Skinovsky

Introduction

Laparoscopic repair of inguinal and femoral hernia is increasingly popular because they offer the potential for less postoperative pain and a quick return to normal activities [1]. When performing laparoscopic inguinal or femoral hernia repair, the hernia defect is approached from its posterior aspect and the repair involves placing mesh in the preperitoneal space. The anatomic approach to the preperitoneal space depends upon the laparoscopic technique used for hernia repair. The two commonly used approaches to laparoscopic repair of inguinal and femoral hernias are the transabdominal preperitoneal hernia repair

(TAPP) and the totally extraperitoneal hernia repair (TEP) approaches.

Laparoscopic transabdominal preperitoneal hernia repair (TAPP) is discussed here.

Patient preference plays perhaps the greatest role in the choice of one type of repair over another; however, surgical expertise plays a key part as well. Data show that the recurrence rate drops significantly as surgeons gain experience with the laparoscopic technique. The learning curve for laparoscopic hernia repair is prolonged with most estimates ranging between 50 and 75 procedures. However, when performed by an experienced surgeon (>75 repairs), hernia recurrence is low [2]. The learning curve of TAPP groin hernia repair is longer than in open procedures and some studies suggest that the learning curve for TEP may be as high as 250 cases [3].

It is generally believed that TAPP is easier to teach and learn, although there is no level 1 evidence in the literature to support this belief.

Both minimally invasive techniques are considered effective approaches to recurrent hernia following open repair; however, adequate experience is recommended [2].

According to several systematic reviews comparing TAPP and TEP, both methodologies seem to be more effective than open hernia repair, although there is not yet sufficient evidence to recommend the use of TAPP rather than TEP [4].

Electronic supplementary material: The online version of this chapter (doi:10.1007/978-3-319-27470-6_43) contains supplementary material, which is available to authorized users.

S. Roll, M.D., Ph.D. (✉)
Division of General Surgery, Center of Abdominal Wall Surgery, Santa Casa of São Paulo, São Paulo, SP, Brazil

School of Medical Science Santa Casa of São Paulo, São Paulo, SP, Brazil
e-mail: sroll@uol.com.br

J. Skinovsky, M.D., Ph.D.
Positivo University, Curitiba, Paraná, Brazil

Surgical Residence of the Red Cross Hospital, Curitiba, Paraná, Brazil

Why Choose the TAPP Procedure

1. TAPP enables a thorough intra-abdominal examination,
2. Provides visualization of both inguinal regions (Occult hernia—For patients in whom a groin hernia is suspected but has been difficult to confirm on imaging studies, a TAPP approach may offer a better view to determine the presence and location of the hernia)
3. As soon as you enter at the abdominal cavity, even without dissecting the peritoneum—you can see the anatomy landmarks
4. Permits thorough exploration of the entire myopectineal orifice
5. Allows visualization of incarcerated hernias and evaluation of possibly strangulated tissue
6. Prior pelvic surgery—In the setting of prior preperitoneal pelvic dissection, it may not be possible to develop the proper exposure purely extraperitoneal
7. Easier in females with indirect inguinal hernia, because the sac is frequently more intimately attached to the round ligament
8. Is easily taught and learned.

Contraindication to the TAPP Technique

Absolute contraindications are few. In general, the inability to tolerate general anesthesia, though there are reports of spinal anesthesia being used for this procedure. Other prohibitive patient factors include coagulopathy and intra-abdominal infections that would preclude the use of a prosthetic mesh [5].

Relative contraindications include previous abdominal surgery, especially pelvic surgery and previous radical prostatectomy (more difficult and carry a higher morbidity). In a large Brazilian Multicenter trial, 8549 TAPP hernias were performed in 6955 patients and with only 2.3% intraoperative complications, with bladder injury being most common.

NOTE: Large inguinoscrotal hernias can be challenging to manage because reducing these indirect sacs laparoscopically can be difficult, so we usually prefer an open Lichtenstein technique [6].

Preoperative Evaluation and Preparation

Preoperative preparation includes thromboprophylaxis and prophylactic antibiotics. To minimize the risk of bladder injury, the bladder should be emptied before surgery. In cases of potential difficult surgery, we place a bladder catheter prior to the beginning of the case [7].

OR Preparation to the Repair

Equipment

Appropriate instrumentation and supplies should be readily available, and the proper functioning of laparoscopic imaging equipment verified prior to initiating anesthesia. In recent years, I have been using a 5-mm 30° laparoscope, two 5-mm trocars, and one 10/12-mm trocar.

Choice of the Mesh

Lightweight mesh has been compared with heavyweight, and the recent data has demonstrated some benefit in lightweight mesh. Lightweight mesh has been shown to result in reduced chronic groin pain, although there was no associated increase in quality of life [8]. My preference is to use a macroporous lightweight polypropylene mesh ($35–45$ g/m^2). The size depends on the anatomy and the type of hernia defect encountered during dissection. The available mesh sizes are 15×15 cm and 30×30 cm. Although in most cases the mesh size used is 15×12 cm, in some recurrent hernia cases, we use a larger mesh (17×14 cm) [9].

The size should be large enough to produce a wide overlap beyond the defect's edges. The mesh can either be flat and rectangular or preformed to fit the myopectineal orifice.

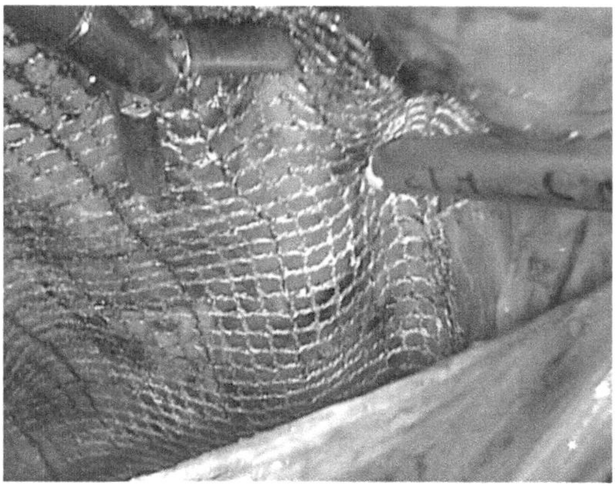

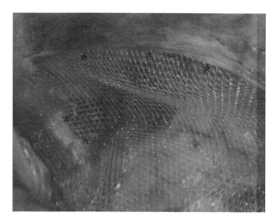

Fig. 43.1 Left side—mesh fixation with absorbable mechanic device

Fig. 43.2 Right Side—mesh fixation (the stars denote attachment points)

In general, a standard polypropylene or polyester uncoated mesh is used for laparoscopic repairs, because the mesh will be covered by peritoneum, and as such isolated from the intra-abdominal cavity. When faced with a thin or brittle peritoneum which is difficult to close and cannot be repaired, a coated polypropylene or polyester meshes or other meshes, approved for intra-abdominal applications, should be used [10].

NOTE: In cases of bilateral hernias, due to the difficulty in handling and positioning the light-weight mesh, a single large mesh covering both defects can be used.

Mesh Fixation

Although some surgeons support nonfixation of mesh, we suggest mesh fixation during TAPP procedure to avoid mesh migration and mesh shrinkage. We utilize absorbable staples or fibrin glue for mesh fixation [11] (Fig. 43.1).

Stapling or tacking injuries to the nerves are the most common source of postoperative neuralgia following laparoscopic hernia repair. This complication should be suspected if severe groin pain develops in the recovery room and during the immediate postoperative period. Although the nerves are essentially never seen during laparoscopic hernia repair, nerve injuries can be prevented by following some strategies: avoid stapling below the ileopubic tract and lateral to

the gonadal vessels (the lateral cutaneous nerve and the femoral branch of genitofemoral nerve are the two nerves vulnerable to trauma) as well as avoiding dissection of the nerves and leaving them in direct contact with the mesh [12].

NOTE: During recent years, with increasing concern for the chronic postoperative pain, we have significantly decreased the number of fixations on the mesh, and today I have used an average of four/five positions tacks (Fig. 43.2).

Technique for Repair

Patient and Team Position

The patient is positioned supine with both arms tucked. During the procedure, the patients are shifted in 15–20° of Trendelenburg position to improve exposure of the working area and to move the small bowel away from the area of dissection.

The surgeon should stand on the opposite side of the defect to be corrected; surgical nurse should be in front of the surgeon, and the assistant with the camera near the patient's head, on the same side of the surgeon. Alternatively, the assistant can stand on the same side as a hernia, provided that the camera is positioned through the port on the ipsilateral side as well. The monitor is placed at the foot of the operating bed (Fig. 43.3).

Fig. 43.3 Patient and time position

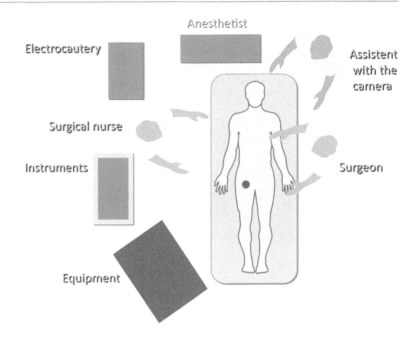

Operative Steps for the Transabdominal Preperitoneal Repair

Access of the peritoneal cavity is achieved using standard techniques with a Veress needle to create the pneumoperitoneum. An incision at the supra umbilicus is then made for placement of a 5 mm trocar (I use a 5 mm 30° laparoscope). Once access to the peritoneal cavity has been established, an inspection of the abdominal cavity is made in search of other affections.

We place two additional trocars bilaterally in a horizontal plane with the umbilicus. This moment requires additional care in order to avoid injury of the superficial epigastric vessels. This can be facilitated through their visualization by means of abdominal wall transillumination [13] (Fig. 43.4).

NOTE: The major advantage of the posterior approach to groin hernias is that all three hernia defects (direct, indirect, and femoral) are well-visualized.

Using a 5 mm, 30-degree angled laparoscope, the groin anatomy is inspected. The inferior epigastric vessels, the internal inguinal ring with the spermatic vessels, and the vas deferens should be

identified. These three structures form the so-called *Mercedes-Benz star*. This easy identification is done by transparency through the peritoneum [14] Fig. 43.5a, b).

The peritoneum is incised 4–5 cm above the hernia defect or internal ring, from the edge of the median umbilical ligament toward the anterior superior iliac spine. Often, at the opening of the peritoneum, we have a tendency to fall toward the region of the nerves. Therefore, before making the incision, mark three points: median umbilical ligament, anterior superior iliac spine, and the line between the two (Figs. 43.6 and 43.7) Dissection is performed in the preperitoneal avascular plane between the peritoneum and the transversalis fascia to provide visualization of the myopectineal orifices. It is very important not to dissect preperitoneal fat from sensitive structures, like psoas muscle and nerves.

After dissection of the preperitoneal space, a surgeon should be able to identify the inferior epigastric vessels, vas deferens, spermatic cord, iliac vessels, bladder, psoas, nerves location, and hernia defects. It is important to make a wide dissection sufficiently above and medial to the hernia defect to allow a 3–4 cm of normal fascia to provide sufficient mesh overlap (Fig. 43.8).

Fig. 43.4   Trocar position

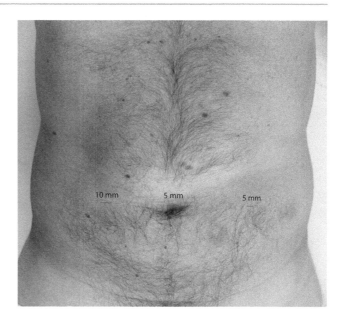

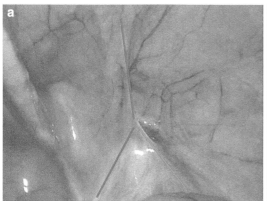

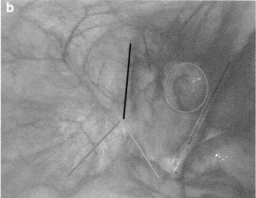

Fig. 43.5 (**a**) Right side—inferior epigastric vessels, spermatic vessels, and the vas deferens ("Mercedes-Benz star"). (**b**) Left side—inferior epigastric vessels, spermatic vessels, vas deferens, median umbilical ligament, and direct hernia

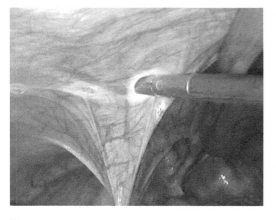

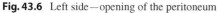

Fig. 43.6   Left side—opening of the peritoneum

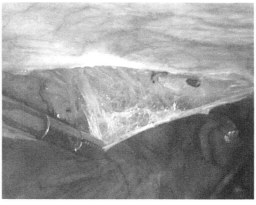

Fig. 43.7   Left side—opening of the peritoneum

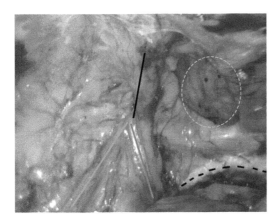

Fig. 43.8 Left side—preperitoneal space dissected

For an indirect hernia, the cord structures are isolated and dissected free from the surrounding tissues. In the process, the indirect hernia sac is identified, usually found on the anterolateral side of the cord and adherent to it. When separating the sac from the cord, it is important to handle the vas deferens and the spermatic vessels with care to minimize trauma. If the sac is sufficiently small, it should be completely dissected free from the cord and returned to the peritoneal cavity. Occasionally, a large sac will be encountered, in which case it should be dissected and may be divided beyond the internal ring, with the resultant peritoneal defect closed with a suture or endoloop. The distal end of the transected sac should be left open to avoid formation of a hydrocele or hematic cyst [15].

Direct hernia sacs are typically easier to reduce than indirect sacs. Once the preperitoneal space has been dissected out laterally, the direct hernia defect is addressed by separating the peritoneum from the overlying myopectineal orifice. When reducing the direct hernia sac, a "pseudosac" may be present, which is transversalis fascia that overlies and adheres to the peritoneum and invaginates into the preperitoneal space during the dissection. This layer must be separated from the true hernia sac in order for the peritoneum to be released back fully into the peritoneal cavity. Once the pseudosac is freed, it will typically retract anteriorly into the direct hernia defect. We must always alert surgeons who are starting in the TAPP technique, that the "pseudosac" is the

"sick" transversalis fascia and not the true hernia sac. At this time, before placing the mesh, I fix the transversalis fascia ("pseudosac") in the anterior abdominal wall in order to prevent seroma formation at this site postoperatively (Fig. 43.9a–c).

The mesh (sized at least 15×12 cm) is then rolled and placed in the preperitoneal space to cover the entire myopectineal orifices, including the direct, indirect, and femoral hernia spaces. For the direct hernias, my concerns about recurrences is greater and I dissect further toward the midline and I also have a tendency to use large meshes and additional fixation (Fig. 43.10).

NOTE: Some surgeons slit the mesh longitudinally or vertically to accommodate the cord structures, however, I prefer to simply place the mesh over the cord.

I always fixate the mesh, most often with absorbable staples and some cases with fibrin glue. The landmarks for fixation of the mesh are the pubic tubercle, Cooper's ligament, posterior rectus sheath, and the transversalis fascia at least 3 cm above the hernia defect and the anterior superior iliac spine to prevent movement of the mesh. When fixating the mesh laterally with tacks or staples, it is important to feel the tip of the device on the outside of the abdomen with the opposite hand to ensure that fixation occurs above the inguinal ligament. The mesh should cover the entire posterior floor of the groin and since it can shrink between 10 and 30%, the mesh should not be fully stretched, but having a little "slack" [16].

NOTE: Do not tack or staple the mesh below the iliopubic tract lateral to the spermatic cord and the epigastric vessels to minimize the chance of damaging nerves and vascular structures. This area contains the "triangle of pain," which contains the lateral cutaneous nerve of the thigh and the femoral branch of the genitofemoral nerve, and the adjacent "triangle of doom," which contains the external iliac artery and vein defined medially by the vas deferens and laterally by the spermatic vessels (Fig. 43.11).

After the mesh is positioned, the peritoneum is re-closed with a running suture or tacks. It is important to leave no gaps in the peritoneum to isolate the mesh from the viscera and to minimize the risk of small bowel herniation and obstruc-

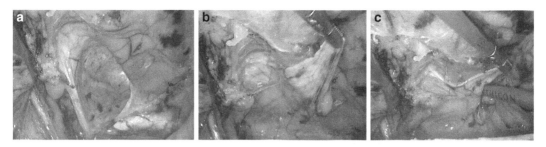

Fig. 43.9 (**a**) Left side—direct hernia. (**b**) Left side—"Pseudosac" is the "sick" transversalis fascia. (**c**) Left side—fixation the transversalis fascia ("pseudosac") in the anterior abdominal wall

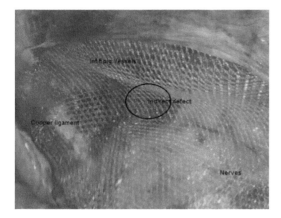

Fig. 43.10 Right side—mesh position and visualization of anatomy by transparency

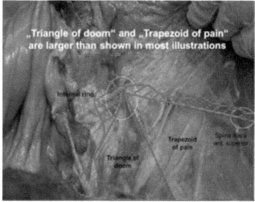

Fig. 43.11 Right side—triangle of doom and trapezoid of pain. Posterior anatomy of the inguinal nerves – a study on 30 fixed cadavers Wolfgang Reinpold, M.D., Wilhelmsburg Gross Sand Hospital and Hernia Center, Hamburg, Germany (in press).

tion in the gaps/peritoneal fenestrations [17] (Fig. 43.12a, b).

The mechanism of recurrences after TAPP is inferiorly, due to insufficient coverage of the inferior edge of the myopectineal orifice or due to mesh migration. It is thus very important to confirm mesh positioning during closure and desufflation, because it can fold on itself by the inferior peritoneal flap during suturing. The ports are removed under direct vision and the abdominal cavity is decompressed. The fascia at the 10 mm cannula should be sutured to reduce the chance for future incisional hernia.

Postoperative Care and Follow-up

Most laparoscopic hernia repairs are performed on an outpatient basis. Postoperative pain is usually well-controlled using nonsteroidal anti-inflammatory agents (NSAIDS), if not contraindicated, with or without low-dose narcotic agents. I recommend an ice pack to be used four times a day, in the inguinal region, for 2 days and local heat for the next 2 days. I maintain the use of a groin hernia support (Tensor) for up to a month.

Complications

As with any hernia repair, postoperative complications are possible. There are two sorts of complications: corresponding to the laparoscopic technique and procedure-correlated.

Morbidity is usually low after a TAPP procedure. R. Bittner in his article, Laparoscopic transperitoneal procedure for routine repair of groin hernia, published at BJS, 2002 reported a rate of 2.6% [18].

Between February 1991 and April 2001, I treated 803 patients: 445 (55.4%) with TAPP and 358 (44.6%) with TEP. The incidence of intraop-

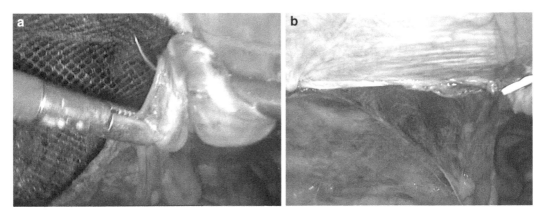

Fig. 43.12 (**a**) Right side—start closure of the peritoneal flap (running suture). (**b**) Right side—final aspect of running suture

erative complications was 2.8%, and the most serious complication was injury of the bladder in one case. The postoperative complications were present in 235 (29.6%) patients. There were 10 (1.2%) relapses; 9 cases in the TAPP, and one in the TEP group.

NOTE: In my experience, inguinoscrotal hernias show a significantly higher rate of complications such as seromas, postoperative pain, bleeding, injury to the deferens, and orchiditis.

Recommendation

	TAPP	TEP
Routine		X
Prior Abdominal Surgery		X
Bilateral Hernia		X
Inguinoscrotal hernia	X	
Incarcerated hernia	X	
Hernia & Diagnosis	X	
Recurrent hernia	X	
Hernia and cholecystectomy		X
Prior preperitoneal surgery	X	
Contraindication–general anesthesia		X

TAPP is an effective and safe technique. It can be performed in a standard way for all inguinal and femoral hernias. It is simple to learn and easy to teach.

References

1. Kavic M, Roll S. Laparoscopic transabdominal preperitoneal hernia repair (TAPP). In: Bendavid R, Abrahamson J, Arregui M, Flament J, Phillips E, editors. Abdominal wall hernias—principles and management. New York: Springer; 2001. p. 454–63.
2. Bittner R, Arregui ME, Bisgaard T, Dudai M, Ferzli GS, Fitzgibbons RJ, et al. Surg Endosc. 2011;25(9): 2773–843.
3. Edwards CC, Bailey RW. Laparoscopic hernia repair: the learning curve. Surg Laparosc Endosc Percutan Tech. 2000;10(3):149–53. (Neumayer L, Giobbie-Hurder A, Jonasson O, Fitzgibbons R Jr, Dunlop D, Gibbs J, et al. Open mesh versus laparoscopic mesh repair of inguinal hernia. N Engl J Med. Apr 29 2004;350(18):1819-27.
4. Cavazzola LT, Rosen MJ. Surg Clin N Am. 2013;93: 1269–79.
5. Zacharoulis D, Fafoulakis F, Baloyiannis I, Sioka E, Georgopoulou S, Pratsas C, Hantzi E, Tzovaras G. Laparoscopic transabdominal preperitoneal repair of inguinal hernia under spinal anesthesia: a pilot study. Am J Surg. 2009;198(3):456–9.
6. Agresta F, Mazzarolo G, Balbi P, Bedin N. Inguinal-scrotal hernias in young patients: is laparoscopic repair a possible answer? Preliminary results of a single-institution experience with a transabdominal preperitoneal approach. Hernia. 2010;14(5):471–5.
7. McCormack K, Wake BL, Fraser C, et al. Transabdominal pre-peritoneal (TAPP) versus totally extraperitoneal (TEP) laparoscopic techniques for inguinal hernia repair: a systematic review. Hernia. 2005;9(2):109–14.
8. Nikkolo C, Lepner U, Murrus M, Vaasna T, Seepter H, Tikk T. Randomised clinical trial comparing light-weight mesh with heavyweight mesh for inguinal hernioplasty. Hernia. 2010;14(3):253–8.

9. Cobb WS, Kercher KW, Heniford BT. The argument for lightweight polypropylene mesh in hernia repair. Surg Innov. 2005;12(1):63–9.

10. Hatzitheofilou C, Lakhoo M, Sofianos C, Levy RD, Velmahos G, Saadia R. Laparoscopic inguinal hernia repair by an intraperitoneal onlay mesh technique using expanded PTFE: a prospective study. Surg Laparosc Endosc. 1997;7(6):451–5.

11. Kapiris S, Mavromatis T, Andrikopoulos S, et al. Laparoscopic transabdominal preperitoneal hernia repair (TAPP): stapling the mesh is not mandatory. J Laparoendosc Adv Surg Tech A. 2009;19:419.

12. Drake RL, Vogl AW, Mitchell AWM. Gray's Anatomy for Students. Philadelphia: Churchill-Livingstone; 2004. p. 258–65.

13. Roll S, dePaula A, Miguel P, Carim J, Campos FG, Hashiba K. Transabdominal laparoscopic hernioplasty using preperitonial mesh. In: Radcliffe R, editor. Inguinal hernia advances or controversies? Oxford: Oxford University Press; 1994. p. 261–4.

14. Spaw AT, Ennis BW, Spaw LP. Laparoscopic hernia repair: the anatomic basis. J Laparoendosc Surg. 1991;1(5):269–77.

15. Bittner R, Leibl BJ, Jäger C, Kraft B, Ulrich M, Schwarz J. TAPP—Stuttgart technique and result of a large single center series. J Minim Access Surg. 2006;2(3):155–9.

16. Richards SK, Vipond MN, Earnshaw JJ. Review of the management of recurrent inguinal hernia. Hernia. 2004;8(2):144–8.

17. Ross SW, Oommen B, Kim M, Walters A, Augenstein V, Heniford BT. Tacks, staples, or suture: method of peritoneal closure in laparoscopic transabdominal preperitoneal inguinal hernia repair effects early quality of life. Surg Endosc. 2015; 29(7):1686–93.

18. Bittner R, Schmedt C-G, Schwarz J, Kraft K, Leibl BJ. Laparoscopic transperitoneal procedure for routine repair of groin hernia. Br J Surg. 2002;89(8): 1062–6.

Tammy Kindel and Dmitry Oleynikov

Introduction to Total Extra-peritoneal Inguinal Hernia Repair

Laparoscopic total extra-peritoneal (TEP) has gained popularity over the past 15 years as an acceptable alternative to the open Lichtenstein repair for the surgical treatment of initial, unilateral inguinal hernias given the similar recurrence risk and decreased post-operative pain, early ambulation and return to work [1, 2]. Initial results of both TEP and TAPP compared to an open, tension-free repair for inguinal hernias were disappointing due to higher recurrence and complication rates with a laparoscopic (10.1 and 39%) compared to open repair (4.9 and 33.4%) at 2 years [4]. However, further studies looking specifically at TEP have shown a similar recurrence rate to the open, Lichtenstein repair [5, 6]. A recent meta-analysis using bias evaluation and trial sequence analysis of randomized controlled trials found no difference in recurrent rates between TEP and the open approach [6]. Early post-operative pain as well as long-term moderate and severe chronic pain is reduced when a TEP is performed compared to an open, tension-free repair [7–9].

It is now believed that one of the primary reasons for inferior early results with TEP compared to open or TAPP repairs is due to the steep learning curve required in TEP [10, 11]. There is an initial critical learning curve of approximately 30–50 cases with TEP due to the unfamiliar anatomic orientation encountered in the pre-peritoneal space as well as limited working space [12, 13]. Even after 50 cases, while the recurrence rate and number of intraoperative complications are not significantly affected, the operative time, conversion rate, and post-operative complications may continue to improve up to 250 cases [14]. Beyond operating with an experienced laparoscopic inguinal hernia surgeon, novices may be able to shorten their learning curve with the use of simulation-based training as well as using a Stoppa's pre-peritoneal approach, if converting to open, to increase anatomic familiarity [13, 15]. Further, careful patient selection may be advised for the surgeon gaining experience with TEP including selection of young, thin male patients with a unilateral, non-scrotal hernia and without prior abdominal surgery [16].

Electronic supplementary material: The online version of this chapter (doi:10.1007/978-3-319-27470-6_44) contains supplementary material, which is available to authorized users.

T. Kindel, M.D., Ph.D. (✉) • D. Oleynikov, M.D.
Department of Surgery, University of Nebraska Medical Center, 986245 Nebraska Medical Center, Omaha, NE 68198-6245, USA
e-mail: tammy.kindel@unmc.edu; doleynik@unmc.edu

Patient Selection for TEP Repair

Indications

As mentioned previously, TEP is an excellent option for a recurrent inguinal hernia following an open repair or for bilateral inguinal hernias. Given surgeon preference, TEP is also an appropriate choice for an initial, unilateral inguinal hernia as long as the patient can tolerate general anesthesia and has no contraindications, as discussed below, with the added advantage of exploring for an occult, contralateral inguinal hernia [3].

Contraindications

Any patient who cannot tolerate general anesthesia and would be better served with local, sedation, or a spinal anesthetic is not an appropriate candidate for TEP. Chronically incarcerated and scrotal hernias have traditionally been a contra-indication to laparoscopic repair. However, these hernias can be repaired successfully by TEP in experienced hands. Modifications from a traditional TEP should include mandatory Foley catheter placement to allow for full development of the space of Retzius as well as surgeon comfort with ligating the epigastric vessels, if needed, as well as knowledge on how to incise the transversalis fascial sling to aid in indirect hernia sac reduction [17].

For acute incarcerations, high suspicion of ischemia is a contraindication for the TEP approach. If there are no concerning signs of bowel compromise, a TEP approach can be considered. Similarly to treatment of other chronically incarcerated hernias, the use of a relaxing incision is often needed in the acute situation for sac content reduction. For direct hernias, an anteriomedial incision can be directed toward the rectus, carefully avoiding injury to the epigastric and iliac vessels. The relaxing incision for the indirect space is performed in the transversalis fascial sling and in the lacunar ligament and/or anteriomedial iliopubic tract for femoral hernias [18]. We advocate opening the sac in all cases of acute incarceration or new obstruction to ensure bowel viability and inspect the transition point if present. The sac and peritoneum can then be closed and the intra-peritoneal gas evacuated to maintain pre-peritoneal visualization.

We also recommend an open approach over TEP-IHR for patients who have had prior violation of the pre-peritoneal space such as occurs after prostatectomy [19].

Technical Considerations of TEP-IHR

(a) *Development of the pre-peritoneal space.* The patient is positioned on the operating table supine with both arms tucked and appropriately padded. A Foley catheter is placed, if it is a known recurrent hernia or large scrotal hernia; otherwise, the patient can void just prior to entering the operating room and avoid Foley catheter insertion. An infra-umbilical, curvilinear incision is made in the midline. This is extended to the anterior rectus sheath. The anterior rectus sheath is divided just off the midline of the affected side with reflection of the rectus muscle proper laterally. With this, the posterior sheath is exposed and the initial blunt dissection can be performed with a finger sweeping the rectus muscle laterally and anteriorly. Care should be taken to enter the retro-rectus space at the most medial aspect of the rectus belly to prevent muscle bleeding. A curved S or Army–Navy retractor can then be placed within the pre-peritoneal space to aid in passage of a lubricated dissecting balloon. The dissecting balloon should be inserted with only gentle force in the direction of the pubis. Once the pubis is reached, we place the balloon just inferior to the bone and insufflate the dissecting balloon under camera visualization. The dissector is then removed with the trocar left in place with an inflatable balloon tip and the pre-peritoneal space insufflated with carbon dioxide to an insufflating pressure of 15 mmHg. A 45° 10-mm laparoscope aids in enhancing the view of the pre-peritoneal inguinal space. Two 5 mm trocars are then placed in the midline. The first is placed in the supra-pubic location and the second just inferior to the trocar balloon.

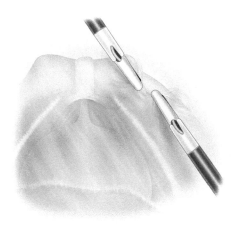

Fig. 44.1 Blunt dissection of the bladder and alveolar tissue inferiorly to expose the pubis and Cooper's ligament

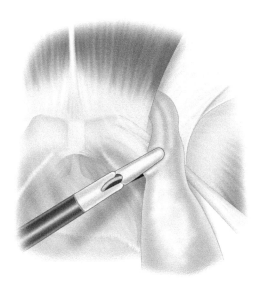

Fig. 44.2 Once Cooper's ligament is exposed laterally reaching the femoral vessels, any fibro-fatty tissue remaining superior to Cooper's represents a direct hernia

(b) *Exposure of the pubic tubercle and Cooper's ligament*. Initial dissection is done with blunt graspers to expose the pubic bone in the midline and Cooper's ligament (Fig. 44.1). The bladder should be gently dissected posteriorly off the pubic bone to avoid injury during mesh placement. Caution should be made for the crossing blood vessels over the pubic bone to prevent significant venous bleeding.

(c) *Identification of a Femoral and Direct Hernia*. If a hernia is identified before reaching the femoral vein while traveling laterally on Cooper's ligament, this represents a femoral hernia. At times, lacunar's ligament will need to be divided medio-superiorly to allow for femoral content reduction. If no femoral hernia is identified, as shown in Fig. 44.2, any fibro-fatty tissue remaining superior to Cooper's ligament lies within the direct space and may represent a direct hernia. This tissue should be cleared and the transversalis fascia identified. If a large direct hernia is found, the pseudo-sac of the weak transversalis fascia can be secured to Cooper's ligament with a tack to potentially reduce the occurrence of a post-operative seroma.

(d) *Identification of an Indirect Hernia*. The lateral space is fully dissected to allow for future mesh placement. Exposure of the abdominal wall muscle may result in bleeding and care should be taken to stay within the alveolar space to minimize muscle and nerve injury leaving pre-peritoneal fat on the anterior abdominal wall. With completion of dissection both medial and lateral to the internal ring, the cord contents are grasped and retracted laterally. This allows for early identification and protection of the vas deferens and spermatic cord vessels, which will be found medially (Fig. 44.3). The vas and vessels are fully separated from the indirect hernia sac. Once the indirect hernia sac has been isolated, both graspers are placed on the hernia sac and the contents fully reduced with the medial hand applying counter traction to the internal ring.

(e) *Mesh placement*. We prefer to use a lightweight, macro-porous, permanent mesh sized to cover the direct, indirect, and femoral hernia spaces. After insertion through the 12 mm umbilical trocar, the mesh is unrolled and positioned within the pre-peritoneal space. The medial aspect of the mesh should be positioned along the pubic bone at least 1 cm off the midline to the opposite side to give adequate coverage of the direct space.

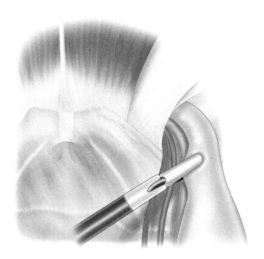

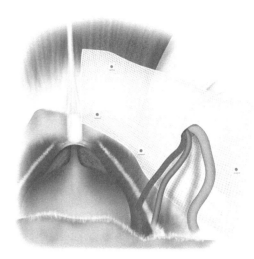

Fig. 44.3 The cord contents are retracted laterally with identification of the vas deferens and cord vessels medially

Fig. 44.5 The mesh is positioned laterally to accommodate the spermatic cord at the medial aspect of the cut slit in mesh with the two tails overlapping laterally and secured to prevent an indirect recurrence. A slit is made in the mesh before insertion for approximately half the distance of the long end of a 10 × 15 cm mesh with one-third of the mesh below the slit and two-thirds above the slit. For direct hernias only, a non-slitted mesh may be used ensuring the peritoneal edge is below the inferior border of the mesh

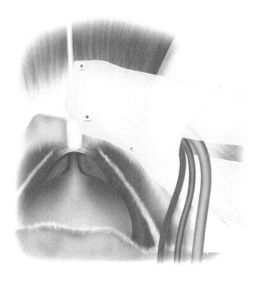

Fig. 44.4 The mesh is secured to Cooper's ligament with non-absorbable tacks

The mesh is then secured with non-absorbable tacks to Cooper's ligament and the rectus muscle anteriorly (Fig. 44.4). The vas and vessels are positioned within the slit, the mesh rolled laterally so that it lies flat without bunching, and the lower flap secured overlying the upper flap slightly with a tack at least

1 cm above the anterior superior iliac spine (Fig. 44.5). Care must be taken to avoid the branches of the lateral femoral cutaneous nerve and genito-femoral and femoral nerve.

(f) *Occult bilateral inguinal hernias.* Our group performed a prospective study of patients undergoing TEP repairs with a pre-operative diagnosis of a unilateral hernia only [3]. 22% of patients had an occult bilateral inguinal hernia. For this reason, we advocate routine exploration of the contralateral side to evaluate for an occult, contralateral inguinal hernia and immediate repair when identified. This is done in a similar manner to the ipsilateral (symptomatic) side; however, the space is selectively dissected to include identification of cooper's ligament for inspection of the direct space, followed by identification of the internal ring and cord contents. The peritoneal reflection can be followed medial to lateral and if found to enter the internal ring, an indirect hernia is assumed and full dissection is

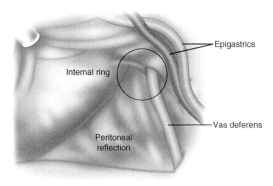

Fig. 44.6 The contralateral side is inspected for an occult inguinal hernia by exposing the direct and indirect space. The cord contents are seen within the indirect space and the peritoneal reflection is noted to not enter the internal ring; therefore, a contralateral indirect hernia is not present

then undertaken (Fig. 44.6). We have found that such inspection of the contralateral side does not significantly increase the difficulty of a contralateral repair, if required later compared to unilateral TEP only.

Conclusions

TEP is an excellent option for the repair of not only recurrent and bilateral inguinal hernias, but also for initial unilateral inguinal hernias. The long-learning curve and complicated, posterior inguinal anatomy associated with TEP limit its application for those surgeons who are not comfortable with dissection of the pre-peritoneal space. However, we find TEP to be our procedure of choice due to the minimal post-operative complication profile, the ability to intra-operatively inspect the opposite inguinal region, and excellent long-term durable outcomes.

References

1. Heikkinen TJ, Haukipuro K, Koivukangas P, Hulkko A. A prospective randomized outcome and cost comparison of totally extra-peritoneal endoscopic hernioplasty versus Lichtenstein operation among employed patients. Surg Laprosc Endosc. 1998;8:338–44.

2. Pawanindra L, Kajla RK, Chander J, et al. Randomized controlled study of laparoscopic total extra-peritoneal versus open Lichtenstein inguinal hernia repair. Surg Endosc. 2003;17:850–6.

3. Bochkarev V, Ringley C, Vitamvas M, Oleynikov D. Bilateral laparoscopic inguinal hernia repair in patients with occult contralateral inguinal defects. Surg Endosc. 2007;21(5):734–6.

4. Neumayer L, Giobbie-Hurder A, Jonasson O, et al. Open mesh versus laparoscopic mesh repair of inguinal hernia. N Engl J Med. 2004;350:1819–27.

5. Pokorny H, Klingler A, Schmid T, et al. Recurrence and complications after laparoscopic versus open inguinal hernia repair: results of a prospective randomized multicenter trial. Hernia. 2008;12:385–9.

6. Koning GG, Wettersley J, van Laarhoven CJ, Keus F. The totally extraperitoneal method versus Lichtenstein's technique for inguinal hernia repair: a systematic review with meta-analyses and trial sequential analyses of randomized clinical trials. PLoS One. 2013;8:e52599.

7. Aigner F, Augustin F, Kaufmann C, Schlager A, Ulmer H, Pratschke J, Schmid T. Prospective, randomized-controlled trial comparing postoperative pain after plug and patch open repair with totally extraperitoneal inguinal hernia repair. Hernia. 2014;18(2):237–42.

8. Eklund A, Montgomery A, Bergkvist L, Rudberg C, et al. Chronic pain 5 years after randomized comparison of laparoscopic and Lichtenstein inguinal hernia repair. Br J Surg. 2010;97(4):600–8.

9. Bracale U, Melillo P, Pignata G, et al. Which is the best laparoscopic approach for inguinal hernia repair: TEP or TAPP? A systematic review of the literature with a network meta-analysis. Surg Endosc. 2012;26:3355–66.

10. Gass M, Banz VM, Rosella L, et al. TAPP or TEP? Population-based analysis of prospective data on 4,552 patients undergoing endoscopic inguinal hernia repair. World J Surg. 2012;36:2782–6.

11. Eker HH, Langeveld HR, Klitsie PJ, et al. Randomized clinical trial of total extraperitoneal inguinal hernioplasty vs Lichtenstein repair: a long-term follow-up study. Arch Surg. 2012;147:256–60.

12. DeTurris SV, Cacchione RN, Mungara A, et al. Laparoscopic herniorrhaphy: beyond the learning curve. J Am Coll Surg. 2002;194:65–73.

13. Pawanindra L, Kajla RK, Chander J, Ramteke VK. Laparoscopic total extraperitoneal (TEP) inguinal hernia repair: overcoming the learning curve. Surg Endosc. 2004;18:642–5.

14. Schouten N, Simmermacher RKJ, van Dalen T, et al. Is there an end of the "learning curve" of endoscopic totally extraperitoneal (TEP) hernia repair? Surg Endosc. 2013;27:789–94.

15. Kurashima Y, Feldman LS, Kaneva PA, et al. Simulation-based training improves the operative performance of totally extraperitoneal (TEP) laparoscopic inguinal hernia repair: a prospective randomized controlled trial. Surg Endosc. 2014;28:783–8.

16. Schouten N, Elshof JWM, Simmermacher RKJ, et al. Selecting patients during the "learning curve" of endoscopic totally extraperitoneal (TEP) hernia repair. Hernia. 2013;17:737–43.

17. Ferzli G, Kiel T. The role of the endoscopic extraperitoneal approach in large inguinal scrotal hernias. Surg Endosc. 1997;11(3):299–302.

18. Ferzli G, Shapiro K, Chaudry G, Patel S. Laparoscopic extraperitoneal approach to acutely incarcerated inguinal hernia. Surg Endosc. 2004;18:228–31.

19. Dulucq JL, Wintringer P, Mahajna A. Totally extraperitoneal (TEP) hernia repair after radical prostatectomy or previous lower abdominal surgery: is it safe? A prospective study. Surg Endosc. 2006;20(3):473–6.

The Extended-View Totally Extraperitoneal (eTEP) Technique for Inguinal Hernia Repair

Jorge Daes

Introduction

Five laparoscopic techniques are currently available for repairing an inguinal hernia: totally extraperitoneal (TEP) repair, extended view totally extraperitoneal (eTEP), transabdominal preperitoneal (TAPP), intra-peritoneal onlay mesh (IPOM), and reduction of the sac with or without closure of the ring. It is our philosophy that surgeons interested in a laparoscopic approach should be skillful in all of the available techniques to accommodate the needs of all patients and to be able to convert to a different technique when necessary.

Since 1996, we have favored the endoscopic extraperitoneal approach for the repair of nearly all inguinal hernias [1]. The major advantage of this approach is that it does not involve entry in the abdominal cavity, thus lessening the risk of intestinal and vascular injuries as well as herniation at the trocar sites [2, 3]. This approach may even allow hernia repair under local anesthesia with intravenous sedation or under regional anesthesia [4, 5], and provides a great view of the local structures.

Electronic supplementary material: The online version of this chapter (doi:10.1007/978-3-319-27470-6_45) contains supplementary material, which is available to authorized users.

J. Daes, M.D., F.A.C.S. (✉)
Department of Minimally Invasive Surgery,
Clinica Bautista, Carrera 58 no. 79-223 PH B,
Barranquilla, Colombia
e-mail: jorgedaez@gmail.com

The extraperitoneal approach is based on the time-tested Rives-Stoppa technique. However, the classical TEP technique has several drawbacks, including the limited space for dissection and mesh placement, restricted port placement, possible intolerance of pneumoperitoneum, and difficulty in teaching and learning the technique. These disadvantages may explain the low implementation of the technique outside the circle of experts [6].

We have noticed the difficulties our trainees experienced in learning TEP, and this inspired us to modify the TEP technique based on the principle that the preperitoneal space can be reached from virtually anywhere in the anterior abdominal wall. We named this modified protocol eTEP; the small "e" stands for "extended view." The technique has been standardized since its first publication in *Surgical Endoscopy* [7].

The most salient features of the eTEP technique are:

1. Fast and easy creation of the extraperitoneal space.
2. A large surgical field.
3. A flexible port setup adaptable to many clinical situations.
4. Unencumbered parietalization of the cord structures (proximal dissection of the sac and peritoneum).
5. Easier management of the distal sac in cases of large inguinoscrotal hernias [8].
6. Improved tolerance of pneumoperitoneum, which is a common complication.

Y.W. Novitsky (ed.), *Hernia Surgery*, DOI 10.1007/978-3-319-27470-6_45

Indications for eTEP

We use the eTEP technique to repair most cases of inguinal hernias; however, there are cases for which eTEP is especially useful.

1. For the novel surgeon: eTEP is easier to master for surgeons new to the technique. In our clinical immersion courses, most of the trainees are surgeons who have only performed TAPPs and have no TEP experience. Notably, in follow-up surveys, most of the surgeons (80%) incorporated the eTEP technique in their practices.
2. Obese or post-bariatric patients: eTEP allows the surgeon to avoid the difficulties caused by the pannus; in addition, the subcutaneous tissue is thinner higher in the abdomen.
3. When the distance between the umbilicus and pubic tubercle is short.
4. In patients with previous pelvic surgeries.
5. Wide variety of indications: with experience, surgeons can expand the indications for eTEP for inguinal hernia repair to cases of large inguinoscrotal, sliding, or incarcerated hernias. This may require combination with a 5 mm laparoscopic intraperitoneal approach to verify the viability of the intestine or assist in reducing the incarcerated content.

Key Technical Aspects of eTEP

High Camera Port Placement

In most unilateral hernias, a 10–12 mm incision is placed high in the upper lateral quadrant of the abdomen approximately 5 cm cephalad and 4 cm lateral to the umbilicus on the same side of the hernia (Fig. 45.1). This incision serves as the camera port, but the incision can alternatively be placed on the hemi-abdomen opposite to the hernia side, especially in patients with previous pelvic surgeries interfering with this setup (Fig. 45.2), patients with large inguinoscrotal, incarcerated, or sliding hernias, or according to surgeon preference. For bilateral hernias, the camera port can be placed on either side. Figure 45.3 shows the camera port location in the

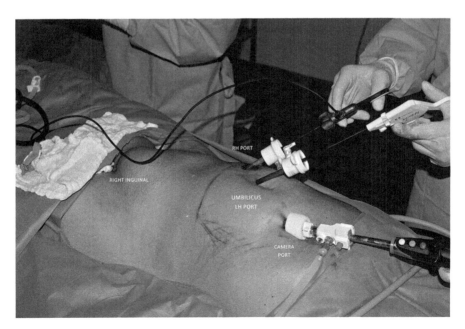

Fig. 45.1 Port setup for a unilateral left inguinal hernia. The camera port is placed high in the upper abdominal quadrant ipsilateral to the hernia. The working port for the left hand is placed at the umbilicus. The surgeon and camera assistant always stand opposite the hernia side

Fig. 45.2 Because of a previous surgery at the right lower abdominal quadrant, the camera port was placed in the left flank. Working ports are placed in triangulation

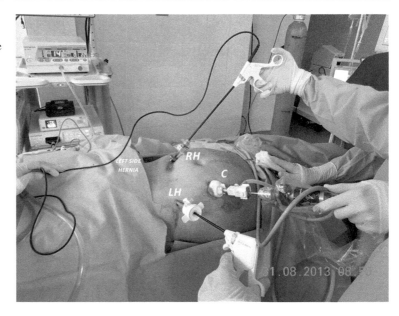

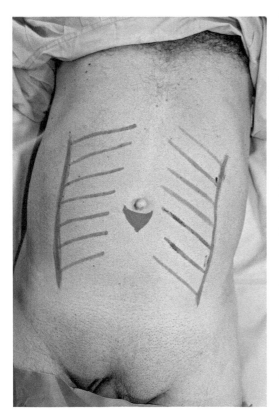

Fig. 45.3 The location of the camera port in the classic TEP approach is shown (*red*). The semilunar lines (*solid blue vertical lines*) and the possible locations for the camera port (*blue stripes*) in the eTEP technique are indicated

classical TEP approach (highlighted in red); the semilunar lines marked under ultrasound guidance are indicated with solid vertical blue lines, and possible sites for the camera port in the eTEP technique are highlighted by blue stripes. The camera port can also be positioned lateral to the semilunar lines, as shown in Fig. 45.4.

The initial incision is then extended to the anterior fascia, and the fascia is exposed and incised with an inverted 11 blade. This allows a finger to be introduced through the fascia and muscle to reach the posterior fascia, which is thick at this location, and the retro-rectus space is manually dissected. The balloon trocar is then introduced along the same path to reach the pubic spine, and the balloon is inflated to create a working space. The surgeon and camera operator stand on the side opposite to the hernia.

Flexible Port Distribution

Two additional working ports can be placed according to each individual case. In a unilateral hernia, we often use the umbilicus as one working port and place the second port high in the lower abdominal quadrant opposite to the hernia (Fig. 45.5). The working ports can also be placed with one port lateral to the umbilicus and the

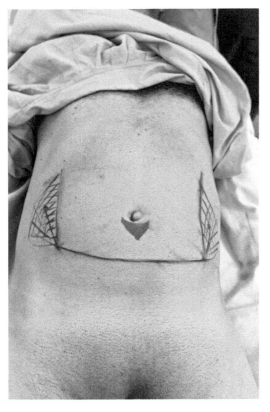

Fig. 45.4 The eTEP enables access to the preperitoneal space outside of the semilunar lines, as shown. This maneuver is rarely necessary

other port slightly lower and lateral to the first. When the camera is opposite the hernia site, we use the distribution shown in Fig. 45.6, which allows for perfect triangulation. For bilateral hernia cases, we use the distribution shown in Figs. 45.7 and 45.8. Placement of a second port in these cases allows for a more ergonomic repair.

Division of the Posterior Fascia (Douglas's Line)

Occasionally, the posterior fascia descends enough to reduce visibility within the preperitoneal space. In such cases of a low-lying arcuate line, we usually divide it. This can be done while maintaining visibility if a 5 mm camera is used through the lowest working trocar. The posterior fascia and peritoneum are firmly adhered at midline, but the peritoneum can be dissected free from the fascia laterally. Usually, we divide the Douglas's line blindly using laparoscopic scissors introduced through one of the working trocars, though this can risk dividing the peritoneum and generating a pneumoperitoneum.

The key technical aspects of the eTEP technique can be observed in the supplemental video.

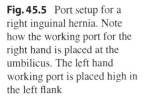

Fig. 45.5 Port setup for a right inguinal hernia. Note how the working port for the right hand is placed at the umbilicus. The left hand working port is placed high in the left flank

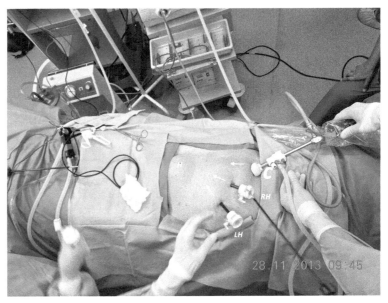

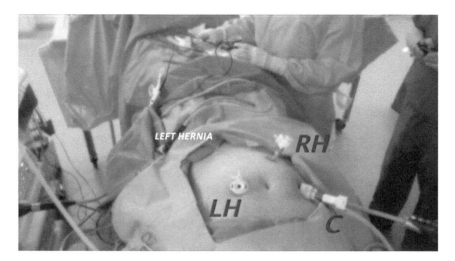

Fig. 45.6 Port distribution for a left inguinoscrotal hernia. The camera port is located at the right flank, and the working ports are placed to obtain a perfect triangulation

Fig. 45.7 Port distribution for a bilateral inguinal hernia case showing setup of the camera and working ports for the right hernia

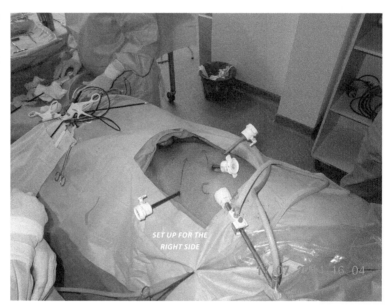

Fig. 45.8 Port distribution for a bilateral inguinal hernia case showing setup of the camera and working ports for the left hernia. An additional trocar can be placed to allow a more ergonomic repair, although this is not strictly necessary

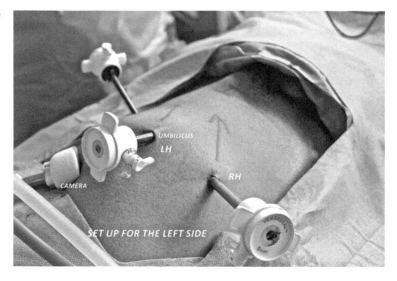

Hernia Repair

Once the extraperitoneal space is created, pubic tubercle and Cooper's ligament are exposed, epigastric vessels are identified and the space of Bogros is fully developed. When a direct hernia is present, lax transversalis fascia is freed from the hernia content. In case of an indirect hernia, the indirect sac is retracted medially while elements of the cord are dissected free laterally, being careful not to grasp them. Dissection is completed when the indirect sac is separated from cord structures by a bluish transparency. The sac can be reduced completely in most cases. When indirect sac extends deep into the scrotum in a large inguinoscrotal hernia, we ligate the sac and divide it distal to the ligation. The ligated sac and peritoneum are dissected as proximally as possible to achieve parietalization of cord elements and ensure correct positioning of the mesh at the end of the procedure. Failure to deal with the distal sac carries the risk of formation of large and sometimes cumbersome seromas, hematomas, and pseudohydroceles. We grasp the lateral edge of the divided distal sac, which is exposed with the help of external pressure applied to the ipsilateral scrotum. We pull the edge of the divided sac upwards and laterally and fix it with tacks (and sometimes sutures) to the abdominal wall well above the ileopubic tract. This maneuver has been helpful to avoid cumbersome seromas (8). In cases of large direct hernias, the lax transversalis fascia is reduced and fixed with tacks to Cooper's ligament to reduce the dead space. Lipomas of the cord are sought for and dissected out. When a complete dissection of the space is achieved, a mesh is introduced, unrolled and placed over the posterior inguinal wall. We use a 15–17 cm by 10–12 cm, midweight, macroporous polyester mesh. Fixation is optional for small hernias. We usually fix the mesh with a few tacks placed on Cooper's ligament and on the upper border of the mesh well above the ileopubic tract/inguinal ligament. Finally, we instill diluted bupivacaine into the space, make sure sac and peritoneum lie behind the mesh and keep the inferior lateral border of the mesh under pressure with a dissector while slowly releasing CO_2 from the space.

Clinical Experience with eTEP

Between October 2010 and September 2014, we performed 307 eTEP repairs in 276 patients. This unselected series included all patients with inguinal hernias. Six cases were converted to TAPP, and none were converted to open surgery. The hernia recurred in two cases. There was one bladder lesion that was corrected during the procedure and five self-limiting seromas. None of the patients have experienced chronic pain.

Conclusions

The eTEP technique has a place in the armamentarium of hernia surgeons. Residents and surgeons early in their experience will find this technique easier to master than the classic TEP method. It can expand the traditional indications of the extraperitoneal approach to patients with a difficult body habitus, a short umbilicus-pubis distance, and previous pelvic surgery. As the surgeon's experience increases, the indications for the traditional TEP technique can be expanded to more complex cases.

References

1. Daes J. Reparo laparoscopico de la hernia inguinal. Experiencia de la Unidad de Laparoscopia. Clinica Bautista, Barranquilla, Colombia. Rev Colomb Circ. 1999;14:97–103.
2. Wake BL, McCormack K, Fraser C, Vale L, Perez J, Grant AM. Transabdominal preperitoneal (TAPP) vs totally extraperitoneal (TEP) laparoscopic techniques for inguinal hernia repair. Cochrane Database Syst Rev. 2005. doi:10.1089/lap.2008.0212
3. Leibl BJ, Jager C, Kraft B, Swartz J, Ulrich M, Bittner R. Laparoscopic hernia repair—TAPP or/and TEP? Langenbecks Arch Surg. 2005;390:77–8.
4. Ferzly G, Sayad P, Vasisht B. The feasibility of laparoscopic extraperitoneal hernia repair under local anesthesia. Surg Endosc. 1999;13:588–90.
5. Ismail M, Garg P. Laparoscopic inguinal total extraperitoneal hernia repair under spinal anesthesia without mesh fixation in 1,220 hernia repairs. Hernia. 2009;13:115–9.
6. Daes J. The enhanced view- totally extraperitoneal technique for repair of inguinal hernia, answer to letter to the editor. Surg Endosc. 2012;26:3693–4.
7. Daes J. The enhanced view- totally extraperitoneal technique for repair of inguinal hernia. Surg Endosc. 2012;26:1187–88.
8. Daes J. Endoscopic repair of large inguinoscrotal hernias: management of the distal sac to avoid seroma formation. Hernia. 2014;18:119–22.

Brian P. Jacob

The Problem

Employing a minimally invasive versus open inguinal hernia repair for a primary inguinal hernia remains debatable. It has been clearly established that in experienced hands, both the open and laparoscopic techniques can produce excellent short- and long-term results. All inguinal hernia operations carry a small risk of chronic pain and recurrences. Weighing the benefits of open versus laparoscopic repair for any new patient presenting with a primary inguinal hernia will remain an academic pursuit, but practical focus needs to shift to establishing the best technique to utilize at different times, depending on the patient, with the goal being outcome optimization. Treatment algorithms for the many different types of patients presenting with inguinal hernias can help guide surgeons toward this objective. These algorithms do require that surgeons feel comfortable performing both open and laparoscopic techniques, but assuming this is the case, following them can help build a complete surgical arsenal.

History and Surgical Work Up

The work-up for a primary inguinal hernia includes a detailed history, a focused physical exam, and in certain situations some further imaging. All

B.P. Jacob, M.D., F.A.C.S. (✉)
Icahn School of Medicine at Mount Sinai,
New York, NY, USA
e-mail: bpjacob@gmail.com

treatment decision trees for patients with primary inguinal hernias should start with the patient and not be limited to one approach. Knowing there is no single "best" approach to every patient; surgeons must pay careful attention to the patient's history and try to match their procedure choice to each patient's specific goals and expectations, as well as any intraoperative findings.

The first question all patients should be asked is, "why do you want your hernia fixed?" "What bothers you about your hernia?" An attempt to document the precise symptoms (whether it is simply a bulge, some bulge and some intermittent pain, or concern for an emergent scenario) related to the patient's hernia will be an important factor to help decide if this patient even needs surgery at all. Patients with completely asymptomatic hernias who have been referred by a physician when the patient themselves did not even know they had a primary inguinal hernia can be safely watched non-operatively, if the patient chooses, to do so and once they have been educated [1]. Even after education, patients with only rare symptoms from a palpable and easily reducible hernia can also be offered non-operative strategies, assuming they are compliant and will return for follow-up if symptoms arise or become more frequent. My words of wisdom are, "if you cannot document a clear reason why you are repairing the hernia, don't repair the hernia."

Sometimes, patients have a chief complaint of groin pain (with or without a bulge). It cannot be stressed enough how important it is to document any preoperative groin pain complaints, and then do a full pain history and physical on these patients. Groin pain can be the result of an extensive differential diagnosis, and if there is any doubt that the patient's complaint of pain is not related directly to the hernia bulge, then they should not be operated on initially.

Groin pain complaints should be fully evaluated by those experienced in narrowing down that vast differential and should not be initially assumed to be related to an inguinal hernia, even if a hernia is obvious on exam. Additionally, it is well accepted that there is a higher incidence of postoperative hernia pain complaints in patients who complained of pain preoperatively. Documenting the patient's goals for seeking surgery will help a surgeon choose the best procedure. Patients who want the hernia fixed with the fastest recovery and return to work option should be advised that, in experienced hands, laparoscopy has been shown to offer this advantage.

Once the decision to operate is made, navigating the inguinal hernia repair algorithm can be facilitated by taking and processing a detailed patient history that includes the patient's body mass index (BMI), prior medical history (PMH), prior surgical history (PSH), current medications, and social history to evaluate for tobacco smoking. It is well accepted that a history of smoking and/or obesity can increase recurrence and infection rates, and thus surgical options known to minimize these risks should be employed. Documenting the details of a previous inguinal hernia repair can aid in deciding whether an open or laparoscopic repair is preferable. Some recurrences after an open Lichtenstein or tissue repair may be better diagnosed and treated with a laparoscopic technique; and a previous laparoscopic repair recurrence may be best repaired by an anterior approach in some hands, but by a laparoscopic method in others. It will truly depend on the history and the surgeon's experience. A surgical history that involves a previous lower midline incision may violate otherwise avascular tissue planes, and thus could be a reason to proceed with an open (anterior) repair. Medications such as blood thinners and Aspirin may play a role in choosing between open and laparoscopic methods.

A history of immunosuppression medications may also help direct a surgeon down a particular pathway. Advanced patient age is not an absolute contraindication to performing a laparoscopic procedure, but the ability for each patient to tolerate general anesthesia must be evaluated carefully. That being said, some patients simply do not want to undergo general anesthesia. Since an open repair can be performed safely under local anesthesia, and epidural, or with IV sedation only, this may be the best option for those patients.

Management Options

The current list of available, well-described, and commonly utilized inguinal hernia repair techniques is extensive (Table 46.1).

Surgeons who wish to embrace inguinal hernia repair as a practice sub-specialty should be familiar with all of these techniques, and be able to perform both open as well as laparoscopic TEP, TAPP, eTEP, and IPOM inguinal repairs. However, at some point in their training, many surgeons become more comfortable with one specific technique over others. Consequently, once training is complete, surgeons trained on open techniques tend to have limited exposure to advanced laparoscopic training, and are therefore likely to avoid adopting such methods. However, in order to accommodate all hernia patients, a surgeon should have a variety of weapons in his or her armamentarium.

Table 46.1 Common hernia repair surgical options

Open techniques	Laparoscopic techniques
Tissue repair—no mesh	TEP (total extraperitoneal)
Lichtenstein (tension-free) (Mesh onlay, no plug)	TAPP (Transabdominal preperitoneal)
Transinguinal preperitoneal (TIP)	IPOM (intraperitoneal onlay mesh)
Mesh plug (alone)	Robotics
Mesh plug and patch	
Prolene™ Hernia System (single mesh device with an intraperitoneal and extraperitoneal layer)	

Robotic surgery is an emerging minimally invasive tool that surgeons are choosing to use to repair inguinal hernias. Robotics, like laparoscopy, is a minimally invasive option, and in this chapter when I mention the use of laparoscopy to perform TEP or TAPP, it can be easily exchanged with the use of a robot to perform a TAPP or TEP, if the surgeon is experienced with and performs a majority of their cases with the robot. In other words, whether a robot or laparoscopy is used, the procedure itself is still a TAPP or a TEP. Until comparative data is available, a robotic inguinal hernia repair is certainly feasible, but has not been shown to be superior or inferior to an open inguinal approach by an open hernia expert or to a laparoscopic approach by a laparoscopic expert, when considering measurable patient outcome metrics.

Author's Preference

While most surgeons with extensive experience in hernia repair techniques have optimized their outcomes, randomized prospective trials are still beneficial in helping to direct surgeons to choose to master operations with proven and optimized success rates. The outcomes after TEP, TAPP, and Open repairs have been scientifically studied in large databases [2]. For instance, in the open technique debate, a Cochrane review of 20 randomized trials comparing open Lichtenstein to open-tissue repair revealed shorter hospital stays, quicker return to activities of daily living, less chronic pain, and lower recurrence rates for the Lichtenstein [3]. That being said, in the open versus laparoscopic debate, the LEVEL-trial concluded that the laparoscopic total extraperitoneal (TEP) procedure, when compared to the Lichtenstein repair, was associated with less-reported acute pain and a slightly faster recovery time [4]. Several other randomized prospective studies have also demonstrated better quality of life and chronic pain outcomes for laparoscopic hernia repair compared to open Lichtenstein repair [5, 6]. For an experienced laparoscopic trained surgeon, recurrence rates following laparoscopic repair are no different than those following an open repair and might be even better, while, if inexperienced, recurrence rates will be higher [7]. Finally, within the laparoscopic repair options debate, when comparing TAPP and TEP, a large 12,000 patient review showed no significant differences in operating times, vascular injuries, recurrence rates, or chronic pain complaints [8]. The TEP repair was associated with more intraoperative conversions to other techniques, and it may be harder for trainees to learn. At the same time, TAPP procedures led to slightly more trocar site hernias, transperitoneal hernias, and visceral injuries, as well as increased intra-abdominal adhesive disease leading to bowel obstruction (0.5%, vs. 0.07% for TEP). Most importantly, after a TEP is complete, there is no peritoneum to close at the end of the procedure. Thus, any morbidity related to this peritoneal closure is eliminated. A large 19,582 patient review found that both laparoscopic and open preperitoneal mesh placement were associated with significantly lower re-recurrence rates than the same repairs of a recurrent hernia using an open technique [9]. However, TAPP has been shown to increase incidence of postoperative obstruction [10]. Combined with TAPP in certain scenarios, TEP's diagnostic ability is superior to an open alternative in patients with, for example, a missed femoral hernia during a plug repair of a direct hernia. Given all of these facts, I routinely rely on the TEP repair for the majority of my patients including all primary unilateral and bilateral inguinal hernias. For the TAPP surgeon advocates, there are not many contraindications to using a TAPP other than the routine contraindications to performing intra-abdominal laparoscopy, like in patients with a history of peritonitis or previous laparotomy with known extensive adhesive disease. The question they may need to answer is why choose an operation where the peritoneum is cut and then sewn together when there is a technique available that can avoid that step.

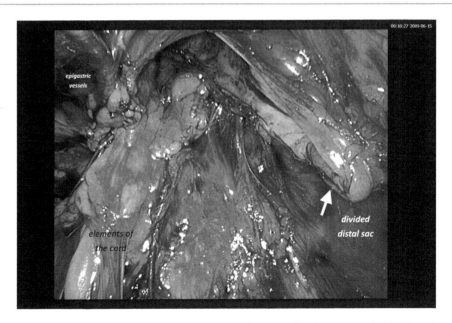

Fig. 46.1 Reduction of excess indirect right hernia sac. Used with permission from personal files of Dr. Jorge Daes

Caveats and Pearls

While TEP appears to be an ideal operation for all unilateral and bilateral primary inguinal hernias, as well as recurrence after an open inguinal hernia, a TAPP remains advantageous for several specific patient scenarios. A standard approach to all patients with an inguinal hernia is presented here in an easy-to-follow algorithm (Fig. 46.1).

Incarcerations and Strangulations

Incarcerations and possible strangulations are a contraindication for the TEP repair. A true TEP repair does not allow easy visualization of the incarcerated tissue, and thus risks leaving behind strangulated or ischemic remnants. If performing a TEP where possible bowel ischemia is suspected, the peritoneal layer should be opened and the bowel inspected. By performing a TAPP repair in these scenarios, the surgeon can evaluate the bowel properly. Should he or she find an ischemic segment of bowel, it can be reduced; but then the patient's primary problem is no longer the hernia, and a bowel resection should be

performed. The use of mesh after finding a true strangulation or bowel ischemia remains at the discretion of the surgeon, though employing a permanent synthetic material in a clean-contaminated or contaminated field carries a risk of chronic mesh infection and is therefore best avoided. An absorbable material is probably the safest choice if the field is clean-contaminated. However, if the field is contaminated, then it is best to stage the repair (if mesh is needed), or perform a primary tissue repair without mesh.

Scrotal Hernias and Large Hernia Sacs

Inguino-scrotal hernias are probably more common than typical reporting might indicate. Small scrotal hernias that are reducible can be approached initially via the TEP procedure; but the larger, more incarcerated or chronic scrotal hernias, especially those with large diameter necks, are sometimes better approached using a TAPP or open technique. Again, it certainly is acceptable to approach these with a TEP, but the number one reason to consider starting with a TAPP repair is that it provides a great view of the incarcerated contents, and usually allows for a straightforward reduction. Often, a TEP repair can be modified (or converted partially) to a TAPP (by opening the peritoneum) to help reduce the incarcerated contents.

In these large hernias, a partial hernia sac can be left in situ in the scrotum (it is not always necessary to excise the entire sac). If sac is left within the canal, an attempt should be made to close the peritoneum on the proximal end (with an endoloop or endoclips or suture) if possible, but you can leave the end within the canal open and patent. Some surgeons leave the rents in the peritoneum open, and report no issues, though I tend (and highly recommend) to close them.

One trick we like to employ for direct defects to reduce seroma rates is to take the retained peritoneum hernia sacs within the canal and pull them intrapreperitoneally and tack its lateral edge to the anterior abdominal wall to reduce the volume of sac in the canal. This will decrease the incidence and size of seroma formation. Nonetheless, patients with these types of hernias should also be forewarned about seromas, as they are fairly common (Fig. 46.2).

Inguinodynia

Chronic groin pain is a complex topic covered in another chapter. The choice of operation will depend on the previous surgery, as well as the patient's response to local and regional nerve blocks, which can be performed for diagnostic purposes, as indicated above. The TAPP is very useful as a diagnostic, and possibly therapeutic, tool for patients presenting with groin pain. Patients should be educated that there is a chance the surgery will not resolve their pain, but can still contribute greatly to the workup, with the goal being an eventual diagnosis and resolution. Before the TAPP, the patient should mark the spot with the maximal pain. He or she should understand that if a TAPP exploration fails to identify the etiology of the pain, an additional surgery requiring neurectomy might be needed. But he or she should also be made aware that proceeding in a staged fashion is the logical and appropriate course of action. During the TAPP procedure, potential pain-inducing tacks and mesh can be removed, adhesions can be identified and lysed, and the femoral, direct, and indirect

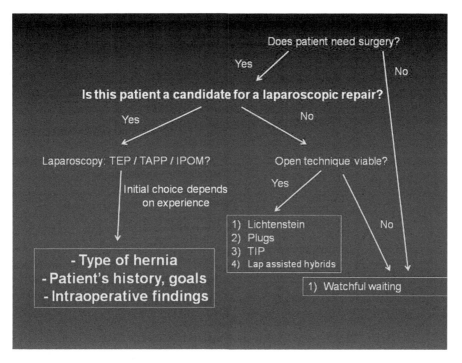

Fig. 46.2 Algorithmic approach to a patient with an inguinal hernia

spaces can be carefully examined for missed, new, or recurrent hernias. Simply stated, a TEP may miss many etiologies and is therefore not as useful as a TAPP for approaching inguinodynia.

Recurrence After a TEP or TAPP

For experienced laparoscopists, a recurrence after a previous TEP or TAPP approach demands a TAPP, or even an IPOM repair. Some surgeons will always resort to an open anterior approach for a patient with a recurrence, but compared to the diagnostic ability of the laparoscope, I find an open approach (used alone) limited. During the laparoscopic dissection, an additional open incision may help with mesh removal or cord preservation, and it may be added at this point. Choosing which procedure is best to perform after a recurrence has been extensively evaluated in the literature and is beyond the scope of this chapter; but it is clearly dependent on surgeon experience.

Using laparoscopy for a recurrence after an open tissue or Lichtenstein repair allows for a precise diagnosis under magnified vision, minimizing untoward outcomes. Preoperatively, if palpable, the recurrence should be marked or prepped into the field. A urinary catheter should be inserted, which can be used to distend the bladder, if necessary, during the dissection. The first step during a recurrent hernia repair is to perform an adequate diagnostic laparoscopy, to survey the entire region and assess the possible etiology of the recurrence. In general, I start with a detailed diagnostic laparoscopy, where I survey the nearby viscera, and then examine the direct, femoral, and indirect spaces. It is important to be particularly careful taking the previous mesh off the myopectineal orifice to avoid injury. It is important to be particularly careful to avoid injury to the cord structures, epigastric vessels, bladder, lateral femoral cutaneous nerve, and iliac vessels (and Genitofemoral nerve, if posterior dissection is needed). The dissection should continue until the recurrence is identified. Usually there is a small defect medially near the Cooper's ligament and pubic tubercle, where the previous

mesh pulled away from the periosteum of the tubercle. Less commonly, the indirect hernia may have recurred or a femoral hernia may have been missed. If no defect is found, the patient's symptoms may be the result of a cord lipoma, which then needs to be ruled out.

Old mesh can be left in situ if it is densely adherent to vital structures and not causing pain. New mesh may be implanted in standard fashion, or, in specific case scenarios, laparoscopically sutured to the old mesh as needed. If the peritoneum is destroyed during the dissection, a two-sided mesh with a barrier coating (also known as tissue separating mesh) can be inserted as an intraperitoneal onlay (IPOM). Laparoscopic sutures may then be used to fix the new mesh to the peritoneum overlying vital structures, to avoid injury by tacks. Adhesive glues are also useful for this purpose.

Women with Previous Pfenensteil

Some women with previous Pfenensteil incisions will not have a peritoneal layer and thus are not candidates for a TEP repair. In such situations, a TAPP or IPOM repair is required. In addition, some Pfenensteil incisional hernias will be felt on palpation like inguinal hernias, when indeed the defect is in the midline. A preoperative CT scan can help differentiate between the two. Also, using a laparoscopic approach allows for an accurate diagnosis and remedy to be achieved concomitantly.

Previous Surgical History Involving Lower Midline Skin Incisions (Prostatectomy)

As with women who have previous Pfenensteil incisions, patients with previous lower midline skin incisions may have an obliterated retrorectus plane. This is most significant in patients who have had open or laparoscopic radical prostatectomies. The history of a prostatectomy deserves specific mention, because, although rare (0.04%), bladder injuries can still occur. An open repair, on the other hand, avoids this risk completely. An open approach should always be considered in this scenario if the surgeon is not completely comfortable with laparoscopy, or if during laparoscopy there are dense and extensive adhesions found. If a laparoscopic technique is used, a urinary catheter is mandatory. The bladder can be distended with methylene blue for easy identification and protection. The surgeon can then perform the laparoscopic dissection more safely. Remember, the patient just wants his or her hernia fixed, and an open Lichtenstein repair almost completely avoids the possibility of a bladder injury.

Obesity (BMI > 35)

Significant obesity can be a relative contraindication for a TEP, given the physical girth of the lower abdominal wall or pannus. A TAPP repair can be more straightforward than a TEP in these patients. However, if the lower abdomen allows entry into the retrorectus space, then an eTEP repair may be utilized in standard fashion. This decision can be made at the time of surgery.

Seroma minimization: Large cavernous defects, both direct and indirect, run the risk of forming large seromas. While these are self-limited, they can last many months and be uncomfortable for patients. Once trick to minimize these is to take the redundant attenuated transversalis fascia and pull it into the preperitoneal space and fixate it to the Cooper's ligament with a permanent tack.

Conclusions

There are many surgical approaches that are appropriate for repairing an inguinal hernia depending on the patient. It is imperative to understand the known outcomes of each, and fine-tune or evolve one's technique to minimize postoperative chronic pain and recurrence rates. Surgeons should stay in touch with the evolving techniques and technology in order to provide

optimized outcomes. Learning the treatment algorithms for the many different types of patients presenting with inguinal hernias can help guide surgeons toward this objective.

References

1. Fitzgibbons RJ, Giobbie-Hurder A, Gibbs JO, Dunlop DD, Reda DJ, McCarthy Jr M, Neumayer LA, Barkun JS, Hoehn JL, Murphy JT, Sarosi Jr GA, Syme WC, Thompson JS, Wang J, Jonasson O. Watchful waiting vs. repair of inguinal hernia in minimally symptomatic men: a randomized clinical trial. JAMA. 2006; 295(3):285–92.
2. Belyansky I, Tsirline VB, Klima DA, Walters AL, Lincourt AE, Heniford TB. Prospective, comparative study of postoperative quality of life in TEP, TAPP, and modified Lichtenstein repairs. Ann Surg. 2011; 254(4):709–14.
3. Scott NW, McCormack K, Graham P, Go PM, Ross SJ, Grant AM. Open mesh versus non-mesh for repair of femoral and inguinal hernia. Cochrane Database Syst Rev. 2002;4:CD002197.
4. Langeveld HR, van't Riet M, Weidema WF, Stassen LP, Steyerberg EW, Lange J, Bonjer HJ, Jeekel J. Total extraperitoneal inguinal hernia repair compared with Lichtenstein (the LEVEL-trial): a randomized controlled trial. Ann Surg. 2010;251(5):819–24.
5. Myers E, Browne KM, Kavanagh DO, Hurley M. Laparoscopic (TEP) versus Lichtenstein inguinal hernia repair: a comparison of quality of life outcomes. World J Surg. 2010;34(12):3059–64.
6. Eklund A, Montgomery A, Bergkvist L, Rudberg C. Chronic pain 5 years after randomized comparison of laparoscopic and Lichtenstein inguinal hernia repair. Swedish Multicentre Trial of Inguinal Hernia Repair by Laparoscopy (SMIL) study group. Br J Surg. 2010; 97(4):600–8.
7. Neumayer L, Giobbie-Hurder A, Jonasson O, Fitzgibbons Jr R, Dunlop D, Gibbs J, Reda D, Henderson W. Open mesh versus laparoscopic mesh repair of inguinal hernia. N Engl J Med. 2004;350(18):1819–27.
8. Wake BL, McCormack K, Fraser C, Vale L, Perez J, Grant AM. Transabdominal pre-peritoneal (TAPP) vs totally extraperitoneal (TEP) laparoscopic techniques for inguinal hernia repair. Cochrane Database Syst Rev. 2005;25(1):cd004703.
9. Sevonius D, Gunnarsson U, Nordin P, Nilsson E, Sandblom G. Recurrent groin hernia surgery. Br J Surg. 2011;98(10):1489–94.
10. Bringman S, Blomqvist P. Intestinal obstruction after inguinal and femoral hernia repair: a study of 33,275 operations during 1992–2000 in Sweden. Hernia. 2005;9(2):178–83.

Martin F. Bjurstrom, Parviz K. Amid, and David C. Chen

Introduction

Chronic postherniorrhaphy inguinal pain (CPIP) is today recognized as the most significant severe complication following inguinal hernia repair. Globally over 20 million inguinal hernia repairs are conducted every year, and in the USA alone about 800,000 procedures are performed [1, 2]. The risk of developing moderate-to-severe chronic pain for those undergoing inguinal herniorrhaphy is 10–12% [3], and a conservative estimate of chronic pain adversely affecting daily life or employment (0.5–6.0%) [2] translates into 4,000–48,000 new cases annually in the USA. Over the last decades, herniorrhaphy techniques have been considerably refined, which has resulted in open and laparoscopic tension-free approaches utilizing advanced prosthetic mesh-material as the gold standard. Consequently, hernia recurrence rates have decreased dramatically (1–5%) [4], but chronic pain remains a tangible challenge, and now constitutes the most relevant outcome measure. Chronic postsurgical pain (CPSP) is defined as pain that develops after a surgical procedure, and temporally lasts more than 2 months, with other causes of pain

M.F. Bjurstrom • P.K. Amid • D.C. Chen (✉)
Department of Anesthesiology, Lichtenstein Amid Hernia Clinic at UCLA, Santa Monica, CA, USA

Department of Surgery, Lichtenstein Amid Hernia Clinic at UCLA, Santa Monica, CA, USA
e-mail: dcchen@mednet.ucla.edu

excluded [5]. For CPIP, the duration of pain should be at least 3 months, since postoperative mesh-related inflammatory processes may take a few months to subside [2]. CPIP patients suffer not only from painful symptoms, but also detrimental psychological and physical consequences, and an overall reduced quality of life [6]. The exact socioeconomic burden has not been calculated for CPIP, but total annual direct and indirect costs may be around US$40,000 per patient, as determined for cases of severe postsurgical neuropathic pain [7]. Prevention and skilled treatment of this serious and complex condition is of utmost importance.

Etiology and Clinical Presentation

Due to multiple pathophysiological mechanisms underlying the development of CPIP, the clinical presentation is complex and heterogeneous. Iatrogenic damage or trauma to inguinal nerves is generally considered the most important pathological mechanism with pain developing in the sensory distribution of the affected nerve(s). The major inguinal nerves vulnerable for damage during or after inguinal herniorrhaphy are the iliohypogastric nerve (IHN), the ilioinguinal nerve (IIN), the genital branch of the genitofemoral nerve (GFN), and more rarely, the femoral branch of the GFN or the lateral femoral cutaneous nerve. Intraoperatively, nerves can be damaged by surgical manipulation, stretching, crushing, electrical/thermal effects, partial or

© Springer International Publishing Switzerland 2016
Y.W. Novitsky (ed.), *Hernia Surgery*, DOI 10.1007/978-3-319-27470-6_47

complete transection, through entrapment in suture during an open repair, or entrapment in tacks, suture or fixation during a laparoscopic repair. Postoperatively, nerves can be damaged due to envelopment within a meshoma [8], irritation secondary to an excessive fibrotic reaction, or inflammatory processes such as granuloma or neuroma formation.

The symptomatology involves several types of pain, including neuropathic, nociceptive (inflammatory non-neuropathic), somatic and visceral pain, which are overlapping in presentation and often hard to discern clinically. The non-neuropathic pain is typically deep, dull, constant, and localized over the entirety of the groin area, while neuropathic pain can be either constant or intermittent, and characterized by negative sensory phenomena, dysesthesia, allodynia, or hyperalgesia. Neuropathic pain may radiate to the scrotum, labium, and/or upper thigh, and occasionally a trigger point can reproduce the neuropathic pain symptoms. The symptoms are often aggravated by ambulation, stooping, hyperextension of the hip, and sexual intercourse, and can be decreased by lying down, and flexion of the thigh. Somatic pain, characterized by maximum tenderness localized to the pubic tubercle area, is most commonly caused by deeply placed anchoring or periosteal anchoring of the mesh near the pubic tubercle (periostitis pubis) [9]. Finally, visceral pain may arise from intestinal involvement with recurrence, incarceration, or mesh adherence or may be related to the spermatic cord (funiculodynia) or other periurethral structures, including venous congestion of the spermatic cord, dyssynergia of the ejaculatory effector muscles, stricture of the spermatic duct, or twisting of the spermatic cord. Visceral pain in CPIP is generally related to sexual dysfunction or ejaculatory pain in the region of the superficial ring or the testicular/labial region.

The relative role of peripheral versus central mechanisms in CPIP has not yet been elucidated, but the mechanisms triggering and driving the transition from acute to chronic pain may encompass intraoperative long-lasting, high frequency injury discharge from damaged nerves, early postoperative ectopic activity in injured nerves, collateral sprouting from neighboring intact nociceptive Aδ afferents, excitotoxic destruction of antinociceptive inhibitory interneurons in the spinal dorsal horn, neuroimmune alterations and maladaptive neuronal plasticity [10–12]. CPIP is also, importantly, influenced and modulated by emotional, cognitive, social, and genetic factors. Evidence from genetic research indicates an important role of an individual's genetic susceptibility to both generation and experience of pain, and response to analgesics [13].

Risk Factors

Several preoperative, perioperative, and postoperative factors related to the development and intensity of CPSP and CPIP have been identified [3, 14, 15]. Table 47.1 provides a complete list of risk factors for CPIP [11]. A high magnitude of pre- and postoperative pain consistently predicts future chronic pain across CPSP conditions, and it is also one of the strongest risk factors for development of CPIP [3, 10, 16]. The optimal type of anesthesia

Table 47.1 Risk factors for chronic postherniorrhaphy inguinal pain [11]

Preoperative factors
Young age
Female sex
High pain intensity level (inguinal/elsewhere)
Lower preoperative optimism
Impairment of everyday activities
Operation for a recurrent hernia
Genetic predisposition
Experimentally induced pain
High-pain intensity to tonic heat stimulation
Perioperative factors
Less experienced surgeon/not dedicated hernia center
Open repair technique
Mesh type: heavyweight (open, laparoscopic)
Mesh fixation: suture (open), staple (laparoscopic)?
IIN neurolysis in Lichtenstein repair
Postoperative factors
Postoperative complications (hematoma, infection)
High early postoperative pain intensity
Lower perceived control over pain
Sensory dysfunction in the groin

Note: ?=conflicting opinions/mixed evidence
IIN ilioinguinal nerve, *HLA* human leukocyte antigen

has not been extensively researched in connection to CPIP, but it is not recommended to utilize regional anesthesia (epidural, spinal) for inguinal herniorrhaphy, especially among older patients, due to an increased risk of urinary retention and other rare, but severe, medical complications [17]. For open repairs, local infiltration anesthesia is the preferred method, providing advantages such as early recovery and discharge, few complications, and improved early pain relief [18, 19]. However, there are no published results regarding the role of local anesthesia on the development of CPIP. Although laparoscopic approaches may result in less chronic pain [3, 16, 20], the incidence of significant pain equilibrates over time, and pain after laparoscopic repair remains a significant challenge due to positioning of the mesh and proximal injury to the inguinal nerves [2, 21, 22].

Mesh is often implicated as a contributing factor in CPIP. Systematic reviews and meta-analyses have demonstrated significant reduction of CPIP using lightweight mesh in both open and laparoscopic settings [23, 24]. This effect is likely mediated through greater biocompatibility, less inflammatory response, and reduced foreign body sensation through greater elasticity. While results are mixed, it is a reasonable assertion that avoidance of sutures and tacks may reduce the incidence of CPIP. In one meta-analysis, glue fixation of mesh in open repair reduced CPIP, hematoma, acute postoperative pain, and time to return to daily activities [25], but in another meta-analysis only the latter and early CPIP (3–6 months) were significantly improved [26]. As concluded in two other systematic reviews [27, 28], glue mesh fixation is an interesting alternative, but more data is needed regarding several important end points, such as CPIP and risk of recurrences in relation to size and type of hernia. Based upon available publications, self-gripping and sutured mesh demonstrate similar CPIP rates [29].

Evaluation

A detailed history and structured clinical examination are essential components of the diagnostic evaluation of chronic groin pain. Imaging modalities, such as ultrasonography, cross-sectional computed tomography (CT) or magnetic resonance imaging (MRI), are used to detect recurrence or meshoma, and exclude a wide spectrum of differential diagnostic entities [30, 31]. Currently, MRI is considered the best valid diagnostic imaging tool for differentiating causes of uncertain inguinal pain [32, 33]. The evaluation should aim to characterize the cause and type of pain, and administration of validated pain, function, and comorbidity assessment instruments may contribute to the diagnostic process and future research. Due to overlapping sensory innervations, it is difficult to precisely ascertain which nerves are involved in the neuralgic pain. Diagnostic peripheral nerve block or paravertebral root block with a local anesthetic are helpful for differentiating neuropathic from non-neuropathic pain, but it is often inconclusive in identifying the specific neuralgias. When results of nerve blocks are equivocal, needle electromyogram may provide additional information [34], and magnetic resonance neurography may identify peripheral nerve compression or injury [35].

Treatment

There is a paucity of high-quality, controlled, randomized trials examining non-interventional, pharmacological, and interventional pain management strategies in CPIP and the best current conclusions are based on small CPIP studies, case series, empiric evidence, and extrapolation of evidence from other neuropathic and CPSP conditions. Once established, CPIP is often complex and refractory to treatment, necessitating multidisciplinary and comprehensive pain management strategies.

Pharmacological Pain Management

At present, it is not possible to definitely rank the pharmacological alternatives for the individual patient, and it is thus important to choose treatment not only based on expected pain-reduction efficacy, but also potential side effects, concomitant treatments, drug interactions, risk of abuse, and cost. Recent guidelines on pharmacological treatment of neuropathic pain provide systematic analyses of treatment options based on randomized clinical trials [36–39]. If basic analgesics (e.g., acetaminophen, non-steroid anti-inflammatory drugs) provide insufficient pain relief, either a calcium channel α2-δ ligands (gabapentin or pregabalin) or antidepressants with both norepinephrine and serotonin reuptake inhibition (SSNRIs, e.g., duloxetine and venlafaxine, and tricyclic antidepressants [TCAs]) may be started. Opioids and tramadol are considered second-line treatment alternatives for neuropathic pain, but can be utilized as first-line during episodic exacerbations of severe neuropathic pain, or during titration of α2-δ ligands, TCAs or SSNRIs. There is often a need for combination therapy, and the strongest evidence supports TCA-gabapentin or gabapentin-opioids. There is no firm evidence to support the use of lidocaine or capsaicin patches for CPIP but these may be used adjunctively [40, 41]. In our practice, all patients considered for operative remediation should have undergone a trial of gabapentin, pregabalin, and/or an atypical antidepressant. A short trial of lidocaine patches may be helpful for mild superficial neuropathic hypersensitivity, especially for patients that are sensitive to the systemic side effects of narcotics and neuropathic agents.

Interventional Pain Management

Nerve blocks of the IHN, IIN, and/or GFN have been used for diagnostic and therapeutic purposes for decades, but there is no robust scientific evidence of analgesic efficacy, or consensus regarding best technique. Ultrasound guidance enables direct visualization of peripheral nerves, which improves accuracy and reduces intraperitoneal needle placement. Most evidence on peripheral nerve blocks in CPIP is based on case reports or case series, and there is only one randomized, double-blind, placebo-controlled study published to date, evaluating the efficacy of ultrasound-guided IIN/IHN blocks in the treatment of CPIP [42]. This study by Bischoff et al.

failed to provide evidence for analgesic efficacy of local anesthetic nerve block in CPIP. In our experience, nerve blocks play an important role in predicting the efficacy of neurectomy for patients with inguinodynia. Improvement with blocks help to distinguish neuropathic pain from nociceptive causes and helps patients to separate these two entities. Failure of blocks to relieve pain, however, is not necessarily predictive of a lack of effect with neurectomy as there is significant operator dependence with blocks and extensive individual neuroanatomic variability.

If nerve blocks provide significant analgesia, neuroablative techniques such as chemical neurolysis, cryoablation, and pulsed radiofrequency (PRF) ablation may be considered for longer-lasting effect. Cryoablation is neurodestructive by means of Wallerian degeneration and selectively destroys axons and myelin sheaths while leaving the epineurium and perineurium intact. The affected axons treated with cryoablation are very unlikely to form neuromas, and patients are less likely to develop deafferentation pain, both of which have been associated with neurectomy or thermal non-PRF ablation. PRF delivers pulses of electromagnetic energy in or near nerve tissues, at the peripheral or vertebral level, which allows for heat (typically 42 °C) to dissipate during the latent phase so that neurodestructive temperatures are not obtained, thus lowering the risk of neuroma formation, neuritis-type reaction, and deafferentation pain. It is hypothesized that this moderate heating of nerve tissue temporarily blocks nerve conduction. A systematic review of PRF ablation for CPIP concluded that the current evidence base is limited, and that the strength of recommendation for this treatment modality is weak to moderate [43]. Neuromodulation techniques utilizing implantable devices, such as peripheral nerve field stimulation (PNFS), dorsal root ganglion (DRG) stimulation, and spinal cord stimulation (SCS) may also be considered when all other conventional treatments have failed. Case reports and case series provide promising results [11], but the scientific evidence for these treatments in CPIP is low quality at present.

Surgical Pain Management

Despite advanced multimodal pain management strategies, a minority of patients will still suffer from intractable, refractory pain. Failure of conservative measures, is however not an indication for further surgery, and successful outcomes are entirely dependent upon choosing patients with discrete, neuroanatomic problems that may be corrected with surgery [1, 2, 44]. There is no level 1 or 2 evidence and best available recommendations are derived from reviews of case series and expert consensus [2, 45, 46]. Development of chronic inguinodynia is largely independent of the method of hernia repair, but an in-depth understanding of the causes of pain, groin neuroanatomy, and technical aspects of the initial operation are necessary to successfully manage these patients, and determine the operative options [2, 21, 47, 48].

The neuroanatomy of the groin is complex and highly variable from the retroperitoneal lumbar plexus to the terminal branches exiting through the inguinal canal. Understanding the location of potential nerve injury is crucial [49].

In front of the transversalis fascia, the IIN, the visible and intramuscular segment of the IHN, and the inguinal segment of the genital branch of the GFN must be considered (Fig. 47.1). These structures may potentially be injured during open anterior repairs (tissue repair, Lichtenstein, PHS [prolene hernia system], and plug) and from mesh fixation during laparoscopic repair (TEP [totally extraperitoneal] and TAPP [transabdominal preperitoneal]). Behind the transversalis fascia within the preperitoneal space, the main trunk of the genitofemoral and the preperitoneal segment of the genital branch of the GFN are at risk (Fig. 47.2). These must be considered during open preperitoneal repair (plug, PHS, and Kugel) and laparoscopic repair (TEP and TAPP). Injury to the nerves within the retroperitoneal space including the main trunk of the GFN over the psoas muscle and the lateral femoral cutaneous nerve must also be considered after open and laparoscopic posterior repair [47, 50].

The recommended timing for surgical treatment of CPIP not responding to nonsurgical management is a minimum of 6 months after the original repair [1, 2]. A systematic and thorough

Fig. 47.1 Inguinal neuroanatomy: classic course and location of the ilioinguinal, iliohypogastric, and genital Branch of the Genitofemoral nerve within the inguinal canal

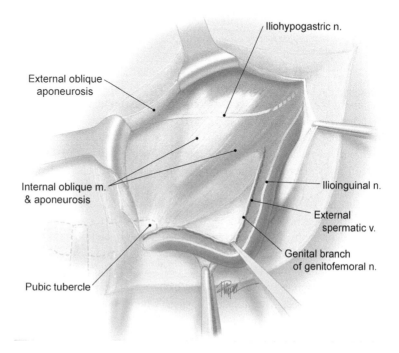

Iliohypogastric n.

External oblique aponeurosis

Internal oblique m. & aponeurosis

Ilioinguinal n.

External spermatic v.

Genital branch of genitofemoral n.

Pubic tubercle

Fig. 47.2 Retroperitoneal neuroanatomy: normal course of the iliohypogastric, ilioinguinal, and genitofemoral nerve trunks within the retroperitoneal lumbar plexus

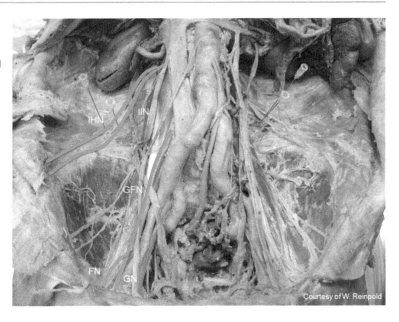

preoperative evaluation is imperative, and should always include review of prior operative reports (specifically, type of repair, type of mesh used, position of the mesh, method of fixation, and nerve handling), and response to prior interventions [2]. Neuropathic pain isolated to the inguinal distribution, that was not present prior to the original operation, and with improvement from diagnostic and therapeutic nerve blocks, has the highest likelihood of improvement with operative neurectomy. In our practice, in the absence of recurrence, infection, or an overt anatomic cause for pain, we require all patients to be at least 6 months out from their initial operation. We ensure that they have exhausted all appropriate conservative measures including pharmacologic management, physical therapy, and interventional nerve blocks prior to consideration for operative neurectomy.

Selective IIN, IHN, and GFN neurolysis or neurectomy, removal of mesh and fixation material, and revision of the prior herniorrhaphy are common options for treatment [51–54]. Neurolysis does not address ultrastructural changes of nerve fibers, and has limited efficacy, and simple removal of entrapping sutures or fixating devices while leaving the injured nerve behind is also inadequate [2]. Selective single or double neurectomy may be

effective for some patients but does not address ultrastructural changes of seemingly normal appearing nerves during reoperation, and discerning which nerve is involved can be extremely difficult [51–53]. The use of preoperative dermatomal mapping and clinical expertise may improve the likelihood of success with selective neurectomy. Anatomically, the significant variation and cross-innervation of the inguinal nerves in the retroperitoneum and inguinal canal make selective neurectomy less reliable [2, 49].

Triple neurectomy of the IIN, IHN, and GFN, pioneered in our institute in 1995, is currently a universally accepted surgical treatment for neuropathic pain refractory to conservative measures and is arguably the most effective option [2, 21, 47, 48, 50]. Our experience has included over 700 patients, 650+ utilizing an open approach with an over 85% success rate and 42 cases using a laparoscopic retroperitoneal approach with a 93% success rate [50]. Operative neurectomy in conjunction with removal of meshoma, when present, provides effective relief in the majority of patients with refractory inguinodynia [2, 50]. Triple neurectomy can be performed through an open approach using the groin incision of the original hernia operation or through a laparoscopic approach particularly for pain after preperitoneal repair or after failed remedial surgery. With open surgery, the IIN can be identified lateral to the internal ring, between the ring and the anterior superior iliac spine. The IHN is identified within the anatomic cleavage between the external and internal oblique aponeurosis. The nerve is then traced proximally within the fibers of the internal oblique muscle to a point lateral to the field of the original hernia repair. Failure to do so may leave the injured intramuscular segment of the nerve behind. In those instances where the IHN has a subaponeurotic course, the internal oblique aponeurosis is split to visualize and address the hidden nerve. The inguinal segment of the genital branch of the GFN can be identified between the cord and the inguinal ligament and traced laterally to the internal ring where it is severed. Alternatively, the nerve may be visualized within the internal ring through the lateral crus of the ring. The nerves should be resected proximal to the field of original hernia repair. Although there are no specific data available, we recommend ligation of the cut ends of the nerves to avoid neuroma formation and insertion of the proximal cut end into the muscle to keep the nerve stump away from the future scarring of the operative field [2, 21, 47]. Advantages of the open approach are a single stage operation, simultaneous plug/meshoma removal, repair of recurrent hernias, extension if needed to include the GFN trunk, and resection of paravasal nerves in case of orchialgia. The disadvantage of the approach is its complexity and technical difficulty operating within the scarred field which places the spermatic cord, testicle, and vascular structures at higher risk of compromise.

Laparoscopic retroperitoneal triple neurectomy may be performed through a transabdominal or extraperitoneal approach [50]. The IIN and IHN can be identified within the retroperitoneal space over the quadratus lumborum muscle and the GFN over the psoas muscle proximal to the scarred operative field. Advantages of the laparoscopic approach are the ability to access the nerves proximal to the mesh-material used during the original herniorrhaphy, more consistent neuroanatomy within the lumbar plexus, and its technical simplicity. Disadvantages include not being able to remove plugs, if any, not being able to resect the lamina propria of the vas in case of associated orchialgia, and potential laxity of the abdominal muscles caused from proximal denervation. It is critical to clearly explain potential benefits and consequences of operative intervention to manage patient expectations. In addition to the usual operative risks, specific considerations include permanent numbness, the inability to access or identify three nerves, abdominal wall laxity from partial denervation of the oblique muscles, testicular atrophy, numbness in the labia in females that can interfere with sexual sensation, and loss of a cremasteric reflex in male patients [2, 47, 50]. Patients are specifically advised of the potential for ongoing pain and disability despite successful neurectomy due to the nociceptive component of pain, maladaptive neuroplasticity, and centralization of pain. The development and course of deafferentation hypersensitivity is unpredictable but typically diminishes over time. These issues require serious consideration and should be discussed with the patient and adequately recorded.

Hernia recurrence and meshoma are obvious anatomic pathologies amenable to surgical correction. When recurrence is identified, surgical correction is typically recommended using an alternative approach (i.e., laparoscopic repair after initial open repair or vice versa). However, if accompanied by neuropathic pain, an anterior, open approach allows for correction of the hernia as well as access to the nerves [47]. Meshoma may cause neuropathic pain from nerve entrapment, direct contact with mesh, or compressive effects [8]. It may also cause nociceptive pain from compression of adjacent structures and foreign body sensation. Operative removal of the meshoma is indicated with the need for simultaneous neurectomy directed by the type of mesh, approach, symptoms, imaging, and anatomy. If coexisting neuropathic pain is present, all nerves within the reoperative field should be addressed, as neuropathy cannot be assessed visually, and mesh removal will often compromise unaffected nerves within the inguinal canal [2]. In patients with groin pain associated with orchialgia, segmental resection of the lamina propria of the vas together with triple neurectomy has improved outcomes and helped in the management of testicular pain [47]. In our experience, we have performed vas neurolysis on over 40 patients with refractory orchialgia in conjunction with triple neurectomy with success in over 80% of patients. Orchialgia, however, is a complex entity and remedial surgery to correct it is less predictable and less effective.

Our personal algorithm for operative remediation depends on whether the pain is neuropathic or nociceptive and is tailored to the initial operation and potential pathologies associated with the initial repair. Neuropathic pain without evidence of recurrence or meshoma may be addressed with triple neurectomy alone either through an open or laparoscopic approach leaving the mesh and prior repair intact. If the initial operation was performed as an open anterior repair, we will typically offer an open triple neurectomy via the inguinal canal. If the initial operation was an open or laparoscopic preperitoneal repair, the neurectomy is best performed through a laparoscopic retroperitoneal approach. Neuropathic pain associated with meshoma will require mesh removal at the time of triple neurectomy and can be performed through an inguinal re-exploration. This is common for problems related to initial PHS and plug and patch repair where mesh traverses both the anterior and posterior planes. Pain caused by an isolated plug may be removed open, laparoscopic, or at times via a hybrid approach to access the mesh and nerves. Our preference to treat neuropathic inguinodynia with triple neurectomy, given the neuroanatomic considerations and efficacy rates. However, selective neurectomy is appropriate at times with isolated nerve injuries that do not overlap in dermatomal distribution, such as an isolated lateral femoral cutaneous nerve (lateral thigh) or femoral branch of the genitofemoral nerve (anterior thigh) injuries. While general principles exist, remedial surgery for inguinodynia remains a challenge and must be tailored for each individual patient requiring creativity, a thorough understanding of inguinal and retroperitoneal neuroanatomy, and an armamentarium of different open, laparoscopic, mesh, and tissue repairs.

Conclusion

Chronic pain after hernia repair is a dreaded, heterogeneous pain syndrome representing a substantial diagnostic and therapeutic challenge. In-depth knowledge of groin neuroanatomy is critical, as the best measure to address this debilitating pain state remains prevention by refining the technique of hernia repair. Meticulous adherence to surgical principles with three nerve identification, preservation, or pragmatic neurectomy during open anterior repair decreases the incidence of CPIP. Avoidance of the preperitoneal nerves below the iliopubic tract and limited or no mesh fixation decreases the risk of pain after laparoscopic herniorrhaphy. Preventive analgesia and anesthesia should be considered for patients at high risk of developing CPIP. Evaluation by a pain specialist is mandatory, and patients should undergo multidisciplinary treatment, including behavioral, pharmacological, and interventional pain management modalities. For patients with pain refractory to conservative measures, operative neurectomy, meshoma removal, and repair of recurrence may provide relief. A multidisciplinary, logical, stepwise approach to CPIP will afford patients the greatest opportunity to minimize symptoms, manage pain, decrease further morbidity, and improve quality of life.

References

1. Aasvang E, Kehlet H. Surgical management of chronic pain after inguinal hernia repair. Br J Surg. 2005;92:795–801.
2. Alfieri S, et al. International guidelines for prevention and management of post-operative chronic pain following inguinal hernia surgery. Hernia. 2011;15: 239–49.
3. Aasvang E, Kehlet H. Chronic postoperative pain: the case of inguinal herniorrhaphy. Br J Anaesth. 2005;95: 69–76.
4. Bittner R, Schwarz J. Inguinal hernia repair: current surgical techniques. Langenbeck's archives of surgery. Deutsche Gesellschaft für Chirurgie. 2012;397: 271–82.
5. Macrae WA, Davies HTO. Chronic postsurgical pain. In: Crombie IK, Croft PR, Linton SJ, LeResche L, Von Korff M, editors. Epidemiology of pain. Seattle: IASP Press; 1999. p. 125–42.

6. Kalliomaki ML, Sandblom G, Gunnarsson U, Gordh T. Persistent pain after groin hernia surgery: a qualitative analysis of pain and its consequences for quality of life. Acta Anaesthesiol Scand. 2009;53:236–46.

7. Parsons B, et al. Economic and humanistic burden of post-trauma and post-surgical neuropathic pain among adults in the United States. J Pain Res. 2013;6: 459–69.

8. Amid PK. Radiologic images of meshoma: a new phenomenon causing chronic pain after prosthetic repair of abdominal wall hernias. Arch Surg. 2004; 139:1297–8.

9. Loos MJ, Roumen RM, Scheltinga MR. Classifying post-herniorrhaphy pain syndromes following elective inguinal hernia repair. World J Surg. 2007; 31:1760–5. discussion 1766-1767.

10. Katz J, Seltzer Z. Transition from acute to chronic postsurgical pain: risk factors and protective factors. Expert Rev Neurother. 2009;9:723–44.

11. Bjurstrom MF, Nicol AL, Amid PK, Chen DC. Pain control following inguinal herniorrhaphy: current perspectives. J Pain Res. 2014;7:277–90.

12. Bjurstrom MF, Giron SE, Griffis CA. Cerebrospinal fluid cytokines and neurotrophic factors in human chronic pain populations: A comprehensive review. Pain Pract. 2014.

13. Dominguez CA, et al. The DQB1 *03:02 HLA haplotype is associated with increased risk of chronic pain after inguinal hernia surgery and lumbar disc herniation. Pain. 2013;154:427–33.

14. Kehlet H, Jensen TS, Woolf CJ. Persistent postsurgical pain: risk factors and prevention. Lancet. 2006; 367:1618–25.

15. Aasvang EK, et al. Predictive risk factors for persistent postherniotomy pain. Anesthesiology. 2010;112: 957–69.

16. Kalliomaki ML, Meyerson J, Gunnarsson U, Gordh T, Sandblom G. Long-term pain after inguinal hernia repair in a population-based cohort; risk factors and interference with daily activities. Eur J Pain. 2008;12: 214–25.

17. Bay-Nielsen M, Kehlet H. Anaesthesia and postoperative morbidity after elective groin hernia repair: a nation-wide study. Acta Anaesthesiol Scand. 2008;52:169–74.

18. Kehlet H, Aasvang E. Groin hernia repair: anesthesia. World J Surg. 2005;29:1058–61.

19. Nordin P, Zetterstrom H, Gunnarsson U, Nilsson E. Local, regional, or general anaesthesia in groin hernia repair: multicentre randomised trial. Lancet. 2003; 362:853–8.

20. Nienhuijs S, et al. Chronic pain after mesh repair of inguinal hernia: a systematic review. Am J Surg. 2007;194:394–400.

21. Amid PK, Hiatt JR. New understanding of the causes and surgical treatment of postherniorrhaphy inguinodynia and orchalgia. J Am Coll Surg. 2007;205:381–5.

22. Kalkman CJ, et al. Preoperative prediction of severe postoperative pain. Pain. 2003;105:415–23.

23. Sajid MS, Leaver C, Baig MK, Sains P. Systematic review and meta-analysis of the use of lightweight versus heavyweight mesh in open inguinal hernia repair. Br J Surg. 2012;99:29–37.

24. Sajid MS, Kalra L, Parampalli U, Sains PS, Baig MK. A systematic review and meta-analysis evaluating the effectiveness of lightweight mesh against heavyweight mesh in influencing the incidence of chronic groin pain following laparoscopic inguinal hernia repair. Am J Surg. 2013;205:726–36.

25. Colvin HS, Rao A, Cavali M, Campanelli G, Amin AI. Glue versus suture fixation of mesh during open repair of inguinal hernias: a systematic review and meta-analysis. World J Surg. 2013;37:2282–92.

26. de Goede B, et al. Meta-analysis of glue versus sutured mesh fixation for Lichtenstein inguinal hernia repair. Br J Surg. 2013;100:735–42.

27. Ladwa N, Sajid MS, Sains P, Baig MK. Suture mesh fixation versus glue mesh fixation in open inguinal hernia repair: a systematic review and meta-analysis. Int J Surg. 2013;11:128–35.

28. Sanders DL, Waydia S. A systematic review of randomised controlled trials assessing mesh fixation in open inguinal hernia repair. Hernia. 2014;18:165–76.

29. Zhang C, et al. Self-gripping versus sutured mesh for inguinal hernia repair: a systematic review and meta-analysis of current literature. J Surg Res. 2013;185: 653–60.

30. Ferzli GS, Edwards ED, Khoury GE. Chronic pain after inguinal herniorrhaphy. J Am Coll Surg. 2007;205:333–41.

31. Bradley M, Morgan D, Pentlow B, Roe A. The groin hernia — an ultrasound diagnosis? Ann R Coll Surg Engl. 2003;85:178–80.

32. van den Berg JC, de Valois JC, Go PM, Rosenbusch G. Detection of groin hernia with physical examination, ultrasound, and MRI compared with laparoscopic findings. Invest Radiol. 1999;34:739–43.

33. Aasvang EK, Jensen KE, Fiirgaard B, Kehlet H. MRI and pathology in persistent postherniotomy pain. J Am Coll Surg. 2009;208:1023–8; discussion 1028–1029.

34. Knockaert DC, Boonen AL, Bruyninckx FL, Bobbaers HJ. Electromyographic findings in ilioinguinal-iliohypogastric nerve entrapment syndrome. Acta Clin Belg. 1996;51:156–60.

35. Filler A. Magnetic resonance neurography and diffusion tensor imaging: origins, history, and clinical impact of the first 50,000 cases with an assessment of efficacy and utility in a prospective 5000-patient study group. Neurosurgery. 2009;65:A29–43.

36. Dworkin RH, et al. Pharmacologic management of neuropathic pain: evidence-based recommendations. Pain. 2007;132:237–51.

37. Attal N, et al. EFNS guidelines on pharmacological treatment of neuropathic pain. Eur J Neurol. 2006; 13:1153–69.

38. Attal N, et al. EFNS guidelines on the pharmacological treatment of neuropathic pain: 2010 revision. Eur J Neurol. 2010;17:1113–88.

39. Moulin DE, et al. Pharmacological management of chronic neuropathic pain—consensus statement and guidelines from the Canadian Pain Society. Pain Res Manag. 2007;12:13–21.

40. Bischoff JM, et al. Lidocaine patch (5%) in treatment of persistent inguinal postherniorrhaphy pain: a randomized, double-blind, placebo-controlled. Anesthesiology: Crossover Trial; 2013.

41. Bischoff JM, et al. A capsaicin (8%) patch in the treatment of severe persistent inguinal postherniorrhaphy pain: a randomized, double-blind, placebo-controlled trial. PLoS One. 2014;9, e109144.

42. Bischoff JM, Koscielniak-Nielsen ZJ, Kehlet H, Werner MU. Ultrasound-guided ilioinguinal/iliohypogastric nerve blocks for persistent inguinal postherniorrhaphy pain: a randomized, double-blind, placebo-controlled, crossover trial. Anesth Analg. 2012;114:1323–9.

43. Werner MU, Bischoff JM, Rathmell JP, Kehlet H. Pulsed radiofrequency in the treatment of persistent pain after inguinal herniotomy: a systematic review. Reg Anesth Pain Med. 2012;37:340–3.

44. Kehlet H. Chronic pain after groin hernia repair. Br J Surg. 2008;95:135–6.

45. Werner MU. Management of persistent postsurgical inguinal pain. Langenbecks Arch Surg. 2014;399: 559–69.

46. Lange JF, et al. An international consensus algorithm for management of chronic postoperative inguinal pain. Hernia. 2014;19(1):33–43.

47. Amid PK, Chen DC. Surgical treatment of chronic groin and testicular pain after laparoscopic and open preperitoneal inguinal hernia repair. J Am Coll Surg. 2011;213:531–6.

48. Amid PK. Causes, prevention, and surgical treatment of postherniorrhaphy neuropathic inguinodynia: triple neurectomy with proximal end implantation. Hernia. 2004;8:343–9.

49. Klaassen Z, et al. Anatomy of the ilioinguinal and iliohypogastric nerves with observations of their spinal nerve contributions. Clin Anat. 2011;24: 454–61.

50. Chen DC, Hiatt JR, Amid PK. Operative management of refractory neuropathic inguinodynia by a laparoscopic retroperitoneal approach. JAMA Surg. 2013;148:962–7.

51. Aasvang EK, Kehlet H. The effect of mesh removal and selective neurectomy on persistent postherniotomy pain. Ann Surg. 2009;249:327–34.

52. Zacest AC, Magill ST, Anderson VC, Burchiel KJ. Long-term outcome following ilioinguinal neurectomy for chronic pain. J Neurosurg. 2010; 112:784–9.

53. Loos MJ, Scheltinga MR, Roumen RM. Tailored neurectomy for treatment of postherniorrhaphy inguinal neuralgia. Surgery. 2010;147:275–81.

54. Keller JE, et al. Combined open and laparoscopic approach to chronic pain after inguinal hernia repair. Am Surg. 2008;74:695–700; discussion 700–691.

Scott Roth and John E. Wennergren

Introduction

Treatment of inguinal hernia disease is as old as recorded time itself with descriptions of the ailment affecting fifteenth century Egyptians as written on papyrus. It is the second most common general surgical procedure performed annually. Over the centuries, its treatment was really one of symptom control with very poor results. It has only been within the last hundred years or so, with the advent of Bassini's repair in the late 1800s to modern day mesh repairs, where treatment of inguinal hernias has gone from one of little recourse to one with treatment strategies where complications and recurrence rates are low. With that said, anywhere from 1 to 10% of repairs, depending on operative method used, will unfortunately develop a recurrence during their lifetime. This rate is much higher for primary/meshless repairs [1]. Approximately 10–15% of all inguinal hernias performed in a Danish study involve recurrent inguinal hernias [2]. In the USA, this is estimated to be around 100,000 recurrent inguinal hernia repairs annually with a

S. Roth (✉)
Department of Surgery/General Surgery,
A.B. Chandler Medical Center, University of
Kentucky, Lexington, KY, USA
e-mail: jsroth2@uky.edu

J.E. Wennergren
Department of Surgery, University of Kentucky
Chandler Hospital, Lexington, KY, USA
e-mail: john.wennergren@uky.edu

cost of approximately $40,000,000 [2]. The advent of mesh repairs has added another layer of complexity, one in which a surgeon requires extensive knowledge of inguinal anatomy and surgical skill to attempt repair of recurrences with obliterated planes and unclear anatomic structures. Failure rates of attempted anterior repairs of recurrent hernias are estimated in some studies to be as high as 36% [3]. Since inguinal hernia surgery is one of the most common general surgical procedures performed annually, this is a problem every general surgeon will deal with during his or her practice. It is with this in mind that we present various options and methodology in dealing with this complex problem.

Pathophysiology

Etiology of inguinal hernias is complex and likely multifactorial. To evaluate this further a group using Danish data wanted to see if there was a difference in recurrence rates between Indirect (IIH) and Direct (DIH) inguinal hernias. Over a 4 year follow-up period and approximately 85,000 patients, they found a recurrence rate of 3.8% for all-comers. When subdivided into IDH and DIHs and controlled for operative technique, the recurrence rates were 2.7% and 5.2%, respectively ($p < 0.001$). At reoperation, 93% were found to be recurrent inguinal hernias while 7% were found to be either femoral hernias, pantaloons hernias, or negative for any hernia. The most significant risk

© Springer International Publishing Switzerland 2016
Y.W. Novitsky (ed.), *Hernia Surgery*, DOI 10.1007/978-3-319-27470-6_48

factor identified was DIH at initial operation compared to IIH. In fact, not only was it a major risk factor leading to increased rates of recurrence but was also found to lead to earlier recurrences compared to IIHs [1].

There is no concrete evidence to explain this discrepancy. Many have argued that the reason this occurs is technical in nature, due to insufficient overlap of mesh at the pubic tubercle. Another explanation may be that while one (IIH) may be due to a developmental disorder, the other (DIH) may be due to a systemic disorder of collagen synthesis. For a long time it has been argued that inguinal hernias were a direct result of structural defects, but, as has been shown recently, there is a rising body of evidence to suggest that deficiencies in connective tissue metabolism may very well likely play a larger role in their development. Recently, a group released findings of a positive correlation between not only family history and increased risk for development of inguinal hernias, but found that mutations within the COL1A1 gene (responsible for transcription of 1(I) protein chain of type I collagen which has been shown to be involved in connective tissue disorders such as Ehlers–Danlos and osteogenesis imperfect) was also implicated in increased risk for development of inguinal hernias [4]. The implications of this understanding knowledge are only just being understood, but ultimately may modify our practice on operative approach and usage of mesh.

Preoperative Evaluation

Evaluation of a patient for a recurrent inguinal hernia is not quite as straightforward as one might think. Postoperative complication rates, mainly defined as recurrence, long-term pain and overall patient comfort, range from 4 to 40% [5]. The previous operative planes, depending on the operative approach used, may be obliterated and the anatomy made unclear. As several randomized control trials have demonstrated, use of tension-free mesh repair has revolutionized treatment of the disease with overall decrease in recurrence rates. However, with this also comes the unfortunate consequence of inflammatory

reaction caused by the mesh, thereby making repeat dissection much more difficult and potentially leading to increased risk of injury to nerves and increased pain. Indeed, one must be certain of the decision to reoperate on a patient for a recurrent inguinal hernia.

In this regard, the surgeon must evaluate the patients' potential risk factors which first will determine whether or not the patient is an optimal surgical candidate and if so, then address modifiable risk factors to maximize outcomes. These risk factors include age >50, smoking, family history, type of hernia, and obesity [6].

In situations where a diagnosis of a hernia is difficult to make clinically, imaging may be required. These hernias, in the literature defined as *occult hernias*, typically present with chronic pain without evidence of recurrence or palpable bulge clinically. It is these circumstances where either US, CT, or MRI may be used, however, data as to the usefulness of each modality is widely variable. A recent meta-analysis demonstrated a sensitivity and specificity for each modality of 86% and 77%, 80% and 65%, 91% and 83%, respectively [7]. Another retrospective study found a sensitivity and specificity of each to be 56% and 0%, 77% and 25%, 91% and 92%, respectively for all-comers [8]. These numbers are even worse if used in patients with the diagnosis of *occult hernias*: 33% and 0%, 54% and 25%, 91% and 92%, respectively [8]. Classically, US has been used as a first-line strategy in the diagnosis of inguinal hernias because of its availability and low cost. However, it's been noted that in the case of *occult hernias*, US and CT may not suffice thus leaving MRI as the mainstay of diagnosis. It has been our practice in cases where it is clinically difficult to confirm the diagnosis to begin with an US followed by CT, if uncertainty remains. However, in cases of chronic pain or occult hernia, we proceed straight to MRI which is more sensitive in identifying neuromas or problems with the mesh.

In deciding when to operate, it appears that time is on our side. A randomized multicenter trial performed in 2006 found that watchful waiting was an acceptable option in management of both first time and recurrent inguinal hernias in men that were asymptomatic or minimally symptomatic. Their study found that the risk of strangulation was extremely rare and that postoperative complication rates were not affected by watchful waiting [9]. Therefore, there is no rush to take an asymptomatic patient back to surgery. Rather, care and planning should precede any operative intervention, operating only on those patients symptomatic enough to warrant therapy in order to avoid potential complications.

Once the decision is made to reoperate, one must then decide which method to use. It is important at this juncture to review the patients' previous surgical history and whenever possible obtain operative reports where one can learn about what previous types of mesh, if any, have been used. These options can be broken down broadly into two categories: Open vs Laparoscopic. Although not entirely prohibitive, in patients with a history of pelvic radiation one may find that a laparoscopic approach may be difficult and therefore opt for an anterior open repair. In those patients who have undergone a prostatectomy, excision of the peritoneum makes a laparoscopic repair difficult making an open repair likely a better-suited repair.

The use of mesh is generally required in patients undergoing recurrent repair due to a high likelihood of wound healing abnormalities such as collagen abnormalities. Rare cases involving infected hernia mesh may preclude placement of a mesh and require special consideration. While recent studies have begun to show no significant difference between biologic and synthetic mesh with regard to quality of life, complication rates and rates of recurrence, use of biologic mesh has been customarily reserved for use in contaminated cases [10, 11]. Lightweight polypropylene mesh (LWPPM) is advantageous due to decreased pain, decreased mesh sensation, and theoretical greater ingrowth of the mesh to provide a more durable repair [12]. However, in situations where a wide bridged repair would be required, such as a large direct inguinal hernia, the use of standard weight polypropylene mesh should be considered to minimize the risk of postoperative mesh eventration or recurrence [13].

Operative Approach

Determining the operative approach is generally predicated upon the patient's medical and surgical history. Those patients with previous open repairs generally benefit from a laparoscopic repair. We prefer a totally extraperitoneal approach, as this minimizes the potential for intra-abdominal adhesions, although transabdominal preperitoneal repairs (TAPP) are also utilized in these situations. The type of prior open repair should be considered as several techniques for hernia repair with placement of preperitoneal mesh through an anterior incision have been described (i.e., Kugel repair, Prolene Hernia System, Plug and patch repairs). The extent of prior preperitoneal dissection will determine the feasibility of a totally extraperitoneal approach. In our experience, the extent of preperitoneal dissection associated with the open preperitoneal repairs does not prevent a totally extraperitoneal approach. As the most commonly performed anterior inguinal hernia repair is the Lichtenstein approach, a totally extraperitoneal repair is generally feasible and is no more difficult than a laparoscopic repair for a primary inguinal hernia. Following a Lichtenstein repair, the preperitoneal space has not been violated, the prior mesh is anterior to the abdominal musculature, and few traces of a prior surgical repair are evident. Unless prior mesh has resulted in chronic pain or other complications, removal is not required. In the event mesh removal is desired, a combined anterior and laparoscopic approach may be required. Additional benefits of a laparoscopic approach for recurrent hernias include the ability to explore the contralateral groin and repair bilateral hernias when necessary. Whether for primary or recurrent inguinal hernias, laparoscopic repair results in more rapid recovery for patients requiring bilateral repairs [14, 15].

For patients with large recurrent hernias, or inguinoscrotal recurrences, laparoscopic repair can be more challenging. Identification and visualization of the contents of a chronically incarcerated recurrent inguinal hernia may be limited through an extraperitoneal approach. A TAPP approach allows for direct visualization of the incarcerated contents and serial reduction of the contents while visualizing the contents of the hernia sac. In the event the hernia sac is not fully reducible, the hernia sac may be dissected from the cord structures and divided leaving the distal hernia sac open while the proximal hernia sac is later closed with the peritoneal flaps. While division of challenging hernia sacs is feasible, we reserve this technique for the most challenging situations, as there is a potential for development of postoperative hydrocele as a result of the remnant hernia sac within the inguinal canal and scrotum. In the event of postoperative hydrocele formation, we would advocate observation for months prior to consideration for excision. As a matter of practice, we will typically utilize a TEP approach for recurrent inguinal hernias following prior anterior repairs when the hernia is reducible following induction of anesthesia. If the hernia remains non-reducible following anesthetic induction, a TAPP approach is preferred.

When trying to decide between using a TEP or a TAPP repair, other than in select situations, the choice is often based upon surgeon experience. A recent randomized prospective study tried to identify any differences between the two operative approaches. While there was significantly higher acute pain postoperatively and longer operative times associated with a TAPP repair, there was no difference between the two procedures when looking at quality of life, chronic groin pain and resumption of normal activities or cost [16].

In addition, a previous history of laparoscopic hernia repair, either TEP or TAPP, doesn't necessarily eliminate the ability to address the recurrence with another attempt laparoscopically. A retrospective study found that out of 51 patients with recurrent inguinal hernias after laparoscopic repair (70% TAPP, 23% TEP, 7% other), 49 underwent successful redo TAPP repair with the other two converting to open anterior repairs due to dense adhesions. There was a 32% post-op complication rate including hematoma/seroma formation and one port site infection. There was also one case where the vas deferens was ligated due to dense adhesions to the mesh and four patients with complaints of persistent chronic

pain. However, there were no recurrences at 70 month follow-up. Of interest, in about two thirds of these patients, the location of the recurrence was found to happen either caudal or medial to previous mesh placement [17].

How about cases where the patient has had both open and laparoscopic repairs? What if you find yourself doing a TAPP repair only to realize that there isn't enough peritoneum to close over the mesh? In such instances, the use of an Intraperitoneal Onlay Mesh (IPOM) can be used. This mesh is customarily a permanent mesh with anti-adhesive barrier, much like one used in laparoscopic ventral hernia repairs (Fig. 48.1). While reports of such repair are uncommon with regard to inguinal hernia surgery, it does appear that when compared to Lichtenstein repair, there is no significant difference in chronic pain [18]. Other studies have shown no difference in seroma formation, recurrence, mesh migration, bowel obstruction, or fistula [19]. It is our practice to reserve IPOM for such situations where TEP, TAPP, or open repairs are unavailable due to concerns of increased adhesion rates. One must keep in mind, and as will be discussed later, tacks

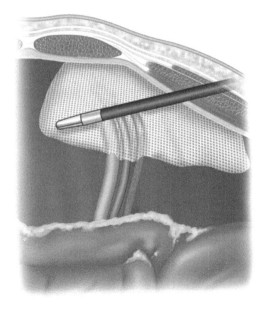

Fig. 48.1 IPOM—Placement of mesh covering an internal hernia. The cord structures are visible along the underside of the mesh

used to secure mesh in this fashion must be done with extreme caution so as to avoid bladder and/ or neurovascular injury. Therefore, tacks are placed above the ileopubic tract, with the use of fibrin glue along the lower edge of the mesh for fixation to prevent bowel migration behind the mesh. If possible, a small peritoneal flap can be raised to cover the lower edge of the mesh and secured to the mesh above the ileopubic tract.

Additionally, there is the scenario where a patient has had both open and laparoscopic repairs but is known to have a "hostile" abdomen, leaving an open repair the only safe option.

Mesh Fixation

The role of mesh fixation in laparoscopic inguinal hernia repair is an area of continuous debate. While some believe that fixation is necessary in order to prevent mesh migration and to minimize recurrence rates, others feel that mesh fixation unnecessarily increases risk of postoperative pain due to injury to nerves. A randomized control trial from the Mayo clinic looked at whether fixation should be used at all and found that in those patients where no fixation was used, there was less analgesic usage in the PACU, less urinary retention, and shorter hospital length of stay but no difference in postoperative pain [20]. A more recent study found that there was no difference in pain scores at 1 day, 1 week, 1 month, 1 year, and 2 year follow-up. There was no difference in length of hospital stay, resumption of normal activity, seroma formation, and recurrence rates (no recurrences in either group at 2 years) [6].

Our Approach

Recurrent inguinal hernias are approached in our practice by utilizing an algorithm. While most patients may be treated utilizing this standardized strategy, certain patient characteristics may occasionally require individualization. The decision as to the best approach is based upon a combination of surgical history, comorbidities, ability to tolerate an operation, as well as patient preferences.

Although inguinal hernia repair can be safely performed in most individuals, there may be some patients that are best managed non-operatively, recognizing the small risk of incarceration and strangulation resulting in emergent repair. Examples of situations in which nonoperative treatment for recurrent hernias include medical conditions limiting a patient's ability to tolerate anesthesia, uncorrected coagulopathies, advanced liver disease, or severe cardiopulmonary conditions. Occasionally, patients will not be suitable for general anesthesia, yet will be considered a reasonable risk for a procedure under local anesthesia. While it is technically feasible to perform a recurrent inguinal hernia repair under a local anesthesia, we favor a nonoperative approach in these individuals, as a recurrent inguinal hernia repair can be quite involved and unanticipated difficulties may necessitate conversion from a local to general anesthetic.

Among patients suitable for a general anesthetic, the decision for recurrent repair type is made based upon the prior surgical history. Patients with a previous anterior repair (Lichtenstein, McVay, Plug and Patch, Bassini, etc.) will undergo a laparoscopic repair. We favor a totally extraperitoneal approach for our laparoscopic inguinal hernia repairs in the majority of patients. However, patients with a history of prior abdominal surgery involving an incision below the umbilicus are approached transabdominally (TAPP). On the other hand, patients with prior laparoscopic abdominal surgery or limited prior open procedures (i.e., appendectomy) are considered for an extraperitoneal approach. We always obtain prior operative notes to determine the details of prior operations as occasionally patients will have undergone a prior open operation involving placement of a mesh in the preperitoneal space such as a Kugel or plug repair. Repairs involving prior mesh in the preperitoneal space can be more challenging, particularly when the preperitoneal space has been widely dissected. We will occasionally place a port in the left upper quadrant to allow visualization of the peritoneal cavity in situations in which dissection of the peritoneum from the prior plug is challenging;

however, in most cases the peritoneum is easily dissected from the plug. In patients with a prior open preperitoneal repair such as a Kugel repair, we will generally perform a laparoscopic transabdominal preperitoneal inguinal hernia repair. Removal of the prior mesh is performed, if feasible, to facilitate new mesh placement. If prior mesh is unable to be removed, we will remove as much as possible while avoiding injury to the vas deferens, gonadal vessels, and other structures. If the peritoneum is not amenable to closure following dissection, a tissue separating mesh is utilized with the barrier placed adjacent to the viscera. We will then affix the mesh to the abdominal wall with fibrin glue along the inferior most edge and subsequently glue the peritoneum over the inferior aspect of the mesh to prevent bowel from migrating behind the inferior aspect of the mesh.

Patients with a prior history of a laparoscopic inguinal hernia repair (TAPP, TEP, or IPOM) with an ipsilateral recurrence will undergo an open mesh hernia repair through an anterior approach (i.e., Lichtenstein repair). Patients with a contralateral inguinal hernia following a prior laparoscopic repair are approached laparoscopically. Although the prior preperitoneal space has been dissected, as long as mesh has not been placed into the space, it is generally feasible to dissect the peritoneum from the abdominal wall without difficulty.

Patients with multiple recurrent inguinal hernias with prior repairs from both an anterior and laparoscopic approach represent unique challenges. The details of the prior operations are carefully considered and a repair is tailored to the patient. Our approach is to generally utilize a TAPP repair, with conversion to an open repair if necessary. When conversion is required, we will perform either a Lichtenstein hernia repair or an open preperitoneal repair (i.e., Stoppa). We will make every attempt feasible to remove prior mesh to allow for maximal integration of the newly placed prosthetic into the abdominal wall. A careful informed consent discussion is mandatory in these situations as there is a significant risk for injuries to the cord structures and testicle, which may result in the need for orchiectomy.

References

1. Burcharth J, Andresen K, Pommergaard HC, Bisgaard T, Rosenberg J. Recurrence patterns of direct and indirect inguinal hernias in a nationwide population in Denmark. Surgery. 2014;155(1):173–7.
2. Sgourakis G, Dedemadi G, Gockel I, Schmidtmann I, Lanitis S, Zaphiriadou P, Papatheodorou A, Karaliotas C. Laparoscopic totally extraperitoneal versus open preperitoneal mesh repair for inguinal hernia recurrence: a decision analysis based on net health benefits. Surg Endosc. 2013;27(7):2526–41.
3. Saber A, Ellabban GM, Gad MA, Elsayem K. Open preperitoneal versus anterior approach for recurrent inguinal hernia: a randomized study. BMC Surg. 2012;12:22.
4. Sezer S, Şimşek N, Celik HT, Erden G, Ozturk G, Düzgün AP, Çoşkun F, Demircan K. Association of collagen type I alpha 1 gene polymorphism with inguinal hernia. Hernia. 2014;18(4):507–12.
5. Lundström KJ, Sandblom G, Smedberg S, Nordin P. Risk factors for complications in groin hernia surgery: a national register study. Ann Surg. 2012;255(4):784–8.
6. Junge K, Rosch R, Klinge U, Schwab R, Peiper C, Binnebösel M, Schenten F, Schumpelick V. Risk factors related to recurrence in inguinal hernia repair: a retrospective analysis. Hernia. 2006;10(4):309–15.
7. Robinson A, Light D, Kasim A, Nice C. A systematic review and meta-analysis of the role of radiology in the diagnosis of occult inguinal hernia. Surg Endosc. 2013;27(1):11–8.
8. Miller J, Cho J, Michael MJ, Saouaf R, Towfigh S. Role of imaging in the diagnosis of occult hernias. JAMA Surg. 2014;149(10):1077–80.
9. Fitzgibbons Jr RJ, Giobbie-Hurder A, Gibbs JO, Dunlop DD, Reda DJ, McCarthy Jr M, Neumayer LA, Barkun JS, Hoehn JL, Murphy JT, Sarosi Jr GA, Syme WC, Thompson JS, Wang J, Jonasson O. Watchful waiting vs repair of inguinal hernia in minimally symptomatic men: a randomized clinical trial. JAMA. 2006;295(3):285–92.
10. Bellows CF, Shadduck P, Helton WS, Martindale R, Stouch BC, Fitzgibbons R. Early report of a randomized comparative clinical trial of Strattice™ reconstructive tissue matrix to lightweight synthetic mesh in the repair of inguinal hernias. Hernia. 2014;18(2):221–30.
11. Bochicchio GV, Jain A, McGonigal K, Turner D, Ilahi O, Reese S, Bochicchio K. Biologic vs synthetic inguinal hernia repair: 1-year results of a randomized double-blinded trial. J Am Coll Surg. 2014;218(4):751–7.

12. Post S, Weiss B, Willer M, Neufang T, Lorenz D. Randomized clinical trial of lightweight composite mesh for Lichtenstein inguinal hernia repair. Br J Surg. 2004;91(1):44–8.

13. Lintin LA, Kingsnorth AN. Mechanical failure of a lightweight polypropylene mesh. Hernia. 2014;18(1):131–3.

14. Chan KL, Hui WC, Tam PK. Prospective randomized single-center, single-blind comparison of laparoscopic vs open repair of pediatric inguinal hernia. Surg Endosc. 2005;19(7):927–32.

15. Celebi S, Uysal AI, Inal FY, Yildiz A. A single-blinded, randomized comparison of laparoscopic versus open bilateral hernia repair in boys. J Laparoendosc Adv Surg Tech A. 2014;24(2):117–21.

16. Bansal VK, Misra MC, Babu D, Victor J, Kumar S, Sagar R, Rajeshwari S, Krishna A, Rewari V. A prospective, randomized comparison of long-term outcomes: chronic groin pain and quality of life following totally extraperitoneal (TEP) and transabdominal preperitoneal (TAPP) laparoscopic inguinal hernia repair. Surg Endosc. 2013;27(7):2373–82.

17. van den Heuvel B, Dwars BJ. Repeated laparoscopic treatment of recurrent inguinal hernias after previous posterior repair. Surg Endosc. 2013;27(3):795–800.

18. Hyllegaard GM, Friis-Andersen H. Modified laparoscopic intraperitoneal onlay mesh in complicated inguinal hernia surgery. Hernia. 2015;19(3):433–6.

19. Olmi S, Scaini A, Erba L, Bertolini A, Croce E. Laparoscopic repair of inguinal hernias using an intraperitoneal onlay mesh technique and a Parietex composite mesh fixed with fibrin glue (Tissucol). Personal technique and preliminary results. Surg Endosc. 2007;21(11):1961–4.

20. Koch CA, Greenlee SM, Larson DR, Harrington JR, Farley DR. Randomized prospective study of totally extraperitoneal inguinal hernia repair: fixation versus no fixation of mesh. JSLS. 2006;10(4):457–60.

Nonoperative Treatment of Sports Hernia

Terra Blatnik

Introduction

Groin pain is an extremely common complaint among athletes of all ages. Incidence of groin pain ranges from 0.5% to as high as 43% in a group of elite Finnish hockey players [1, 2]. The anatomy of this area is extremely complex and can make diagnosis and treatment challenging. Pain in the setting of no appreciable hernia can result from something as simple as an adductor strain or can be more complex involving several structures or even the hip joint itself.

The term "sports hernia" has been used to describe a number of complaints in the groin of athletes. Other terms such as "athletic pubalgia," "Gilmore groin," and "sportsman's hernia" have all been used to describe the same entity. A consensus definition does not exist and the term is used to describe a wide variety of pathology in the groin area of athletes. In 2014, the British Hernia Society developed a position statement on treatment of sportsman's groin [3]. This position statement labeled this type of injury an "inguinal disruption" and defined it as pain in the groin area near the pubic tubercle where "no other pathology exists to explain the symptoms." Several other studies advocate for the use of five signs and symptoms that indicate a likely sports hernia: (1) deep groin or lower abdominal pain, (2) that worsens with sports-specific activity, (3) tenderness on palpation over the pubic ramus or the conjoint tendon, (4) pain with resisted hip adduction, and (5) pain with resisted abdominal sit-up [4]. Regardless the terminology, sports hernia is a common complaint in active individuals that participate in high-risk sports and this chapter will discuss its diagnosis and treatment.

Epidemiology

Sports hernia is most common in sports like soccer, ice hockey, and Australian rules football (similar to American rugby). Any sport that requires a twisting motion of the torso places an athlete at increased risk. Traditionally, sports hernias happened predominately in men, but over the last 5 years women are making up a larger proportion of those athletes diagnosed, with estimates of up to 15.2% in one study [5]. Sports hernia is most common in athletes in their mid-20s.

There are numerous areas in the groin that can be potential sources of pathology in athletes with groin pain. The pubic symphysis seems to be the central location of pathology in this condition, as this area is the central point for several tendinous attachments from the adductor musculature. The internal and external obliques, rectus abdominus, and transversus abdominus also insert in this region. In men, these muscles extend from the spermatic fascia which, if injured, can lead to

T. Blatnik (✉)
Cleveland Clinic, Twinsburg, OH, USA
e-mail: Terra.blatnik@yahoo.com

© Springer International Publishing Switzerland 2016
Y.W. Novitsky (ed.), *Hernia Surgery*, DOI 10.1007/978-3-319-27470-6_49

pain that radiates into the testicular region. In addition to the complex muscle crossings in this area, the hip joint can also contribute to groin pain. The labrum in the hip and issues from femoral acetabular impingement have often been identified as potential sources of pain [7].

The common consensus is that sports hernia may result from imbalance between the strong adductor muscles of the leg and the weaker muscles of the abdomen [6, 8, 9]. Athletes use their adductor muscles to stabilize the leg during single leg support, and this imbalance in strength between the adductor leg muscles and core muscles leads to tears and other pathology in this region. Chronic groin pain in athletes has also been correlated with reduced hip abduction and internal/external rotation [6]. The restricted motion may lead to additional stress on the attachments of the musculature.

Presentation/Physical Exam

The presentation for sports hernia can be quite variable, but most athletes will complain of an insidious onset of unilateral or bilateral groin pain. Pain may radiate to the scrotum and testicles in men [6]. On rare occasions, there will be an acute precipitating event for the onset of pain. Athletes will complain that the pain worsens with activity, but improves with rest. Rest will tend to resolve the pain, but it will often worsen again once sports are resumed.

Physical exam of patients with exercise-associated groin pain needs to include the groin, hip, and lower back regions. During passive palpation, patients may have tenderness over the inguinal canal and/or pubic tubercle, hip adductor origin (at the pubic symphysis), or a dilated superficial inguinal ring. In addition to these areas, the examiner needs to palpate the obliques, transversus abdominus, and the pubic symphysis, to see if pain can be reproduced [3]. On active exam, a resisted sit-up or abdominal crunch may cause pain in the distal rectus abdominus insertion. Valsalva maneuvers may also reproduce groin pain in patients who have a sports hernia.

Resistance testing of the hip flexors or adductors on the affected side may also demonstrate weakness compared with the contralateral muscle group [6].

There should not be any pain on palpation of the lumbosacral spine or sacroiliac joint region unless a concomitant injury is occurring. A full hip exam including testing of internal hip rotation, FABER (flexion, abduction, and external rotation), and FADIR (flexion, adduction, and internal rotation) can help identify any intra-articular pathology (Fig. 49.1). Testicular exam should also be conducted along with exam looking for true inguinal hernias.

Figure 49.2 demonstrates the additional areas that should be points of focus during physical exam in athletes with groin pain. Each of these areas can be the source of pain or occur concurrently with a diagnosis of sports hernia.

Imaging

Imaging for sports hernia has evolved significantly over the last 5–10 years. Plain radiographs including an AP pelvis and a lateral view of the femur should be done on the affected side initially to exclude obvious bony pathology [7]. This may show a femoral neck stress fracture, degenerative hip disease, femoral acetabular impingement, osteitis pubis, or apophyseal avulsions. Ultrasound was initially touted as being important but it was found to be very operator-dependent, and thus difficult to interpret the findings. Non-contrast magnetic resonance imaging (MRI) has become the most important imaging modality for identifying the underlying pathology of sports hernia. Many institutions have developed MRI protocols specifically for sports hernia. These include large-view sequences of the bony pelvis and smaller field-of-view sequences of the pubic symphysis [10]. A number of abnormalities have been found on MRI that may occur with sports hernia (Fig. 49.3). Several studies have shown that there are potentially two signs identifiable on MRI, the "superior cleft sign" and the "secondary cleft sign,"

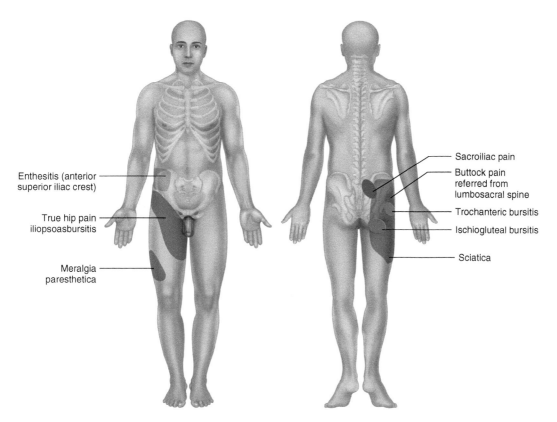

Fig. 49.1 Other areas of pathology causing pain in and around the groin. *Left*: anterior locations of pain. *Right*: posterior locations of pain

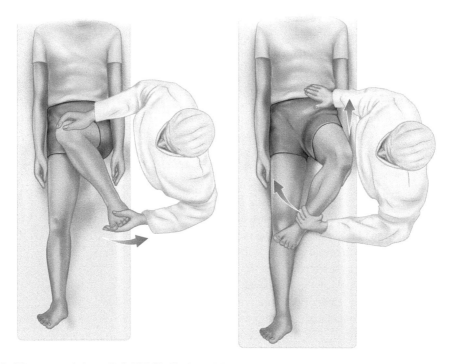

Fig. 49.2 Hip exam techniques *Left*: FADIR (flexion, adduction, internal rotation). *Right*: FABER (flexion, abduction, external rotation)

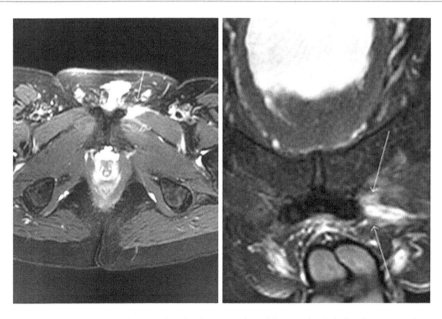

Fig. 49.3 MRI (non-contrast): Hyperintense signal adjacent to the pubic symphysis indicating tear to the rectus abdominus — common finding in sports hernia

that are found in patients diagnosed with sports hernia [3, 6, 10, 11]. The secondary cleft is a space between the rectus abdominus/adductor aponeurosis and the pubic bone indicating a tear at the insertion. This sign appears as a hyperintensity on coronal STIR images at the inferior margin of the inferior pubic ramus. One study showed that this was the most common finding in athletes experiencing pain from a sports hernia. The "superior cleft sign" is a similar sign that appears as a hyperintense area at the inferior margin of the superior pubic ramus [11]. This sign represents a tear of the rectus abdominus or adductor longus attachment. Another study looking at 100 pelvic MRIs showed that the most common finding overall was unilateral rectus abdominus/adductor injury [5]. Other abnormalities on MRI include pubic plate lesions, osteitis pubis, or tears of the adductor muscles. MRI may show minimal changes or reveal another cause for pathology, such as a stress fracture. It is extremely important to look at the hip because Meyers et al., found that 15% of patients with sports hernia on MRI also had hip pathology [5]. If intra-articular hip pathology is suspected, an MR arthrogram should be done to look for labral tears or evidence of femoral acetabular impingement (Fig. 49.4).

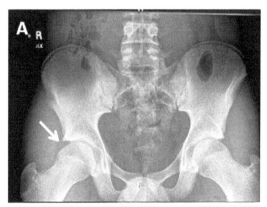

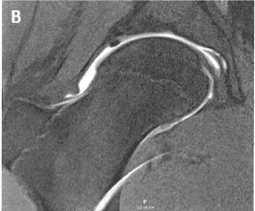

Fig. 49.4 15-Year-old soccer player with groin/hip pain, (**a**) AP pelvis radiograph showing some evidence of potential femoroacetabular impingement. (**b**) MRI arthrogram right hip; evidence of labral tear

Treatment

Treatment of sports hernia or chronic groin pain in athletes has been as controversial as the definition of this entity. The two avenues of treatment include conservative/physical therapy and surgical intervention. The surgical technique and indications for sports hernia will be discussed in a subsequent chapter, with this chapter focusing on conservative techniques.

Conservative Therapy

Many clinicians will advocate for an initial trial of physical therapy for sports hernia prior to surgical intervention. In general, physical therapy should be tried for a minimum of 6–8 weeks prior to moving on to surgical intervention. Occasionally high-level (i.e., NFL) athletes will go straight to surgical repair because of concerns regarding the length of absence from the game.

In general, most physical therapy for sports hernia focuses on strengthening the core muscles and the adductors along with manual techniques and gentle stretching. The goal of therapy is to fix what is believed to be deficient or out of balance musculature and is a cause for sports hernia. This includes strengthening the lower abdominal muscles to meet the strength of the adductors, in order to correct pelvic misalignment and improve the limited mobility of the hip capsule. Most physical therapists will use some variation of the following three studies when trying to rehabilitate an athlete with sports hernia.

Holmich et al. published a study in 1999 on the use of adductor strengthening for treatment of groin pain in athletes [8]. Patients were randomized to either an active therapy group or physiotherapy group without active training for at least 8 weeks. The subjects in this group were male aged 18–50 years and had groin pain related to sports for at least 2 months. Active therapy consisted of static adduction of the legs, sit-ups, balance training on a wobble board, and slide board exercises. Additionally, this group also performed abduction and adduction strength exercises. The physiotherapy group underwent laser treatments, friction massage, stretching, and nerve stimulation. It was found that 79% of the patients in the active therapy group had no residual groin pain and had returned to sport, while only 14% in the passive therapy group had the same improvement. This study showed that active improvement in adductor and core strength can improve groin pain in athletes.

Kachingwe and Grech proposed an algorithm for the conservative treatment of sports hernia. They performed a case series with 6 patients (4 males and 2 females, ages 19–22 years) [4]. The treatment algorithm in this study was a combination of manual/manipulation techniques and active exercise. Three times per week patients received manual therapy which included soft-tissue mobilization to improve muscle tightness in the pelvic musculature, manipulation of the pelvic musculature to improve sacroiliac joint and pelvic alignment, and neuromuscular reeducation and gradual stretching. In addition to this, three to five times per week the athletes participated in a supervised exercise program. This program consisted of dynamic flexibility, trunk stabilization exercises, and dynamic exercises. Dynamic flexibility consisted of active stretching of the iliopsoas, quadriceps, hamstrings, internal and external rotators, and adductors. Trunk stabilization exercises function to improve core and hip strength included cardio activity, such as swimming or elliptical trainer. The final portion, initiated around 3–6 weeks, included dynamic exercises to strengthen the adductors, core, and upper leg muscles. Three of the 6 athletes were able to return to sport within 6 weeks, while the other three underwent surgical repair for sports hernia. All three of these athletes utilized the above program for rehabilitation following surgical repair and all six returned to pre-injury level of play. This study did have some limitations. The sample size was extremely small and the algorithm employed was quite complex. This complexity may make it difficult to fully follow in a typical physical therapy office.

Most recently, Yuill, et al. published a case series in 2012 involving soccer players that underwent conservative treatment for chronic groin pain [12]. The treatment for these athletes was similar to other previously mentioned studies and included manual therapy and active rehabilitation. Manual therapy in this study consisted of manual soft-tissue therapy (massage), microcurrent stimulation, laser therapy, and acupuncture. Active therapy included strengthening exercises for the hip adductors, squats to strengthen upper thighs, and pelvic bridges to strengthen the core. Plyometric training (jump training) was also included. Therapy was undertaken for 8 weeks and all three athletes in this study were able to return to full sport participation at the conclusion of conservative therapy.

All of the methods of conservative therapy listed above have similar objectives, with the ultimate goal being to improve hip and core strength after reducing pain and inflammation in the groin region. When evaluating a new patient suspected of a sports hernia, our protocol is to bring them in for history and physical to see if we can determine alternative causes for groin pain and the need for further intervention. Each patient will have initial plain radiographs to exclude stress fracture and hip derangement. If plain films are negative, then we will send the patient for physical therapy. It is important to work with local physical therapists that are familiar with the rehabilitation of athletes and have the equipment to perform functional rehabilitation. The athlete should abstain from sports and begin a program that lasts 6–8 weeks. This program should have both active and passive elements. Passive elements should include soft-tissue mobilization/massage and techniques to

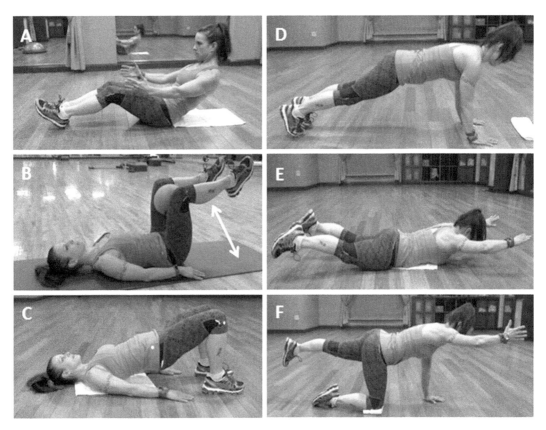

Fig. 49.5 Hip and core strengthening exercises: (**a**) partial sit-up, (**b**) abdominal and adductor strength—squeeze ball and lower and lift legs, (**c**) pelvic bridge, (**d**) plank, (**e**) "Superman" pose—lift arms and legs while lying on abdomen, (**f**) quadriped—opposite arm and opposite leg lifted

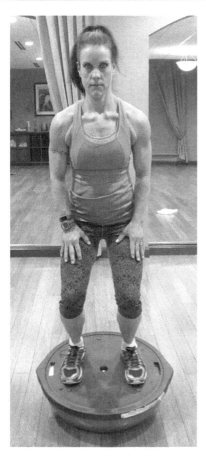

Fig. 49.6 Using overturned balance ball to work on core strength and balance

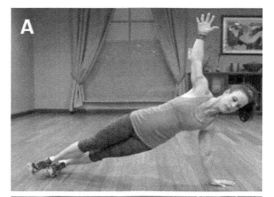

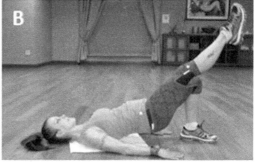

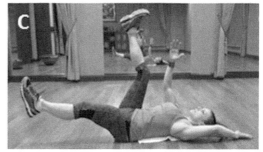

Fig. 49.7 Advanced core exercises: (**a**) side plank, (**b**) bridge with leg extended, (**c**) "Dead Bug" with arm movement

ensure proper alignment of the pelvis and SI joints. Alongside this, an intense program for hip and core strength should be used. Core exercises work to strengthen not only the abdominal muscles, but also the lower back and hips. Figure 49.5 demonstrates a series of core exercises to be integrated into therapy. Using an overturned balance ball can also improve core strength and balance (Fig. 49.6) and once the basic moves have been mastered, the athlete can move on to more advanced core conditioning (Fig. 49.7). Figure 49.8 shows hip adductor strengthening moves and abductor strengthening moves. Side lunges and squats can also be used to strengthen the upper legs and core along with other dynamic moves (Fig. 49.9). Along with this, the athlete should also be given the option for electrical stimulation or other

modalities described in the next section. Sports medicine-trained physicians are most likely to offer these services and would be the appropriate referral for more complex procedures. The patient should be seen in the office for follow-up 6–8 weeks after beginning therapy. If at that time the patient is still having significant pain, they should have advanced imaging (non-contrast MRI) done. If results are consistent with a sports hernia, the patient can resume therapy for another 4 weeks and abstain from sports/exercise. If after the additional month of rehabilitation the patient still has pain, then referral to a surgeon is warranted. The

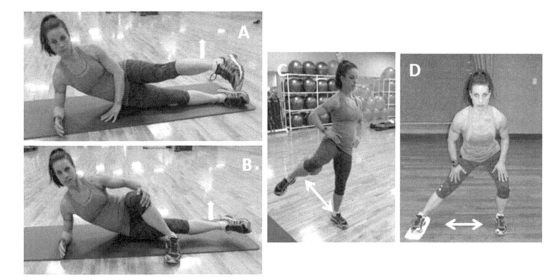

Fig. 49.8 Adductor/abductor strengthening exercises, (**a**) abductor lift, (**b**) adductor lift, (**c**). adductor/abductor standing lift with ball, (**d**) side slide lunges

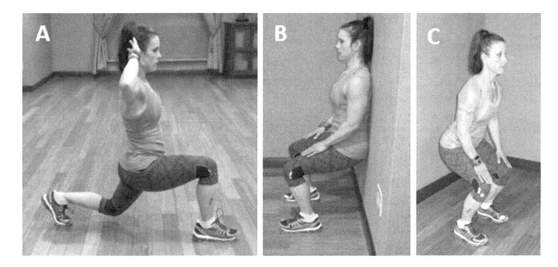

Fig. 49.9 Dynamic strength: (**a**) front lunge, (**b**) wall sit, (**c**) squats

only exception to this should be high-level athletes (i.e., NFL, NBA) that do not have time for extensive rehabilitation or for athletes that had a distinct injury that felt like a pop or tear that may benefit from earlier surgical intervention.

It is important to note that a shortened version of those protocols above should be used after surgery has been done. Hip and core strength is important postoperatively and patients should be started into 3–4 weeks of physical therapy when the surgeon deems appropriate (depending on scar healing time and degree of surgical intervention).

Alternative Treatment

Comin et al. performed a pilot study in 2012 looking at radiofrequency denervation of the inguinal ligament for treatment of sports hernia [13]. The basis behind this treatment is that desensitizing the nerves in the groin area will relieve pain, regardless of its source. All patients in the study had pain greater than 6 months and had failed conservative therapy. Patients were randomized to either the radiofrequency ablation or steroid injection. Both groups had improvement in pain scores with the ablation group getting slightly more relief. At 6 months post-procedure, the difference was slightly more pronounced with more in the ablation group still having improved pain scores. A smaller pilot group received denervation after a failed surgical intervention and this group also had improved pain scores. Although this is a small study, it does have promise for a noninvasive treatment for those with refractory and long-standing groin pain.

A variety of injection techniques have also been explored. Local anesthestic, cortisone, platelet-rich plasma, and autologous blood have all been tried; however, there are very few studies that currently examine these techniques. These injections have proven efficacy for tendinopathy and for joint pain for various reasons, so they may also show promise in the treatment of sports hernia [3].

Prevention

As mentioned at the beginning of this chapter, groin pain is extremely common in athletes and can cause loss of playing time and mean changes in affect revenues for professional teams. If these injuries could be prevented, it could save athletes months of rehabilitation and potentially surgery. Tyler, et al., published a prospective study in 2002 examining the use of an adductor strengthening program in preventing groin strains in NHL players [9]. Players that were found to have an imbalance of adductor to abductor strength were enrolled in a strengthening program three times per week for 6 weeks during the preseason. By using this program in "at-risk" athletes, the incidence of adductor strains was significantly reduced from 3.2 strains per 1000 player-game exposures to 0.71 strains per 1000 player-game exposures. This study demonstrates that programs for athletes in the preseason time period could prevent future strains and lower incidence of sports hernia.

Conclusion

Sports hernia is a complex issue for athletes that generally presents as unilateral groin pain that gets worse with physical activity, improves with rest, and resumes once activity has restarted, if proper treatment is not completed. Physical exam can often be inconclusive, but can reveal other concurrent pathology, including intra-articular hip derangements or stress fractures. Imaging can be helpful in both ruling in and ruling out sports hernia and has become increasingly useful as radiologists develop improved protocols looking for sports hernia. There is continued debate about appropriate treatment, most commonly involving surgical repair vs. conservative management. This author would advocate for rest from sport and an aggressive rehabilitation program for 6–8 weeks, except in cases where a player cannot take this amount of time out from sport. Newer emerging therapies, including nerve ablation, may provide additional avenues in the future. Advocating for preseason strengthening of hip adductors may be beneficial in all athletes, even for the highest level professionals. If the conservative approach is not effective after an appropriate amount of time (minimum 8 weeks), then surgical consultation should be the next step in management.

References

1. Molsa J, Airaksinen O, Naisam O, Torstila I. Ice hockey injuries in Finland: a prospective epidemiologic study. Am J Sports Med. 1997;25(4):495–9.
2. Tyler T, Silvers H, Gerhardt M, Nicholas S. Groin injuries in sports medicine. Sports Health. 2010;2(3):231–6.
3. Sheen A, Stephenson B, Lloyd D, et al. 'Treatment of sportsman's groin': British Hernia Society's 2014 position statement based on the Manchester Consensus Conference. Br J Sports Med. 2014;48:1079–87.

4. Kachingwe A, Grech S. Proposed algorithm for the management of athletes with athletic pubalgia (sports hernia): a case series. J Orthop Sports Phys Ther. 2008;38(12):768–81.

5. Meyers W, McKechnie A, Philippon M, Horner M, Zoga A, Devon O. Experience with "sports hernia" spanning two decades. Ann Surg. 2008;248(4): 656–65.

6. Caudill P, Nyland J, Smith C, Yerasimides J, Lach J. Sports hernias: a systematic literature review. Br J Sports Med. 2008;42:954–64.

7. Larson C. Sports hernia/athletic pubalgia: evaluation and management. Sports Health. 2014;6(2):139–44.

8. Holmich P, Uhrskou P, Ulnits L, et al. Effectiveness of active physical training as treatment for long standing adductor-related groin pain in athletes: randomized trial. Lancet. 1999;353(9151):439–43.

9. Tyler T, Nicholas S, Campbell R, Donellan S, McHugh M. The effectiveness of preseason exercise program to prevent adductor muscle strains in professional ice hockey players. Am J Sports Med. 2002;30(5):680–3.

10. Palisch A, Zoga A, Meyers W. Imaging of athletic pubalgia and core muscle injuries. Clin J Sports Med. 2013;32:427–47.

11. Murphy G, Foran P, Murphy D, Tobin O, Moynagh M, Eustace S. "Superior cleft sign" as a marker of rectus abdominus/adductor longus tear in patients with suspected sportsman's hernia. Skeletal Radiol. 2013;42:819–25.

12. Yuill E, Pajaczkowski J, Howitt S. Conservative care of sports hernias within soccer players: a case series. J Bodyw Mov Ther. 2012;16(4):540–8.

13. Comin J, Obaid H, Lammers G, Moore J, Wotherspoon M, Connell D. Radiofrequency denervation of the inguinal ligament for the treatment of 'Sportsman's Hernia:' a pilot study. Br J Sports Med. 2013;47:380–6.

The Surgical Approach to Sports Hernia

Thomas J. Wade and L. Michael Brunt

Sports hernia refers to a condition in which there is chronic exertional lower abdominal/inguinal pain that limits athletic performance. The term sports hernia, although firmly ingrained in the lexicon, is a misnomer since it does not involve a true herniation on internal contents, but rather broadly refers to conditions in which there are various injuries to structures associated with the pubis or pubic joint. As a result, the term athletic pubalgia has been recommended to more accurately reflect the various clinical and anatomic presentations and pathophysiology of this condition [1]. The pattern of injury may be primarily to the abdominal wall including the distal rectus [1], posterior inguinal floor [2], external oblique [3], and the associated attachments to the pubis. Additionally, Meyers et al. included the concept of shearing force injury to the muscular attachments to the pubis in the definition of athletic pubalgia [4]. This injury may be primarily associated with either the rectus abdominus attachment or the adductor compartment, or a combination of the two, or other associated attachments to the pubis. For the purposes of this review, the terms sports hernia and athletic pubalgia will be used interchangeably. Groin injuries are prevalent in sport and particularly in those associated with athletes that frequently perform explosive cutting, pivoting, kicking, and twisting movements. Sports including football, soccer, and ice hockey, in particular, are associated with significant risk of groin injury. Ekstrand and Hilding reported that groin injuries occur in 5–23% of soccer players and account for 8% of all injuries over one season [5]. A study of elite soccer players in the Union of European Football Associations revealed that groin injuries accounted for 12–16% of all injuries in a season [6]. Additionally, a Swedish study revealed that groin injuries account for approximately 10% of injuries in elite hockey players [3]. A number of risk factors have been identified in professional hockey players for groin injury that include preseason or training camp, prior history of groin injury, and veteran player status [7]. Tyler and colleagues also have shown that reduced adductor to abductor strength ration can also result in a high risk for adductor muscle strain injuries [8]. Unlike many other sport injuries, groin injuries may not be associated with direct physical contact. Most of these injuries are muscular or tendinous strains and resolve with conservative management, and so sports hernia represents a

Electronic supplementary material: The online version of this chapter (doi:10.1007/978-3-319-27470-6_50) contains supplementary material, which is available to authorized users.

T.J. Wade, M.D. • L.M. Brunt, M.D. (✉)
Section of Minimally Invasive Surgery, Department of Surgery, Washington University School of Medicine, St. Louis, MO, USA
e-mail: bruntm@wustl.edu

Fig. 50.1 Schematic illustration of the anatomy of the lower abdominal/inguinal region and proximal thigh musculature. (**a**) Anterior view, (**b**) Sagittal view

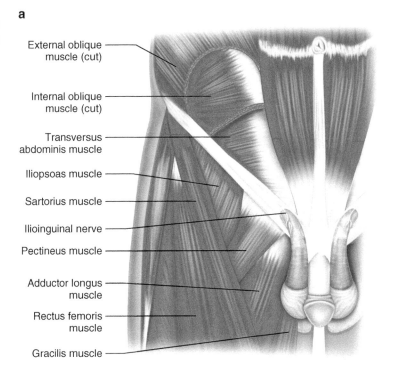

a

External oblique muscle (cut)

Internal oblique muscle (cut)

Transversus abdominis muscle

Iliopsoas muscle

Sartorius muscle

Ilioinguinal nerve

Pectineus muscle

Adductor longus muscle

Rectus femoris muscle

Gracilis muscle

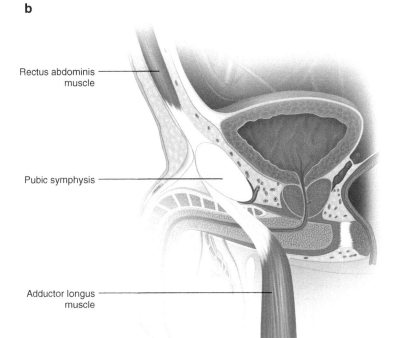

b

Rectus abdominis muscle

Pubic symphysis

Adductor longus muscle

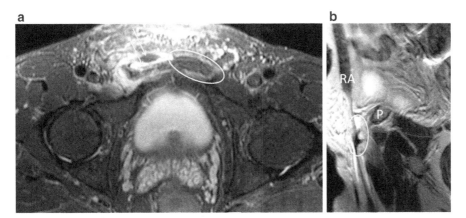

Fig. 50.2 MRI showing right rectus tear (**a**) axial view— *arrows* point to tear in rectus aponeurosis on the right side. *Circle* denotes the normal rectus on the left; and (**b**) sagittal view with the circle denoting the area of tear from the pubis. *RA* rectus abdominus, *P* pubis. Photographs courtesy of Dr. David Rubin, Mallinckrodt Institute of Radiology, Washington University School of Medicine

small subset of injuries that fail to resolve with conservative treatment measures. The persistence of symptoms more than 3 months in duration increases the odds of a sports hernia diagnosis that may require surgical intervention.

Anatomy and Pathophysiology

A thorough understanding of the groin and pelvic anatomy is essential to the evaluation of groin pain and sports hernia. The pelvis functions as a fulcrum for the abdominal and thigh muscles attachments (Fig. 50.1). The external oblique muscle attaches to the rectus and inferiorly forms the inguinal canal through which the spermatic cord and ilioinguinal and genital nerves pass. The rectus abdominus attaches to the superior pubic rami and its aponeurosis is in continuity with the adductor longus attachment. The transversus abdominus and internal oblique aponeuroses may combine to form the "conjoined tendon," which inserts on the pubis although a true conjoined tendon is present in only about 10% of patients. The adductor complex includes six muscles (adductor longus, adductor brevis, adductor magnus, pectineus, gracilis, and obturator externus), the most frequently injured of which is the adductor longus.

The relative strength of the thigh adductor muscle complex at the pubis may result in instability and shear forces that lead to injury. This imbalance may lead to excessive stress and tension on the abdominal muscles that attach to the pubis. In some cases, a visible tear or separation in the rectus aponeurosis is present on imaging (Fig 50.2). In most cases, a consistent finding is a weakened posterior inguinal floor/transversalis fascia. A true inguinal hernia is infrequently present. Others have postulated that tension on the inguinal ligament is the primary pathology.

Additionally, some groups have postulated that ilioinguinal or genital nerve involvement accounts for main components of a patient's symptoms [9, 10]. The nerve involvement is postulated to be from ilioinguinal or iliohypogastric nerve entrapment through tears in the external oblique aponeurosis [9], or from pressure on the genital nerve from a bulging weakened floor during Valsalva [10], although there is no consensus about the extent to which these findings play a role in the athletic pubalgia pain syndrome.

Approach to Evaluation

Differential Diagnosis

The differential diagnosis for groin pain in an athlete is extensive, including injury associated with the bony pelvis, muscles, hip, or even non-sport related causes. Pelvic injuries that may cause chronic groin pain include osteitis pubis, stress or other fracture, and muscular contusions. Most injuries in the groin are muscular and consist of abdominal or thigh strains that typically resolve with conservative management. The adductor muscle group is a common source of groin pain and most commonly involves the adductor longus. A true inguinal hernia must be considered in the differential diagnosis as well although this is infrequently present. Hip-related etiologies include labral tears, femoral acetabular impingement and, in older athletes, osteoarthritis. Finally, non-musculoskeletal related causes such as gynecologic disorders in females, should be considered if symptoms are atypical for a sports-related injury.

History and Physical Examination

A detailed history and physical is essential in the evaluation of athletic groin pain. The history should include onset of pain and potential mech-anism of injury, precise location, pain radiation, aggravating and alleviating factors, and prior history of injury to the area. Patients' response to attempted therapy including rest, nonsteroidal anti-inflammatory drugs (NSAIDS), and ice should also be elicited. Finally, the presence of recurrent pain symptoms with return of activity should be noted. Classically, sports hernia will present with chronic lower abdominal or inguinal pain worsened by explosive movements. It is unusual for it to occur at rest or with sitting. The pain may also be aggravated by sprinting, cutting movements, kicking, and coughing/sneezing. As a result, the pain limits athletic performance and can negatively impact success in competition.

Physical exam should include a focused inguinal hernia exam, assessment of the pubic symphysis for tenderness or instability, resisted trunk movements and rotation, lower extremity muscle evaluation, and hip examination. The inguinal exam includes palpation through the external inguinal ring to assess for bulging. The pubic symphysis evaluation includes palpation of the medial inguinal floor and rectus insertion at rest and during a resisted sit-up. (Fig 50.3) Pain at this location is most characteristic of a sports hernia diagnosis. Lower extremity testing includes resisted straight leg raise, hip flexion, and resisted adduction in both extended and frog leg positions. Finally, hip evaluation is performed to rule out a hip etiology of the pain.

Fig. 50.3 Abdominal crunch during palpation of the inguinal floor during examination for sports hernia

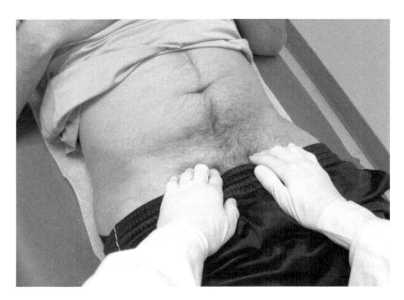

Diagnostic Imaging

The preferred imaging modality at our institution is a pelvic MRI utilizing a pubalgia protocol, which has been previously described [11]. This study utilizes a multi-coil pelvic array coil centered over the lower pelvis. The MRI sequences include coronal TI and short T1 inversion recovery, transverse T1 and T2 with fat suppression, and sagittal high resolution sequences through the pubic bones and symphysis. Injuries that support the diagnosis of sports hernia include a tear in the rectus abdominus aponeurosis insertion, parasymphyseal edema, combined adductor or rectus-adductor tear, and a secondary cleft. In one large series, a rectus tendon abnormality was seen in 2/3 of athletes with a clinical diagnosis of sports hernia [12]. In part, the MRI is also useful to exclude other injuries such as osteitis pubis, stress fracture, congenital pelvis anomalies, and hip pathology (femoroacetabular impingement, labral tears, hip arthritis). A limitation of MRI is that it does not image the posterior inguinal floor weakness and, therefore, a negative MRI does not necessarily exclude the diagnosis of a sports hernia.

In some centers, dynamic ultrasound testing is utilized preferentially to assess for this condition [13, 14]. The advantages of ultrasound are that the testing can be done during Valsalva to assess for bulging in the posterior inguinal floor/transversalis fascia, and it is readily available and portable. The limitations of ultrasound are that it is very operator dependent and does not provide as much structural information as MRI about the rest of the musculoskeletal anatomy in the pubic region. In the author's experience, CT has a limited role in the evaluation of athletic groin pain unless intra-abdominal pathology is suspected. Radionuclide bone scanning may be useful in demonstrating increased activity in the pubis in cases of suspected osteitis pubis.

Nonoperative Management

Nonoperative management of athletic groin injuries should initially consist of a period of rest from athletic activity, ice, and nonsteroidal anti-inflammatory medications. If the injury does not resolve quickly, then imaging should be considered to define the nature and extent of it. Physical therapy is an important component of a nonoperative management strategy and should be oriented toward progressive range of motion exercises, balanced training and graduated strengthening, and thermal modalities such as ultrasound or e-stim therapy. Core strengthening and stabilization is also an important component of therapy for any groin injury. Deep tissue massage including active release technique may be useful for isolated muscle tightness and therapies. The goal should be to achieve balance in strength and flexibility across the pelvis with a graduated return to sports-specific activity.

For patients who present with well-localized inguinal or lower abdominal pain, an injection with local anesthetic and steroid may be attempted to break the cycle of pain and inflammation, especially if the occurrence is in-season, and may, in some cases, provide long-term relief. Some groups have utilized platelet-rich plasma injections for recalcitrant groin injuries with some success, but controlled data are lacking on the effectiveness of this approach. An initial trial of nonoperative management is important as one randomized trial reported return to sport in 23 of 29 patients at 4 months [15]. The exception would be if a rectus tear is demonstrated on MRI, which increases the likelihood of failure of conservative management and supports earlier surgical intervention.

Surgical Management

Indications

The indications for surgical intervention for sports hernia include three primary criteria: (1) symptoms and exam findings consistent with a sports hernia diagnosis; (2) alternative diagnoses excluded by imaging; and (3) failure of nonoperative management for a period of at least 6–8 weeks. The period of nonoperative management may vary according to whether the athlete is professional/elite high school/college or recreational. Two prospective, randomized trials have been carried out to assess the value of conservative treatment versus surgery for this condition. Ekstrand and colleagues prospectively randomized 66 soccer players with groin pain who had failed nonoperative treatment to surgery vs. continued conservative management or no treatment [16]. All athletes in this study had groin pain of >3 months duration. Only the surgical group showed substantial and statistically significant improvement over the observation period. Paajanen et al. randomized 60 patients with suspected sports hernia and 3–6 months of groin symptoms to surgery (laparoscopic posterior mesh repair) or conservative management (physical therapy, NSAIDS, and corticosteroid injections) [17]. Outcome measures were visual pain scores and return to sports at 1, 3, 6 and 12 months and return to sport. At 3 months, return to sport was 90% in the operative group compared to only 27% in the conservative treatment group. Pain scores were significantly different in the two groups at each time point evaluated. These studies indicate that surgery provides superior results to conservative management in appropriately selected athletes.

Operative Approaches

A variety of operative approaches have been described for the management of sports hernia. These include open primary inguinal floor repairs, open tension-free mesh repairs, and laparoscopic posterior mesh repairs.

Open Primary Tissue Repairs

The two primary repairs that have been most employed are the "pelvic floor repair" described by Meyers and the "minimal repair technique" described by Muschawek [14, 18]. Although the details of the technique described by Meyers are not fully reported, the general description involves suture plicating the inferolateral border of the rectus abduminus fascia to the pubis and inguinal ligament. The goal of this approach is to tighten and stabilize the attachments of the rectus

around the pubis. A partial adductor release is often performed, if there is associated adductor pathology. Meyers has reported the largest series of sports hernia repairs with operation performed on 5218 athletes out of 8490 patients evaluated (61.4%) [18]. The return to sport rate was reported as 95.3% at 3 months after surgery.

Muschawek's technique involves stabilizing the posterior inguinal floor with a minimal tension suture technique [14]. A part of the strategy of this procedure is to repair the transversalis fascia weakness and reduce tension on the genital nerve. In this approach, only the area of posterior inguinal floor bulging is opened, and it is then resutured to the inguinal ligament and pubis to restore more normal alignment. In a significant percentage of cases, the genital nerve is resected. This group reported on 132 procedures performed in 128 patients. At 4 weeks after surgery, 83.7% of patients had returned to sport [14, 19].

Open Tension-Free Mesh Repairs

The open anterior tension-free mesh repair that is utilized in the management of sports hernia is similar to the well-known Lichtenstein repair. The proposed advantages of this approach include improved durability of the repair due to mesh reinforcement and potential for earlier return to activity due to the tension-free aspects of the repair. In this approach, a lightweight polypropylene mesh is sutured to the transversalis fascia and rectus sheath medially and to the inguinal ligament laterally (described in more detail under the "Step-by-step approach" section below). This provides support of the inguinal floor and distal rectus and increased strength across the pubis. Our group has utilized an individualized approach to sports hernia repair but, most commonly has performed an open tension-free mesh repair. Over the last 13 years, a total of 209 athletes have undergone repair in our center [20]. The mean duration of symptoms prior to repair was 9.2 months. Return to sport was successfully sustained in approximately 92% of athletes over a mean follow-up of 11.4 months.

An alternative mesh based repair has been described by the Montreal group [3, 9]. The details of this approach include placement of a polytetrafluoroethylene (PTFE) mesh patch below the external oblique aponeurosis and a primary repair of any external oblique tears. The group reported on 98 hockey players over an 18-year period with a total of 107 repairs. They reported only 3 recurrences and 97 of 98 returned to sport activities [3]. The selective addition of ilioinguinal and/or iliohypogastric neurectomies may be indicated in either of the tension-free

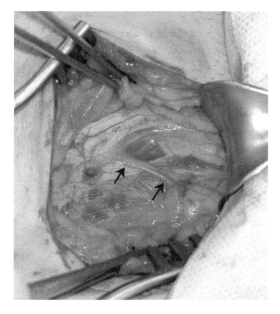

Fig. 50.4 Acute angulation of the ilioinguinal nerve as it exits a slit in the external oblique aponeurosis (*arrows*). The nerve would be resected in such cases

mesh based repairs, but especially if the nerve is acutely angulated through a slit in the external oblique aponeurosis (Fig. 50.4).

Laparoscopic Posterior Mesh Repair

Some groups have preferentially utilized the laparoscopic approach for sports hernia repair [17, 21, 22]. The approach is identical to that utilized for a standard inguinal hernia repair, and includes both total extraperitoneal and transabdominal preperitoneal techniques. This allows for a tension-free reinforcement of the entire posterior inguinal floor (Fig. 50.5). Potential advantages, as with standard inguinal hernia repair, include decreased postoperative pain and more rapid return to activity. Genitsaris et al. reported on 131 patients that failed nonoperative management [21]. All patients underwent bilateral mesh repair and all returned to sport at 3 weeks after surgery. Evans reported on 278 athletes who underwent laparoscopic repair with 90% return to play at 4 weeks [23].

An alternative laparoscopic approach has been described by Lloyd who postulates tension in the inguinal ligament as a mechanism for the pain. He carries out a release of the inguinal ligament at its attachment to the pubis and then reinforces the posterior inguinal floor with mesh [24]. In his early experience, 73% of patients were pain free at 4 weeks after surgery and overall symptoms were improved compared to preoperatively in

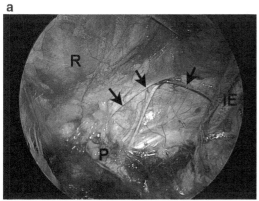

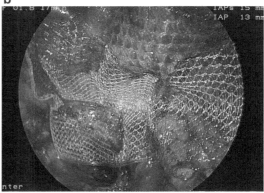

Fig. 50.5 Laparoscopic operative view of left inguinal floor (extraperitoneal approach). (**a**) Weakened posterior inguinal floor and distal rectus (*right side*). *R* rectus, *P* pubis, *IE* inferior epigastrics. (**b**) Mesh positioned to cover the entire inguinal floor

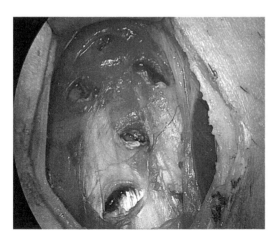

Fig. 50.6 Operative photo demonstrating partial release of adductor longus

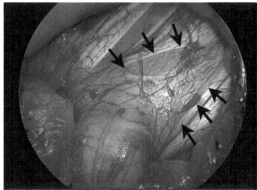

Fig. 50.7 Operative view of attenuated external oblique aponeurosis (*arrows*)

97%. Further validation of this approach is needed before it can be widely recommended.

Adductor Release

Patients with a significant component of adductor tendinopathy may benefit from the addition of a partial adductor release procedure. For this procedure, the patient's leg is positioned with the thigh flexed and abducted. The partial release consists of a small 2.5 cm incision over the upper adductor tendon in the groin crease. Multiple incisions in the anterior epimysial fibers of the adductor longus tendon are created approximately over a distance of 3–4 cm from its insertion on the pubis. In general, five to seven incisions are required to release the compartment while leaving the adductor muscle and the tendon attachments to the pubis intact (Fig. 50.6). The leg is then returned to the neutral position for the abdominal component of the procedure.

Author's Step-by-Step Approach

Our preferred approach for most athletes is an open anterior tension-free repair with lightweight polypropylene mesh. The procedure is performed with local anesthesia and intrave-

nous sedation. A slightly oblique incision is made over the inguinal canal after administration of local anesthetic. Dissection is performed to identify the external oblique aponeurosis, which is often markedly attenuated (Fig. 50.7) The external oblique is opened and the cremaster fibers within the cord are opened medially to exclude an indirect hernia. The ilioinguinal nerve is identified and left within its sheath to avoid exposing it to the mesh. The posterior inguinal floor is often weak and markedly attenuated (Fig. 50.8). The floor is reconstructed with tension-free mesh placement suturing it to the transversalis aponeurosis and rectus sheath medially and to the inguinal ligament laterally (Fig. 50.9). The mesh should be positioned to lie evenly across the inguinal floor. In some cases, the internal oblique is brought over the mesh to minimize contact between the mesh and the spermatic cord. The external oblique aponeurosis is closed with a running 2-0 absorbable suture.

Special Circumstances

The ilioinguinal nerve is generally left in place, however, if it takes an acute turn through the external oblique or appears at risk of becoming tethered to the mesh repair it is resected. The genital nerve is left protected within the cord. In young athletes who are still in their growth

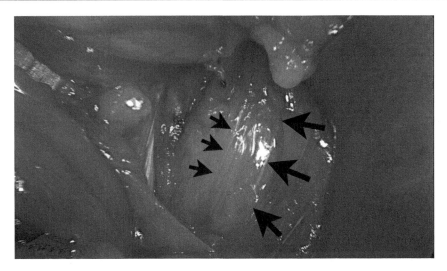

Fig. 50.8 Operative view of weakened posterior floor weakness in a sports hernia case (*arrows*). Note the stranding in some of the fibers in the posterior wall of the canal (*small arrows*)

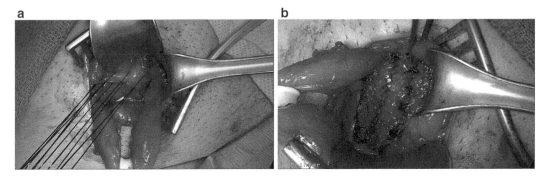

Fig. 50.9 Technique of open mesh repair of the inguinal floor. (**a**) Sutures are anchored in the healthy transversalis fascia medially with 0 gauge nonabsorbable sutures. (**b**) Completed mesh repair

phase, a primary repair analogous to a Bassini type repair is used and mesh is avoided. In athletes who have undergone prior open inguinal hernia repair, especially if there is evidence of a rectus tear on MRI, a laparoscopic posterior mesh repair will be utilized and we have used this approach selectively in other athletes with a demonstrable rectus tear as well with good outcomes.

The addition of an adductor release is performed in selected athletes with significant adductor symptoms and findings on exam. The release is almost always performed in addition to the inguinal floor repair but in some cases may be performed as an isolated procedure.

Postoperative Management and Recovery

A structured postoperative rehabilitation program is essential to a successful return to athletic activity after surgical management of sports hernia. Our group utilizes a program that is focused on core abdominal and lower body strength, flexibility, and balance. Particular attention is placed on strength and flexibility of the adductor and related muscle groups. It should be noted that the rehabilitation program should be individualized to each athlete's recovery progression and not tied to a rigid timetable. Our program starts with normal activities and walking for the first 5–7 days progressing to light running and stationary cycling at 7–14 days [25]. Passive stretching is initiated on postoperative day one for patients with an adductor release. Activity is then increased in a stepwise fashion beginning with aerobic conditioning including light jogging and stationary biking. Activity can then be advanced as pain symptoms allow to include sport-specific training, generally by week 3. The final step in the program is return to play with physical contact. The goal of return to play is generally accomplished by weeks 5–7. Scar mobilization and massage therapy to the hip musculature may be incorporated throughout the program. An important concept has been put forth by Muschawek who emphasizes the potential for earlier return to conditioning and sport. Athletes are allowed to lift up to 20 kg within days of surgery and return to running and training as soon as comfort allows. Return to sport within 3 weeks of surgery has been achieved in some cases [10].

Summary

With experience, the diagnosis of sports hernia/athletic pubalgia can be made with confidence. A multidisciplinary approach that includes sports medicine orthopedist/specialists, athletic trainer, and hernia surgeon with an interest in this condition is recommended. A variety of surgical approaches have been successfully employed for this problem, and all achieve success provided the athlete has been appropriately selected for operation. Postoperative rehabilitation is an important component of management and successful return to sport.

References

1. Meyers W, Yoo E, Devon O, et al. Understanding "sports hernia" (athletic pubalgia): The anatomic and pathophysiologic basis for abdominal and groin pain in athletes. Oper Tech Sports Med. 2007;15(4):13.
2. Swan Jr KG, Wolcott M. The athletic hernia: a systematic review. Clin Orthop Relat Res. 2007; 455:78–87.
3. Brown RA, et al. An 18-year review of sports groin injuries in the elite hockey player: clinical presentation, new diagnostic imaging, treatment, and results. Clin J Sport Med. 2008;18(3):221–6.
4. Meyers WC, Greenleaf R, Saad A. Anatomic basis for evaluation of abdominal and groin pain in athletes. Oper Tech Sports Med. 2005;13(1):55–61.
5. Ekstrand J, Hilding J. The incidence and differential diagnosis of acute groin injuries in male soccer players. Scand J Med Sci Sports. 1999;9(2):98–103.
6. Werner J, et al. UEFA injury study: a prospective study of hip and groin injuries in professional football over seven consecutive seasons. Br J Sports Med. 2009;43(13):1036–40.
7. Emery CA, Meeuwisse WH. Risk factors for groin injuries in hockey. Med Sci Sports Exerc. 2001; 33(9):1423–33.
8. Tyler TF, et al. The association of hip strength and flexibility with the incidence of adductor muscle strains in professional ice hockey players. Am J Sports Med. 2001;29(2):124–8.
9. Irshad K, et al. Operative management of hockey groin syndrome: 12 years of experience in National Hockey League players. Surgery. 2001;130(4):759–64; discussion 764–6.
10. Minnich JM, et al. Sports hernia: diagnosis and treatment highlighting a minimal repair surgical technique. Am J Sports Med. 2011;39(6):1341–9.
11. Rubin DA. Imaging of athletic groin pain. In: Diduch DR, Brunt LM, editors. Sports hernia and athletic pubalgia: diagnosis and treatment. New York: Springer; 2014.
12. Zoga AC, et al. Athletic pubalgia and the "sports hernia": MR imaging findings. Radiology. 2008;247(3):797–807.
13. Orchard JW, et al. Groin pain associated with ultrasound finding of inguinal canal posterior wall deficiency in Australian Rules footballers. Br J Sports Med. 1998;32(2):134–9.
14. Muschaweck U, Berger L. Minimal repair technique of sportsmen's groin: an innovative open-suture repair to treat chronic inguinal pain. Hernia. 2010; 14(1):27–33.
15. Holmich P, et al. Effectiveness of active physical training as treatment for long-standing adductor-related groin pain in athletes: randomised trial. Lancet. 1999;353(9151):439–43.
16. Ekstrand J, Ringborg S. Surgery versus conservative treatment in soccer players with chronic groin pain : a prospective randomised study in soccer players. Eur J Sports Traumatol Relat Res. 2001;23:141–5.
17. Paajanen H, et al. Laparoscopic surgery for chronic groin pain in athletes is more effective than nonoperative treatment: a randomized clinical trial with magnetic resonance imaging of 60 patients with sportsman's hernia (athletic pubalgia). Surgery. 2011;150(1):99–107.
18. Meyers WC, et al. Experience with "sports hernia" spanning two decades. Ann Surg. 2008;248(4): 656–65.
19. Muschaweck U, Berger LM. Sportsmen's groin-diagnostic approach and treatment with the minimal

repair technique: a single-center uncontrolled clinical review. Sports Health. 2010;2(3):216–21.

20. Brunt LM. Surgical treatment of sports hernia: open mesh approach. In: Diduch DR, Brunt LM, editors. Sports hernia and athletic pubalgia: diagnosis and treatment. New York: Springer; 2014. p. 133142.

21. Genitsaris M, Goulimaris I, Sikas N. Laparoscopic repair of groin pain in athletes. Am J Sports Med. 2004;32(5):1238–42.

22. Paajanen H, Syvahuoko I, Airo I. Totally extraperitoneal endoscopic (TEP) treatment of sportsman's hernia. Surg Laparosc Endosc Percutan Tech. 2004;14(4):215–8.

23. Evans DS. Hunterian lecture. Laparoscopic transabdominal pre-peritoneal (TAPP) repair of groin hernia: one surgeon's experience of a developing technique. Ann R Coll Surg Engl. 2002;84(6):393–8.

24. Lloyd DM, et al. Laparoscopic inguinal ligament tenotomy and mesh reinforcement of the anterior abdominal wall: a new approach for the management of chronic groin pain. Surg Laparosc Endosc Percutan Tech. 2008;18(4):363–8.

25. Brunt LM, Barile R. My approach to athletic pubalgia. In: Byrd JWT, editor. Operative hip arthroscopy. New York: Springer; 2013. p. 55–65.

ERRATUM TO

Emergent Surgical Management of Ventral Hernias

Phillip Chang

© Springer International Publishing Switzerland 2016
Y.W. Novitsky (ed.), *Hernia Surgery*, DOI 10.1007/978-3-319-27470-6

DOI 10.1007/978-3-319-27470-6_51

The original version of the book contained error which has been corrected.
The correction is given below:

Chapter 39

Levi D. Procter is co-author of this chapter along with Phillip Chang which was not included in the book.

The updated online version for this chapter can be found at
DOI 10.1007/978-3-319-27470-6_39

The updated online version of the original book can be found at
http://dx.doi.org/10.1007/978-3-319-27470-6

Index

A

Abdominal compartment syndrome (ACS), 365, 412
Abdominal fascial defect, 307
Abdominal laxity, 325
Abdominal wall
  clinical anatomy and physiology
    arcuate line, 9
    boundary, 1–2
    EO, 9
    extraperitoneal space, 10
    IOM, 7–8
    linea alba, 2–4
    midline and anterolateral groups of muscles, 2
    nerve supply, 11–12
    pyramidalis muscles, 5
    RA, 4–5
    TAM, 5–7
    vascular supply, 10
  eventration (*see* Pseudoherniation)
  hernias, 207
  reconstruction, 261
    algorithm hypogastric defects, 315
    by region, 315–316
    local flaps, 316
    perforator flaps, 316
    using TE, 309–311
  repair (*see* Negative pressure wound therapy (NPWT))
  spaces (*see* Abdominal wall spaces)
  transplantation, 319, 321
  wounds
    etiology, 351
    surgical treatment, 353, 355
Abdominal wall reconstructions (AWR)., 232
Abdominal wall repair. *See* Negative pressure wound
    therapy (NPWT)
Abdominal wall spaces
  mesh placement
    laparoscopic repair, 82
    onlay, 79–80
    randomized trials, 82
    retrorectus repair, 82
    sublay repair, 80–81
    underlay, 81–82
  positioning, 83
  surgical site infection, 83

Abobotulinum toxin A (Dysport®), 425
ABRA abdominal wall closure system, 418, 419
Absorbable tacks, 287–288
Acute kidney injury (AKI), 215
Adhesives, 288–291
AirSeal™ port, 150
Anterior rectus sheath
  excisional techniques, 328
  resorbable/non-resorbable mesh, 330
  thickness of, 323
Antibiotic prophylaxis, 35

B

Bard's Phasix Mesh, 73
Bassini technique, 439
Beer classification, 327
Biodegradable meshes
  Bard's Phasix Mesh, 73
  CDC wound classification, 76
  Ethicon Vicryl Mesh, 71
  Gore Bio-A, 71, 74
  infected surgical field, 74–75
  Phasix Mesh, 71
  TAR, 76
  Tigr Matrix, 71, 73
  UCSD algorithm, 76
  Vicryl (polyglactin 910) woven mesh, 72
Biologic mesh
  characterization, 63–64
  decellularization process, 63
  enzymatic degradation, 64–65
  hernia repair applications, 61
  implantation, in human subjects, 66, 68
  long-term packaging and storage, 63
  porcine model, 65, 66
  repetitive loading, 64
  species and type of tissue, 63
  variables, 63
  XenMatrix™ AB Surgical Graft, 61
  xenogeneic meshes, 63
Bioprosthetic matrices, 390
Bioprosthetic mesh, 314, 318
Blunt dissection, 174
Body mass index (BMI), 396

Bone anchors, 265, 268
Botulinum toxin
  abdominal wall hernia
    antinociceptive effects, 428
    paralyzing effects, 427–428
    porcine model, 427
    toxin-induced paralysis, 427
  administration, 424
  C. botulinum, 424
  clinical studies, 429–430
  complex midline incisional hernia, 433, 434
  evidence-based medicine, 423
  formulation, 424
  generic names, 425
  immunological considerations, 424
  inguinal hernia, 435
  personal comprehension, 428–435
  potential indications, 436
  temporary abdominal closure, 435
  tolerability and contraindications, 426
  treatment of neurological conditions, 424
Botulinum toxin types A (BoNT-A), 424
Botulinum toxin types B (BoNT-B), 424

C
Cautery, 175
Central mesh failure (CMF), 217
Chemical component separation (CCS).
        See Botulinum toxin
Chest wall, posterior, 317
Chronic mesh infections, 213
Chronic postherniorrhaphy inguinal pain (CPIP)
  etiology andclinical presentation, 483–484
  evaluation, 485
  history, 483
  inguinal neuroanatomy, 487
  interventional pain management, 486
  pharmacological pain management, 485
  retroperitoneal neuroanatomy, 488
  risk factors, 484–485
  surgical pain management
    hernia recurrence and meshoma, 489
    laparoscopic retroperitoneal triple neurectomy, 489
    meshoma, 489
    neuroanatomy, 487
    neurolysis, 488
    personal algorithm, 490
    recommended timing, 487
    triple neurectomy, 488
  treatment, 485
Clinical quality improvement (CQI) principles, 59
CollaMend™, 64
Complex abdominal wall defect reconstruction, 344–347
Complications, ventral hernia repair, 208–213
Component separation, 314, 321
Concomitant panniculectomy
  complications management, 305
  postoperative care, 304–305
  ventral hernia repair (*see* Panniculectomy)
Congenital epigastric defects, 253

D
Damage control laparotomy (DCL), 431
Decellularization process, 63, 64
Decontamination process, 64
Deep inferior epigastric arteries (DIEAs), 5
Diastasis. *See* Pseudoherniation
Diastasis recti
  abdominoplasty, 328
  anterior abdominal wall, 323
  classification systems, 327
  complications, 332, 333
  diagnosis, 325
  endoscopic technique, 331
  etiology, 325
  exercise, 328
  indications, 327, 328
  initial consultation, 327
  laparoscopic reinforcement, 332
  midline plication, 328
  sheath plication, 334
  structural anatomic deformity, 323
  suture techniques, 334
  treatment, 328
Dynamic fascial closure systems, 418

E
Early Recovery After Surgery (ERAS) protocol, 34
Electrocautery, 174
Emergency care
  abdominal wall defect, 403
  complex hernias, 403
  femoral hernia, 404–405
  groin hernias, 403
  inguinal hernias, 404
  morbidity and mortality, 403
  umbilical hernias, 405–406
  ventral hernias, 403
  ventral incisional hernia
    anatomic information, 406
    bowel viability and bowel obstruction, 406
    laparoscopic repair, 406
    mesh prosthesis, 407
    open surgery, 407
    SBO, 406
    urgent/emergent scenario, 406
Endoscopic component separation (ECS)
  access and muscle separation, 150
  complications, 158
  external oblique division, 153–157
  hernia repair, 157
  indications, 149
  limitations, 157–158
  muscle separation, 156
  outcomes, 158
  patient position, 150
  port placement, 150–152
  space, 157
  subcutaneous fascial division, 153–156
  troubleshooting, 152–153
Enteroatmospheric fistula, 419, 420

Enterocutaneous fistula
    definition, 381
    definitive hernia repair, 384
    definitive herniorrhaphy, 383–384
    hernia defect, 384–386
    permanent prosthetic material, 386
    preoperative considerations
        extensive adhesiolysis, 382
        GI surgical approach, 382
        optimal outcomes, 382
        SOWATS approach, 381
    surgical principles, 382
Enterocutaneous fistula (ECF) formation, 212
Enterotomy
    adhesiolysis, 374
    adhesion characteristics, 376
    incidence of EBR, 375
    laparoscopic ventral hernia repair, 375
    management, 376–378
    morbidity and mortality, 374
    previous laparotomies, 373
    prospective evaluation, 376
    risk factors, 373
    small bowel resection, 374
    traction/counter-traction technique, 376
    ventral hernia repair repairs, 375
Enterotomy, with planned bony fixation, 193
Expanded polytetrafluoroethylene (ePTFE), 390
Extended-view totally extraperitoneal (eTEP) technique
    clinical experience, 474
    endoscopic extraperitoneal approach, 469
    features, 469
    flexible port distribution, 471
    hernia repair, 474
    high camera port placement, 470, 471
    IPOM, 469
    port distribution, 473
    port setup, 470
    posterior fascia, 472
    preperitoneal space outside, 472
    TAPP, 469
    TEP, 469
    working ports, 471
Expander
    abdominal wall fascia, 309
    capsulotomies/capsulectomies, 311
    internal/external, 308
External oblique (EO), 9
External oblique aponeurosis, 174

F
Femoral hernia, 26, 404–405
Fixation device, 287–290, 292
Flank hernia
    definition and anatomy, 261
    descriptions, 263
    epidemiology, 263
    patient counseling, 271
    patient positioning, 266
    preoperative approach, 264–266

preoperative preparation, 271
    repairs (see Flank hernia repairs)
    trocar positioning, 267
Flank hernia repairs
    anatomy, 184
    durable repair, 184
    native blood supply, 184
    operative technique
        abdominal wall closure, 192–193
        mesh selection and insertion, 189–192
        patient positioning, 187–188
        postoperative care, 193
        preperitoneal space dissection, 188
    patient morbidity and wound complications, 184
    preoperative planning
        large fascial defect, 184, 186
        patient optimization, 186–187
        pseudoherniation, 184
        small fascial defect, 184
    reconstruction, 184
    unplanned complications
        enterotomy, with planned bony
            fixation, 193
        fascial closure, 193
        multiple fenestrations, 193
        pseudohernia, with true fascial defect, 194
Flap reconstruction
    abdominal wall musculofascia, 314
    bioprosthetic and synthetic meshes, 314
    hernia repair, 314
    recipient vessels, 319
    reconstructive algorithm, skin coverage, 315
Free flap, 317–318

G
Glucose control, 32–33
Gore Bio-A, 74

H
Hematomas, 211, 212
Hernia classification
    EHS classification schemes, 19
    incisional hernia, 18
    TNM-like classification, 19–21
    wound morbidity and outcomes, 16–18
Hernia repair
    adhesive fixation, 104
    anecdotal evidence, 105
    application, 104
    Chevrel repair, 100
    Chevrel's technique, 100
    clinical data, 100–102
    fibrin glue fixation, 102
    light weight polypropylene, 103
    medialization, 102
    post-operative, 104
    principles, 104
    semilunar line, 102
    skin flap creation, 102

Hernia surgery
   diagnostic testing, 23–24
   femoral hernias, 26
   inguinal hernia
      CT, 24
      herniography, 25
      MRI, 24
      ultrasound, 24
   obturator hernias, 26
   ventral hernia
      CT, 28
      MRI, 29
      ultrasound, 27–28
Herniography, 25
Hypothermia, 36

I

Iatrogenic hernia formation, 218–219
Incisional hernia
   abdominal aneurysms repair, 41
   abdominal binders, 45
   connective tissue, 41
   continuous *vs.* interrupted sutures, 42
   development, 41
   Dutch PRIMA trial, 47
   fascial dehiscence, 48
   fascial redehiscence, 48
   incidences, 41
   mass *vs.* layered closures, 42
   minimally invasive techniques, 48
   polypropylene mesh, 48
   primary mesh augmentation, 45–47
   reconstructive options
      laparoscopic repair with mesh reinforcement,
         94–97
      open repair with/without mesh reinforcement,
         93–94
      rectus diastasis, 97
   repair (*see* Incisional hernia repair)
   risk factor, 42
   small bites technique, 48
   suture length to wound length ratio, 43–45
   suture materials, 42
Incisional hernia repair
   antibiotic prophylaxis, 35
   antibiotic-impregnated sutures, 36
   cross-sectional imaging, 34
   glucose control, 32–33
   intraoperative wound protectors, 36
   metabolic manipulation, 33, 34
   nutritional intervention, 33
   obesity, 32
   perioperative oxygenation, 36
   perioperative warming, 36
   preoperative skin preparation and decolonization
      protocols, 35–36
   smoking, 31, 32
Incisional negative pressure wound therapy, 304
Incisional/traumatic hernias, 264

Incisional/ventral hernia defects, 293
Incobotulinum toxin A (Xeomin®), 425
Infected mesh
   biologic mesh, 390
   CT scan, 392
   ePTFE mesh floating, 392
   granulation tissue, 392
   hernia working group grading system, 391
   mesh explantation, 393
   mesh salvage, 391–392
   mesh selection and wound classification,
      390–391
   partial salvage, 392
   risk factors and prevention, 393
   ventral hernia, 389
Inguinal hernia
   algorithmic approach, 479
   caveats and pearls, 478
   CT, 24
   groin pain complaints, 476
   hernia repair surgical options, 476
   incarcerations and strangulations, 478
   inguinodynia, 479
   inguino-scrotal hernias, 478
   Lichtenstein repair, 477
   management options, 476
   MRI, 24
   non-operative strategies, 475
   obesity, 481
   Pfenensteil incisions, 480
   recurrence, 480
   reduction of excess, 478
   repair, 292, 293
   risk of chronic pain and recurrences, 475
   seroma minimization, 481
   TEP repair, 477
   TEP's diagnostic ability, 477
   ultrasound, 24
Inguinal recurrences
   algorithmic approach, 497
   mesh fixation, 497
   operative approach, 495–497
   papyrus, 493
   pathophysiology, 493–494
   preoperative evaluation, 494–495
   preperitoneal repair, 498
   preperitoneal space, 497, 498
Inguino-scrotal hernias, 478
Instillation therapy, 341
Insufflation system, 150
Internal oblique muscle (IOM), 7–8
Interventional pain management, 486
Intestinal function (ileus), hernia
      surgery, 214
Intra-abdominal hypertension, 215–216
Intraperitoneal onlay mesh (IPOM), 398, 469, 496

K

Keyhole technique, 170, 242

L
Laparoscopic defect closure
   dead space obliteration, 234
   EndoStitch device, 237
   fascial tension, 237
   functional, dynamic repair, 232, 233
   multimodal analgesia, 239
   patient selection, 233
   reduced recurrence rate, 233
   smaller mesh, 233
Laparoscopic hernia repair
   adhesiolysis, 267
   factors affecting operative approach, 265
   intra-abdominal placement, 267
   mesh fixation, 267, 455
   mesh position and visualization, 459
   opening of peritoneum, 457
   OR preparation
      equipment, 454
      lightweight mesh, 454
      mesh fixation, 455
   patient and time position, 456
   patient preference, 453
   peritoneal flap, 460
   postoperative care and quality of life,
      270, 271
   preperitoneal space, 458
   primary closure, 270
   quality of life, 271
   TAPP, 453, 454
   technique
      complications, 459
      patient and team position, 455
      post operative care, 459
      recommendation, 460
      transabdominal preperitoneal
         repair, 456
   TEP, 453
   transfascial sutures and tacks, 267
   transversalis fascia, 459
   trapezoid of pain, 459
   trocar position, 457
Laparoscopic repair, 82
Laparoscopic shoelace closure
   access, 234
   anaglgesia, 237
   buttressing sutures, 236
   hernia defect closure, 236
   mesh placement, 236
   pneumoperitoneum, 236
   setup, 234
   stab incision, 235
Laparoscopic sleeve gastrectomy, 208
Laparoscopic total extra-peritoneal inguinal hernia repair
      (TEP-IHR)
   bladder and alveolar tissue, 465
   Cooper's ligament, 465, 466
   cord contents, 466
   non-slitted mesh, 466
   occult inguinal hernia, 467

   patient selection
      contra-indications, 464
      femoral and direct hernia, 465
      indications, 464
      indirect hernia identification, 465
      mesh palcement, 465
      pre-peritoneal space, 464
      pubic tubercle and Cooper's ligament, 465
   TEP and TAPP, 463
Laparoscopic umbilical hernia repair
   open mesh repair, 198, 200, 203
   primary repair (sutures), 196, 198
Laparoscopic ventral hernia repair (LVHR)
   abdominal wall mechanics, 231–232
   complications
      adhesiolysis, 225
      contralateral trocar, 225
      decreased perioperative pain, 230
      first-generation cephalosporin, 224
      hernia recurrence, 229
      intra-operative complications, 229
      minimal wound morbidity, 230
      peritoneal cavity, 224
      pneumoperitoneum, 224
      postoperative care, 228
      reduced hospital stay, 230
      seroma formation, 229
      suture fixation, 228
      trocar placement, 224
      wound and mesh infections, 228
   defect closure (*see* Laparoscopic defect closures)
Laparoscopic ventral/incisional hernia repair, 291, 292
Laser angiography, indocyanine green, 304
Lichtenstein technique, 439, 448
Lightweight polypropylene mesh (LWPPM), 495
Linea semilunaris, 218–219
Loss of domain (LOD)
   definition, 363
   patient's preparation, 367
   physics
      broken cylinder, 364
      cylinder, 363–364
      morbidity of, 364
      repairing, 365
   postoperative care and complications
      ACS and pulmonary complications, 370
      intestinal complications, 371
      wound complications, 371
   presentation
      emergency surgery' s role, 365
      obesity role, 366
      recurrent hernia role, 366
   surgeon preparation, 366
   surgical strategies
      drains placement and management, 369
      mesh choice, 369
      Novitsky technique, 368
      pre-operative pneumoperitoneum, 370
      Ramirez technique, 368
Lumbar hernia, 264

M
Mechanical ventilation, 179
Mesh
  complications
    erosion, 216, 217
    fracture, 217
    infection, 216
  onlay and plication, 330–331
  retrorectus repair, 331
  techniques, 415
Mesh erosion, 181
Mesh fixation
  absorbable tacks, 287
  categorisation, 287
  nonabsorbable tacks, 287
  sutures and glues, 287
  ventral and inguinal hernia repair, 287
Mesh infections, 213, 216
Mesh repair
  dissection and tissue division, 198
  hemostasis, 199
  intra-peritoneal mesh placement, 198
  laparoscopic techniques, 203–204
  pneumoperitoneum, 202
Mesh salvage, 391–392
Methicillin-resistant *Staphylococcus aureus* (MRSA), 390
Modified grading system, 18
Morbidity, hernia repair, 207
Morbidly obese patient
  BMI, 396
  body morphology, 397, 398
  mesh choice, 399
  mesh location, 398
  operative approach, 397
  preoperative preparation and planning, 400
  previous repairs, 398
  size of defect, 397
  ventral hernia repair, 400
Muschawek's technique, 516

N
National Surgery Quality Improvement Program
    (NSQIP) database, 36
Negative pressure wound therapy (NPWT)
  abdominal wall reconstruction
    full-thickness abdominal defect, 341–342
    partial-thickness abdominal defects, 342
  biofilm, 357
  clinical indications, 347
  closed surgical wounds, 343
  foam *vs.* gauze, 338–339
  mechanism of action, 337, 338
  mechanisms of action, 337
  mesh salvage, 344
  skin grafts, 344
  subatmospheric pressure, 339–341
  wound healing, 337
Nonabsorbable tacks, 287
Nonsteroidal anti-inflammatory agents (NSAIDS), 459

Novitsky technique, 368
Nutritional intervention, 33

O
Obesity, 32
Obturator hernias, 26
Onabotulinum toxin A (Botox®), 425
Onlay technique, 174
Open anterior component separation
  algorithms and technique
    postoperative management, 145
    preoperative evaluation, 140–141
    surgical technique, 142–145
  external oblique relaxing incisions, 137
  minimal dissection technique, 138
  outcomes, 138
  with perforator preservation
    acute failure, 161
    chronic failures, 161
    history, 160–161
    laminar *vs.* pulsatile blood flow, 159–160
    outcomes, 164–165
    patient preoperative evaluation, 162
    subacute failures, 161
    surgery technique, 162–164
  "sandwich" repair, 140
  synthetic *vs.* biologic, 138–140
Open hernia repair complications. *See* Ventral
    hernia repair
Open techniques
  Bassini technique, 439
  Lichtenstein technique, 439
  prosthetic mesh repairs
    bilayer mesh, 446
    bilayer PHS, 447
    EHS guidelines, 448
    Lichtenstein tension-free repair, 443–445
    modified Lichtenstein repair, 444
    open preperitoneal repair, 446
    PHS, 446
    pluig and patch technique, 445
    prolene hernia system, 446
    TIPP repair, 447
    TREPP repair, 448
  tissue approximation repairs
    Bassini repair, 440
    Desarda repair, 442
    Desarda technique, 443
    McVay repair, 441, 442
    Shouldice repair, 440, 441

P
Panniculectomy
  abdominal wall reconstruction, 297
  and abdominoplasty operation, 297
  aesthetic and functional benefits, 297
  ambulation and decreased rashing, 297
  descriptions, 301, 303

excess abdominal contents, 298
  indications/contraindications, 298
  nicotine, 298
  open cholecystectomy incision, 298
  patient markings, 301
  preoperative evaluation, 299
  smoking tobacco, 298
  soft tissue and muscular anatomy, 299
  transverse upper abdominal incisions, 298
  transverse waistline incision, 297
  vascular anatomy, 299
Parastomal hernia (PH) repair
  classification, 241
  complications, 242
    stoma, 180, 181
    wound infections, 180
  cruciate pairs, 170
  definition, 241
  diagnosis, 242
  formation, 169
  incidence, 242
  laparoscopic approach, 242
  keyholere pairs, 170
  operative approach, 172, 242, 245, 248
  outcomes, 242, 243
  patient selection, 172, 173
  post-operative care, 179–180
  prevention, 169, 249, 250
  primary repair vs. mesh repair, 170
  risk factors, 169, 241
  stoma closure, 171
  stoma creation, 241
  stoma relocation/in situ position, 171
  sugarbaker repair, 170
  surgical techniques
    anterior component separation, 174
    Foley catheter, 173
    open vs. laparoscopic, 170
    posterior component separation,
      174–176
    PPHR, 176–179
    sugarbaker, 173
  synthetic vs. biologic mesh, 171
  types, 180
Partial salvage, 392
Pauli parastomal hernia repair (PPHR), 176–179
Pedicled flap, 315–317
Peri-umbilical perforator sparing (PUPS), 174
Permacol™, 64
Pharmacological pain management, 485
Polyethylene terephthalate (PET), 56
Polytetrafluoroethylene (PTFE), 56
Posterior component separation herniorraphies, 219
Posterior component separation (PCS) technique, 281
Posterolateral abdominal wall, 261–263
Postoperative complications, 317
Postpartum women, 325
Prehabilitation strategy, elective open ventral hernia
      repairs, 208
Pre-peritoneal mesh reinforcement, 204

Primary repair
  intravenous antibiotics, 198
  with permanent suture, 198
  transverse orientation, 196
Prior medical history (PMH), 476
Prior surgical history (PSH), 476
Prolene hernia system (PHS), 439, 446
Prosthetic mesh repair failure, 249
Pseudoherniation, 184
Pseudohernia, with true fascial defect, 194
Pulmonary complications, 214
Pulmonary medicine, 208
Pyramidalis muscles, 5

R
Ramirez technique, 368
Reconstructive options
  epigastric hernias, 92
  incisional hernias
    laparoscopic repair with mesh reinforcement,
      94–97
    open repair with/without mesh reinforcement,
      93–94
    rectus diastasis, 97
  open/laparoscopic approach
    adequate skin/soft tissue coverage, 90
    factors, 90
    inadequate skin/soft tissue coverage, 90
    mesh placement, location of, 91
    static/functional classification, 90
  patient selection, 89–90
  umbilical hernias, 91–92
Rectus abdominis, 317
Rectus abdominus muscles (RA), 4–5
Rectus diastasis, endoscopic technique, 335
Recurrent PH, 248
Regional flap, 317
Retrorectus dissection, 175
Retrorectus repair, 82, 335
Rives-Stoppa retromuscular repair
  anterior tension assessment, 112–113
  biomechanical principles, 108
  history, 107
  lateral defects, 113
  limitations, 113
  operative steps
    hernia sac, 108
    mesh fixation, 112
    midline abdominal wall reconstruction, 112
    posterior rectus sheath dissection, 110–111
    visceral sac closure, 111
  parastomal hernia, 113
  postoperative care, 113–114
Robotic incisional hernia repair
  accessory port location, 275
  direct bowel handling, 276
  docking, 274–275
  fascial defect, 284
  hemostasis, 276

Robotic incisional hernia repair (*cont.*)
  instrumentation, 276
  intra-abdominal access, 275
  intraperitoneal onlay mesh, 274–277
  mesh placement and fixation, 277
  patient positioning, 274–275
  primary closure, defect, 276
  trocar placement, 274–275
Robotic Rives-Stoppa repair. *See* Transversus abdominis
     muscle release (TAR)
Robotic transabdominal preperitoneal (TAPP) VHR
  bowel erosion, fistula/severe adhesions, 277
  conventional laparoscopy, 277
  docking and instrumentation, 277, 279
  fixation, 278
  mesh placement, 278
  patient positioning, trocar placement and docking, 279
  preperitoneal fat, 278
  primary closure, defect, 278
  reperitonealization, 278
  subxiphoidal hernias, 278
  tissue separating mesh, 277
  trocar placement, 277, 279
Robotic ventral hernia repair (RVHR)
  intracorporeal suturing, 273
  laparoscopic repair, 273
  limitations, 274
  postoperative pain, 273
  preoperative considerations, 274
  Rives-Stoppa repair, 273
  tacking/stapling devices, 273
  tissue and nerve entrapment, 273

S
Sandwich technique, 242
Seroma formation, 210, 211, 305
Skin grafting, 355, 360
Small bowel obstruction (SBO), 406
Smoking, 31, 32
Soft-tissue flap reconstruction, 313
Sports hernia
  abdominal crunch, 514
  adductor/abductor strengthening exercises, 508
  advanced core exercises, 507
  anatomy and pathophysiology, 513
  anatomy of lower abdominal/inguinal region, 512
  areas of pathology, 503
  definition, 501
  diagnosis, 514
  diagnostic imaging, 515
  dynamic strength, 508
  epidemiology, 501–502
  external oblique aponeurosis, 518
  groin injuries, 511
  groin pain, 501
  hip and core strengthening exercises, 506
  hip exam techniques, 503
  history and physical examination, 514
  imaging, 502–505

  laparoscopic operative view, 517
  nonoperative management, 515
  open mesh repair, 519
  overturned balance ball, 507
  partial release of adductor longus, 518
  presentation/physical exam, 502
  rectus abdominus, 504
  rectus tear, 513
  surgical management
    adductor release, 518
    author step-by-step- approach, 518
    indications, 515
    laparoscopic posterior mesh repair, 517
    open anterior tension-free mesh repair, 516, 517
    open primary tissue repairs, 516
    postoperative management and recovery, 519
    special circumstances, 518
  treatment
    alternative, 509
    conservative therapy, 505–507
    prevention, 509
  weakened posterior floor weakness, 519
Standard LVHR technique, 277
Strattice™, 64
Subxiphoid hernia repair
  adhesiolysis, 254, 255
  cardio-pulmonary injuries, 255
  congenital/incisional, 253
  falciform ligament, 255
  incidence, 253
  mesh orientation and fixation, 255–257
  preoperative considerations, 253–254,
     (*see also* Suprapubic hernia repair)
  xiphoid process, 255
Sugarbaker technique, 170, 242, 249, 250
Superior epigastric arteries (SEAs), 5
Suprapubic hernia repair
  absorbable tacks/sutures, 280
  bladder injuries, 256
  bladder mobilization, 257, 279
  fascial defect, 255
  intra-operative bladder infusion, 256
  mesh orientation and fixation, 257–259
  partial desufflation, abdominal cavity, 280
  patient positioning, trocar placement and
    docking, 279
  postoperative management, 259
  retroinguinal space (space of Bogros), 279
  standard intravenous infusion tubing, 256
  steep Trendelenburg positioning, 256
    (*see also* Subxiphoid hernia repair)
Surgical debridement, 355, 357
Surgical site infection (SSI), 74, 208, 209
Surgical site occurrence (SSOs)
  empiric antibiotics, 212
  granulation disuse formation, 212
  management strategies, 213
  rates, open ventral hernia repair, 209
  wound erythema, 212
  wound ischemia, 212

Synthetic mesh
    clinical background, 53–54
    coated polypropylene/polyester prostheses, 58
    complexity science tools, 59
    contaminated/potentially contaminated field, 57
    decision-making process, 59
    design, 57
    direct viscus exposure, 57
    "ideal" mesh, 58
    medical and legal aspects, 58
    nonlinear data analytics, 59
    PET, 56
    polypropylene, 54
    PTFE, 56
    randomly generated fibers/non-woven material, 58

T
Temporary abdominal closure
    abdominal compartment syndrome/damage control
        surgery, 411, 412
    abdominal wall reconstruction, 413
    ABRA abdominal wall closure system, 418, 419
    Bogota bag closure, 414
    damage control principles, 411
    decision-making, 420
    dynamic fascial closure systems, 418
    enteroatmospheric fistula, 419, 420
    ePTFE mesh, 417
    intra-abdominal hypertension, 412
    mesh based techniques, 415
    negative pressure therapy, 416
    open abdomen, 419
    open packing/planned ventral heria, 412
    silastic closure/bogota bag, 414
    towel clip closure, 413, 414
    V.A.C., 421
    Wittmann Patch™, 415, 416
    Zipper-based closures, 414
Tension-free repair of incisional and inguinal hernias, 195
Thromboembolic complications, 218
Thromboembolic prophylaxis, 142
Tigr matrix, 73, 74
Tissue expansion (TE)
    congenital defects, lower abdominal wall, 307
    effects, 308
    indications, 309, 311
    physiology, 308
    techniques, 311–312
Totally extraperitoneal hernia repair (TEP), 453, 469
Transabdominal preperitoneal hernia repair (TAPP),
        453, 469
Transversus abdominis muscle (TAM), 5–7
Transversus abdominis muscle release (TAR)
    abdominal wall reconstruction, 281
    anatomy, 118
    anterior component separation techniques, 117
    anterior sheath closure, 282
    drain placement, 284
    history, 117–118

laparoscopic access, 281
limitations, 281
mesh placement, 283
minimally invasive modifications, 117
patient positioning, 282
    anterior fascia and skin closure, 131
    exposure and division, 121–124
    extraperitoneal space and TAP block, 130
    incision/adhesiolysis, 120
    inferior dissection, 124–125
    lateral/retroperitoneal dissection, 124
    mesh fixation, 130
    mesh placement, 130
    mesh selection, 130
    outcomes, 134
    posterior layers, closure of, 127–130
    rectus sheath release/retro-rectus dissection,
        120–121
    superior dissection, 125–127
patient selection, 119
physiologic function, 118
posterior component separation, 117
posterior sheath closure, 283
posterior sheath incision, 282
post-operative care, 131–134
pre-operative planning, 119–120
relative contraindications, 119
transversus abdominis release, 282
trocar placement and docking, 282
wound complications, 281
Transversus abdominis muscles release (TAR), 76
Transversus abdominis release (TAR), 173–176

U
Umbilical hernia, 405–406
    cirrhotic patients, 195
    congenital, 195
    fascial defects, adults, 195
    laparoscopic port placement, 195
    management algorithms, 195, 204–205
    primary/recurrent, 195
    repair studies, 196
    wound/infectious complications, 195
Umbilicoplasty, 303

V
Ventral hernia, 313, 389
    CT, 28
    MRI, 29
    ultrasound, 27–28
Ventral hernia repair (VHR)
    large abdominal incisions, 223
    porcine model, 65
    risk factors of complications, 207–208
    tension-free repairs, 223
    ventral herniorrhaphies, 223
    wide tissue dissection, 223
Ventral Hernia Risk Score (VHRS), 18

Ventral Hernia Working Group (VHWG), 16, 18, 391
Vicryl (polyglactin 910) woven mesh, 72

W
Wittmann patch, 415, 416
Wound care, 357, 360, 361
Wound cellulitis, 16
Wound closure. *See* Incisional hernia
Wound dehiscence, 212
Wound healing
    biofilm, 353
    cellular interactions, 351
    closure of abdominal wound, 303
    fibroproliferative phase, 351

    and flap necrosis, 305
    inflammatory phase, 351
    remodeling phase, 351
    transverse incision, 303
Wound infections, 180
Wound-related complications, 208
Wound vac systems, 386

X
XenMatrix™, 64

Z
Zipper-based closures, 414

Printed by Printforce, the Netherlands